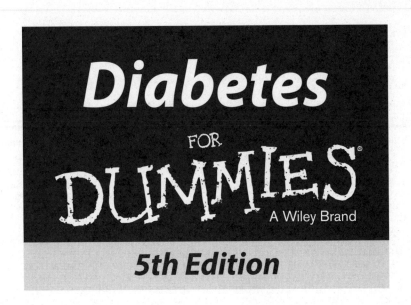

Diabetes

FOR DUMMIES®

A Wiley Brand

5th Edition

by Alan L. Rubin, MD

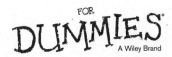

Diabetes For Dummies®, 5th Edition

Published by: **John Wiley & Sons, Inc.,** 111 River Street, Hoboken, NJ 07030-5774, www.wiley.com

Copyright © 2015 by John Wiley & Sons, Inc., Hoboken, New Jersey

Published simultaneously in Canada

For general information on our other products and services, please contact our Customer Care Department within the U.S. at 877-762-2974, outside the U.S. at 317-572-3993, or fax 317-572-4002. For technical support, please visit www.wiley.com/techsupport.

Wiley publishes in a variety of print and electronic formats and by print-on-demand. Some material included with standard print versions of this book may not be included in e-books or in print-on-demand. If this book refers to media such as a CD or DVD that is not included in the version you purchased, you may download this material at http://booksupport.wiley.com. For more information about Wiley products, visit www.wiley.com.

Library of Congress Control Number: 2015945230

ISBN 978-1-119-09072-4 (pbk); ISBN 978-1-119-09076-2 (ebk); ISBN 978-1-119-09077-9 (ebk)

Manufactured in the United States of America

10 9 8 7 6 5 4 3 2

Contents at a Glance

Table of Contents

Introduction

You're reading the 5th edition of *Diabetes For Dummies,* and you may be wondering why another edition is necessary. The previous edition (published in 2012) had everything you needed to know to reverse the plague of diabetes, yet the problem seems to be increasing, not decreasing. Following are some of the possible explanations for this situation:

- ✔ Not enough people bought the last edition of the book.
- ✔ Even if they bought it, not enough people followed the recommendations in the book.
- ✔ Too many people aren't even aware that this book exists.
- ✔ No book or books can stop an avalanche after the snow starts rolling downhill.
- ✔ Some new information, not available three years ago, may be able to make a major difference toward reversing diabetes, especially the information in Chapter 9.

The real answer is actually all of the above (and probably more reasons).

The Centers for Disease Control and Prevention recently suggested that as many as one in three adults in the United States will have diabetes by the year 2050. The International Diabetes Federation reports that 387 million people had diabetes in 2014 and that 552 million will have the disease by 2030 — that's one in every ten people on the earth. In a previous edition of this book, I set this figure at 366 million by 2030, so you can see that today's predictions are even more dire than those of four years ago. This increase is because the population is aging, minority groups who have a higher risk for diabetes are increasing, and, fortunately, people with diabetes are living longer. However, these numbers are based on past trends. The prediction will not turn out to be true if people improve their lifestyle choices through the means discussed in this book.

Over the last decade, a large study was performed in Germany to see if lifestyle change could make a difference. Four major factors were evaluated in over 23,000 Germans. The factors were

- ✔ Never smoking
- ✔ Body-mass index less than 30

    ✔ Exercising for three and a half hours or more a week

    ✔ Following healthy dietary principles: high intake of fruits and vegetables, eating whole-grain bread, and low meat consumption

The happy finding was that the more factors a person followed, the lower the risk of major chronic diseases, including heart disease, diabetes, and cancer. People who followed all four had a 78 percent lower risk of those diseases than people who had no healthy factor. People with three factors were a little less protected, with two a bit less and with one even less but still better than no factors at all.

About This Book

So much has changed in the three years since the fourth edition of *Diabetes For Dummies* was written that a fifth edition was clearly necessary. I need to tell you about new medicines (see Chapter 11), new glucose meters (Chapter 7), and new ideas about diet and exercise and curing diabetes with surgery (Chapters 8, 9, and 10). I also need to share new information about diabetes in children (Chapter 13) and the occupational and insurance problems of people with diabetes (Chapter 15). Just about every chapter has something new, especially (obviously) Chapter 16, which deals specifically with what's new in diabetes care.

A new edition also gives me the opportunity to thank the thousands of people who have thanked me for *Diabetes For Dummies.* You have given me a sense of enormous gratification for writing this book. You have shared your stories with me, permitting me to laugh and cry with you. One of the best is the following from Andrea in Canada:

> *My 3-year-old daughter was recently diagnosed with diabetes type 1. It has been a rough time. To help us out, my brother and his wife bought us your book,* Diabetes For Dummies. *One day my daughter saw this bright yellow book and asked what I was reading. I told her Diabetes For Dummies. As soon as the words came out of my mouth, I regretted it. I didn't want her to think that dummies got diabetes so I quickly added, "I am the dummy." Without missing a beat, she then asked, "Am I the diabetes?"*

> *The story doesn't just end there. The other day she was relaxing on the couch. She looked at me and said, "I don't want to have diabetes anymore." Feeling terrible, I responded, "I know sweetie; I don't want you to have it anymore either." I then explained that she would have diabetes for the rest*

of her life. With a very concerned look she then asked, "Will you be the dummy for the rest of your life?"

*As sad as it is, I guess you're right, **one must look for humor in everything;** otherwise we would have broken down by now.*

You're not required to read this book from cover to cover, although if you know nothing about diabetes, reading straight through may be a good approach. This book is designed to serve as a source for information about the problems that arise over the years. You can find the latest facts about diabetes and the best sources to discover any information that comes out after the publication of this edition.

Throughout this book I use some specific conventions to make the text clearer, to highlight information, and to make your read as effortless as possible. These conventions are important to know, so I list them here:

- ✔ **Sugar versus glucose:** Diabetes, as you may know, is all about sugar. But sugars come in many types. So doctors avoid using the words *sugar* and *glucose* interchangeably. In this book (unless I slip up), I use the word *glucose* rather than *sugar.* (You may as well get used to it.)

- ✔ **Emphasis on type 2 diabetes:** There are a number of different types of diabetes (see my explanation in Chapter 3), and the most common are type 1 diabetes and type 2 diabetes. Because I recently published *Type 1 Diabetes For Dummies* (John Wiley & Sons, Inc.), most of what you read here is about type 2 diabetes.

- ✔ **Abbreviations:** To save time, I use the following abbreviations:

  - **T1DM:** Type 1 diabetes mellitus (formal name of type 1 diabetes)

  - **T2DM:** Type 2 diabetes mellitus (formal name of type 2 diabetes)

- ✔ **Pharmaceutical drug names:** When I mention a drug used in the treatment of diabetes, I give the generic name. I provide the trade name in parentheses if relevant.

Foolish Assumptions

The book assumes that you know nothing about diabetes. So you won't have to face a term that you've never heard of before and that is not explained. For those who already know a lot about diabetes, you can find more in-depth explanations in this book as well. You can pick and choose how much you want to know about a subject, but the key points are clearly marked.

Icons Used in This Book

The icons alert you to information you must know, information you should know, and information you may find interesting but can live without.

When you see this icon, it means the information is essential and you should be aware of it.

This icon points out when you should see your doctor (for example, if your blood glucose level is too high or you need a particular test done).

This icon marks important information that can save you time and energy.

I use this icon whenever I tell a story about patients.

This icon gives you technical information or terminology that may be helpful, but not necessary, to your understanding of the topic.

This icon warns against potential problems (for example, if you don't treat a complication of diabetes properly).

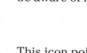

I use this icon to direct you to supplemental information online, including a glossary, at www.dummies.com/extras/diabetes.

Beyond This Book

In addition to the content of this book, you can access some related material online. I have posted the Cheat Sheet at www.dummies.com/cheatsheet/diabetes. It contains important information that you may want to refer to on a regular basis. I also share some additional bits of information and pointers at www.dummies.com/extras/diabetes that can help you navigate this medical condition. You can find a glossary as well as a reference guide for additional help you can find online to deal with your diabetes.

Where to Go from Here

Where you go from here depends on your needs. If you already have basic knowledge of diabetes and want to know more about complications, go to Chapter 3. If you are a novice, start at Chapter 1. If you want to know more about the medications you are taking, go to Chapter 11. Each chapter title clearly tells you what you can find there, so check the table of contents to find what you need rapidly.

As you'll find out, keeping a positive attitude and finding some humor in your diabetes can help you a great deal. At times you'll feel like doing anything but laughing. But scientific studies are clear about the benefits of a positive attitude. In a very few words: He who laughs, lasts. Another point is that people learn more and retain more when humor is part of the process.

Part I
Getting Started with Diabetes

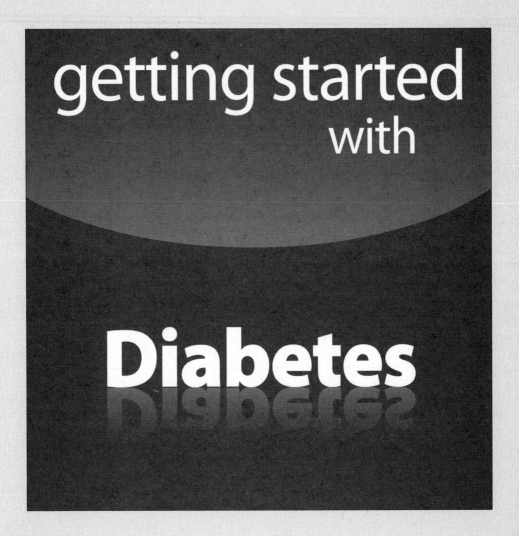

 Check out www.dummies.com/cheatsheet/diabetes for a handy Cheat Sheet chockfull of important information about diabetes that you can refer to on a regular basis.

In this part . . .

- ✔ Deal with the diagnosis of diabetes so you can take appropriate action with your doctor to create a treatment and action plan.

- ✔ Obtain an in-depth understanding of the definition of diabetes so you can determine the severity of your condition.

- ✔ Clarify the types of diabetes to form a foundation for your understanding of the various treatment options.

- ✔ Get to know your pancreas and all it does for you, allowing you to appreciate what it means when it isn't working appropriately.

Chapter 1

Dealing with Diabetes

. . . .

In This Chapter

▶ Discovering successful people with diabetes

▶ Coping with the initial diagnosis

▶ Upholding your quality of life

. . . .

If you have diabetes, in the course of a year you live with that diagnosis for about 8,760 hours. During that time, you spend perhaps one hour with a physician. In Chapter 12, I introduce you to many of the other people who may help you to manage your disease. Clearly, however, the ball is in your hands alone practically all the time. How you deal with your diabetes determines whether you score or are shut out.

One of my patients told me about working at her first job out of college, where each employee birthday was celebrated with cake. She came to the first celebration and was urged to eat a slice. She refused and refused, until finally she had to say, "I can't eat the cake because I am diabetic." The woman urging her said, "Thank God. I thought you just had incredible willpower." Twenty years later, my patient clearly remembers being told that having diabetes is better than having willpower. Another patient told me the following: "The hardest thing about having diabetes is having to deal with doctors who do not respect me." Several times over the years, she had followed her doctor's recommendations exactly, but her glucose control hadn't been satisfactory. The doctor blamed her for this "failure."

Unless you live alone on a desert island (in which case I'm impressed that you got your hands on this book), your diabetes doesn't affect just you. How you deal with your diabetes affects your family, friends, and co-workers. This chapter shows you how to cope with diabetes and how to understand its impact on your important relationships.

Achieving Anything . . . Or Everything!

Diabetes has become such a common disease in the United States that in any group of ten people, one will probably have it. Is it any wonder that successful people have diabetes in every walk of life? In this chapter, I tell you of the accomplishments of just a few of them. Just like them, I can promise you that if you follow the advice in this book, your diabetes will never prevent you from accomplishing your goals. In fact, your success in managing diabetes may lead to success in other areas of your life.

Keeping good company

If you have diabetes, you're not alone. Quite a few famous people live with diabetes every day, just like you. Here are just a few actors that you may recognize:

- **Tom Hanks:** This actor has played numerous roles since he was diagnosed with type 2 diabetes in 2013, including *Captain Phillips, Saving Mr. Banks,* and others. Diabetes hasn't slowed his career at all. In addition to acting, he also produces, directs, and writes screenplays.

- **Wendell Pierce:** If you enjoyed *The Wire* on TV, you enjoyed watching this actor, who played Detective Bunk Moreland. He has been in more than 30 movies and has played many roles on TV including *Treme.* Pierce has tried to help others with his disease by starting a chain of groceries that sell quality food in low-income areas.

- **Sharon Stone:** No one could say that this actress with type 1 diabetes has failed to obtain any roles or to play them with the greatest skill.

People with diabetes also successfully perform in every professional sport. Here are a few sports and the athletes who live with diabetes and still perform at high levels: (To read about the role of sports and exercise in your life, see Chapter 10.)

- **Football:** Kyle Love of the Carolina Panthers and Jake Byrne, who played with the San Diego Chargers, are football players who don't let their diabetes slow them down. Love has type 2 diabetes, and Byrne has type 1 diabetes.

- **Baseball:** Sam Fuld plays baseball for the Oakland Athletics and Brandon Marrow plays baseball with the San Diego Padres.

- **Basketball:** Gary Forbes plays basketball for the Toronto Raptors and Adam Morrison recently retired from professional basketball after playing for the Los Angeles Lakers and the Charlotte Bobcats.

If you think that diabetes might prevent you from a career in the sciences, just consider these modern day researchers with diabetes performing at the highest level in every field:

- **David Cummings, MD:** A professor at the University of Washington, he is exploring the place of metabolic surgery in type 2 diabetes.

- **Martin Gillis, DDS:** He is clarifying the effect of diabetes on the oral cavity.

- **Nicholas Mayall:** He added to science's knowledge of nebulae, supernovae, spiral galaxies, and the age of the universe, and he's in no way limited by his diabetes. And neither should you be.

Realizing your potential

The names in the preceding paragraphs are just a few examples of people with diabetes who have achieved greatness. Here is my point: *Diabetes shouldn't stop you from doing what you want to do with your life.* If you follow the rules of good diabetic care, as I describe in Chapters 7 through 12, you will actually be healthier than people without diabetes who smoke, overeat, and/or don't exercise enough.

Reacting to Your Diagnosis

Do you remember what you were doing when you found out that you had diabetes? Unless you were too young to understand, the news was quite a shock. Suddenly you had a condition from which people can die. In fact, many of the feelings that you went through were exactly those of a person learning that he or she is dying. The following sections describe the normal stages of reacting to a diagnosis of a major medical condition such as diabetes.

Experiencing denial

Your first response was probably to deny that you had diabetes, despite all of the evidence. Your denial mindset may have begun when your doctor tried to sugarcoat (forgive the pun) the news of your condition by telling you that you had just "a touch of diabetes," (an impossibility equivalent to "a touch of pregnancy"). You probably looked for any evidence that the whole thing was a mistake. Perhaps you even neglected to take your medication, follow your diet, or perform the exercise that is so important to maintaining your body. But ultimately, you had to accept the diagnosis and begin to gather the information you needed to help yourself.

When you accepted the diabetes diagnosis, I hope you also shared the news with your family, friends, and people close to you. Having diabetes isn't something to be ashamed of, and you shouldn't hide it from anyone. You need the help of everyone in your community: your co-workers who need to know not to tempt you with treats that you can't eat, your friends who need to know how to give you *glucagon* (a treatment for low blood glucose) if you become unconscious from a severe insulin reaction (see Chapter 4), and your family who needs to know how to support and encourage you to keep going.

Your diabetes isn't your fault — nor is it a form of leprosy or some other disease that carries a social stigma. Diabetes also isn't contagious; no one can catch it from you.

Feeling anger

When you pass the stage of denying that you have diabetes, you may become angry that you're saddled with this "terrible" diagnosis. But you'll quickly find that diabetes isn't so terrible and that you can do something to rid yourself of the disease. Anger only worsens your situation, and being angry about your diagnosis is detrimental in the following ways:

- ✔ If your anger becomes targeted at a person, he or she is hurt.
- ✔ You may feel guilty that your anger is harming you and those close to you.
- ✔ Anger can prevent you from successfully managing your diabetes.

As long as you're angry, you are not in a problem-solving mode. Diabetes requires your focus and attention. Use your energy positively to find creative ways to manage your diabetes. (For help managing your diabetes, see Part III.)

Bargaining for more time and feeling depressed

The stage of anger often transitions into a stage when you become increasingly aware of your mortality and bargain for more time. Even though you probably realize that you have plenty of life ahead of you, you may feel overwhelmed by the talk of complications, blood tests, and pills or insulin. When you realize that bargaining doesn't work, you may even experience depression, which makes good diabetic care all the more difficult.

Studies have shown that people with diabetes suffer from depression at a rate that is two to four times higher than the rate for the general population.

People with diabetes also experience anxiety at a rate three to five times higher than people without diabetes.

If you suffer from depression, you may feel that your diabetic situation creates problems for you that justify being depressed. You may rationalize your depression in the following ways:

- ✔ You can't make friends as easily because diabetes hinders you.
- ✔ You don't have the freedom to choose your leisure activities.
- ✔ You're too tired to overcome difficulties.
- ✔ You dread the future and possible diabetic complications.
- ✔ You don't have the freedom to eat what you want.
- ✔ You're constantly annoyed by all of the minor inconveniences of dealing with diabetes.

All of the preceding concerns are legitimate, but they also are all surmountable. How do you handle your many concerns and fend off depression? Following are a few important methods:

- ✔ Try to achieve excellent blood glucose control (see Part III).
- ✔ Begin a regular exercise program (Chapter 10).
- ✔ Tell a friend or relative how you are feeling; get it off your chest (Chapter 20).
- ✔ Recognize that every abnormal blip in your blood glucose is not your fault (Chapter 7).

If you can't overcome the depression brought on by your diabetic concerns, you may need to consider therapy or antidepressant drugs. But you probably won't reach that point.

Moving on

You may experience the various stages of reacting to your diabetes in a different order than I describe in the previous sections. Some stages may be more prominent for you, and others may be hardly noticeable.

Don't think that any anger, denial, and depression are wrong. These feelings are natural coping mechanisms that serve a psychological purpose for a brief time. Allow yourself to have these feelings — and then drop them. Move on and discover how to live normally with your diabetes.

These phases of coping may not occur in the order given, may not occur at all, and/or may last a long time. If one phase inhibits your ability to cope with your diabetes for more than a few months, you may need outside help.

Here are some key steps you can take to manage the emotional side of diabetes:

- **Focus on your successes.** Some things may go wrong as you find out how to manage diabetes, but most things will go right. As you concentrate on your successes, you will realize that you can cope with diabetes and not let it overwhelm you.

- **Involve the whole family in your diabetes.** A diabetic lifestyle is a healthy lifestyle for everyone. For instance, the exercise you do is good for the whole family. By doing it together, you strengthen the family ties while everyone gets the health benefits. Also, should you need your family to help you, for instance, during a particularly severe case of low blood glucose, their early involvement in learning about diabetes will give them the peace of mind to know they are helping you, not hurting you. (See Chapter 20 for ways to enlist help from people around you.)

- **Develop a positive attitude.** A positive attitude gives you a can-do mindset, whereas a negative attitude leads to low motivation preventing you from doing all that is necessary to manage your diabetes.

- **Find a great team, pinpoint problems, and set goals.** Determine the most difficult problems that you have with your diabetes and then consider how you can solve them by yourself or with a great team of supporting players like a primary care physician, a diabetes specialist, a diabetes educator, a dietitian, an eye doctor, a foot doctor, and so forth. Set realistic goals to get past your problems. (Chapter 12 tells you everything you need to know about getting help from the supporting players.)

- **Don't expect perfection.** Although you may feel that you're doing everything right, you may experience blood glucose levels that are too high or too low. This uncontrollable situation happens to every person with diabetes, and it's one of the biggest frustrations of the disease. Don't beat yourself up over something you can't control. Keep doing the things I suggest in the treatment section, and you will be very gratified at the end.

Maintaining a High Quality of Life

You may assume that a chronic disease like diabetes leads to a diminished quality of life, but you don't have to settle for anything less than a full and fulfilling life.

Many studies have evaluated the quality-of-life question, and the following sections not only describe what these studies found but also describe my hope that you can take control and ensure that you maintain a high quality of life.

Exercising regularly

People who do regular exercise often describe it as addictive. They find it so pleasurable that they look forward to the next session. And the benefits for the person with diabetes are enormous.

In one long-term study on quality of life for people with diabetes, a factor that contributed to a lower quality of life rating was a lack of physical activity, which is one negative factor that you can alter immediately. Physical activity is a habit that you must maintain on a lifelong basis. (See Chapter 10 for advice on exercise.) The problem is that making a long-term change to a more physically active lifestyle is difficult; most people become more active for a time but eventually fall back into inactive routines.

Another study demonstrated the tendency for people with diabetes (and for people in general) to abandon exercise programs after a certain period of time. This information was reported in the *New England Journal of Medicine* in July 1991. In this study, a group of people with diabetes received professional support for two years to encourage them to increase physical activity. For the first six months, the study participants responded well and exercised regularly, resulting in improved blood glucose, weight management, and overall health. After that, participants began to drop out and not come to training sessions. At the end of the two-year study, most participants had regained their weight and slipped back into poor glucose control. However, the few people who didn't stop their exercise maintained the benefits and continued to report an improved quality of life.

Factoring in the (minimal) impact of insulin treatments

If you're in the small group of diabetics who require intensified insulin treatment, perhaps you're afraid that intensified insulin treatment, which involves three or four daily shots of insulin and frequent testing of blood glucose, will keep you from doing the things that you want to do and will diminish your daily quality of life. (See Chapter 11 for more information about intensified insulin treatment.) Your fears are not justified by the facts.

A study published in *Diabetes Care* in 1998 explored whether the extra effort and time consumed by such diabetes treatments had an adverse effect on people's quality of life. The study compared people with diabetes to people with other chronic diseases, such as gastrointestinal disease and hepatitis (liver infection). The diabetic group reported a higher quality of life than the other chronic illness groups. Interestingly, the people in the diabetic group were not so much concerned with the physical problems of diabetes, such as intense and time-consuming tests and treatments, as they were concerned with the social and psychological difficulties.

Another report in *Diabetes Care* in 1998 stated that insulin injections don't reduce the quality of life; the person's sense of physical and emotional well-being remains the same after beginning insulin injections as it was before injections were necessary.

Teenagers who require insulin injections don't always accept the treatment as well as adults do, so teenagers more often experience a diminished quality of life. However, a study of more than 2,000 such teenagers, published in *Diabetes Care* in 2001, showed that as their diabetic control improved, teens felt like they were in better health, experienced greater satisfaction with their lives, and therefore believed themselves to be less of a burden to their families.

Managing stress

A study described in *Diabetes Care* in January 2002 showed that lowering stress lowers blood glucose. Patients were divided into two groups, one of which received diabetes education alone and the other of which received diabetes education plus five sessions of stress management. The latter group showed significant improvement in diabetic control versus the former group.

Whether stress raises the blood glucose directly by causing the release of stress hormones or raises it indirectly by causing overeating, under-exercising, and failure to take medications, managing stress certainly helps to manage your diabetes. Here are some of the things you can do to help manage stress in your life:

- ✔ **Identify the source of the stress.** Are you adding to stress yourself by accepting it as an unchanging part of your life or blaming others or outside events that you can't control?

- ✔ **Examine the way that you cope with stress now.** Do you smoke, drink too much, overeat, spend too much time in front of screens, sleep too much, or overschedule yourself so you have no time?

✔ **Replace unhealthy coping mechanisms with healthy ones.** Avoid the stress you've identified or make a change in your life. Adapt to the stress or accept it. You can't avoid your diabetes, but you can make it less stressful by following my recommendations in Part III.

✔ **Take time out for fun and relaxation.** Here are some of the things you might do:

- Have a picnic lunch

- Get a massage

- Take a long bath

- Work in a garden

- Play with a pet or go to the zoo

- Listen to your favorite music

- Go to a comedy show or rent a funny movie

- Stay in bed with your significant other

Considering other key quality-of-life factors

Many other studies have examined the different aspects of diabetes that affect quality of life. These studies show some useful information on the following topics:

✔ **Family support:** People with diabetes greatly benefit from their family's help in dealing with their disease. But does having a close family help people with diabetes maintain better diabetic control? One study in *Diabetes Care* in February 1998 addressed this question and found some unexpected results. Having a supportive family didn't necessarily mean that the person with diabetes would maintain better glucose control. But a supportive family did make the person with diabetes feel more physically capable in general and much more comfortable with his or her place in society.

✔ **Quality of life over the long term:** How does a person's perception of quality of life change over time? As they age, do most people with diabetes feel that their quality of life increases, decreases, or persists at a steady level? The consensus of several studies is that most people with diabetes experience an increasing quality of life as they get older. People feel better about themselves and their diabetes after dealing with the disease for a decade or more. This report shows the healing property of time.

Following are some other factors that improve quality of life for people with diabetes. Though I can't cite any particular studies here, doctors and patients alike can vouch for their importance.

- **Blood glucose levels:** Keep your blood glucose as normal as possible (see Part III for tips).

- **Continuing education:** Stay aware of the latest developments in diabetes care.

- **Your attitude:** Maintain a healthy attitude. Remember that someday you will laugh about things that bug you now, so why wait?

When you're having trouble coping

You wouldn't hesitate to seek help for your physical ailments associated with diabetes, but you may be reluctant to seek help when you can't adjust psychologically to diabetes. The problem is that sooner or later your psychological maladjustment will ruin any control that you have over your diabetes. And, of course, you won't lead a very pleasant life if you're in a depressed or anxious state all the time. The following symptoms are indicators that you're past the point of handling your diabetes on your own and may be suffering from depression:

- You can't sleep or you sleep too much.

- You have no energy when you're awake.

- You can't think clearly.

- You can't find activities that interest or amuse you.

- You feel worthless.

- You have frequent thoughts of suicide.

- You have no appetite.

- You find no humor in anything.

If you recognize several of these symptoms in your daily life, you need to get some help. Your sense of hopelessness may include the feeling that no one else can help you — but that's simply not true. First, go to your primary physician or endocrinologist (diabetes specialist) for advice. He or she may help you to see the need for some short-term or long-term therapy. Well-trained therapists — especially therapists trained to take care of people with diabetes — can see solutions that you can't see in your current state. You need to find a therapist whom you can trust so that when you're feeling low you can talk to this person and feel assured that he or she is very interested in your welfare.

Your therapist may decide that you would benefit from medication to treat the anxiety or depression. Currently, many drugs are available that are proven safe and free of side effects. Sometimes a brief period of medication is enough to help you adjust to your diabetes.

You can also find help in a support group. The huge and continually growing number of support groups shows that positive things are happening in these groups. In most support groups, participants share their stories and problems, helping everyone involved cope with their own feelings of isolation, futility, or depression.

Chapter 2

Making the Diagnosis with Glucose and Hemoglobin A1c

The Greeks and Romans knew about diabetes. The way they tested for the condition was — prepare yourself — by tasting people's urine. In this way, the Romans discovered that the urine of certain people was *mellitus,* the Latin word for *sweet.* (They got their honey from the island of Malta, which they called *Mellita.*) In addition, the Greeks noticed that when people with sweet urine drank, the fluids came out in the urine almost as fast as they went in the mouth, like a siphon. The Greek word for *siphon* is *diabetes.* Thus we have the origins of the modern name for the disease, *diabetes mellitus.*

In this chapter, I cover some not-so-fun stuff about diabetes — the big words, the definitions, and so on. If you really want to understand what's happening to your body when you have diabetes — and I know I would — then you won't want to skip this chapter.

Realizing the Role of Glucose

The body has three sources of energy: protein, fat, and carbohydrates. I discuss the first two sources in greater detail in Chapter 8, but I tackle the third one now. Sugar is a carbohydrate. Many different kinds of sugars exist in nature, but glucose, the sugar that has the starring role in the body, provides a source of instant energy so that muscles can move and important chemical reactions can take place. Table sugar, or *sucrose,* is actually two different kinds of sugar — glucose and fructose — linked together. Fructose is the type of sugar found in fruits and vegetables. Because fructose is sweeter than glucose, sucrose (the combination of fructose and glucose) is sweeter than glucose alone as well. Therefore, your taste buds don't need as much sucrose or fructose to get the same sweet taste of glucose.

For many years, scientists have debated the role of sugar in the causation of diabetes. Now the evidence seems conclusive. Too much sugar leads to diabetes. In a study of 175 countries over the last decade, increased sugar in the food supply was linked to higher diabetes rates, regardless of obesity. The greater the level of sugar in the food supply, the higher the level of diabetes. The longer a high level of sugar persisted in the food supply, the higher the level of diabetes. The incidence of diabetes decreases as the sugar in the food supply decreases. Increased consumption of sugar precedes diabetes. How much is too much? Researchers haven't established this amount, but the US Department of Agriculture recommends no more than 10 teaspoons of added sugar (sugar not normally found in fruits, vegetables, and dairy) per day. One 12-ounce can of soda has that much added sugar. Most Americans eat more than twice that amount.

In order to understand the symptoms of diabetes, you need to know a little about the way the body normally handles glucose and what happens when things go wrong. A hormone called *insulin* finely controls the level of glucose in your blood. A *hormone* is a chemical substance made in one part of the body that travels (usually through the bloodstream) to a distant part of the body where it performs its work. In the case of insulin, that work is to act like a key to open a cell (such as a muscle, fat, or liver cell) so that glucose can enter. If glucose can't enter the cell, it can provide no energy to the body.

Insulin is essential for growth. In addition to providing the key to entry of glucose into the cell, insulin is considered the *builder hormone* because it enables fat and muscle to form. It promotes the storage of glucose in a form called *glycogen* for use when fuel is not coming in. It also blocks the breakdown of protein. Without insulin, you do not survive for long.

With this fine-tuning, your body keeps the level of glucose pretty steady at about 60 to 100 mg/dl (3.3 to 6.4 mmol/L) all the time.

Your glucose starts to rise in your blood when you don't have a sufficient amount of insulin or when your insulin is not working effectively (see Chapter 3). When your glucose rises above 180 mg/dl (10.0 mmol/L), glucose begins to spill into the urine and make it sweet. Up to that point, the kidneys, the filters for the blood, are able to extract the glucose before it enters your urine. The loss of glucose into the urine leads to many of the short-term complications of diabetes. (See Chapter 4 for more on short-term complications.)

Understanding the Hemoglobin A1c

Your *blood glucose level* is the level of sugar in your blood, a key measure of diabetes. Individual blood glucose tests are great for deciding how you're doing at that moment and what to do to make it better, but they do not give the big picture. They are just a moment in time. Glucose can change a great deal even in 30 minutes. What you need is a test that gives an integrated picture of many days, weeks, or even months of blood glucose levels. The test that accomplishes this important task is called the *hemoglobin A1c.*

Hemoglobin is a protein that carries oxygen around the body and drops it off wherever it's needed to help in all the chemical reactions that are constantly taking place. The hemoglobin is packaged within red blood cells that live in the bloodstream for 60 to 90 days. As the blood circulates, glucose in the blood attaches to the hemoglobin and stays attached. It attaches in several different ways to the hemoglobin, and the total of all the hemoglobin attached to glucose is called *glycohemoglobin.* Glycohemoglobin normally makes up about 6 percent of the hemoglobin in the blood. The largest fraction, two-thirds of the glycohemoglobin, is in the form called *hemoglobin A1c,* making it easiest to measure. The rest of the hemoglobin is made up of hemoglobin A1a and A1b.

The more glucose in the blood, the more glycohemoglobins form. Because red blood cells carrying glycohemoglobin remain in the blood for two to three months, glycohemoglobin is a reflection of the glucose control over the entire time period and not just the second that a single glucose test reflects.

Hemoglobin A1c has a number of advantages over the variety of glucose tests for diagnosing diabetes, which I discuss in the later section "Diagnosing diabetes through testing." Hemoglobin A1c is now as well standardized as glucose testing, and it has the following benefits:

- ✔ A1c reflects chronic high blood glucose rather than a few seconds in time.
- ✔ A1c has been found to reflect future complications (see Chapter 5) better than fasting glucose.
- ✔ Fasting isn't necessary, and acute changes like diet and exercise don't affect A1c.
- ✔ A1c is not as affected by sample delays on the way to or in the lab.
- ✔ A1c is also used to follow the course of diabetes, so the level of treatment needed is immediately understood.
- ✔ A1c is cost-effective, because no further testing is immediately necessary when results are abnormal (whereas an abnormal glucose test requires another glucose or A1c as the next test).

Following are some disadvantages of hemoglobin A1c:

- Abnormal glucose after eating is a better predictor of heart disease than A1c.

- Some subjects with anemia, a recent blood transfusion, and abnormal hemoglobin types (there are several types of hemoglobin) produce an unreliable A1c result.

- Different ethnic groups have different levels for their abnormal A1c.

According to one study, in the United States, hemoglobin A1c detects that diabetes is present in one in every five people admitted to a hospital for any reason without a diagnosis of diabetes.

Getting a Wake-Up Call from Prediabetes

Diabetes doesn't suddenly appear one day without previous notification from your body. For a period of time, which may last up to ten years, you may not quite achieve the criteria for a diagnosis of diabetes but not be quite normal either. During this time, you have what's called *prediabetes*.

A person with prediabetes doesn't usually develop eye disease, kidney disease, or nerve damage (all potential complications of diabetes, which I discuss in Chapter 5). However, a person with prediabetes has a much greater risk of developing heart disease and brain attacks than someone with entirely normal blood glucose levels. Prediabetes has a lot in common with insulin-resistance syndrome, also known as the *metabolic syndrome,* which I discuss in Chapter 5. The following two sections take the mystery out of whether you may have prediabetes by giving you some guidelines on when to get tested as well as explaining what testing for prediabetes involves.

Knowing whether you should get tested

Approximately 90 million people in the United States have prediabetes, although most of them don't know it. Testing for prediabetes is a good idea for everyone over the age of 45. I also recommend getting tested if you're under 45 and overweight or eat more than ten teaspoons of added sugar daily and have one or more of the following risk factors:

- A high-risk ethnic group: African American, Hispanic, Asian, or Native American

- High blood pressure

- Low HDL ("good" cholesterol)

- High triglycerides

- A family history of diabetes

- Diabetes during a pregnancy or giving birth to a baby weighing more than 9 pounds

A study in the journal *Diabetes Care* in November 2007 showed that testing for prediabetes in overweight or obese people older than age 45 is highly cost effective if they then undergo lifestyle modification (see Chapters 7 through 12) or take medication if necessary. A study published in *Diabetes Care* in February 2014 showed that physically fit individuals with prediabetes have a lower death rate than unfit people with prediabetes, regardless of obesity.

Testing for prediabetes

Testing for prediabetes involves finding out your blood glucose level, the level of sugar in your blood. Prediabetes exists when the body's blood glucose level is higher than normal but not high enough to meet the standard definition of diabetes mellitus (which I discuss in the section "Diagnosing diabetes through testing," later in this chapter). Testing measures a random capillary blood glucose. If the level is greater than 100 milligrams per deciliter (mg/dl), a fasting plasma glucose or oral glucose tolerance test is performed. As of 2010, the American Diabetes Association recommends that the hemoglobin A1c (see the next section) can also be used for the definition. Table 2-1 shows the hemoglobin A1c and glucose levels that indicate prediabetes:

- If the glucose before the test (the fasting plasma glucose) is between 100 and 125 mg/dl, the person has impaired (abnormally high) *fasting glucose,* the glucose before eating (see Table 2-1). The glucose in the fasting state (no food for eight hours) is not normal, but it's not high enough to diagnose diabetes.

- If the glucose is between 140 and 199 mg/dl at two hours after eating 75 grams of glucose, the person has impaired glucose tolerance. Both impaired fasting glucose and impaired glucose tolerance may be present.

- A hemoglobin A1c between 5.7 and 6.4 percent suggests prediabetes.

Table 2-1	Diagnosing Prediabetes		
Condition	Glucose Before Eating	Glucose Two Hours After Eating 75 gm Glucose	Hemoglobin A1c
Normal	Less than 100 mg/dl (5.5 mmol/L)	Less than 140 mg/dl (7.8 mmol/L)	Less than 5.7 percent
Prediabetes	100–125 mg/dl (5.5–7 mmol/L)	140–199 mg/dl (7.8–11.1 mmol/L)	5.7–6.4 percent

Mg/dl, or *milligrams per deciliter,* is the unit of measurement commonly used in the United States. The rest of the world uses the International System (SI), where the units are mmol/L, which means *millimoles per liter.* To get mmol/L, you divide mg/dl by 18. Therefore, 200 mg/dl equals 11.1 mmol/L.

Diagnosing prediabetes can be the best thing that ever happened to a person. It could be the wake-up call that he or she needs. The diagnosis may motivate a person to make crucial lifestyle changes, especially in diet and exercise, which have been shown to prevent the onset of diabetes in people with prediabetes. And for people whose prediabetes doesn't respond to lifestyle changes, medication may accomplish the same thing.

After a diagnosis of prediabetes is made, all the techniques described in Chapters 7 through 12 can help prevent the onset of clinical diabetes. If patients with prediabetes are left untreated, large numbers of these patients will develop diabetes over time. Preventing diabetes saves a person almost $13,700 in annual costs for the treatment of diabetes. And properly responding to a diagnosis of prediabetes prevented almost 20 percent of people with prediabetes from becoming diabetic.

Detecting Diabetes

When prediabetes becomes diabetes, the body's blood glucose level registers even higher. In this section, I discuss the evidence for diabetes and the symptoms you may experience with diabetes.

Diagnosing diabetes through testing

The standard definition of diabetes mellitus is *excessive glucose in a blood sample.* For years, doctors set this level fairly high. The standard level for normal glucose was lowered in 1997 because too many people were experiencing complications of diabetes even though they did not have the disease by the then-current standard. In November 2003, the standard level was modified again. In 2009, the International Expert Committee on Diagnosis and Classification of Diabetes Mellitus recommended using the hemoglobin A1c as a diagnostic criterion for diabetes, and the American Diabetes Association subsequently accepted the recommendation.

After much discussion, many meetings, and the usual deliberations that surround a momentous decision, the American Diabetes Association published the new standard for diagnosis, which includes any *one* of the following four criteria:

- ✔ **Hemoglobin A1c equal to or greater than 6.5 percent.**

- ✔ **Casual plasma glucose concentration greater than or equal to 200 mg/dl, along with symptoms of diabetes.** *Casual plasma glucose* refers to the glucose level when the patient eats normally prior to the test. I discuss symptoms in the section "Examining the symptoms of diabetes" later in this chapter.

- ✔ **Fasting plasma glucose (FPG) of greater than or equal to 126 mg/dl or 7 mmol/L.** *Fasting* means that the patient has consumed no food for eight hours prior to the test.

- ✔ **Blood glucose of greater than or equal to 200 mg/dl (11.1 mmol/L) when tested two hours (2-h PG) after ingesting 75 grams of glucose by mouth.** This test has long been known as the *oral glucose tolerance test*. Although this time-consuming, cumbersome test is rarely done, it remains the gold standard for the diagnosis of diabetes.

Following is another way to look at the criteria for diagnosis:

- ✔ FPG less than 100 mg/dl (5.5 mmol/L) is a normal fasting glucose.

  FPG greater than or equal to 100 mg/dl but less than 126 mg/dl (7.0 mmol/L) is impaired fasting glucose (indicating prediabetes).

  FPG equal to or greater than 126 mg/dl (7.0 mmol/L) gives a provisional diagnosis of diabetes.

- ✔ 2-h PG less than 140 mg/dl (7.8 mmol/L) is normal glucose tolerance.

  2-h PG greater than or equal to 140 mg/dl but less than 200 mg/dl (11.1 mmol/L) is impaired glucose tolerance.

  2-h PG equal to or greater than 200 mg/dl gives a provisional diagnosis of diabetes.

- ✔ Hemoglobin A1c equal to or greater than 6.5 percent gives a provisional diagnosis of diabetes. As the hemoglobin A1c rises from normal, the occurrence of diabetes rises with it. If the hemoglobin A1c is equal to or greater than 5.6, the patient has a threefold chance of developing diabetes in the next six years.

Testing positive for diabetes one time isn't enough to confirm a diagnosis. Any one of the tests must be positive on another occasion to make a diagnosis of diabetes. I've had patients come to me with a diagnosis of diabetes after being tested only once, and a second test has shown the initial diagnosis to be incorrect.

Examining the symptoms of diabetes

The following list contains the most common early symptoms of diabetes and how they occur. One or more of the following symptoms may be present when diabetes is diagnosed:

- **Frequent urination and thirst:** The glucose in the urine draws more water out of your blood, so more urine forms, making you feel the need to urinate more frequently. As the amount of water in your blood declines, you feel thirsty and drink much more frequently.

- **Blurry vision:** As the glucose level shifts from normal to very high, the lens of the eye swells due to water intake. This swelling prevents the eye from focusing light at the correct place, and blurring occurs.

- **Extreme hunger:** Inability to get energy in the form of glucose into the muscle cells that need it leads to a feeling of hunger despite all the glucose that is floating in the bloodstream. Such hunger is called "starvation in the midst of plenty."

- **Fatigue:** Without sufficient insulin, or with ineffective insulin, glucose can't enter cells (such as muscle and fat cells) that depend on insulin to act as a key. (The most important exception here is the brain, which does not need insulin to extract glucose from the blood.) As a result, glucose can't be used as a fuel to move muscles or to facilitate the many other chemical reactions that have to take place to produce energy. A person with diabetes often complains of fatigue and feels much stronger after treatment allows glucose to enter his or her cells again.

- **Weight loss:** Weight loss occurs among some people with diabetes because they lack insulin, the builder hormone. When the body lacks insulin for any reason, the body begins to break down. You lose muscle tissue. Some of the muscle converts into glucose even though the glucose can't get into cells. It passes out of your body in the urine. Fat tissue breaks down into small fat particles that can provide an alternate source of energy. As your body breaks down and you lose glucose in the urine, you often experience weight loss. However, most people with diabetes are heavy rather than skinny. (I explain why in Chapter 3.)

Similar symptoms; different diseases

Frequent thirst and urination are the most commonly recognized symptoms of diabetes, but diabetes mellitus is not the only condition that causes these symptoms. Another condition in which fluids go in and out of the body like a siphon is called *diabetes insipidus.* With this condition, the urine is not sweet. Diabetes insipidus is an entirely different disease that you should not mistake for diabetes mellitus.

Diabetes insipidus results when a hormone in the brain called *antidiuretic hormone* is missing or when the kidneys can't properly respond to antidiuretic hormone. This hormone normally helps the kidneys prevent the loss of a lot of the water in the body. Other than the name *diabetes,* this condition has nothing to do with diabetes mellitus.

✔ **Persistent vaginal infection among women:** As blood glucose rises, all the fluids in your body contain higher levels of glucose, including the sweat and body secretions such as semen in men and vaginal secretions in women. Many bugs, such as bacteria and yeast, thrive in the high-glucose environment. Women begin to complain of itching or burning, an abnormal discharge from the vagina, and sometimes an odor.

A study in the November 2007 issue of *Diabetes Care,* however, showed that in a group of over 15,000 people being treated for diabetes, 44 percent of people with type 2 diabetes reported not one of the symptoms above in the previous year when given a questionnaire. It is no wonder that a third of people with diabetes don't know they have it.

Tracing the History of Diabetes Treatment

More than 2,000 years ago, people writing in China and India described a condition that must have been diabetes mellitus. The description is the same one that the Greeks and Romans reported — urine that tasted sweet. Scholars from India and China were the first to describe frequent urination. But not until 1776 did researchers discover the cause of the sweetness — glucose. And it wasn't until the 19th century that doctors developed a new chemical test to actually measure glucose in the urine.

Later discoveries showed that the pancreas produces a crucial substance that controls the glucose in the blood: insulin. Since that discovery was made, scientists have found ways to extract insulin and purify it so it can be given to people whose insulin levels are too low.

After insulin was discovered, diabetes specialists, led by Elliot Joslin and others, recommended three basic treatments for diabetes that are as valuable today as they were in 1921:

✔ Diet (see Chapter 8)

✔ Exercise (see Chapter 10)

✔ Medication (see Chapter 11)

Although the discovery of insulin immediately saved the lives of thousands of very sick individuals for whom the only treatment had been starvation, it did not solve the problem of diabetes. As these people aged, they were found to have unexpected complications in the eyes, the kidneys, and the nervous system (see Chapter 5). And insulin didn't address the problem of the much larger group of people with diabetes now known as type 2 (see Chapter 3). Their problem was not lack of insulin but resistance to its actions. (Fortunately, doctors do have the tools now to bring the disease under control.)

The next major leap in the effort to treat diabetes, occurring in 1955, was the discovery of the group of drugs called *sulfonylureas* (see Chapter 11), the first drugs that could be taken by mouth to lower blood glucose levels. But even while those drugs were improving patient care, the only way to know if someone's blood glucose level was high was to test the urine, which was entirely inadequate for good diabetic control (see Chapter 7).

Around 1980, the first portable meters for blood glucose testing became available. For the first time, doctors and patients could relate treatment to a measurable outcome. This development has led, in turn, to the discovery of other great drugs for diabetes, such as metformin, exenatide, and others yet to come.

If you are not using these wonderful tools for your diabetes, you are missing the boat. You can find out exactly how to use portable meters in Part III.

Tracking diabetes around the world

Diabetes is a global health problem. Type 2 diabetes is especially prevalent where obesity is common. In 2008, more than 1.5 billion people were overweight (body-mass index greater than 25 kilograms/meter squared — see Chapter 7) and 500 million people were obese (body-mass index greater than 30) in the world. Currently 366 million people have diabetes. Diabetes is most concentrated in areas where large food supplies allow people to eat more calories than they need, causing them to develop excessive fat. Several different types of diabetes exist, but the type usually associated with obesity, called *type 2 diabetes* (see Chapter 3), is far more prevalent than the other types.

Another reason diabetes cases have continued to grow in number throughout the world is that the life span of the population is increasing. What's the connection? Well, as a person ages, his or her chances of developing diabetes increases greatly. Along with obesity, age is a major risk factor for diabetes. (See Chapter 3 for more risk factors.) So as other diseases are controlled and the population in general gets older, more diabetes is being diagnosed.

One very interesting study traced people of Japanese ancestry as they went from living in Japan to living in Hawaii to living in the United States mainland. In Japan, where people customarily maintain a normal weight, they tended to have a very low incidence of diabetes. As they moved to Hawaii, the incidence of diabetes began to rise along with their average weight. On the U.S. mainland, where food is most available, these Japanese had the highest rate of diabetes of all.

In general, as people migrate to areas of the world consuming a Western diet, not only the number of calories they consume but also the composition of their diets changes. Before they migrate, they tend to consume a low-fat, high-fiber diet. After they reach their destination, they adopt the local diet, which tends to be higher in fat and lower in fiber. The carbohydrates in the new diet are from high-energy foods, which do not tend to be filling, which in turn promotes more caloric intake.

Explaining the Obesity (and Diabetes) Epidemic

Many changes explain the epidemic of obesity and diabetes that began to explode in the 1950s and '60s. Here are some of them:

- The availability of fast-food restaurants and vending machines
- The frequency of television commercials for foods filled with fats and sugar
- The large number of screens watched passively all day, from TVs to smartphones

- ✔ The larger, higher-calorie meals that tend to be eaten, both at home and at restaurants

- ✔ The dependence on vehicles for much movement

- ✔ The huge increase in mass-produced, high-calorie convenience foods

What steps can people take to reverse this trend? Some of the ideas developed to reverse the high rate of cigarette smoking can be recycled, but the process takes years for the whole population. What you can do immediately is contained in Part III. Some of the population-wide measures include the following strategies:

- ✔ A tax on low-nutrition foods like sweetened beverages

- ✔ Better labeling of foods; for example, a red label for low-nutrition, high-calorie foods; a yellow label for intermediate foods; and a green label for low-calorie, high-nutrition foods

- ✔ A ban on or reduction of advertising of junk foods

- ✔ School-based programs promoting healthier eating and elimination of soft drinks and sugared juices

- ✔ A low, fixed amount of screen time for children

Putting Faces to the Numbers: Sharing Some Real Patient Stories

The numbers that are used to diagnose diabetes don't begin to reflect the human dimensions of the disease. People end up with test results after days, months, or even years of minor discomforts that reach the point where they can no longer be tolerated. The next few stories of real (though renamed) patients can help you understand that diabetes is a disease that happens to real people — people who are working, relaxing, traveling, sleeping, and doing many other things that make life so complex.

Sal Renolo was a 46-year-old black-belt judo instructor. Despite his very active lifestyle, he was not careful about his diet and had gained 16 pounds in the last few years. He was more fatigued than he had been in the past but blamed this fatigue on his increasing age. His mother had diabetes, but he assumed that his physical fitness would protect him from this condition. However, he could barely get through a one-hour class without excusing himself for a bathroom break. One of his new students had diabetes, and he suggested to Sal that he ought to have the problem checked, but Sal insisted that he could not possibly have diabetes with all his activity. The symptoms of fatigue and frequent urination got worse, and Sal finally made an appointment with the doctor. Blood tests revealed a random blood glucose level of 264 mg/dl (14.7 mmol/L). The following week, another random blood glucose was 289 (16.0 mmol/L). The doctor told Sal he had diabetes, but Sal refused to believe it. He left the doctor's office angry but vowed to lose weight and did so successfully. On a repeat visit to the doctor, a random glucose was 167 mg/dl (9.3 mmol/L). Sal told the doctor that he knew he didn't have diabetes, but his resolve to eat carefully didn't last, and he was back six weeks later with a glucose of 302 mg/dl (16.8 mmol/L). Finally, Sal accepted the diagnosis and started treatment. He rapidly returned to his usual state of health, and the fatigue disappeared.

Debby O'Leary's active sex life with her husband was continually being interrupted by vaginal yeast infections, which resulted in an unpleasant odor, redness, and itching. Over-the-counter preparations promptly cured the condition, but it always rapidly returned. Finally, after three of these infections in two months, she decided to see her gynecologist. The gynecologist told her she needed a prescription drug. The cure lasted a little longer this time, but the infection promptly returned. On a return visit, the gynecologist did a urinalysis and found glucose in her urine. A random blood test showed a glucose of 243 mg/dl (13.5 mmol/L). He sent her to an internist, who ordered a variety of tests including a fasting blood glucose, which was 149 mg/dl (8.3 mmol/L). The doctor told her she had diabetes and recommended exercise and diet change to start with. She followed his advice, and as a result she not only lowered her blood glucose to the point that she no longer developed yeast infections but also lost weight and increased her energy, making her sex life with her husband even more satisfying.

Chapter 3

Recognizing the Various Types of Diabetes

In This Chapter

▶ Paying attention to your pancreas

▶ Comparing type 1 and type 2 diabetes

▶ Being aware of other types of diabetes

*L*adies and gentlemen, I'd like to introduce you to your pancreas. This shy little organ — to which you've probably never given any attention — can rear its lovely head at entirely unexpected moments. (You probably didn't even know that your pancreas has a head and a tail, but it does. Now you've broken the ice!) Most of the time, your pancreas hides behind your stomach, quietly doing its work by assisting with digestion first and then helping to make use of the digested food. The information in this chapter should put you on closer terms with your pancreas, which is good, because you need your pancreas as much as it needs you. In one way or another, the pancreas plays a role in all of the various types of diabetes.

Here's the good news: You can prevent diabetes. Here's the bad news: You can't do so quite as easily as you may like. Your best method for preventing diabetes is to pick your parents carefully, but that method is slightly impractical, even with modern technology.

In general, you can prevent a disease if it meets two requirements. First, you have to be able to identify if you are at high risk for getting the disease. Second, some treatments or actions must exist that can definitely reduce the occurrence of the disease. This chapter shows you how to identify whether you're at risk for type 1 or type 2 diabetes, and it covers definite actions that you can take to prevent both of these types of diabetes.

This chapter helps you get a clear understanding of your type of diabetes, how it relates to the other types of diabetes, and how the failure of your friendly pancreas to do its assigned job can lead to a host of unfortunate consequences. (I cover these consequences in detail in Part II.)

Getting to Know Your Pancreas and Its Role in Diabetes

You don't see your pancreas very often, but you hear from it all the time. It has two major functions. One is to produce *digestive enzymes,* which are the chemicals in your small intestine that help to break down food. The digestive enzymes don't have much relation to diabetes. Your pancreas's other function is to produce a hormone of major importance, *insulin,* and to secrete it directly into the blood. The following sections explore the ins and outs of your pancreas and insulin so that you're well acquainted with both.

Examining your pancreas

Figure 3-1 shows the microscopic appearance of the pancreas. The following list explains the different cells found in the pancreas as well as their functions:

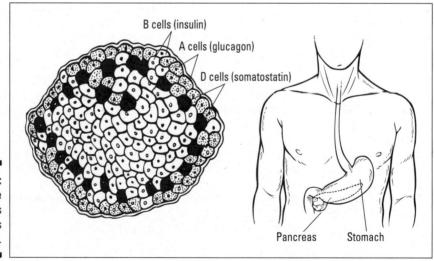

Figure 3-1: The pancreas and its parts.

Illustration by Kathryn Born

✔ **B cells:** The insulin-producing pancreas cells (also called *beta* cells) are found in groups called *Islets of Langerhans.*

✔ **A cells:** These cells produce *glucagon,* a hormone that's very important to people with diabetes because it raises blood glucose when the glucose level gets too low. A cells are present in the Islets of Langerhans.

✔ **D cells:** These cells make *somatostatin* (a hormone that blocks the secretion of other hormones but doesn't have a use in diabetes because it causes high blood sugar and increased ketones by blocking insulin as well). Like the cells described above, D cells are also found in the Islets of Langerhans.

Understanding insulin

If you understand only one hormone in your body, insulin should be that hormone (especially if you want to understand diabetes). Over the course of your life, the insulin that your body produces or the insulin that you inject into your body (as I describe in Chapter 11) affects whether or not you control the glucose levels in your blood and avoid the complications of the disease.

Think of your insulin as an insurance agent who lives in San Francisco (which is your pancreas) but travels from there to do business in Seattle (your muscles), Denver (your fat tissue), Los Angeles (your liver), and other places. This insulin insurance agent is insuring your good health.

Wherever insulin travels in your body, it opens up the cells so that glucose can enter them. After glucose enters, the cells can immediately use it for energy, store it in a storage form of glucose (called *glycogen*) for rapid use later on, or convert it to fat for use even later as energy.

After glucose leaves your blood and enters your cells, your blood glucose level falls. Your pancreas can tell when your glucose is falling, and it turns off the release of insulin to prevent *hypoglycemia,* an unhealthy low level of blood glucose (see Chapter 4). At the same time, your liver begins to release glucose from storage and makes new glucose from amino acids in your blood.

If your insurance agent (insulin, remember? — stick with me here!) doesn't show up when you need him (meaning that you have an absence of insulin, as in type 1 diabetes) or he does a poor job when he shows up (such as when you have a resistance to insulin, as in type 2 diabetes), your insurance coverage may be very poor (in which case your blood glucose starts to climb). High blood glucose is the beginning of all your problems.

Doctors have proven that high blood glucose is bad for you and that keeping the blood glucose as normal as possible prevents the complications of diabetes (which I explain in Part II). Most treatments for diabetes are directed at restoring the blood glucose to normal.

Understanding Type 1 Diabetes and You

John Phillips, a 6-year-old boy, was always very active, and his parents became concerned when the counselors at summer camp told them that he seemed to not have much energy. When he got home from camp, John's parents noticed that he was thirsty all the time and running to the bathroom. He was very hungry but seemed to be losing weight, despite eating more than enough. John's parents took him to the pediatrician, who did several blood glucose tests and diagnosed their son with *type 1 diabetes mellitus* (T1DM), which used to be called *juvenile diabetes* or *insulin-dependent diabetes.*

This story has a happy ending because John's parents were willing to do the necessary things to bring John's glucose under control. John is just as energetic as ever, but he has had to get used to a few inconveniences in his daily routine. (I cover such daily lifestyle changes in Part III.) The following sections touch on the symptoms and causes of this type of diabetes.

Note: Type 1 diabetes is covered extensively in my book *Type 1 Diabetes For Dummies* (John Wiley & Sons, Inc.). Because this book is mainly about type 2 diabetes, I simply point out where the two types are the same and where they differ.

Identifying symptoms of type 1 diabetes

Following are some of the major signs and symptoms of type 1 diabetes. If you find you have any of these symptoms and haven't already been diagnosed with diabetes, call your doctor.

- ✔ Frequent urination
- ✔ Increase in thirst
- ✔ Weight loss
- ✔ Increase in hunger
- ✔ Weakness

Type 1 diabetes used to be called *juvenile diabetes* because it occurs most frequently in children. However, so many cases are found in adults that doctors don't use the term *juvenile* any more. Some children are diagnosed early in life, and other children have a more severe onset of the disease as they get a little older.

With children over age 10 and adults, the early signs and symptoms of diabetes may have been missed. These people have a great deal of fat breakdown in their bodies to provide energy, and this fat breakdown creates other problems. *Ketone bodies,* products of the breakdown of fats, begin to accumulate in the blood and spill into the urine. Ketone bodies are acidic and lead to nausea, abdominal pain, and sometimes vomiting.

At the same time as fat is breaking down, the child's blood glucose rises higher. From a normal level of 80 mg/dl (4.4 mmol/L), blood glucose can rise to the unhealthy level of 300 mg/dl (16 mmol/L) and even up to the dangerously high levels of 400 to 600 mg/dl (22.2 to 33.3 mmol/L). At high levels, the child's blood is like thick maple syrup and doesn't circulate as freely as normal. The large amount of water leaving the body with the glucose depletes important substances such as sodium and potassium. Vomiting causes the child to lose more fluids and body substances. All these abnormalities cause the child to become very drowsy and possibly lose consciousness. This situation is called *diabetic ketoacidosis,* and if it isn't identified and corrected quickly, the child can die. (See Chapter 4 for more details on the symptoms, causes, and treatments of ketoacidosis.)

A few special circumstances affect the symptoms that you may see in persons with type 1 diabetes. Remember the following factors:

- ✔ **The *honeymoon* period, a natural occurrence, is a time after the diagnosis of diabetes when the person's insulin needs decline for one to six months and the disease seems to get milder.** The honeymoon period is longer when a child is older at the time of diagnosis, but the apparent diminishing of the disease is always temporary.

- ✔ **Males and females get type 1 diabetes to an equal degree.**

- ✔ **Warm summer months are associated with a decrease in the occurrence of diabetes compared to the winter months, particularly in children older than 10.** The probable reason for this occurrence is that a virus is involved in bringing on diabetes (which I discuss in "Getting type 1 diabetes"), and viruses spread much more when children are learning and playing together inside in the winter.

Investigating the causes of type 1 diabetes

When your doctor diagnoses you with type 1 diabetes, you almost certainly will wonder what could have caused you to acquire the disease. Did someone with diabetes sneeze on you? Did you eat so much sugary food that your body reacted by giving you diabetes? Rest assured that the causes of diabetes aren't so simple.

Type 1 diabetes is an *autoimmune disease,* meaning that your body is unkind enough to react against — and in this case, destroy — a vital part of itself, namely the insulin-producing *beta (B) cells* of the pancreas. One way that doctors discovered that type 1 diabetes is an autoimmune disease is by measuring proteins in the blood, called *antibodies,* which are literally substances directed against your body — in particular, against your islet cells. Another clue that type 1 diabetes is an autoimmune disease is that drugs that reduce autoimmunity also delay the onset of type 1 diabetes. Also, type 1 diabetes tends to occur in people who have other known autoimmune diseases.

You may wonder how doctors can know in advance that certain people will develop type 1 diabetes. The method of prediction isn't 100 percent accurate, but people who get type 1 diabetes more often have certain abnormal characteristics on their genetic material, their *chromosomes,* that are not present in people who don't get type 1 diabetes. Doctors can look for these abnormal characteristics on your DNA. But having these abnormal characteristics doesn't guarantee that you'll get diabetes.

Another essential factor in predicting whether you will develop type 1 diabetes is your exposure to something in the environment, most likely a virus. I discuss this factor in detail in the next section.

Getting type 1 diabetes

To develop diabetes, most people also have to come in contact with something in the environment that triggers the destruction of their beta cells, the cells that make insulin. Doctors think that this environmental trigger is probably a virus. This type of virus can cause diabetes by attacking your pancreas directly and diminishing your ability to produce insulin, which quickly creates the diabetic condition in your body. The virus can also cause diabetes if it is made up of a substance that is also naturally present in your pancreas. If the virus and your pancreas possess the same substance, the antibodies that your body produces to fight off the virus will also attack the shared substance in your pancreas, leaving you in the same condition as if the virus itself attacked your pancreas.

A small number (about 10 percent) of patients who develop type 1 diabetes don't seem to need an environmental factor to trigger the diabetes. In them, the disease is entirely an autoimmune destruction of the beta cells. If you fall into this category of people with diabetes, you may have other autoimmune diseases, such as autoimmune thyroid disease.

Although genetics plays a role in developing type 1 diabetes, the connection is relatively minor. An identical twin has only a 20 percent chance of developing type 1 diabetes if his identical twin (who has the exact same genetic material) has it.

Preventing type 1 diabetes

The most important study of prevention of diabetes complications ever done for type 1 diabetes is called the Diabetes Control and Complications Trial (DCCT), published in 1993. The DCCT showed that keeping very tight control over your blood glucose is possible but difficult. The difficult part of keeping your blood glucose close to normal is that you increase your risk of having low blood glucose, or hypoglycemia (see Chapter 4). The DCCT study showed that you can prevent many of the complications of diabetes — including eye, kidney, and nerve disease — by keeping your blood glucose as close to normal as possible. If you already suffer from such complications, improving your blood glucose control very significantly slows the progression of the complications. Since the DCCT, doctors generally treat type 1 diabetes by keeping the patient's blood glucose as close to normal as is possible and practical.

If you would like to read much more on the subject of type 1 diabetes, please see my book *Type 1 Diabetes For Dummies* (John Wiley & Sons, Inc.).

Having Type 2 Diabetes

Edythe Fokel, a 46-year-old woman, has gained about 10 pounds in the last year, so that her 5-foot 5-inch body now weighs about 155 pounds. Edythe doesn't do much exercise. She has felt somewhat fatigued recently, but she blames her age and approaching menopause. She also blames the fact that she now gets up several times a night to urinate, which she didn't used to do. She is disturbed because her vision is blurry and her job requires working on a computer. Finally, Edythe goes to her gynecologist after developing a rash and discharge in her vagina. When Edythe describes her symptoms, her gynecologist decides to do a blood glucose test. He refers her back to her primary physician when Edythe's blood glucose level registers at 220 mg/dl (12.2 mmol/L).

Edythe's primary doctor asks her whether other members of her family have had diabetes, and she replies that her mother and a sister are both being treated for it. The doctor also asks Edythe about any tingling in her feet, and she admits that she has noticed some tingling for the past few months but didn't think it was important. The primary doctor repeats the random blood glucose test, which comes back at 260 mg/dl (14.4 mmol/L). He informs Edythe that she has type 2 diabetes (T2DM).

The signs and symptoms that Edythe manifests in this scenario, along with the results of the two blood glucose tests, provide a textbook picture of type 2 diabetes. (Type 2 diabetes used to be known as *adult-onset diabetes* or *non-insulin-dependent diabetes.*) But be aware that people with type 2 diabetes may have few or none of these symptoms. Because of the varying symptoms, your doctor needs to check your blood glucose level on a regular basis. (I discuss how often you should do this test in Chapter 7.)

Most people with type 2 diabetes are over the age of 40, but I am seeing more and more cases in children and young adults. Your chances of getting type 2 diabetes increase as you get older. Type 2 diabetes is a disease of gradual onset rather than the severe emergency that can herald type 1 diabetes. Because the symptoms are so mild at first, you may not notice them. You may ignore these symptoms for years before they become bothersome enough to consult your doctor. No autoimmunity is involved in type 2 diabetes, so no antibodies are found. Doctors believe that no virus is involved in the onset of type 2 diabetes.

Recent statistics show that ten times more people worldwide have type 2 diabetes than type 1 diabetes. Although type 2 is much more prevalent, those with type 2 diabetes seem to have milder severity of complications (such as eye disease and kidney disease) from diabetes. (See Part II for details about the possible complications of diabetes. See Part III for treatments that can help you prevent these complications.)

Identifying symptoms of type 2 diabetes

A fairly large percentage of the U.S. population (approximately 26 million people) has type 2 diabetes. The numbers are on the rise, and one reason is an increase in the incidence of obesity, a major risk factor for T2DM. If you're obese, you are considerably more likely to acquire T2DM than you would be if you maintained your ideal weight. (See Chapter 7 for the details on how to figure out your weight classification.)

The following signs and symptoms are good indicators that you have type 2 diabetes. If you experience two or more of these symptoms and haven't already been diagnosed with diabetes, call your doctor:

- ✓ **Fatigue:** Type 2 diabetes makes you tired because your body's cells aren't getting the glucose fuel that they need. Even though your blood has plenty of insulin, your body is resistant to its actions. (See the "Getting to Know Your Pancreas and Its Role in Diabetes" section for more explanation.)

- ✓ **Frequent urination and thirst:** As with type 1 diabetes, you find yourself urinating more frequently than usual, which dehydrates your body and leaves you thirsty.

- ✓ **Blurred vision:** The lenses of your eyes swell and shrink as your blood glucose levels rise and fall. Your vision blurs because your eyes can't adjust quickly enough to these lens changes.

✔ **Slow healing of skin, gum, and urinary infections:** Your white blood cells, which help with healing and defend your body against infections, don't function correctly in the high-glucose environment present in your body when it has diabetes. Unfortunately, the bugs that cause infections thrive in the same high-glucose environment. So diabetes leaves your body especially susceptible to infections.

✔ **Genital itching:** Yeast infections also love a high-glucose environment, so diabetes is often accompanied by the itching and discomfort of yeast infections.

✔ **Numbness in the feet or legs:** You experience numbness because of a common long-term complication of diabetes called *neuropathy.* (I explain the details of neuropathy in Chapter 5.) If you notice numbness and neuropathy along with the other symptoms of diabetes, you probably have had the disease for quite a while, because neuropathy takes more than five years to develop in a diabetic environment. Occasionally numbness occurs earlier when extreme elevations of the glucose happen.

✔ **Heart disease, stroke, and peripheral vascular disease:** Heart disease, stroke, and peripheral vascular disease (blockage of arteries in the legs) occur much more often in type 2s than in the nondiabetic population. But these complications may appear when you are merely glucose-intolerant (which I explain in the next section), before you actually have diagnosable diabetes.

The signs and symptoms of type 2 diabetes are similar in some cases to the symptoms of type 1 diabetes (which I cover in the "Identifying symptoms of type 1 diabetes" section, earlier in this chapter), but in many ways they are different. The following list shows some of the differences between symptoms in type 1 and type 2 diabetes:

✔ **Age of onset:** People with type 1 diabetes are usually younger than those with type 2 diabetes. However, the increasing incidence of type 2 diabetes in overweight children is making this difference less useful for separating type 1 and type 2 diabetes.

✔ **Body weight:** Those with type 1 diabetes are usually thin or normal in weight, but obesity is a common characteristic of people with type 2 diabetes.

✔ **Level of glucose:** People with type 1 diabetes have higher glucose levels at the onset of the disease. Type 1 diabetics usually have blood glucose levels of 300 to 400 mg/dl (16.6 to 22.2 mmol/L), and people with type 2 diabetes usually have blood glucose levels of 200 to 250 mg/dl (11.1 to 13.9 mmol/L).

✔ **Severity of onset:** Type 1 diabetes usually has a much more severe onset, but type 2 diabetes gradually shows its symptoms.

Investigating what causes (and what doesn't cause) type 2 diabetes

If you've been diagnosed with type 2 diabetes, you're probably shocked and curious about why you developed the disease. Doctors have learned quite a bit about the causes of type 2 diabetes. For example, they know that T2DM runs in families.

Usually, people with type 2 diabetes can find a relative who has had the disease. Therefore, doctors consider T2DM to be much more of a genetic disease than T1DM. In studies of identical twins, when one twin has type 2 diabetes, the likelihood that it will develop in the other twin is nearly 100 percent.

Insulin resistance

People with type 2 diabetes have plenty of insulin in their bodies (unlike people with type 1 diabetes), but their bodies respond to the insulin in abnormal ways. Type 2 diabetics are *insulin-resistant,* meaning that their bodies resist the normal, healthy functioning of insulin. This resistance, combined with not having enough insulin to overcome the insulin resistance, causes the disease.

Most people who develop type 2 diabetes are born with the genes for insulin resistance. Before diabetes is present, future T2DM patients already show signs of insulin resistance. First, the amount of insulin in their blood is elevated compared to normal people. Second, a shot of insulin doesn't reduce the blood glucose in these insulin-resistant people nearly as much as it does in people without insulin resistance. (See Chapter 11 to find out more about insulin shots in diabetes.)

When your body needs to make extra insulin just to keep your blood glucose normal, your insulin is, obviously, less effective than it should be — which means that you have insulin resistance. If your insulin resistance worsens to the point that your body can't produce enough insulin to keep your blood glucose normal, or if your pancreas starts to get "tired" of making so much extra insulin, your blood sugars become abnormal. This condition is prediabetes, because your blood glucose is still lower than the levels needed for a diagnosis of diabetes (see Chapter 2). When you add other factors such as weight gain, a sedentary lifestyle, certain medications, and aging, your pancreas can't keep up with your insulin demands, and you develop prediabetes, followed by diabetes.

Another factor that comes into play when doctors make a diagnosis of type 2 diabetes is the release of sugar from the glycogen stored in your liver, known as your *hepatic glucose output.* People with T2DM have high glucose levels in the morning after having fasted all night. You would think that your glucose would be low in the morning if you haven't eaten any sugar. But your liver is a storage bank for a lot of glucose, and it can make even more from other substances in the body. As your insulin resistance increases, your liver begins to release glucose inappropriately, and your fasting blood glucose level rises.

Mistaken beliefs about type 2

People often think that the following factors cause type 2 diabetes, but they actually have nothing to do with the onset of the disease:

- ✔ **Emotions:** Changes in your emotions do not play a large role in the development of type 2 diabetes, but they may be very important in dealing with diabetes mellitus and subsequent control.

- ✔ **Stress:** Too much stress isn't a major factor that causes diabetes.

- ✔ **Antibodies:** Antibodies against islet cells are not a major factor in type 2 diabetes (see the section "Investigating the causes of type 1 diabetes," earlier in this chapter). Type 2 diabetes isn't an autoimmune disease like type 1.

- ✔ **Gender:** Males and females are equally as likely to develop type 2 diabetes. Gender doesn't play a role in the onset of this disease.

- ✔ **Diabetic ketoacidosis:** Type 2 diabetes isn't generally associated with diabetic ketoacidosis (see Chapter 4). People with type 2 diabetes are ketosis resistant, except under extremely severe stress caused by infections or trauma. (See Chapter 4 for a discussion of *hyperosmolar syndrome,* a related condition in which people with type 2 diabetes have extremely high glucose but don't have the fat breakdown that leads to ketoacidosis.)

Getting type 2 diabetes

Genetic inheritance is necessary in type 2 diabetes, but environmental factors such as obesity and lack of exercise trigger the disease. People with type 2 diabetes are insulin-resistant before they become obese or sedentary. Aging, poor eating habits, obesity, and failure to exercise combine to worsen insulin resistance and bring out the disease.

Inheritance seems to be a much stronger factor in type 2 diabetes than in type 1 diabetes. Consider the following facts:

- ✔ If your father has type 2 diabetes but your mother doesn't, you have about a 4 percent chance of getting the disease.

- ✔ If your mother has type 2 diabetes but your father doesn't, your chances of getting it leap to about 10 percent.

- ✔ If your identical twin has type 2 diabetes, you have a nearly 100 percent chance of eventually getting the disease.

- ✔ If your brother or sister (*not* an identical twin) gets type 2, you have about a 40 percent chance of doing the same.

Here's an interesting fact: Spouses of people with type 2 diabetes are at higher risk of developing diabetes and should be screened just like relatives of people with diabetes. Why? Because they share the environmental risk factors for diabetes, such as poor diet and a sedentary lifestyle. If your wife is a good cook and you have a big-screen TV, watch out!

Preventing the causes of type 2 diabetes

Doctors can predict type 2 diabetes years in advance of its actual diagnosis by studying the close relatives of people who have the condition. This early-warning period offers plenty of time to try techniques of primary prevention. After a doctor discovers that someone's blood glucose levels are high and diagnoses type 2 diabetes, complications such as eye disease and kidney disease (see Chapter 5) usually take ten or more years to develop in that person. During this time, doctors can apply secondary prevention techniques (the various treatments I discuss in Part III).

Because so many people suffer from type 2 diabetes, doctors have had a wealth of people to study in order to determine the most important environmental factors that turn a genetic predisposition to type 2 diabetes into a clinical disease. Following are the major environmental factors:

✓ **High body-mass index:** The *body-mass index (BMI)* is the way that doctors look at weight in relation to height. BMI is a better indicator of a healthy weight than just weight alone, because taller people tend to weigh more. For instance, a person who weighs 150 pounds and is 62 inches tall is overweight, but a person who weighs 150 pounds and is 70 inches tall is thin.

You can easily determine your BMI by using the following formula: Multiply your weight (in pounds) by 703, and then divide that number by your height (in inches). Divide that result by your height (in inches) again. If you use the metric system, divide your weight in kilograms by your height in meters and divide that result by your height in meters again. Using this formula, the 150-pound person with a height of 62 inches has a BMI of 27.5, whereas the person with the height of 70 inches has a BMI of 21.6.

Current guidelines state that a person with a BMI from 25 to 29.9 is overweight, and a person with a BMI of 30 or greater is obese. A BMI between 18.5 and 25 is considered normal. A person with a BMI of 40 or higher has morbid obesity.

Many studies have verified the great importance of the BMI level in determining who gets diabetes. For example, a large study of thousands of nurses in the United States showed that nurses with a BMI greater than 35 had diabetes almost 100 times more often than nurses with a BMI less than 22. Even among the women in this study considered to be lean, those with the higher BMI, though still in the category of normal, had three times the prevalence of diabetes compared to those with lower BMI. Another large study of U.S. physicians found the same relationship of high BMI to high levels of type 2 diabetes. The same study showed that the length of time that you're obese is important; participants who were obese for ten years were more likely to have diabetes than those who had become obese more recently.

✔ **Physical inactivity:** Physical inactivity has a high association with diabetes, as evidenced in many studies. Former athletes have diabetes less often than nonathletes. The same study of nurses' health that I cite in the preceding bullet showed that women who were physically active on a regular basis had diabetes only two-thirds as often as the couch potatoes. A study conducted in Hawaii, which did not include any obese people, showed that the occurrence of diabetes was greatest for people who don't exercise.

✔ **Central distribution of fat:** When people with diabetes become fat, they tend to carry the extra weight as centrally distributed fat, also known as *visceral fat.* You check your visceral fat when you measure your waistline, because this type of fat stays around your midsection. So a person with visceral fat is more apple-shaped than pear-shaped. Visceral fat also happens to be the type of fat that probably comes and goes most easily on your body, and it is relatively easy to lose when you diet. Visceral fat seems to cause more insulin resistance than fat in other areas, and it is also correlated with the occurrence of coronary artery disease. If you have a lot of visceral fat, losing just 5 to 10 percent of your weight may very dramatically reduce your chance of diabetes or a heart attack.

Even when the BMI is within the normal range (less than 25), people with a greater waist circumference have an increased mortality. If you are 40 or younger and your waistline measures 39.5 inches (100 centimeters) or greater, or you are between the ages of 40 and 60 and your waistline measures 35.5 inches (90 centimeters) or more, you have a significantly increased risk of a heart attack. Try to shrink your waistline as well as your weight.

Asians tend to develop visceral fat at a lower weight than non-Asians and are therefore more prone to type 2 diabetes at a lower weight. Asian Indians are particularly susceptible, developing diabetes up to ten years earlier than Chinese and Japanese.

✔ **Low intake of dietary fiber:** Populations with a high prevalence of diabetes tend to eat a diet that is low in fiber. Dietary fiber seems to be protective against diabetes because it slows down the rate at which glucose enters the bloodstream.

If you recognize any of the preceding factors in your body or lifestyle, you can correct them in time to prevent diabetes. Type 2 diabetes allows the high-risk individual or the diagnosed person the time to work toward prevention or control of the disease. In Part III, I show you specific ways to reduce your weight, increase your exercise, improve your diet, and prevent or reverse diabetes and diabetic complications.

Type 2 diabetes begins with insulin resistance and worsens with reduced beta-cell function. An ideal agent that prevents type 2 diabetes would have to

- ✔ Be effective in treating type 2 diabetes
- ✔ Improve sensitivity to glucose or beta-cell function
- ✔ Promote weight loss
- ✔ Improve risk factors for heart disease
- ✔ Not cause low blood glucose
- ✔ Be required only once a day or even once a week
- ✔ Not cause unacceptable side effects

A drug that fulfills all of these requirements has been available for some time. It's called a glucagon-like peptide-1 agonist, and I discuss it extensively in Chapter 11.

Recognizing variants of type 1 and 2 diabetes

Certain groups of patients with diabetes do not follow the classic description of type 1 or 2. They make up a sizable portion of type 2 patients and require individualized treatment (and you could be among them), so I briefly explain their characteristics in this section.

LADA

As many as 10 percent of people diagnosed with type 2 diabetes do not respond well to medications that stimulate the pancreas to release more insulin like the sulfonylurea class of drugs (see Chapter 11). When they are tested, they are found to have glutamic acid decarboxylase (GAD) antibodies similar to those found in T1DM. This condition, called *latent autoimmune diabetes in adults* (LADA), is really adult-onset T1DM rather than T2DM. It is generally milder than type 1 diabetes, with lower blood glucose levels, and it presents without ketosis or weight loss. The treatment is similar to that for T1DM.

If you are having trouble controlling your diabetes with oral drugs that work by causing more insulin release, ask your doctor to test you for GAD antibodies.

MODY

One to five percent of all patients with type 2 diabetes have a condition called *maturity onset of diabetes of the young* (MODY). Although most cases of type 2 diabetes result from abnormalities in multiple genes, MODY results from an abnormality in a single gene of that patient. If one parent has MODY, his or her children have a 50 percent chance of inheriting the disease.

MODY can be diagnosed in any family with a high degree of inheritance of diabetes by doing genetic studies. Clinically, the disease looks like a mild form of type 2 diabetes that begins in early adolescence or early adulthood but is not diagnosed until later in life (unless it is suspected in the family and a glucose tolerance test and genetic testing are done). It generally does not require insulin, and it responds to oral agents (see Chapter 11).

Possibilities for future prevention of diabetes

Researchers have performed many valuable studies on the prevention of type 2 diabetes. The results of these studies suggest that you can prevent diabetes, but probably only by making major lifestyle changes and sticking to them over a long period of time. Here are some important conclusions based on prevention research:

✔ Taking drugs that don't treat your insulin resistance doesn't help to prevent your diabetes or its complications.

✔ Exercising regularly may delay the onset of diabetes.

✔ Maintaining a proper diet can delay the onset of diabetes and slow the complications that may occur.

✔ Controlling both your blood pressure and your blood glucose has substantial benefits for preventing the complications of diabetes.

The results of the Diabetes Prevention Program, a study of more than 3,000 people, were published in the *New England Journal of Medicine* in February 2002. They clearly showed that diet and exercise are effective in preventing type 2 diabetes. Participants who successfully modified their diet and exercise routines reduced their chances of developing type 2 diabetes by 58 percent. They generally did 30 minutes of moderate exercise (like walking) every day and lost between 5 and 7 percent of their body weight during the three-year study period. In contrast, patients who used a drug called *metformin* (see Chapter 10) without modifying their diet and exercise reduced their risk of developing type 2 diabetes by only 31 percent.

Another study, the Finnish Diabetes Prevention Study (reported in *Diabetes Care* in December 2003), shows that lifestyle changes can be accomplished and sustained not only in a research setting (like that of the Diabetes Prevention Program) but in a community setting as well, where patients are taken care of by their own doctors. Study participants worked with a nutritionist to improve their diets and received some advice on exercise. They continue to be successful after three years, with the same 58 percent reduction in the onset of diabetes.

Restoring insulin sensitivity in people at risk for prediabetes (see Chapter 2) was the focus of another study, published in *Diabetes Care* in March 2002. This study compared intensive lifestyle change, both diet and exercise, with moderate lifestyle change. The intensive group ate less fat and did more vigorous exercise than the moderate group, and every member of the intensive group increased his or her insulin sensitivity, which resulted in holding off the development of diabetes.

Dealing with Gestational Diabetes

If you're pregnant (yes, that excludes you men) and you've never had diabetes before, during your pregnancy you could acquire a form of diabetes called *gestational diabetes*. If you already have diabetes when you become pregnant, it's called *pregestational diabetes*. As I discuss in Chapter 6, the difference between pregestational diabetes and gestational diabetes is very important in terms of the consequences for both mother and baby. Gestational diabetes occurs in about 9 percent of all pregnancies. (I discuss diabetes in pregnancy extensively in Chapter 6.)

During your pregnancy, you can acquire gestational diabetes because the growing fetus and the placenta create various hormones to help the fetus grow and develop properly. Some of these hormones have other characteristics, such as anti-insulin properties, that decrease your body's sensitivity to insulin, increase glucose production, and can cause diabetes.

Recognizing Other Types of Diabetes

Cases of diabetes other than type 1 and type 2 are rare and usually don't cause severe diabetes in the people who have them. But occasionally one of these other types is responsible for a more severe case of diabetes, so you should know that they exist. The following list gives you a brief rundown of the symptoms and causes of other types of diabetes:

- **Diabetes due to loss or disease of pancreatic tissue:** If you have a disease, such as cancer, that necessitates the removal of some of your pancreas, you lose your pancreas's valuable insulin-producing beta cells and your body becomes diabetic. This form of diabetes isn't always severe, because you lose glucagon, another hormone found in your pancreas, after your pancreatic surgery. Glucagon blocks insulin action in your body, so when your body has less glucagon, it can function with less insulin, leaving you with a milder case of diabetes.

- **Diabetes due to iron overload:** Another disease that damages the pancreas, as well as the liver, the heart, the joints, and the nervous system, is *hemochromatosis*. This condition results from excessive absorption of iron into the blood. When the blood deposits too much iron into these organs, damage can occur. This hereditary condition is present in 1 of every 200 people in the United States; half of those who have it develop a clinical disease, sometimes diabetes.

Hemochromatosis is less common in younger women, who are protected by the monthly loss of iron that occurs with menstrual bleeding. This finding has led to the current treatment for hemochromatosis, which is removing blood from the patient regularly until the blood iron returns to normal; then repeating the procedure occasionally to keep iron levels normal. If treatment is done early enough (before organs are damaged), complications such as diabetes are avoidable.

✔ **Diabetes due to other diseases:** Your body contains a number of hormones that block insulin action or have actions that are opposed to insulin's actions. You produce these hormones in glands other than your pancreas. If you get a tumor on one of these hormone-producing glands, the gland sometimes produces excessive levels of the hormones that act in opposition to insulin. Usually, this condition gives you simple glucose intolerance rather than diabetes, because your pancreas makes extra insulin to combat the hormones. But if you have a genetic tendency to develop diabetes, you may develop diabetes in this case.

✔ **Diabetes due to hormone treatments for other diseases:** If you take hormones to treat a disease other than diabetes, those hormones could cause diabetes in your body. The hormone that is most likely to cause diabetes in this situation is *hydrocortisone,* an anti-inflammatory agent used in diseases of inflammation, such as arthritis. (Similar drugs are prednisone and dexamethasone.) If you take hydrocortisone and you have the symptoms of diabetes listed in earlier sections of this chapter, talk to your doctor.

✔ **Diabetes due to other drugs**: If you're taking other commonly used drugs, be aware that some of them raise your blood glucose as a side effect. Some antihypertensive drugs, especially hydrochlorothiazide, raise your blood glucose level. Niacin, a drug commonly used for lowering cholesterol, also raises your blood glucose. Even the wonder drugs for lowering cholesterol, the statins, have been implicated. If you have a genetic tendency toward diabetes, taking these drugs may be enough to give you the disease.

Part II
Knowing How Uncontrolled Diabetes Affects Your Body

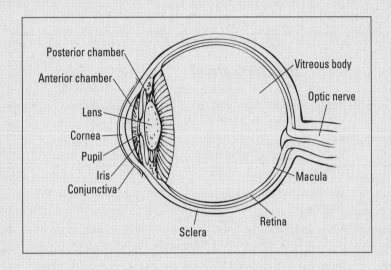

Refer to www.dummies.com/extras/diabetes for a glossary full of terms you need to know related to diabetes.

In this part . . .

✔ Know and avoid short-term complications of diabetes in order to maintain your health on a daily basis.

✔ Prevent long-term complications of diabetes so that you can avoid eye disease, nerve disease, kidney disease, and heart disease.

✔ Continue to enjoy your sexual function for your good health and happiness.

✔ Know that producing a healthy baby and being a healthy mother is difficult with diabetes but very doable if you know how.

✔ Understand your body's physiology to help you fully understand how diabetes affect you.

✔ Realize that you can live a long and healthy life with diabetes if you're willing to put in the effort.

Chapter 4

Avoiding Short-Term Complications

After receiving a diagnosis of type 2 diabetes, you need to understand how the disease can affect you. The previous chapters cover some of the signs and symptoms of diabetes, which you could consider to be the shortest of the short-term complications of the disease because they're generally mild and begin to subside when you start treatment. This chapter covers the more serious forms of short-term complications, which occur when your blood glucose is out of control, reaching dangerously high or low levels.

With the exception of mild *hypoglycemia* (low blood glucose that you can manage yourself), you should treat all the complications in this chapter as medical emergencies. Keep in touch with your doctor and go to the hospital promptly if your blood glucose is uncontrollably high or you're unable to hold down food. You may need a few hours in the emergency room or a day or two in the hospital to reverse your problems.

Solving (and Steering Clear of) Short-Term Complications

Although the complications that I cover in this chapter are called *short-term*, you may experience them at any time during the course of your diabetes. *Short-term* simply means that these complications arise rapidly in your body, as opposed to the long-term complications (discussed in Chapter 5) that take ten or more years to develop. Short-term complications develop in days or even hours, and fortunately they respond to treatment just as rapidly.

Generally, you experience the severe short-term complications associated with high blood glucose when you aren't monitoring your blood glucose levels. Small children and older folks who live alone or have illnesses are most susceptible to lapses in glucose monitoring and, therefore, to short-term complications. If you suffer an acute illness or trauma, you should monitor your glucose even more frequently than usual because you're more vulnerable to short-term complications.

The short-term complications of diabetes affect your ability to function normally. For example, if you're a student, you may have difficulty studying or taking tests. Or you may have trouble driving your car properly. For this reason, you may find that the Bureau of Motor Vehicles and the Federal Aviation Association are extra careful about giving people with diabetes a driver's license or pilot's license. Potential employers may question your ability to perform certain jobs. But most companies and government agencies are very enlightened about diabetes and do everything possible to accommodate you in these situations.

You can control your diabetes, and all the short-term complications are avoidable. If you take your medication at the appropriate time, eat the proper foods at the proper times, and monitor your blood glucose regularly, you're unlikely to suffer from any severe short-term complications. Your blood glucose may drop to lower than normal levels, but closely monitoring it quickly alerts you to the drop so you can treat it before it affects your mental and physical functioning. (See Chapter 7 for all the details on glucose monitoring and other testing.)

Dropping Too Low: Hypoglycemia

The condition of having low blood glucose is known as *hypoglycemia*. If you have diabetes, you can get hypoglycemia only as a consequence of your diabetes treatment.

One of the readers who wrote to thank me for the first edition of this book told me how her son had once gone on a blind date. He and his date went to a bar where they had a drink before dinner. As he sat there, he began to say, "Sugar, baby, sugar, baby, sugar, baby." At first his date was offended until she realized that he had a glazed look in his eyes and found that he was wearing a bracelet identifying him as a person with diabetes. He was suffering from hypoglycemia and needed glucose.

This story is amusing, but the subject is very serious. Hypoglycemia can ruin your day and leave you feeling dazed and exhausted afterwards. You also run the risk of overtreating it, leaving yourself with very high blood glucose.

Hypoglycemia is a barrier that prevents most patients with diabetes from achieving normal blood glucose levels. They can lower their blood glucose enough to prevent long-term complications such as eye disease, kidney disease, and nerve disease, but preventing heart disease requires a lower glucose level that is difficult to sustain because of the threat of hypoglycemia, particularly for people with type 1 diabetes. A normal blood glucose is between 80 and 140 mg/dl. Hypoglycemia begins below 80 mg/dl, but you may not feel symptoms until it goes below 60 mg/dl.

The positive news is that most patients experience complete recovery from the effects of hypoglycemia.

Identifying the signs of hypoglycemia

Your body doesn't function well when you have too little glucose in your blood. Your brain needs glucose to run the rest of your body, as well as to function intellectually. Your muscles need the energy that glucose provides in much the same way that your car needs gasoline. So when your body detects that it has low blood glucose, it sends out a group of hormones that rapidly raise your glucose. But those hormones have to fight the strength of the diabetes medication that has been pushing down your glucose levels.

At what level of blood glucose do you develop hypoglycemia? Unfortunately, the level varies for different individuals, particularly depending on the length of time that the person has had diabetes. But most experts agree that a blood glucose of 70 mg/dl (3.9 mmol/L) or less is associated with signs and symptoms of hypoglycemia in most people. This level is an *alert value* and should probably be repeated in 20 minutes or so. Avoid driving or exercise until it improves.

Doctors usually put the symptoms of hypoglycemia into two categories:

- **Symptoms due to the side effects of the hormones (especially epinephrine) that your body sends out to counter the glucose-lowering effect of insulin:** This category of symptoms is called *adrenergic* symptoms, because epinephrine comes from your adrenal gland. They occur most often when your blood glucose falls rapidly.

  - Whiteness, or pallor, of your skin

  - Sweating

- Rapid heartbeat

- Palpitations, or the feeling that your heart is beating too fast

- Anxiety

- Numbness in the lips, fingers, or toes

- Irritability

- Sensation of hunger

✔ **Symptoms due to your brain not receiving enough fuel, causing your intellectual function to suffer:** This category of symptoms is called *neuroglycopenic* symptoms, which is medicalese for "not enough *(penic)* glucose *(glyco)* in the brain *(neuro)*." (If your brain could speak, it would just say, "Whew, I'm ready for a meal!") These symptoms occur most often when your hypoglycemia takes longer to develop, and they become more severe as your blood glucose drops lower.

- Headache

- Loss of concentration

- Visual disorders, such as double vision or blurred vision

- Fatigue

- Confusion and trouble concentrating

- Trouble hearing

- Poor color vision

- Feeling of warmth

- Slurred speech

- Convulsions

- Coma, or an inability to be awakened

People lose their ability to think clearly when they become hypoglycemic. They make simple mistakes, and other people often assume that they are drunk.

If you take insulin or a *sulfonylurea drug,* which squeezes more insulin out of your reluctant pancreas, you should wear or carry with you some form of identification, in case you unexpectedly develop hypoglycemia. (See Chapter 11 for a full explanation of insulin and the sulfonylurea medications.) You can find a simple bracelet at the MedicAlert Foundation at www.medicalert.org. If you prefer something a little sexier that you will be proud to wear as jewelry, try www.laurenshope.com/.

Categorizing levels of hypoglycemia

The severity of hypoglycemia falls into three categories, defined by the level of the blood glucose:

- ✔ **Mild hypoglycemia:** With this level, corresponding to blood glucose of around 70 mg/dl, patients can easily treat it. It doesn't cause the patients to change their routine, other than taking a little glucose, and in fact is discovered not so much by symptoms as by routine testing of the blood. Treatment may not even be necessary.

- ✔ **Moderate hypoglycemia:** This level is achieved when the blood glucose is around 65 mg/dl. Patients begin to feel the adrenergic symptoms described earlier, especially anxiety and a rapid heartbeat. Patients who have moderate hypoglycemia may not recognize that they need glucose and may have to be helped by someone else.

- ✔ **Severe hypoglycemia:** This level, at which blood glucose is less than 55 mg/dl, leaves patients severely impaired and thus requiring outside assistance to restore their glucose. An emergency injection of glucagon or intravenous glucose solution is necessary.

The level of glucose that causes you to have mild, moderate, or severe hypoglycemia may differ from these numbers. They are only approximate. If you are alert with a blood glucose level of 55 mg/dl, taking glucose by mouth will reverse the hypoglycemia.

Managing the causes of hypoglycemia

Hypoglycemia results from elevated amounts of insulin driving down your blood glucose to low levels, but an extra high dose of insulin or sulfonylurea medication isn't always the culprit. Your blood glucose level is also affected by the amount of food you take in, the amount of fuel (glucose) that you burn for energy, the amount of insulin circulating in your body, and your body's ability to raise glucose by releasing it from the liver or making it from other bodily substances.

On average, hypoglycemia in people with type 1 diabetes causes noticeable symptoms only about twice a week and is severe perhaps once a year. In people with type 2 diabetes, severe hypoglycemia occurs only one-tenth as often. (The medications described in the next section are part of the reason that people with type 1 diabetes have to deal with hypoglycemia more often.) The following sections cover the causes of hypoglycemia and the ways you can manage those factors to keep your blood glucose level in check.

Insulin and sulfonylurea medications

All people with type 1 diabetes (and some with type 2) rely on insulin injections to control the disease. When you take insulin shots, you have to time your food intake to raise your blood glucose as the insulin is taking effect. Chapter 11 explains the different kinds of insulin and the proper methods for administering them. But remember that the different types of insulin are most potent at differing amounts of time (minutes or hours) after you inject them. If you skip a meal or take your insulin too early or too late, your glucose and insulin levels won't be in sync and you'll develop hypoglycemia. If you go on a diet and don't adjust your medication, the same thing happens.

If you take sulfonylurea drugs, you need to follow similar restrictions. You and your doctor must adjust your dosage when your calorie intake falls. Other drugs don't cause hypoglycemia by themselves, but when combined with sulfonylureas they may lower your glucose enough to reach hypoglycemic levels. (Chapter 11 discusses these other drugs.)

Diet

Your diet plays a major role in helping you avoid hypoglycemia if you take medication. You should try to have a snack in the middle of the morning and in the afternoon — in addition to your usual breakfast, lunch, and dinner — especially if you take insulin. A properly timed snack provides you with a steady source of glucose to balance the insulin that you're taking.

You can use your blood glucose level to determine whether to have a snack at bedtime. If your glucose is greater than 180 mg/dL (10 mmol/L), you probably don't need a snack. If your glucose is between 126 and 180 mg/dL (7 to 10 mmol/L), a couple slices of bread and an ounce of cheese will prevent hypoglycemia. If your glucose is less than 126 mg/dL (7 mmol/L), a couple ounces of meat plus a slice of bread will do the trick.

Exercise

Exercise burns your body's fuel, which is glucose, so it generally lowers your blood glucose level. Some people with diabetes use exercise in place of extra insulin to get their high blood glucose down to a normal level. But if you don't adjust your insulin dose or food intake to match your exercise level, exercise can result in hypoglycemia.

One of my patients is dedicated to exercise. He has taken insulin shots for years but requires very little insulin to control his glucose because he burns so much glucose through exercise. He avoids hypoglycemia by measuring his blood glucose level many times a day — especially before vigorous exercise. If his level is low at the beginning of exercise, he eats extra carbohydrates before he starts. Chapter 8 tells you which foods to eat (and when) to achieve the intended effect on your glucose levels.

Nondiabetes drugs

Several drugs that you may take unrelated to your diabetes can lower your blood glucose. One of the most widely used, which you may not even think of as a drug, is alcohol, which can block your liver's ability to release glucose. It also blocks hormones that raise blood glucose and increases the glucose-lowering effect of insulin. If you're malnourished or you simply haven't eaten in a while and you drink alcohol before going to bed, you may experience severe fasting hypoglycemia the next morning. If you take insulin or sulfonyl-urea drugs, don't drink alcohol without eating some food at the same time. Food counteracts some of the glucose-lowering effects of alcohol.

Also, be aware that aspirin (and all of the drugs related to aspirin, called *salicylates*) can lead to hypoglycemia. In adults who have diabetes, aspirin can increase the effects of other drugs that you're taking to lower your blood glucose. In children with diabetes, aspirin has an especially profound effect on lowering blood glucose to hypoglycemia levels. However, the low dose of aspirin taken daily to reduce the risk of heart attacks does not cause hypoglycemia.

More than 160 drugs have been associated with severe hypoglycemia. Usually it is found in a person taking insulin or a drug that works by increasing the body's own insulin. Following are the major drugs that cause hypoglycemia:

- ✔ **Angiotensin-converting enzyme inhibitors:** Blood pressure drugs, most of which end in *-pril*

- ✔ **Beta blockers:** Blood pressure drugs, most of which end in *-olol* (which also block the warning symptoms of hypoglycemia)

- ✔ **Pentamidine:** An antibiotic

- ✔ **Quinine:** Used to treat malaria

- ✔ **Quinolones:** A group of drugs that are antibiotics, most of which end in *-floxacin*

Hormonal changes

As type 1 diabetes progresses, your body produces fewer and fewer hormones that counteract insulin when hypoglycemia is present. This situation leads to more severe hypoglycemia later in type 1 diabetes, especially if you and your doctor don't adjust your insulin injections in response to your lower glucose levels. People with type 2 diabetes who take insulin also develop this loss of protective hormones.

These same hormones also play the role of giving you warning signs when your blood glucose drops, such as sweating, a rapid heartbeat, and anxiety, so you are prompted to eat. When the hormone levels drop, these warning signs don't occur, so you aren't signaled that you need to eat. This situation is called *hypoglycemia unawareness.* If hypoglycemia is avoided, however, the loss of the protective hormones and the development of hypoglycemia unawareness may be reversed.

Understanding the risks of hypoglycemia in special situations

Hypoglycemia is also present in a few special situations. I discuss them in this section.

Hypoglycemia with fasting

When you fast, your body doesn't permit the glucose to fall to hypoglycemic levels. If you take no insulin or oral drug that raises insulin and you become hypoglycemic during fasting anyway, you may have an internal source of excessive insulin, such as a tumor of the beta cells of the pancreas, an *insulinoma.* Insulinoma is easily diagnosed by having a person fast and checking the blood glucose over 72 hours. If it falls, the patient shows symptoms of hypoglycemia, and the insulin is elevated, a tumor of the pancreas is likely.

Hypoglycemia in the critically ill

On the basis of one small study, some doctors believed that keeping the blood glucose of a critically ill person as normal as possible would decrease the possibility of death. The trouble is that in making the blood glucose normal, these patients often suffer severe hypoglycemia. More recent studies have shown that keeping blood glucose normal in certain populations is not only not associated with decreased mortality but also is associated with increased risk of death.

Hypoglycemia and intellectual changes

Occasional severe hypoglycemia in younger people doesn't seem to have long-term consequences. The same is not true for the elderly. An increasing incidence of loss of mental function (dementia) occurs as elderly patients have one, two, or three episodes of severe hypoglycemia. That's all the more reason for frequently checking blood glucose levels (at least once or twice daily with type 2 diabetes and four or more times daily with type 1 or type 2 on multiple shots of insulin per day).

Hypoglycemia and the heart

Recent evidence suggests that hypoglycemia may be the cause of sudden unexplained death in young people with type 1 diabetes. Death may be caused by changes in the electrical rhythm of the heart. Hypoglycemia is often associated with low potassium, which can stop the heart. In patients with known heart disease, the highest death rate due to heart problems occurs at the lowest and highest blood glucose levels.

Treating hypoglycemia

Although hypoglycemia is preventable, you may still experience it at some point. Fortunately, the vast majority of cases are mild. You can treat hypoglycemia with a small quantity of glucose in the form of:

- ✔ Two sugar cubes
- ✔ Three or four glucose tablets (available in any drugstore, and any person with diabetes who may develop hypoglycemia should carry them)
- ✔ A small amount (6 ounces) of a sugary soft drink
- ✔ 8 ounces of milk or 4 ounces of orange juice
- ✔ Anything that has about 15 grams of pure glucose in it

Sometimes you may need a second treatment. Approximately 20 minutes after you try one of these solutions, measure your blood glucose to find out whether your level has risen sufficiently. If it is still low, give a second treatment.

Keep the following in mind to aid in your treatment of hypoglycemia:

- ✔ **You can easily overtreat hypoglycemia,** causing your blood glucose to rise higher than you'd like. However, the high blood glucose resulting from overtreatment of hypoglycemia usually doesn't last long. You're better off not using a drug or insulin to bring it down, because doing so can result in alternate highs and lows.
- ✔ **Make sure that your friends or relatives know in advance what hypoglycemia is and what to do about it,** because your mental state may be mildly confused when you have it. Inform people about your diabetes and about how to recognize hypoglycemia. Don't keep your diabetes a secret. The people close to you will be glad to know how to help you.
- ✔ **Try to eat a snack of carbohydrates and protein every hour if you are doing prolonged exercise,** such as playing a baseball or soccer game that lasts several hours. (For example, half a turkey sandwich would work well.) And carry jelly beans (or any source of pure glucose) at all times, just in case — six or seven are all you need to combat mild symptoms of hypoglycemia.

If you are losing consciousness and can't sit up and swallow properly when you have hypoglycemia, no one should try to feed you. One of the following options should be used:

✔ **Someone helping you can use an emergency kit, such as the kit called "Glucagon for Emergencies."** This kit includes a syringe with 1 mg of *glucagon,* one of the major hormones that raises glucose, which your helper should inject under your skin or into your muscle. The injection of glucagon raises your blood glucose so that you regain consciousness within 20 minutes. Glucagon corrects your hypoglycemic condition for about an hour after you receive an injection.

You need to get a prescription from your doctor for this type of glucagon kit. If you don't use your kit for a long time, make sure the date on the kit indicates that it's still active.

✔ **If your hypoglycemia recurs shortly after you receive glucagon or doesn't respond to the glucagon, the person helping you should call 911.** (Sulfonylurea drugs are most often the cause of such a severe prolonged case of hypoglycemia.) The emergency crew checks your blood glucose and gives you an intravenous (IV) dose of high-concentration glucose. Most likely, you will continue the IV in the emergency room until you show stable and normal blood glucose levels.

Combating Ketoacidosis

In Chapter 3, I talk about the tendency of people with type 1 diabetes to suffer from a severe diabetic complication called *ketoacidosis,* or very high blood glucose with large amounts of acid in the blood. This section explains the symptoms, causes, and treatments of ketoacidosis.

The prefix *keto* refers to *ketones* — substances that your body makes when fat breaks down during ketoacidosis. *Acid* is part of the name because your blood becomes acidic from the presence of ketones.

Occasionally, ketoacidosis is the symptom that alerts doctors that you have type 1 diabetes, but more frequently it occurs after you already know that you have the disease. Although ketoacidosis occurs mostly in people with type 1 diabetes (who develop diabetes at an early age), the person is usually 40 or more years old when ketoacidosis actually begins.

Ketoacidosis occurs mostly in people with type 1 diabetes because they have no insulin in their bodies except what they inject as medication. People with type 2 diabetes (or with other forms of the disease) rarely get ketoacidosis, because they have some insulin in their bodies. People with type 2 diabetes get ketoacidosis mainly when they have severe infections or traumas that put their bodies under great physical stress. Because ketoacidosis is a complication of type 1 diabetes and only very rarely type 2 diabetes, I limit my discussion of ketoacidosis to a few brief remarks. For a much more complete explanation, see my book *Type 1 Diabetes For Dummies* (John Wiley & Sons, Inc.).

The two most common causes of ketoacidosis are the interruption of your insulin treatment and an infection. Your body can't go for many hours without insulin activity before it begins to burn fat for energy and begins to make extra glucose that it can't use.

Whether you have diabetes or not, if you go on a strict diet to lose weight, your body burns some of its fat stores and produces ketones, similar to how it burns fat when you lack insulin. But in this case, your glucose remains low and (unless you have type 1 diabetes) you have sufficient insulin to prevent the excessive production of new glucose or the release of large amounts of glucose from your liver. So a strict diet doesn't generally lead to ketoacidosis but rather a benign condition called *ketosis*.

Most of the time, your doctor can control ketoacidosis with little or no risk to you. But be aware that ketoacidosis is fatal for 10 percent of people with diabetes who get it — mostly elderly people with diabetes and those with other illnesses that complicate treatment. Recognizing the symptoms early and seeking treatment quickly greatly enhance your chances of an uneventful recovery from ketoacidosis.

Managing Hyperosmolar Syndrome

The highest blood glucose condition that you may find yourself in is called *hyperosmolar syndrome*. Like ketoacidosis, hyperosmolar syndrome, referring to the excessive levels of glucose in the blood, is a medical emergency that needs to be treated in a hospital.

Hyperosmolar syndrome is also like ketoacidosis in its effects on your body. It creates ketones in your blood, but it doesn't make your blood as acidic as ketoacidosis does. However, it raises your blood glucose levels considerably higher than ketoacidosis does. (See the "Combating Ketoacidosis" section earlier in this chapter for more information.)

Hyper means "larger than normal," and *osmolar* has to do with concentrations of substances in the blood. So hyperosmolar, in this situation, means that the blood is simply too concentrated with glucose. Other hyperosmolar syndromes occur when other substances are at fault.

The following sections explain hyperosmolar syndrome's symptoms, causes, and treatments.

Heeding the symptoms of hyperosmolar syndrome

Because hyperosmolar syndrome is so similar to ketoacidosis, it has many of the same symptoms as ketoacidosis. The main difference is that with hyperosmolar syndrome, you don't experience rapid breathing called *Kussmaul breathing,* because your blood isn't overly acidic as a part of this complication. Also, the symptoms of hyperosmolar syndrome develop over many days or weeks, unlike the quick and acute development of ketoacidosis in your body.

If you measure your blood glucose on a daily basis, you should never develop hyperosmolar syndrome because you'll notice that your blood glucose is getting high before it reaches the critical complication level.

Following are the most important signs and symptoms of hyperosmolar syndrome:

- ✔ Frequent urination
- ✔ Thirst
- ✔ Weakness
- ✔ Leg cramps
- ✔ Sunken eyeballs
- ✔ Rapid pulse
- ✔ Decreased mental awareness or (if you delay treatment) coma
- ✔ Blood glucose of 600 or even higher if you delay seeing a doctor

You may also develop more threatening symptoms with this complication. Your blood pressure may be low. Your nervous system may be affected with paralysis of the arms and legs, but these problems respond to treatment.

Finding the cause

Hyperosmolar syndrome afflicts mostly elderly diabetes patients who live alone or in nursing homes where they're not carefully monitored. Age and usually some neglect combine to increase the likelihood that a person with diabetes will lose large quantities of fluids through vomiting or diarrhea and then not replace those fluids. These people tend to have mild type 2 diabetes, which is sometimes undiagnosed and untreated.

Another reason why age is a contributing cause of hyperosmolar syndrome is that your kidneys gradually become less efficient as you age. When your kidneys are in their prime, your blood glucose level needs to reach only 180 mg/dl before your kidneys begin to remove some excess glucose through your urine. But as your kidneys grow older and slower, they require a gradually higher blood glucose level before they start to send excess glucose to your urine. If you're at an age (usually 70 or older for people in average health) when your kidneys are really laboring to remove the excess glucose from your body and you happen to lose a large amount of fluids from sickness or neglect, your blood volume decreases, which makes it even harder for your kidneys to remove glucose. At this point, your blood glucose level begins to sky-rocket. If you don't replace some of the lost fluids quickly, your glucose rises even higher.

If you allow your blood glucose to rise and don't get the fluids that you need, your blood pressure starts to fall and you get weaker and weaker. As the concentration of glucose in your blood continues to rise, you become increasingly confused, and your mental state diminishes until you eventually fall into a coma.

Other factors — such as infection, failure to take your insulin, and taking certain medications — can raise your blood glucose to the hyperosmolar syndrome levels, but not replacing lost body fluids is the most frequent cause.

Treating hyperosmolar syndrome

Hyperosmolar syndrome requires immediate and skilled treatment from a doctor. By no means should you try to treat yourself. In fact, you should avoid doctors who are not experienced in treatment of this condition. You need the proper treatment from an experienced doctor — and you need it fast. The death rate for hyperosmolar syndrome is high, in fact ten times higher than that of diabetic ketoacidosis, because most people who suffer from it are elderly and often have other serious illnesses that complicate treatment.

When you arrive at your doctor's office or emergency room with hyperosmolar syndrome, your doctor must accomplish the following tasks fairly rapidly:

- Restore large volumes of water to your body
- Lower your blood glucose level
- Restore other substances that your body has lost, such as potassium, sodium, chloride, and so on

Chapter 5

Warding Off Long-Term Complications

First, the good news: Between the years 1998 and 2010, lower-limb amputations (which are mostly due to diabetes) dropped 37 percent in the United States. At the same time a striking reduction in other long-term complications, including nerve disease, eye disease, and kidney disease, also occurred. Doctors believe that this reduction is due to improved testing of blood glucose (see Chapter 7) and more use of insulin and other medications to lower the glucose (see Chapter 11). Furthermore, benefits in terms of reduction in complications persist for years after a period of tight control of blood glucose.

Now the bad news: The incidence of type 2 diabetes is increasing so rapidly that it will overwhelm improvements in treatment over the next 20 years unless some major improvement in diabetes prevention takes place. Complications will start to rise again.

The complications detailed in this chapter are the problems that occur if you permit your blood glucose to rise and remain high over many years. The point that I stress throughout this book is that you have a choice. Working with your doctor and other helpers, you can keep your blood glucose near normal so that you never have to deal with these long-term complications.

Knowing How Long-Term Complications Develop and How to Avoid Them

For most long-term complications — such as kidney disease, eye disease, and nerve disease — doctors believe that years of high blood glucose levels initiate the complications. (Heart disease is an exception. In that case, high blood glucose levels may make the disease worse or more complicated but not actually cause it.) Most long-term complications require ten or more years to develop, which seems like a long time until you consider that many people with type 2 diabetes have it for five or more years before a doctor diagnoses it.

Often the long-term complication itself (rather than a high blood glucose level) is the clue that leads a doctor to diagnose diabetes in a patient. Therefore, doctors need to look for long-term complications immediately after diagnosing diabetes, because the diabetes and any long-term complications may have been with the patient for quite some time already.

If you're preventing short-term complications (see Chapter 4), you're also preventing long-term complications. But here are the differences you need to remember between short-term and long-term complications:

- ✔ Short-term complications result from the immediate effects of very high and very low blood glucose levels, and they're usually reversible.

- ✔ Long-term complications result from damage done by high blood glucose levels as well as abnormal fat levels and abnormal blood pressure. After a while, long-term complications aren't reversible.

The struggle to live an uncomplicated life with diabetes reminds me of a commercial airplane pilot who took the airplane down for a rough landing. As was his custom, after the plane landed the pilot stood at the exit while passengers departed. A little old lady walked to the exit with her cane and said to the pilot, "Tell me, did we land, or were we shot down?" The choice is yours: You can have a smooth landing, free of complications, that goes relatively unnoticed by you and those around you. Or you can have the feeling that you have been shot down.

Kidney Disease

Your kidneys rid your body of many harmful chemicals and other compounds produced during the process of normal metabolism. Your kidneys act like a filter through which your blood pours, trapping the waste and sending it out in your urine while the normal contents of the blood go back into your bloodstream. They also regulate the salt and water content of your body. When kidney disease (also known as *nephropathy*) causes your kidneys to fail, you must either use artificial means, called *dialysis,* to cleanse your blood and control the salt and water or receive a new working donor kidney, called a *transplant.*

Chronic kidney disease is more prevalent now than it has been in the past, and the major source of all these new cases is diabetes. In the United States today, half the patients who require long-term dialysis require it because of diabetes. Fortunately, the number requiring dialysis is on the decline because of the increasing awareness among people that they need to control their blood glucose. The incidence of kidney disease is only about 5 percent among people with type 2 diabetes, compared to 30 percent among people with type 1 diabetes; however, the absolute number of patients with kidney disease is about the same for the two groups because type 2 diabetes is so much more common than type 1.

How high glucose leads to complications

Although doctors aren't certain about the causes of most long-term complications of diabetes, I mention the current theories about the causes of the complications as I explain each complication in this chapter. However, all long-term complications share some common characteristics.

Advanced glycated end-products (AGEs) are one of the substances that damage tissues. AGEs can damage the eyes, the kidneys, the nervous system, and other organs in your body. You always have glucose in your blood, and some of that glucose attaches to other substances in your bloodstream to form *glycated* (glucose-attached) products. In this way, hemoglobin, which carries oxygen through your blood to cells and tissues throughout your body, attaches to glucose to form hemoglobin A1c. Albumin, a protein in blood, forms glycated albumin. Glucose can attach to red blood cells and white blood cells, as well as to other cells and molecules in the bloodstream. When these normal body substances attach to glucose, they no longer work normally.

Your body handles a certain level of glycated substances. But when your blood glucose is elevated for prolonged periods of time, the level of glycated cells and substances becomes excessive, and the complications I describe in this chapter result.

The polyol pathway is another major source of damage to the body in diabetes. *Polyol pathway* refers to one direction that glucose can take as it is *metabolized* (broken down).

When you have a lot of glucose in your blood, an abnormal amount is metabolized to become a product called *sorbitol,* which accumulates in many tissues where it can damage them in the following ways:

- **Damage from swelling:** Sorbitol causes body water to enter cells, which causes damage and destruction of cells.

- **Damage from chemical reactions:** During the production of sorbitol, other compounds are produced that chemically damage the cells and tissues.

Autoantibodies to autonomic nerves are present in patients with diabetes. Autoimmunity may be yet another mechanism by which diabetes causes long-term complications.

The following sections tell you what you need to know to prevent and manage diabetic kidney disease. I explain how diabetes affects your kidneys, what changes are occurring in your body, and how you can both check for them while they are still reversible and prevent them from getting any worse.

The impact of diabetes on your kidneys

Each kidney consists of about a million units called *nephrons*. Each nephron contains a structure called the *glomerulus* (the plural is *glomeruli*) that filters blood and separates out waste products and some water.

When you first get diabetes, your kidneys are enlarged and seem to function abnormally well, judging by how fast they clear wastes from your body. Your kidneys seem to function so well because you have a large amount of glucose entering your kidneys, which draws a lot of water with it and causes an increase in the pressure inside each glomerulus. This more-rapid transit of blood through the kidneys is known as an increased *glomerular filtration rate* (GFR). Early in the development of your diabetes, the membrane surrounding your glomeruli, called the *glomerular basement membrane,* thickens, as do other adjacent structures. These expanding membranes and structures begin to take up the space occupied by the capillaries inside the glomeruli, so the capillaries are unable to filter as much blood.

Fortunately, you have many more glomeruli than you really need. In fact, you can lose the equivalent of a whole kidney (half of each kidney) and still have plenty of reserve to clean your blood. If your kidney disease goes undetected for about 15 years, damage may become so severe that your blood shows measurable signs of the beginning of kidney failure, called *azotemia.* If the neglect of the disease reaches 20 years, both kidneys may fail entirely.

Not every person with diabetes is at equal risk for kidney disease and kidney failure. This complication seems to be more common in certain families and among certain racial groups, especially African Americans, Mexican Americans, and Native Americans. It is certainly more common when high blood pressure is present. Although doctors and researchers believe that high blood glucose is the major factor leading to nephropathy, only half of the people whose blood glucose has been poorly controlled go on to develop nephropathy.

Early indications of kidney disease

A healthy kidney permits only a tiny amount of *albumin,* a protein in the blood, to enter the urine. However, a kidney being damaged by nephropathy is unable to hold back as much albumin, and the level in the urine increases, causing *microalbuminuria* (the presence of tiny but abnormally high amounts of albumin in your urine). If your kidneys are on their way to being damaged by *diabetic nephropathy* (kidney disease caused by diabetes), doctors can detect microalbuminuria in your urine.

For three-quarters of the patients in the early stages of kidney disease, however, the amount of albumin in your urine is so small that it won't trigger a positive result when the traditional urine dipstick test is used. Therefore, your doctor should perform a more sophisticated test for microalbuminuria. With the test, you collect a 24-hour urine specimen (meaning you save all the urine you produce in 24 hours and have it tested), by taking a random urine sample or by collecting a specimen over a certain time period, usually four hours. If the level of albumin is abnormally high, it needs to be checked once again to be certain, because some factors (such as exercise) can trigger a false positive test. A second positive test should lead to action to protect your kidneys.

Because microalbuminuria can be detected about five years before a urine dipstick would test positive for albumin, you have time to treat the onset. Furthermore, treatment during the stage of microalbuminuria can reverse the kidney disease. After *macroalbuminuria* is found (indicating much larger amounts of protein in the urine) using the dipstick method, the disease can be slowed but not stopped.

If you have had type 1 diabetes for five years or more, or if you've recently been diagnosed with type 2 diabetes, *your doctor must check for microalbuminuria* unless you've already tested positive for albumin with a urine dipstick. If your test comes back negative, you should have it rechecked annually.

As many as 25 percent of patients with no microalbuminuria still have kidney disease, so treatment with drugs that protect your kidneys makes sense.

In June 2003 in the *New England Journal of Medicine,* researchers showed that microalbuminuria doesn't always lead to kidney failure. Patients with type 1 diabetes who improved their blood glucose levels, blood pressure, and abnormal blood fats (which I discuss in the next section) experienced a decline in microalbuminuria and, therefore, a decline in kidney damage.

Progressive changes in the kidneys

If diabetes is poorly controlled for five years or more, your kidney experiences a significant expansion of the *mesangial tissue,* the cells between the capillaries in the kidneys. The amount of microalbuminuria (discussed in the preceding section) correlates to the amount of mesangial expansion. Thickening of the glomerular basement membrane is taking place at the same time but does not correlate as well with the amount of microalbuminuria.

Over the next 15 to 20 years, the open capillaries and tubules are squeezed shut by the encroaching tissues. Less and less filtration of the blood can take place, ultimately ending in *uremia,* a condition in which the kidneys are not doing any cleansing.

Other factors besides high blood glucose contribute to the continuing destruction of the kidneys. They include the following:

- **High blood pressure (hypertension):** This factor may be almost as important as the glucose level. If your blood pressure is controlled by drugs, the damage to your kidneys slows very significantly.

- **Factors of inheritance:** Certain families and ethnic groups have a higher incidence of diabetic nephropathy, as I discuss in the section "The impact of diabetes on your kidneys," earlier in this chapter.

- **Abnormal blood fats:** Research shows that elevated levels of certain cholesterol-containing fats promote enlargement of the mesangium.

Diabetic nephropathy does not occur alone. If you experience kidney disease, you need to be aware that the following complications are associated with it:

- **Diabetic eye disease:** When someone experiences complete failure of the kidneys, called *end-stage renal disease,* diabetic retinopathy (eye disease) is almost always present (see the section "Eye Disease," later in this chapter). As kidney disease gets worse, retinopathy accelerates. But only half the people with retinopathy also have nephropathy.

    If you test positive for microalbuminuria, you will likely also have some retinopathy if diabetes is the cause of your kidney problems. If you have diabetes and have microalbuminuria but retinopathy is not present, your doctor should look for another cause of kidney disease besides diabetes.

- **Diabetic nerve disease (neuropathy):** Fewer than 50 percent of patients with nephropathy also experience diabetic nerve disease, or neuropathy. Neuropathy gets worse as kidney disease gets worse, but after dialysis has begun, some of the neuropathy disappears. This situation indicates that part of the neuropathy may be due to wastes that are retained because of the failing kidney rather than true damage to the nervous system. (For more on this condition, see the section "Nerve Disease, also known as Neuropathy" later in this chapter.)

- **High blood pressure (hypertension):** Hypertension plays an important role in accelerating kidney damage.

- **Edema:** *Edema,* or water accumulation, in the feet and legs occurs as the amount of protein in the urine exceeds one or two grams a day.

Treatment for diabetic nephropathy

If the information in the previous section is making your blood pressure rise, take a deep breath. I'm happy to report that all the inconvenience and discomfort associated with diabetic nephropathy can be avoided. Following are a few key treatments that you can do to prevent the disease or significantly slow it down after it begins:

- ✔ **Control your blood glucose.** This crucial step has been shown to avoid the onset of nephropathy and to slow it down after it starts. Both the Diabetes Control and Complications Trial (DCCT) in the United States, which studied glucose control in type 1 diabetes, and the United Kingdom Prospective Diabetes Study Groups in type 2 diabetes have proved this point. If you keep your blood glucose close to normal, you will not develop diabetic nephropathy. (For information on controlling your blood glucose, see Part III.)

  One of the best findings from the DCCT is that even 20 years after the trial ended, participants experienced persistent benefits of reduced blood pressure and reduced albumin excretion (a marker for kidney damage). Controlling your blood glucose now will pay off years in the future.

- ✔ **Control your blood pressure.** This step protects the kidneys from rapid deterioration. Treatment begins with a low-salt diet, but drugs are usually needed. High blood pressure can be controlled by a variety of drugs, but one class of drugs seems particularly valuable in nephropathy. This class is called the *angiotensin converting enzyme inhibitors,* or ACE inhibitors. (For more on ACE inhibitors, see the sidebar "ACE inhibitors to the rescue.") If ACE inhibitors can't be used for any reason, a similar class of drugs called *angiotensin II receptor blockers* are equally or more effective. Be especially alert for kidney damage if you have *white-coat high blood pressure* (WCH). This condition occurs in patients who have normal blood pressure at home but high blood pressure in the doctor's office. WCH has a high correlation with both kidney damage and eye damage.

- ✔ **Control the blood fats.** Because abnormalities of blood fats seem to make kidney disease worse, you must lower your bad, or LDL, cholesterol and raise your good, or HDL, cholesterol while lowering the other fat that is damaging — the triglycerides. A number of excellent drugs, in a class called *statins,* can accomplish this task. The ACE inhibitors also seem to help the levels of fats. (See the sidebar on ACE inhibitors for more information.)

- ✔ **Avoid other damage to the kidneys.** People with diabetes tend to have more urinary-tract infections, which damage the kidneys. Urinary tract infections must be looked for and treated. People with diabetes also have damage to the nerves that control the bladder, producing a neurogenic bladder. (See the section "Recognizing disorders of automatic [autonomic] nerves," later in this chapter.) When the nerves that detect a full bladder fail, proper emptying of the bladder is inhibited, which can lead to infections.

If you have disease in the urinary system, your doctor may want to do an *intravenous pyelogram* (IVP), a study to observe the appearance and function of your kidneys and the rest of your urinary tract. But people with diabetes with some kidney failure are at high risk for complete failure of the kidneys as a result of an IVP because of the dye used in the test. Your doctor should use another type of study that don't put your kidneys at risk.

If these preventative treatments fail, the patient undergoes dialysis or a kidney transplant.

When the kidneys fail, a main source for the breakdown of insulin is gone, and the patient requires much less or no insulin, so control of blood glucose may actually get easier. Drugs like the sulfonylureas are also reduced or stopped because the failed kidneys no longer eliminate them.

✔ **Dialysis:** Two dialysis techniques are currently in use.

  • **Hemodialysis:** The patient's artery is hooked into a tube that runs through a filtering machine that cleanses the blood and then sends it back into the patient's bloodstream. When the patient is moderately well, hemodialysis is done three times a week in a dialysis center. The potential exists for many complications, including infection and low blood pressure.

  • **Peritoneal dialysis:** A tube is inserted into the body cavity that contains the stomach, liver, and intestines, called the *peritoneal cavity*. A large quantity of fluid is dripped into the cavity, and it draws out the wastes, which are then removed as the fluid drains out of the cavity. Peritoneal dialysis is done at home, often on a daily basis. Peritoneal dialysis requires the use of sugar in the fluid, so people with diabetes have very high blood glucose levels (which is undesirable) unless insulin is added to the bags of dialysis fluid. Alternatively, the patient's subcutaneous insulin doses are increased. Peritoneal dialysis is also associated with a high rate of infection where the tube enters the peritoneal cavity.

✔ Poor control of blood glucose during any form of dialysis is associated with a higher death rate. Make sure you control your glucose!

Little difference exists in the long-term survival of patients treated with hemodialysis compared with peritoneal dialysis, so the choice becomes one of convenience and whether insurance covers one procedure more than the other. People with diabetes do not tolerate kidney failure well, so dialysis tends to be started earlier in them than in people without diabetes.

✔ **Kidney transplant:** Patients who receive a kidney transplant seem to do better than dialysis patients, but in the United States, because of a lack of kidneys, 80 percent of patients have dialysis and 20 percent have a transplant. Obviously, a transplanted kidney is foreign to the person who receives it, and the body tries to reject it. To avoid this result, the patient is given antirejection drugs, some of which make diabetic control more complicated. The kidney that is least rejected is the one from a donor who is most closely related to the patient.

When a healthy kidney enters the body of a person with diabetes, it is subject to the damage done by elevated glucose levels. After a transplant, controlling your blood glucose is crucial. At 85.5 percent, the five-year survival rate for kidney transplants is more than twice the 35.8-percent, five-year survival rate for dialysis patients.

Diabetes-related end-stage kidney disease (total kidney failure) is declining in all age groups thanks to better control of glucose, blood pressure, and fat.

ACE inhibitors to the rescue

The class of drugs called *angiotensin converting enzyme inhibitors,* or ACE inhibitors, has long been known to lower blood pressure. Recent studies show that these drugs also lower the pressure inside the *glomeruli* (the structures inside your kidneys that cleanse your blood). The result is a 50 percent reduction in death due to diabetic nephropathy and an equal reduction in the need for dialysis or a kidney transplant.

Your doctor should prescribe one of these medications if your blood pressure is 140/90 or higher. The target blood pressure is 120/80 in people with kidney disease and even lower in younger people. ACE inhibitors can even be used to reverse early kidney disease if you have microalbuminuria without hypertension, because the microalbuminuria suggests that there is increased pressure within the kidney. When ACE inhibitors are used, the excretion of albumin begins to fall; if you are leaking albumin into the urine, your urine albumin level can be used to monitor the drugs' effectiveness if your blood pressure is normal.

ACE inhibitors aren't perfect: They cause a cough in some patients, which some people find hard to tolerate, but the choice of a particular ACE inhibitor may solve this problem. In addition, ACE inhibitors tend to raise the potassium level in the blood. The potassium level is already an issue with failing kidneys, so a higher potassium level may add to the problem. A very high potassium level can cause abnormalities in the heart. Angiotensin II receptor blockers (ARBs) can replace ACE inhibitors when necessary. They're not associated with the cough but do raise potassium.

Other drugs used for high blood pressure include the calcium channel blockers, which may be as useful as ACE inhibitors. Other antihypertensives that have been standards in the past for hypertension may cause unacceptable side effects. Water pills (diuretics such as hydrochlorothiazide) raise the blood glucose. Beta blockers like propranolol make the abnormal fats worse. They also cause a difficulty in recognizing when the blood glucose has gone down to very low levels.

Eye Disease

The eyes are the second major organ of the body affected by diabetes over the long term. Blurred vision, often present at diagnosis, is reversible with control of the glucose. Some eye diseases, such as glaucoma and cataracts, also occur in the nondiabetic population, though they appear at a higher rate and earlier in people with diabetes. Glaucoma and cataracts respond to treatment very well. Diabetic retinopathy, however — which I explain in the next section — is limited to the diabetic population and may lead to blindness. In the past, blindness was inevitable, but that is not the case today. In fact, after 20 years of diabetes, eye disease occurred in 30 percent of patients with type 1 diabetes before 1979, in 18 percent between 1980 and 1984, and in only 6 percent after 1984.

In the following sections you find out about the normal function of the eye and how diabetes can damage or even eliminate that function. You also discover the importance of early diagnosis by regular eye exams and how you can stop the progress of eye disease should it occur.

Noting common eye problems in diabetics

In order to help you understand how diabetes affects the eyes, Figure 5-1 shows you the different parts of the eye.

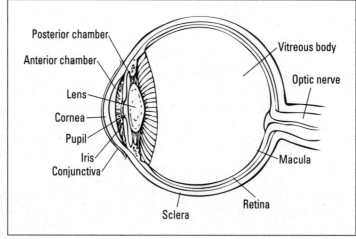

Figure 5-1:
The
structure of
the eye.

Illustration by Kathryn Born

Light enters the eye through the lens, where it is bent and focused on the retina. The place in the retina where the lens focuses is called the *macula*. The retina collects an image and transfers it to the optic nerve, which carries it to the brain, where the image is interpreted. Between the lens and the retina is a transparent material called the *vitreous body*. Many more structures exist within the eye, but they're not important for my purposes in this chapter. The eye muscles surround the eye on all sides and are attached to it. These muscles permit you to look up, down, and sideways without moving your head. These eye muscles are important in the discussion of diabetic nerve damage, called *neuropathy*. (For more on this condition, see the section "Nerve Disease, also known as Neuropathy," later in this chapter.)

Following is a list of common eye diseases found in people with diabetes:

- **Cataracts:** These opaque areas of the lens can block vision if they're large enough. Cataracts tend to be more common in people with diabetes, even at a young age, both as a result of advanced glycated end-products (AGEs) that form within the lens and as a result of the increased concentration of sorbitol in the lens. (I discuss AGEs and sorbitol in the sidebar "How high glucose leads to complications," earlier in this chapter.) Cataracts can be surgically removed by a fairly routine operation. The entire lens is removed, and an artificial lens is put in its place. With removal, you have an excellent chance for the restoration of your vision.

- **Glaucoma:** This condition, high pressure inside the eye, is enough to do damage to the optic nerve. Glaucoma is found more often in people with diabetes than in the nondiabetic population. If left unchecked, the high pressure can destroy the optic nerve and destroy your vision. Fortunately, medical treatment can lower the eye pressure and save the eye. Eye doctors check for glaucoma on a routine basis.

- **Retinopathy:** *Diabetic retinopathy* refers to a number of changes that are seen on the retina of the eye. These changes indicate that the patient has been exposed to high levels of blood glucose over time. If untreated at the appropriate time, retinopathy can lead to blindness. The first changes are seen after ten years of diabetes in both type 1 and 2. Because retinopathy is much more complicated and less treatable than the other two conditions, I discuss it in detail in the next section.

If you have diabetes, you must get an eye examination by an ophthalmologist or optometrist to preserve your vision. If no evidence suggests eye disease, your doctor can repeat it every two years. This situation is one where an expert is definitely needed. Doctors who aren't ophthalmologists or optometrists diagnose retinopathy correctly only 50 percent of the time, whereas ophthalmologists and optometrists are correct more than 90 percent of the time. You need to get an eye examination as soon as you are diagnosed with type 2 diabetes or five years after the diagnosis of type 1 diabetes.

Eyeing the risks of retinopathy

Ophthalmologists break down retinopathy, damage to the retina caused by high blood glucose, into two major types according to their potential to cause visual loss:

✔ **Background retinopathy:** This type is usually benign but can be a predictor of worse problems. The first changes noted by the ophthalmologist are *retinal aneurysms,* which are the result of weakening of the capillaries of the eye; they produce outpocketing of the capillaries, which look like tiny balloons. These aneurysms appear as small red dots on the back of the eye. They are benign and disappear over time.

The weakened capillaries also rupture sometimes and release blood to form *retinal hemorrhages* and *hard exudates.* The hard exudates, which are yellowish and appear round and sharp, are scars from the hemorrhage. If they extend into the macular area, they reduce vision. If the capillaries in the retina allow fluid to flow into the macula, you get *macular edema,* which also causes loss of vision. These exudates and hemorrhages can last for years. As the capillaries close, you have a decreased blood supply to the retina, and *cotton wool spots* or *soft exudates* appear. These spots represent destruction of the nerve fiber layer because of the lack of blood.

These changes usually do not cause complete loss of vision, but in about 50 percent of cases, they go on to the more serious proliferative retinopathy.

✔ **Proliferative retinopathy:** This condition results in vision loss if untreated. Just as in many other parts of the body, when the blood supply in the eye is reduced, new blood vessels form to carry more blood to the retina. This is the stage of proliferative retinopathy. This condition is when some visual loss becomes more certain. The growth of blood vessels takes place into the vitreous body. Hemorrhage into the vitreous body blocks vision. As the hemorrhage forms a clot and contracts, it may pull up the retina to produce *retinal detachment.* Because the lens can no longer focus the light onto the macula, you have a complete loss of vision.

Like diabetic nephropathy, retinopathy has a number of important associations:

✔ Certain ethnic groups as a result of genetic material in their chromosomes are at very high risk for retinopathy, including certain American Indian groups, like the Pima Indians, and Mexican Americans. African Americans may also be at higher risk, but only because of poorer glucose control.

- ✔ Males and females get retinopathy equally.

- ✔ Greater duration of diabetes results in more eye disease.

- ✔ High blood pressure may worsen the eye disease.

- ✔ Nephropathy occurs along with the eye disease. (See the "Progressive changes in the kidneys" section, earlier in this chapter.)

- ✔ Smoking worsens retinopathy, and alcohol abuse causes reduced visual acuity but not increased retinopathy.

- ✔ Patients with severe diabetic retinopathy are at increased risk for heart attacks. An article in *Diabetes Care* in July 2007 strongly confirmed this relationship. People with diabetic retinopathy are twice as likely to have a heart attack as people with diabetes who don't have retinopathy. If they have a heart attack, it's three times as likely to be fatal.

In recent clinical studies, ranibizumab (Lucentis) and other antibodies have been highly effective in treating diabetic retinopathy by reducing fluid leakage and formation of new blood vessels. An ophthalmologist injects it directly into the eye, but it isn't as painful as it sounds. Up to now laser surgery has been an excellent treatment option. And the use of laser surgery to create many burns in the retina has been shown to save many eyes. Only 5 percent of diabetics with proliferative retinopathy who undergo laser treatment develop severe visual loss. Because the retina is being burned, you have some minor loss of vision. You also have a mild decrease in night vision and a minor decrease in the size of the field that your eye can take in at one time. The procedure is done outside the hospital. It is used for treating macular edema with success as well.

Tight control of the blood glucose (maintaining a hemoglobin A1c under 7 percent) is associated with a much better response to laser surgery than loose control.

Laser surgery can't treat a retinal detachment that has already occurred. To do so, a surgical procedure called *vitrectomy* is used. This operation, done under general anesthesia, involves removing the vitreous body and replacing it with a sterile solution. Attachments to the retina are cut, and the retina returns to its place. Any hemorrhages in the vitreous body are removed at the same time. Vitrectomy is successful in restoring some vision about 80 to 90 percent of the time. If a retinal detachment is present in addition to hemorrhage, the amount of improvement depends on the extent and duration of the retinal detachment, with restoration of vision occurring about 50 to 60 percent of the time.

Resources for the blind and visually impaired

A search for resources for the blind and visually impaired must begin with the World Wide Web. One helpful site is the Blindness Resource Center (www.nyise.org/text/blindness.htm), sponsored by the New York Institute for Special Education, which contains a huge list of other sources of information. The site itself uses large print, so a person with impaired vision can easily read it.

Here are some other useful sites regarding blindness (and which you can link to from the Blindness Resource Center's site):

- ✔ Blind Net (www.blind.net) provides useful information about blindness.

- ✔ New York Institute for Special Education's Blindness Resource Center, www.nyise.org/blind.htm, provides programs for children who are blind or visually disabled.

- ✔ *Dialogue* magazine (www.blindskills.com) is written specifically for the blind.

- ✔ Guide Dogs for the Blind (www.guidedogs.com) explains everything you want to know about these amazing animals.

Undoubtedly, one of the best resources is the American Foundation for the Blind (AFB) at www.afb.org. It would take a good part of a lifetime to read all of the resource materials that the AFB provides on thousands of web pages. The AFB is the organization that Helen Keller devoted her life to, and it has every imaginable resource — and some that are unimaginable.

Nerve Disease, Also Known as Neuropathy

The third major part of the body that's attacked by poorly controlled diabetes is the nervous system. Sixty percent of people with diabetes have some abnormality of the nervous system. These patients usually don't realize it, because nerve disease doesn't have any early symptoms. These patients usually have poor glucose control, smoke, and are over age 40. Nerve disease is found most often in the people who have diabetes the longest. Diabetic neuropathy often leads to foot infections, foot ulcerations, and amputation — complications that are all entirely preventable (see the section "Diabetic Foot Disease," later in this chapter). The sections that follow describe the basics of nerve disease as well as disorders associated with nerve disease.

Examining the basics of neuropathy

How high glucose levels damage nerves remains uncertain. Doctors do know that the *axon,* the part of the nerve that connects to other nerves or to muscle, becomes degenerated. The damage may be *vascular* in some cases, resulting from a cut-off of blood to the nerve, and *metabolic* in others, resulting from chemical toxins produced by the metabolism of too much glucose.

Diabetic neuropathy occurs in any situation where the blood glucose is abnormally elevated, usually for ten years or more. It is therefore not limited to type 1 or type 2 diabetes, although it's most commonly paired with these diseases. When the elevated blood glucose is brought down to normal, the signs and symptoms improve. In some cases, the neuropathy disappears.

The fact that intensive control of the blood glucose improves the neuropathy suggests that the disease is a consequence of abnormal metabolism that damages the nerves.

The speed with which a nervous impulse travels down a nerve fiber is called the *nerve conduction velocity.* In diabetic neuropathy, the nerve conduction velocity (NCV) is slowed. This slowing may not be accompanied by any symptoms at first; testing the NCV provides a way of diagnosing neuropathy in people without symptoms. If a patient who has very mild symptoms takes medication to control neuropathy, the improvement that follows may be hard to detect except by doing a nerve conduction velocity study. Medication that helps the neuropathy is expected to speed up the NCV.

In addition to a persistently high blood glucose level, neuropathy is made worse by the following conditions:

- ✔ **Age:** Neuropathy is most common in people over 40.
- ✔ **Height:** Neuropathy is more common in taller individuals, who have longer nerve fibers to damage.
- ✔ **Alcohol consumption:** Even small quantities of alcohol can make neuropathy worse.

Doctors can test nerve function in a variety of ways because different nerve fibers seem to be responsible for different kinds of sensation, such as light touch, vibration, and temperature. The connection between the kind of test and the fiber it tests for is as follows:

- ✔ **Vibration testing:** Using a tuning fork, for example, can bring out abnormalities of large nerve fibers.
- ✔ **Temperature testing:** Uses a warm or cold item tests for damage to small fibers, which are very important in diabetes. When small fibers are damaged, the patient can lose the ability to feel that he is entering a burning hot bath, for instance.

✔ **Light touch testing:** Perhaps the most important test that is done reflects the large fibers, which sense anything touching the skin. This test is done using a filament that looks like a hair. The thickness of the filament determines how much force is needed to bend the filament so that it is felt. For example, a filament that bends with 1 gram of force can be felt by normal feet. If a patient can feel a filament that bends with 10 grams of force, the person is unlikely to suffer damage to the foot without feeling it. If the patient cannot feel any sensation with a filament that requires 75 grams of force to bend, that area is considered to have lost all sensation.

Either you or your doctor can use the 10-gram filament to discover whether you are at risk for damage to your feet because you cannot feel the pain. This test takes a minute to do and can save your feet from amputation. (See the section about the diabetic foot, later in this chapter.)

Recognizing disorders of sensation

Disorders of sensation are the most common and bothersome disorders of nerves in diabetes, because they are often associated with pain. They occur where the sensory nerves are damaged, and they include a number of different conditions that break down into two categories:

✔ **Diffuse neuropathies:** Involve many nerves

✔ **Focal neuropathies:** Involve one or several nerves

This section focuses on the diffuse neuropathies affecting sensation.

Distal polyneuropathy

Distal polyneuropathy is the most frequent form of diabetic neuropathy. *Distal* means far away from the center of the body — in other words, the feet and hands. *Poly* means many, and *neuropathy* is disease in nerves. So this disease concerns many nerves and is noticed in the feet and hands.

Physicians believe that distal polyneuropathy is a metabolic disease (a problem of too much glucose in the blood, specifically) because patients who have other diseases with a general abnormality of metabolism, such as kidney failure or vitamin deficiency, experience a distal polyneuropathy as well.

The signs and symptoms of distal polyneuropathy are

✔ Diminished ability to feel light touch (numbness) or feel the position of a foot, whether bent back or forward, resulting from the loss of the large fibers

✔ Diminished ability to feel pain and temperature from loss of small fibers

- ✔ No significant weakness
- ✔ Tingling and burning
- ✔ Extreme sensitivity to touch
- ✔ Loss of balance or coordination
- ✔ Worsening of symptoms at night

The danger of this kind of neuropathy is that the patient doesn't know, without looking, whether he has trauma to his feet, such as a burn or stepping on a tack. When the small fibers are lost, the symptoms are uncomfortable but not as serious. The patient may feel pain when the bed covers are on his feet or other uncomfortable sensations. The majority of patients with this condition are unaware of the loss of nerve fibers, and the disease is detected by nerve-conduction studies.

The complications of this loss of sensation are preventable. If you can't feel your feet, you must look at them. In the section on feet, later in this chapter, I offer specific techniques to preserve your feet when neuropathy is present.

The most serious complication of loss of sensation in the feet is the neuropathic foot ulcer. A person with normal nerve function feels pains when pressure mounts on an area of the foot. However, a person with diabetic neuropathy doesn't feel this pressure. A callus forms and, with continued pressure, the callus softens and liquefies, finally falling off to leave an ulcer. This ulcer becomes infected. If it isn't promptly treated, it spreads, and amputation may be the only way of saving the patient. In this situation, loss of blood supply to the feet is not an important contributing factor to the ulceration — in fact, the blood supply may be very good.

A less common complication in distal polyneuropathy is *neuroarthropathy,* or Charcot's joint. In this condition, trauma, which isn't felt, occurs to the joints of the foot or ankle. The bones in the foot get out of line, and many painless fractures may occur. The patient has redness and painless swelling of the foot and ankle. The foot becomes unusable and is described as a bag of bones.

Treatment of distal polyneuropathy starts with the best glucose control possible and extremely good foot care. Your doctor should look at your feet during each visit, particularly if you have any evidence of loss of feeling.

Some drugs can help in various ways, but a November 2014 study in the *Annals of Internal Medicine* couldn't conclude that any one of them is significantly better than the others:

- ✔ Nonsteroidal anti-inflammatory agents, like ibuprofen and sulindac, can reduce the inflammation.

- ✔ Antidepressants, such as amitriptyline and imipramine, reduce the pain and other discomfort.

✔ Topical capsaicin creams reduce pain as well, but it may cause a burning sensation and cough.

✔ A drug called *gabapentin* has been found to work more often than many of the older drugs, but it causes dizziness and sleepiness, which may make treatment more complicated.

✔ A spray of isosobide dinitrate or trinitrate patches may be helpful.

✔ Alpha lipoic acid, which has to be injected into a vein, was very successful in improving pain and other symptoms in a large trial study. (The results were reported in *Diabetes Care* in March 2003.)

✔ Duloxetine (Cymbalta) has been effective for diabetic peripheral neuropathy in several clinical trials when compared to a placebo.

The results of these treatments vary and seem to work about 60 percent of the time. However, the longer the pain has been present and the worse the pain, the less likely these drugs are to work.

Polyradiculopathy-diabetic amyotrophy

Polyradiculopathy-diabetic amyotrophy is a mixture of pain and loss of muscle strength in the muscles of the upper leg so that the patient cannot straighten the knee. Pain extends down from the hip to the thigh. This nerve condition is second in occurrence after distal polyneuropathy in the diabetic population. Polyradiculopathy-diabetic amyotrophy generally has a short course but may continue for years and doesn't particularly improve with better diabetic control. Patients often improve only after the passage of time.

Radiculopathy nerve-root involvement

Sometimes a severe pain in a particular distribution suggests that the root of the nerve, as it leaves the spinal column, is damaged. The clinical picture is pain distributed in a horizontal line around one side of the chest or abdomen. The pain can be so severe that it is mistaken for an internal abdominal emergency. Fortunately, the pain goes away after a variable period of time — anywhere from 6 to 24 months. In the meantime, good glucose control and pain management are helpful.

Comprehending disorders of movement

Neuropathy can affect nerves to various muscles. Disorders of movement, called *mononeuropathy,* occur when you lose motor nerves that carry the impulses to muscles to make those muscles move. When you lose those nerves, you lose the ability to move or use those muscles. These disorders are believed to originate as a result of the sudden closing of a blood vessel supplying the nerve. The clinical picture depends on which nerve or nerves are affected. If one of the nerves to the eyeball is damaged, the patient can't turn his eye to the side that nerve is on. If the nerve to the face is affected, the eyelid may droop or the smile on one side of the face may be flat. The patient can have trouble with vision or problems with hearing. Focusing the eye may not be possible. No treatment really exists, but fortunately the disorder goes away on its own after several months.

Recognizing disorders of automatic (autonomic) nerves

Even as you're reading this page, many movements of muscles are going on inside your body, but you're unaware of them. Your heart muscle is squeezing down and relaxing. Your diaphragm is rising up to empty the lungs of air and relaxing to draw air in. Your esophagus is carrying food from the mouth to the stomach and, in turn, the stomach pushes it into the small intestine, which pushes it into the large intestine. All these muscle functions are under the control of nerves from the brain, and diabetic neuropathy can affect all of them. These automatic functions are handled by the *autonomic nerves.* Sensitive tests determine that as many as 40 percent of people with diabetes have some form of autonomic neuropathy.

The clinical presentation of this type of neuropathy depends on the involved nerve. Following are some of the possibilities:

- ✔ **Bladder abnormalities, starting with a loss of the sensation of bladder fullness:** The urine is not eliminated, and urinary-tract infections result. After a while, loss of bladder contraction occurs, and the patient has to strain to urinate or loses urine by dribbling. The doctor can easily diagnose this abnormality by finding out how much urine is left in the bladder after urinating. The treatment is to remember to urinate every four hours or take a drug that increases the force of bladder contraction.

- ✔ **Sexual dysfunction, which occurs in 50 percent of males with diabetes and 30 percent of females with diabetes:** Males cannot sustain an erection, and females have trouble lubricating the vagina for intercourse. (See Chapter 6 for more information on these problems.)

- ✔ **Intestinal abnormalities of various kinds:** The most common abnormality is constipation. In one quarter of all patients with diabetes, nerves to the stomach are involved, so the stomach doesn't empty on time. This condition is called *gastroparesis.* It can lead to what's called *brittle diabetes,* where the insulin is active when there is no food. Fortunately, the drug metocloprimide helps to empty the stomach. A treatment that has worked well is the implantation of a device that stimulates the stomach electrically. It greatly diminishes the symptoms. This treatment was described in a report in *Diabetes Care* from the University of Kansas Medical Center in May 2004.

✔ **Involvement of the gallbladder, which leads to gallstones:** Normally, the gallbladder empties each time you eat, especially if you eat a fatty meal, because the substances in the bile (within the gallbladder) help to break down fat. If disease of the nerve to the gallbladder prevents it from emptying, these same substances form stones.

✔ **Involvement of the large intestine that can result in diabetic diarrhea with as many as ten or more bowel movements in a day:** Accidental loss of bowel contents can occur, and bacteria can grow abnormally in the intestine. This problem responds to antibiotic treatment. Diarrhea is treated with one of several drugs that quiet the large intestine.

✔ **Heart abnormalities:** If loss of nerves to the heart occurs, the heart may not respond to exercise by speeding up as it should. The force of the heart may not increase when the patient stands, and the patient then becomes lightheaded. A fast fixed heart rate also may occur, and the rhythm of the heart may not be normal. Such patients are at risk for sudden death.

✔ **Sweating problems, especially in the feet:** The body may try to compensate for the lack of sweating in the feet by sweating excessively on the face or trunk. Heavy sweating can occur when certain foods, such as cheese, are eaten.

✔ **Abnormalities of the pupil:** The pupil determines the amount of light let in by the eye. As a result of the neuropathy, the pupil is small and does not open up in a dark room.

Entrapment neuropathies

Entrapment neuropathies result from squeezing of individual nerves as they pass through bony or ligamentous areas. Those areas don't allow expansion, so the nerve is trapped if swelling takes place for any reason. The entrapment neuropathies can produce symptoms similar to the mononeuropathies described above, but they differ in several ways:

✔ Onset of mononeuropathies is sudden, whereas entrapment neuropathies have a gradual onset.

✔ Mononeuropathies are self-limited, usually resolving over six weeks, whereas entrapment neuropathies persist unless the nerve is released by surgery.

✔ Mononeuropathies are painful from the start, but entrapment neuropathies gradually get more and more painful.

Entrapment neuropathies are very common in people with diabetes, occurring in one in every three patients.

Following are the entrapment neuropathies:

- **Carpal tunnel syndrome:** Produces reduced sensation in the fingers and weakness touching the thumb to the fifth finger. The median nerve is trapped at the wrist.

- **Ulnar entrapment:** Produces reduced sensation in part of the fourth finger and the entire fifth finger as well as the hand between the fifth finger and the wrist. The ulnar nerve is trapped at the elbow.

- **Radial nerve entrapment:** Produces loss of sensation in the back of the hand and "wrist drop" from weakness of the muscles that straighten up the wrist. The radial nerve is trapped at the elbow.

- **Common peroneal entrapment:** Produces loss of sensation in the side of the leg and top of the foot and "drop foot" from weakness of the muscles that pull up the foot. The common peroneal nerve is trapped as it passes the head of the fibula, one of the two bones that begin at the knee joint and end at the ankle.

- **Tarsal tunnel syndrome:** Produces loss of sensation on both sides of the foot and wasting of the muscles of the foot, resulting in decreased toe movement. It's like carpal tunnel syndrome in the foot and results from trapping of the tibial nerve between two of the small foot bones.

- **Lateral femoral cutaneous nerve entrapment:** Produces loss of sensation on the outside of the thigh but no muscle weakness. It results from trapping of that nerve at the groin.

The entrapment neuropathies respond to rest, splints, drugs that promote water loss, injections of steroids, and surgery if necessary. The important thing is not to confuse them with mononeuropathies.

You can see that you can run into all kinds of problems if you develop diabetic neuropathy. None of them need ever bother you, though, if you follow the recommendations in Part III — the closest you will ever get to a nerve problem will be when you try to get a date with that cute neighbor.

Heart Disease

In the last three decades, the number of deaths due to heart disease has fallen dramatically, thanks to all kinds of new treatments as well as improved diets. However, the tremendous increase in the number of type 2 diabetes patients predicted for the next few decades may reverse this trend. In this section, you find out about the special problems that diabetes brings to the heart.

In the past, diabetic heart disease has been considered disease of the large blood vessels *(macroangiopathy)*. This sets it apart from eye, kidney, and nerve disease, which are considered diseases of the small blood vessels *(microangiopathy)*. This idea was strengthened by the fact that microangiopathy responds to good blood glucose control but macroangiopathy does not. More recently, doctors and researchers believe that both kinds of complications have much in common. The large blood vessels in the heart, brain, arms, and legs are affected by the same metabolic abnormalities (see the sidebar "How high glucose leads to complications," earlier in this chapter) and structural abnormalities that affect the small blood vessels.

Controlling the blood glucose, the blood fats, and the blood pressure early in the disease help to lessen or prevent coronary artery disease. A study in *The Lancet* in November 2014 suggests there is benefit to early control of the blood glucose on heart disease. However, good evidence suggests that intensive control is not nearly as effective after an event such as a heart attack, stroke, or loss of blood flow to the leg has already occurred.

Identifying risks of heart disease to diabetic patients

Coronary artery disease (CAD) is the term for the progressive closure of the arteries, which supply blood to the heart muscle. When one or more of your arteries closes completely, the result is a heart attack (or *myocardial infarction*). In diabetes, the incidence of CAD is increased even in the young type 1 patient. The duration of time with diabetes promotes CAD in type 1 patients. CAD affects males and females with type 1 diabetes in the same way.

Type 2 diabetes is different. CAD is the most common reason for death in type 2 patients. Women with type 2 are at increased risk for CAD compared to men. The following risk factors promote CAD in type 2 patients:

- ✔ **Increased production of insulin,** caused by insulin resistance.
- ✔ **Obesity.**
- ✔ **Central adiposity,** which refers to the distribution of fat, particularly in the waist area.
- ✔ **Hypertension** (high blood pressure).
- ✔ **Abnormal blood fats,** especially elevated LDL (bad) cholesterol. Decreased HDL (good cholesterol) appears to correlate with coronary heart disease as well, but the goal is to lower LDL. The abnormal fats may persist even when the patient's glucose is controlled. People without diabetes but with impaired glucose tolerance may show the same abnormalities.
- ✔ **Sitting time,** especially long stretches of inactivity, such as watching television for a long time.

People with diabetes have more CAD than people without diabetes. When X-ray studies of the heart blood vessels are compared, people with diabetes have more arteries involved than people without diabetes.

If a heart attack occurs, the risk of death is much greater for the person with diabetes. More than half of all people with diabetes die of heart attacks. If people without diabetes have heart attacks, they die 15 percent of the time, but people with diabetes die 40 percent of the time. The death rate is worse for people with diabetes who poorly controlled their glucose before the heart attack. The same poorly controlled people have more complications, such as shock and heart failure, from heart attacks than people without diabetes. After a heart attack occurs, the outlook is much worse for diabetic people. A second heart attack occurs in 50 percent of people with diabetes (as opposed to 25 percent of people without diabetes), and the death rate in five years is 80 percent (versus 25 percent for people without diabetes).

The picture is not a pretty one. The treatment options are the same for people with and without diabetes. Therapy to dissolve the clot of blood that is obstructing the coronary artery can be used, but people with diabetes don't do as well with *angioplasty,* the technique by which a tube is placed into the artery to clean it out and open it up. New techniques using certain chemicals in the tube are making this better therapy. People with diabetes do as well with surgery to bypass the obstruction (called *bypass surgery*) as people without diabetes, but the long-term prognosis for keeping the graft open is not as good.

It has been believed that red wine (but not white wine) is good for your heart. Recent studies suggest that white wine has substances that are heart healthy as well, and both have alcohol, which is healthy in moderate amounts (two drinks daily for men and one for women).

Although low-dose aspirin (81 milligrams) has been effective in protecting the heart of people without diabetes without preexisting heart disease, it has not been proven successful in preventing heart attack in people with diabetes. A higher dose may be needed. Doctors don't recommend it for women with diabetes who are younger than 60 or men with diabetes who are younger than 50 with no major risk factors for a heart attack because the bleeding risk is too great.

Studies indicate that body-mass index is not a good predictor of heart attacks and death in obese diabetic patients. The waist in inches divided by the height in inches is the best predictor (a waist-to-height ratio under 0.5 is considered healthy), followed by the waist circumference (less than or equal to 40 inches in men and 35 inches in women is lower risk), followed by the waist-to-hip ratio (under 0.9 in men and 0.8 in women is healthy).

Metabolic syndrome

The earliest abnormality in type 2 diabetes is insulin resistance, which is found in people even before diabetes can be diagnosed. People with impaired glucose tolerance, and even 25 percent of the population with normal glucose tolerance, have evidence of insulin resistance. The condition, formerly known as *insulin-resistance syndrome,* is now called *metabolic syndrome.* It is particularly worrisome because it is being found in obese children and adolescents, resulting in greater danger of diabetes and an early heart attack in these children. The next 20 years will reveal how these risks play out.

Linking metabolic syndrome and insulin resistance

Several features accompany insulin resistance, which is associated with three times the incidence of coronary artery disease compared to people with normal insulin sensitivity:

- **Hypertension:** High blood pressure may be a consequence of the increased insulin required to keep the glucose normal when a patient is insulin resistant. When people are given insulin to control glucose, a rise in blood pressure often occurs.

- **Abnormalities of blood fats:** The level of triglycerides is elevated, as is the amount of small, dense LDL (a particle in the blood that carries bad cholesterol). At the same time, you see a decline in the amount of HDL, the good cholesterol particle that helps to clean out the arteries.

- **Microalbuminuria:** The presence of microalbuminuria strongly correlates with the development of coronary artery disease. (See the section "Early indications of kidney disease," earlier in the chapter.)

- **C-reactive protein:** This marker for inflammation in the body (easily obtained by a blood test) rises as the severity of the metabolic syndrome increases. It indicates that inflammation plays an important role in coronary artery disease.

- **Increased plasminogen activator inhibitor-1:** This chemical, which blocks the activity of plasminogen activator, prevents the breakdown of blood clots that form in the arteries of the heart and other areas.

- **Increased abdominal visceral fat:** You can lose a lot of this fat, which is found at the waistline, by dieting and losing 5 to 10 percent of your body weight.

- **Obesity:** Many people with metabolic syndrome are obese, but not all. Likewise, many people who are obese don't have the metabolic syndrome.

- **Sedentary lifestyle:** This feature is also often found, but an active lifestyle doesn't preclude metabolic syndrome.

The preceding features, plus others, are found in people who have an increased tendency to have coronary artery disease and heart attacks. Keep in mind that metabolic syndrome may be present even when diabetes is not. Metabolic syndrome is probably a primary abnormality and not a consequence of an elevated blood glucose over time.

Finding out who's at risk

Metabolic syndrome is believed to be present in one-third of all Americans. Overweight males (with a BMI of 25 or greater) are six times as likely to have metabolic syndrome, and obese males (BMI of 30 or greater) were 32 times as likely.

Metabolic syndrome is present when three or more of the following conditions are present:

✔ Waist circumference in men greater than 102 cm and in women greater than 88 cm

✔ Fasting triglyceride greater than or equal to 150 mg/dl

✔ Blood pressure greater than or equal to 130/85

✔ HDL cholesterol less than or equal to 40 in men and 50 in women

✔ Fasting glucose greater than or equal to 110 mg/dl

✔ Abnormal glucose tolerance (glucose level of 140–199 two hours after 75 gm of glucose)

People who are at the top of the normal weight curve and slightly overweight have also been found to have metabolic syndrome. You don't have to be obese.

Unexpectedly, people who consume diet sodas daily have been found to have an increased risk of metabolic syndrome and type 2 diabetes. The explanation is not known.

Although alcohol consumption up to the daily guideline of one drink for women and two drinks for men may be protective against heart disease, drinking more than that or binge drinking one or more days per week is associated with an increased risk of metabolic syndrome and its complication of heart disease.

Treating metabolic syndrome

A number of treatments are available for metabolic syndrome. If you are obese and have a sedentary lifestyle, you should correct these problems. Even a small amount of weight loss or exercise can make a major contribution toward decreasing the risk of a heart attack. An exercise training program has reversed metabolic syndrome in 30 percent of patients.

Many features of metabolic syndrome are dependent on an abnormal blood glucose. Restriction of carbohydrates reverses these features, including elevated triglyceride, elevated blood pressure, reduced HDL cholesterol, fasting glucose, and glucose tolerance.

You can treat elevated triglyceride and reduced HDL with drugs such as the class called *fibric-acid derivatives*.

Use of the DASH (Dietary Approach to Stop Hypertension) diet, which was developed to control high blood pressure, can also be helpful in reversing the features of metabolic syndrome. It consists of mostly fruits and vegetables and can be found extensively discussed in my book *High Blood Pressure For Dummies* (John Wiley & Sons, Inc.).

Studies have found that there is variability in the prevalence of metabolic syndrome by occupation. Food preparation and food service workers have the highest risk. About 30 percent of them have been found to have metabolic syndrome. The groups of writers, artists, entertainers, athletes, engineers, architects, and scientists have the lowest risk, at about 9 percent.

Cardiac autonomic neuropathy

I discuss cardiac autonomic neuropathy briefly in the section on neuropathy earlier in this chapter. Basically, the heart is under the control of nerves, and high glucose levels can damage these nerves. Your doctor can test for this condition in a number of ways:

- **Measure the resting heart rate:** It may be abnormally high (greater than 100).

- **Measure the standing blood pressure:** It may fall abnormally low (a decrease of 20 mm sustained for 3 minutes) compared to the sitting blood pressure.

- **Measure the variation in heart rate when the patient breathes in compared to breathing out:** The variation may be abnormally low (under 10).

The presence of cardiac autonomic neuropathy results in a diminished survival even among patients who don't have coronary artery disease.

Cardiomyopathy

Cardiomyopathy refers to an enlarged heart and scarring of the heart muscle in the absence of coronary artery disease. As a result, the heart does not pump enough blood with each stroke. The patient may be able to compensate by a more rapid heart rate, but if hypertension is present, a stable condition can deteriorate.

The key treatment in this condition is control of the blood pressure as well as control of the blood glucose. Studies in animals in which diabetic cardiomyopathy has been induced have shown healing by controlling the blood glucose.

Diabetic Blood Vessel Disease Away from the Heart

The same processes that affect the coronary arteries can affect the arteries to the brain, producing cerebrovascular disease, and the arteries to the rest of the body, producing peripheral vascular disease. I explain each condition in the following sections.

Peripheral vascular disease

Peripheral vascular disease (PVD) occurs much earlier in people with diabetes and proceeds more rapidly. This clogging of the arteries to parts of your body other than the heart and brain results in the loss of pulses in the feet; after ten years of diabetes, a third of men and women no longer feel a pulse in their feet. The most common symptom of PVD is intermittent pain in the calves, thighs, or buttocks that begins after some walking and subsides with rest. People with PVD have a reduction in life expectancy. When PVD occurs, just as when CAD occurs, it is much worse in people with diabetes because more of their arteries are involved.

The major screening test for peripheral vascular disease is the ankle-brachial index (ABI). The systolic blood pressure in the ankle is divided by the systolic blood pressure in the arm. A result of 0.95 or greater is normal. A result of less than 0.75 suggests serious peripheral vascular disease. Some people with diabetes have a lot of calcium in their arteries and get a higher blood pressure in the ankle than the arm. If the ABI is more than 1 and the systolic blood pressure in the ankle is more than 300 mm mercury or 75 greater than the arm, this condition also suggests PVD.

An ABI in a person with diabetes that is less than 0.9 is associated with a much higher risk of death from a heart attack according to a study published in *Diabetes Care* in March 2006.

In addition to diabetes, certain risk factors increase the severity of PVD. The following risk factors are unavoidable:

- **Genetic factors:** PVD is more common in some families and certain ethnic groups, especially African Americans.
- **Age:** The risk of PVD increases as you age.

The following risk factors are within your control:

- Smoking, which promotes early foot amputation
- Hypercholesterolemia (high cholesterol)
- High glucose
- Hypertension
- Obesity

In addition to controlling the preceding factors as much as possible, you may need to take drugs that help prevent closure of the arteries and loss of blood supply. Aspirin, which inhibits clotting, is among the most useful. Pentoxifylline (Trental) improves the circulation of cells in the blood. In addition, exercise improves blood flow and promotes the development of blood vessels around an obstruction. If none of these measures reverses the symptoms, some form of surgery that opens or bypasses the blocked arteries may be necessary.

Smoking and diabetes

As everyone knows, smoking has a number of ill effects on people without diabetes, but the effects are even worse in people with diabetes. Current smokers and those former smokers who have stopped, but smoked for 15 years or more, have felt these bad effects. Among other things, smoking has the following consequences:

- Reducing blood flow in arteries and blocking increased flow when it is needed
- Increasing pain in the legs in people with peripheral vascular disease and in the heart in people with coronary artery disease

- Increasing *atheromatous plaques,* the changes in arteries in the heart and other areas (like the brain and the legs) that precede closing of the blood vessels
- Increasing clustering of *platelets,* the blood elements that form a plug or clot that blocks the artery
- Increasing blood pressure, which also worsens atheromatous plaques

These problems don't even take into account the effects of smoking on the lungs, the bladder, and the rest of the body.

Cerebrovascular disease

Cerebrovascular disease (CVD) is a disease of the arteries that supply the brain with oxygen and nutrients. What I say about peripheral vascular disease in the preceding section also covers cerebrovascular disease, with some exceptions. The risk factors and the approach to treatment are similar. However, the symptoms are very different because the clogged arteries in CVD supply the brain.

If a temporary reduction in blood supply to the brain occurs, the person suffers from a *transient ischemic attack,* or TIA. This temporary loss of brain function may present itself as slurring of speech, weakness on one side of the body, or numbness. TIA may disappear after a few minutes, but it comes back again some hours to days later. If a major artery to the brain completely closes, the person suffers a stroke. Fortunately, stroke victims who are seen soon enough after the stroke can take advantage of clot-dissolving materials.

People with diabetes are at increased risk for CVD just as they are for PVD. Their disease tends to be worse than the disease in a person without diabetes, and they can have blockage in many small blood vessels in the brain that leads to the loss of intellectual function, a symptom similar to Alzheimer's disease.

The treatable risk factors for CVD are the same as those for PVD (see the preceding section). You should make attempts to improve them, particularly high blood pressure.

Diabetic Foot Disease

If I ever have an opportunity to save people from the consequences of diabetes, it's in this section of the book. About 73,000 amputations occur in the United States each year on people with diabetes. Despite the wonderful surgery to bring more blood into the feet, the number of amputations is actually rising.

Good medical care can prevent amputations. Your doctor should look at your feet as routinely as he or she measures your weight.

In the section on neuropathy, earlier in this chapter, I point out that a filament that requires a pressure of 10 grams to be felt can differentiate a patient who will not suffer damage to the feet under normal walking conditions from a patient who will. All doctors who have patients with diabetes should have this filament to test the feet at least annually. Even better, you should have your own filament and test yourself any time you feel like it. If you can't feel the filament, you had better start looking at your feet every day. See Chapter 7 for where to obtain a filament.

If your feet are dry, you may have loss of sweating. Loss of sweating is usually accompanied by the loss of touch sensation and the development of ulcers. You need to moisturize your feet, first by soaking them in water (which you test with your hand for its temperature), and then by drying them with a towel and applying a moisturizer. Soaking should always be accompanied by drying and moisturizing.

Ulcers of the foot can develop in a number of ways:

- ✔ Constant pressure
- ✔ Sudden higher pressure
- ✔ Constantly repeated moderate pressure

It takes very little pressure, if constantly applied, to damage the skin. If you have diminished sensation, some of the following tips may save your feet:

- ✔ Change your shoes about every five hours.
- ✔ If you have new shoes, change them every two hours at first. Your shoes should not be too tight or too loose.
- ✔ Never walk barefoot.
- ✔ Shake out your shoes before you put them on.
- ✔ Inspect your feet daily, with a mirror if necessary.
- ✔ Do not use a heating pad on your feet.
- ✔ Stop smoking. If you smoke, you are asking for an amputation.

If you do develop an ulcer, the treatment is to take pressure off the site by resting the foot and elevating it. When the infection is localized in a foot with adequate blood supply, a plaster cast is applied to overcome the natural tendency to want to stand or walk. The cast protects the ulcer from slight trauma that could prevent healing.

A product called becaplermin (Regranex Gel) has been shown to speed the healing of deep diabetic foot ulcers when it is combined with good wound care. (Good wound care means carefully removing dead tissue and keeping your weight off the ulcer, along with treating any infection and controlling your blood glucose.) The product is applied to a clean wound bed once daily. You should see significant reduction in the size of the ulcer within 10 weeks and complete healing by 20 weeks. The long duration for healing is a problem, because Regranex Gel is very expensive. However, a typical deep diabetic ulcer is very expensive to treat in any case, and if this product can speed up your healing, it may be worthwhile. Patients with known malignancy shouldn't use Regranex Gel.

I must reiterate that ulcers of the foot, which can lead to amputation in people with diabetes, are entirely preventable. If your feet lack sensation, your doctor must examine them at every visit, and you must examine them daily. At the first sign of a problem, take appropriate action.

Skin Disease in Diabetes

Many conditions involving the skin are unique to diabetic people because of the treatment and complications of the disease. Following are the most common and important skin complications:

- ✔ Bruises occur due to the cutting of blood vessels by the insulin needle.

- ✔ *Vitiligo* (loss of skin pigmentation) is part of the autoimmune aspect of type 1 diabetes and cannot be prevented.

- ✔ *Necrobiosis lipoidica,* which also affects people without diabetes, creates patches of reddish-brown skin on the shins or ankles, and the skin becomes thin and can ulcerate. Females tend to have this condition more often than males. Steroid injections are used to treat this condition, and the areas eventually become depressed and brown.

- ✔ *Xanthelasma,* which are small yellow flat areas called *plaques* on the eyelids, occur even when cholesterol is not elevated.

- ✔ *Alopecia,* or loss of hair, occurs in type 1 diabetes. It's considered an autoimmune disease, like type 1 diabetes.

- ✔ *Insulin hypertrophy* is the accumulation of fatty tissue where insulin is injected. Moving the injection site around can prevent this condition.

- ✔ *Insulin lipoatrophy* is the loss of fat where the insulin is injected. Although the cause is unknown, this condition is rarely seen now that human insulin has replaced beef and pork insulin (see Chapter 10).

- ✔ Dry skin is a consequence of diabetic neuropathy, which leads to a lack of sweating.

- ✔ Fungal infections occur under the nails or between the toes. Fungus likes moisture and elevated glucose. Lowering your glucose and keeping your toes dry prevent these infections. Medications may cure this problem, but it recurs if glucose and moisture are not managed.

- ✔ *Acanthosis nigricans,* a velvety-feeling increase in pigmentation on the back of the neck and the armpits, causes no problems and needs no treatment. This condition is usually found when insulin resistance exists. It is seen in adults and children with type 2 diabetes.

- ✔ Diabetic thick skin, which is thicker than normal skin, occurs in people who have had diabetes for more than ten years.

Gum Disease in Diabetes

The major problem that people with diabetes may have in their mouths is gum disease. This problem develops because the higher concentration of glucose in the mouth promotes the growth of germs, which mix with food and saliva to form plaque on your gums. If you don't brush your teeth twice a day and floss your teeth once a day, the plaque may harden into tartar, which is very hard for you to remove. The gums may develop gingivitis, becoming brittle and bleeding easily. You may experience pain and bad breath, and eventually the gums may become so weakened that they cannot support your teeth.

Controlling your blood glucose is a key step in preventing gum disease. Visiting your dentist for routine cleanings of your teeth twice a year is another important way to keep your gums healthy. Interestingly, people with diabetes do not seem to develop cavities more often than people who do not have the disease.

Sleep Apnea

Sleep apnea is another complication of obesity, and it can lead to metabolic syndrome and type 2 diabetes. Sleep apnea is characterized by recurrent episodes, lasting 10 to 30 second each, of failure to breathe while asleep. These episodes are due to obstruction of the airway due to extra fat in the neck or nerve disturbances. As many as 60 to 90 episodes may occur per hour, during which the oxygen saturation of the blood drops to as low as 50 percent (normal is greater than 95 percent).

In a 2009 study of more than 300 patients with type 2 diabetes and obesity, over 86 percent of the patients had obstructive sleep apnea. Waist circumference was a key indicator of obstructive sleep apnea.

Sleep apnea makes the patient very sleepy the next day, which results in slow reactions, poor memory and concentration, and irritability. Sleep apnea also causes increased blood pressure and increased insulin resistance by unclear mechanisms. Sleep apnea increases the risk of heart disease. The reduction in oxygen in the blood may also increase damage to the kidneys, leading to nephropathy. Finally, the severity of the sleep apnea correlates with the severity of poor glucose control.

When obstructive sleep apnea is due to upper airway obstruction, it can be improved or even cured by treating an underlying condition such as low thyroid function or a tumor of the pituitary gland producing excessive growth hormone (acromegaly) if this is present. Maintaining weight loss may improve the obstructive sleep apnea. If not, then a positive pressure device worn on the face, a CPAP machine, should greatly improve the condition; unfortunately, many patients find it uncomfortable.

Other Conditions Associated with Diabetes That You Should Know

These and the complications that I discuss in this chapter should encourage you to make every effort to avoid getting diabetes or to reverse it if possible.

- ✔ Diabetes increases the risk of death from breast, liver, and colon cancer.
- ✔ Diabetes is associated with a high incidence of arthritis and bone fractures.
- ✔ *Psoriasis,* an autoimmune skin condition of raised, red, scaly patches, has a high incidence of associated diabetes.
- ✔ Older people, especially those on insulin, have a higher incidence of falls requiring hospitalization than those without diabetes.
- ✔ Those diabetics with earlier onset and greater severity have mild cognitive impairment, which includes problems with perception, thinking, reasoning, and remembering.

Chapter 6

Preserving Sexual Function and Protecting Pregnancy

In This Chapter

▶ Treating impotence caused by diabetes

▶ Dealing with female sexual problems

▶ Coping with diabetes in pregnancy

▶ Recognizing polycystic ovarian syndrome

*N*othing is quite so pleasant as walking into the hospital room of a mother with diabetes holding her healthy newborn. Pregnancy associated with diabetes used to be a disaster for both the baby and the mother. No longer. With the proper precautions, diabetic pregnancies can proceed like pregnancies without diabetes. This chapter describes everything you need to know from start to finish, including overcoming obstacles to intercourse, enjoying a healthy pregnancy, and delivering a healthy baby.

Men with diabetes have sexual problems as well. Fortunately, they are manageable, so I get started here with their issues.

Examining Erection Problems

If carefully questioned, up to 50 percent of all males with diabetes admit to having difficulty with sexual function. This difficulty usually takes the form of *erectile dysfunction (ED)*, the inability to have or sustain an erection sufficient for intercourse. It develops 10 to 15 years earlier in men with diabetes than in men without diabetes. After the age of 70, more than 95 percent of men with diabetes have erectile dysfunction. Many factors besides diabetes can cause the same problem, and you should rule them out before blaming diabetes.

After you eliminate the following possibilities for erectile dysfunction, you can feel confident that diabetes is the source of the problem:

- Trauma to the penis

- Medications, such as certain antihypertensives and antidepressants

- Hormonal abnormalities, such as insufficient production of the male hormone testosterone or overproduction of a hormone from the brain called *prolactin.* Note that sildenafil and the other three similar drugs in the treatment section work even with low testosterone.

- Poor blood supply to the penis due to blockage of the artery by peripheral vascular disease (see Chapter 5), which can be treated very effectively by microvascular surgery

- *Psychogenic impotence,* an inability to have an erection for psychological rather than physical reasons (this problem should be managed by a therapist)

In order to understand how diabetes affects an erection, you need to first understand how an erection is normally produced.

Reviewing the erection process

As a result of some form of stimulation — such as touch, sight, or sound — the brain activates nerves in the *parasympathetic nervous system,* which is part of the autonomic nervous system. These nerves cause muscles to relax so that blood flow into the penis greatly increases. As blood flow increases, the veins through which blood leaves the penis compress, and the penis becomes erect. An erect penis contains about 11 times as much blood as a flaccid penis. With sufficient stimulation, muscles contract, propelling semen through the *urethra* (the tube in the penis that normally carries urine from the bladder) to the outside of the body. The pleasant sensation that occurs along with the muscle contractions *(ejaculation)* is called *orgasm.*

Orgasm and ejaculation are the result of stimulation by the other side of the autonomic nervous system, the sympathetic nervous system. As the stimulation causes contraction of the muscles, it closes the muscle over the bladder so that urine does not normally accompany expulsion of semen and the semen does not go back into the bladder.

Diabetes can damage the parasympathetic nervous system so that the male can't get an erection sufficient for sexual intercourse. The sympathetic nervous system is spared, so ejaculation and orgasm can occur, but intercourse may be unpleasant for both partners because of the psychological consequence of not being able to sustain a firm erection.

For diabetes patients, ED is affected by the following factors:

- **Degree of control of the blood glucose:** Better control is associated with fewer problems.
- **Duration of the diabetes:** The longer you have diabetes, the more likely you are to be unable to have an erection.
- **Interaction with your partner:** A positive relationship is important.
- **Use of drugs, tobacco, or alcohol:** Each may prevent erections.
- **State of mind:** A positive frame of mind is associated with more successful erections.

Discussing ED with your doctor

Although sexual intercourse tends to be an embarrassing topic for many men and women, if you have diabetes and have a problem in this key area of life, you need to discuss it with your doctor. Some doctors find this topic just as embarrassing as some patients. Any doctor who treats patients with diabetes should bring the topic up (no pun intended) in the first meeting and annually thereafter. If he or she does not, you should broach the subject yourself.

Erectile dysfunction has been shown to predict coronary artery disease in men with type 2 diabetes. Diabetics with ED who had heart attacks were older and had higher blood pressure, higher total cholesterol, lower HDL cholesterol, and longer duration of diabetes. This fact makes it especially important to discuss the problem with your doctor. In men with erectile dysfunction, the occurrence of heart attacks has been reduced with the use of statins.

Treating for ED

Fortunately for men with diabetes with erectile dysfunction, numerous approaches to treatment exist, beginning with drugs, continuing with external devices to create an erection, and ending with implantable devices that provide a very satisfactory erection. Treatment is successful in 90 percent or more of men, but only 5 percent ever discuss the problem with their doctors. The following sections discuss these treatment options.

Viagra and similar medications

Sildenafil (Viagra) has been specifically studied in males with diabetes and is successful in 70 percent of patients.

Sildenafil doesn't seem to affect diabetic control, but it isn't free of side effects. Some men experience headaches, facial flushing, or indigestion, which generally decline with continued use of the drug. It has also been found to cause a temporary color tinge to a man's vision as well as increased sensitivity to light and blurred vision. These side effects also decline with continued use of the drug.

Sildenafil is taken no more than once a day, about an hour before sexual activity. While the starting dose is 50 milligrams for men, when diabetes is present, 100 mg is often required. The drug itself doesn't cause erections; an erection occurs only as a result of some kind of sexual stimulation. But it does prevent an erection from subsiding, so it lasts longer. The effects of sildenafil begin in 30 to 60 minutes and can last for twelve hours after taking it.

Pfizer, which makes Viagra, could not expect to have the playing field to itself for very long, given that the game is something most men want to play. Bayer Pharmaceuticals and GlaxoSmithKline have now brought vardenafil (Levitra) to the marketplace. Its characteristics are very similar to Viagra but the starting dosage is 10 mg, which probably means 20 mg for men with diabetes. Vardenafil is also marketed as Staxyn.

The absorption of both sildenafil and vardenafil is decreased if taken with fatty foods, resulting in decreased effectiveness, which isn't true for the next two drugs.

Eli Lilly and ICOS Corporation market tadalafil (Cialis), which works like sildenafil and vardenafil but stays active for 36 hours. In addition, its onset of action is 15 minutes, half the time of the competing drugs. Cialis has been nicknamed the "weekender pill" because it permits spontaneous sexual activity from Friday to Sunday. The starting dose for Cialis is 10 mg, but, again, men with diabetes may need to start at twice that amount. Some patients take 2.5 to 5.0 mg daily so they're always ready to go. Tadalafil sometimes causes back and muscle pains.

In 2012, Vivus, Inc. introduced avanafil (Stendra), which has an onset of action of 15 to 30 minutes and stays active for up to six hours. The recommended dosage is 100 mg or up to 200 mg for diabetics.

Some men must not take any of these drugs. Men who have chest pain often take nitrate drugs, the most common of which is nitroglycerine. The combination of any of them and nitrates may cause a significant and possibly fatal drop in blood pressure. Great care must be taken if the patient is on one of the blood pressure drugs called *alpha blockers* for the same reason. Common alpha blockers are doxazosin (Cardura), prazosin (Minipress), and tamsulosin (Flomax).

A very small number of cases have been reported of one-sided hearing loss in men who took any of the above drugs.

Injection into the penis

The patient himself can use an injection to create an erection. It is called alprostadil (Caverject or Edex), a chemical that relaxes the blood vessels in the penis to allow more flow. Alprostadil does not require sexual stimulation in order to work.

The drug is injected about 30 minutes before intercourse and no more than once in 24 hours and three times per week. An injection gives a full erection lasting about an hour in 85 to 95 percent of men, except for those who have the most severe loss of blood flow to the penis.

Complications of injections are rare but include bruising, pain, and the formation of nodules at the injection site. A very rare complication is *priapism,* where the penis maintains its erection for many hours. If the erection lasts more than four hours, the patient must see his doctor to get an injection of a *vasoconstrictor,* a drug that squeezes down the arteries into the penis so that blood flow is interrupted.

Suppository in the penis

Alprostadil — the chemical that can be injected into the penis — also comes in a suppository form. The patient inserts a tube containing this small pill into the opening of the penis after urination. When the tube is fully in the opening, the man squeezes the top so that the pill exits the tube. This preparation, called Muse, comes in several different strengths so that patients can use a higher dose if the lower dose does not result in a satisfactory erection. It may safely be used twice in 24 hours. A few men experience pain with this procedure. Sexual stimulation is unnecessary to achieve an erection.

Vacuum-constriction devices

Vacuum-constriction tubes, which fit over the penis, create a closed space when pressed against the patient's body. A pump draws out the air in the tube, and blood rushes into the penis to replace the air. When the penis is erect, a rubber band is placed around the base of the penis to keep the blood inside it. Sometimes pain and numbness of the penis occur. Because a rubber band is constricting the penis, semen does not get through, so conception can't take place. The rubber band may be kept on for up to 30 minutes.

Implanted penile prostheses

If the patient doesn't like the idea of injecting himself in his penis or using a vacuum device, and if pills don't work for him, a *prosthesis* (an artificial substitute) can be implanted in the penis to give an erection. Prostheses come, in several varieties. A semi-rigid type produces a permanent erection, but some men do not like the inconvenience of a permanent erection. An inflatable prosthesis involves a pump in the scrotal sac that contains fluid. The pump can be squeezed to transfer the fluid into balloons in the penis to stiffen it. When not pumped up, the penis appears normally soft. In the past few years, the surgery to insert these prostheses has become very satisfactory.

Facing Female Sexual Problems

Sexual dysfunction in women is not as visually obvious as it is in men. But as many as half of women with diabetes have problems with sexual function, and the problems can be just as difficult to handle as they are for men. The following problems are associated with diabetes:

- ✔ Dry mouth and dry vagina because of the high blood glucose

- ✔ Irregular menstrual function when the diabetes is out of control

- ✔ Yeast infections of the vagina that make intercourse unpleasant

- ✔ A feeling of being fat and unattractive because type 2 diabetes is usually associated with obesity

- ✔ Discomfort about discussing the problem with a partner or physician

- ✔ Loss of bladder control due to a neurogenic bladder (see Chapter 5)

- ✔ A reduction in estrogen secretion and associated vaginal thinning and dryness due to increasing age made worse by the diabetes

Menopause can cause several of the same difficulties as diabetes-related sexual dysfunction, particularly the dry vagina and irregular menstrual function. You must rule out menopause before assuming that diabetes is the source of the problem.

A female with long-standing diabetes may have several other problems that are specific to her sexual organs. These problems include

- ✔ **Reduced lubrication because of parasympathetic nerve involvement:** Lubrication serves to permit easier entry of the penis, but it also increases the sensitivity of the vagina to touch, thus increasing pleasant sensations.

- ✔ **Reduced blood flow because of diabetic blood vessel disease:** Some of the lubrication comes from fluid within the blood vessels.

- ✔ **Loss of skin sensation around the vaginal area:** This loss reduces pleasure.

Most women who have problems with lubrication, whether due to diabetes or menopause, medicate themselves with over-the-counter preparations. These preparations fall into three categories:

- Water-based lubricants, like K-Y jelly and In Pursuit of Passion, which are probably the easiest to use and clean up

- Oil-based lubricants, like vegetable oils

- Petroleum-based lubricants, which are not recommended because of the possibility of bacterial infection

Estrogen, which can be taken by mouth or placed in the dry vagina in suppository form, also may be useful for menopausal women.

When psychological or interpersonal issues exist, a discussion with a therapist, the use of antidepressant medications (some of which can dry the vagina, by the way), and sex therapy with your partner are important steps to take to improve sexual pleasure.

Striving for a Healthy Pregnancy

About 0.4 percent of pregnancies occur in women with preexisting diabetes, called *pregestational diabetes,* and an additional 9.2 percent develop diabetes sometime in the second half of the pregnancy, called *gestational diabetes.* Four million births occur in the United States annually, and diabetes affects 360,000 or more pregnancies each year.

If you have diabetes and want to become pregnant, you need to talk with an expert in pregnancy and diabetes before you conceive. In the following sections, I explain potential complications you may experience and some steps you should take to ensure the healthiest pregnancy possible.

Realizing the body's reaction to pregnancy

During pregnancy, hormones block insulin action. In a nondiabetic pregnancy, the woman's body makes enough insulin to overcome this effect, and her blood glucose stays normal. But a woman with type 1 diabetes can't make more insulin, and during pregnancy she needs two or three times her usual dose to counteract the effect of her hormones (although in the early first trimester, her insulin needs may decrease). This increased need for insulin in a woman with type 1 diabetes usually begins in the second trimester and stabilizes in the last several weeks of the pregnancy; by the last one or two weeks, the mother-to-be may actually begin to have hypoglycemia. After the baby and the placenta are delivered, her insulin needs plummet immediately.

A woman with type 1 or type 2 diabetes may have some retinopathy (see Chapter 5) before she becomes pregnant. If the condition is severe, her eyes may deteriorate during the pregnancy. The deterioration probably results from rapid improvement of blood glucose control in a woman who has been poorly controlled previously. If glucose control is improved or if laser photocoagulation (see Chapter 5) is carried out before the pregnancy, this deterioration does not take place. After the baby is delivered, her eyes will return to their previous state.

To find out much more about pregnancy in the woman with type 1 diabetes, check out my book *Type 1 Diabetes For Dummies* (John Wiley & Sons, Inc.).

If you're thinking about becoming pregnant and you have diabetes-related eye disease, that condition must be stabilized before you try to conceive.

Kidney disease, or *nephropathy* (see Chapter 5), increases the danger of complications of pregnancy for both the mother and baby. Severe, permanent worsening of the nephropathy is unusual as a result of pregnancy, but a temporary decline in kidney function in the mother may occur. The baby may have to be delivered early and may suffer some growth retardation.

Being proactive before and during pregnancy

You can take a number of steps both before and during the pregnancy to ensure a healthy baby and an uncomplicated pregnancy.

Getting your health in order

You must take action in advance to avoid potential problems by controlling your glucose before conception. (See Part III for more on how to manage your diabetes.) In addition, you need to monitor your diet after you become pregnant.

Following are some other key steps you should take to improve your chances of a problem-free pregnancy:

- ✔ **Lose weight.** Obesity, which is prevalent in type 2 patients, puts a mom-to-be at greater risk for hypertension during pregnancy.

- ✔ **Quit smoking.** Children of mothers who smoke during pregnancy are at much greater risk of developing obesity and diabetes later in life, not to mention numerous other health problems.

✔ **Use insulin for glucose control.** If you have type 2 diabetes and are taking oral agents to lower your glucose, you need to switch to insulin to control your glucose during pregnancy.

✔ **Control your blood pressure.** Elevated blood pressure before and during early pregnancy is associated with increased risk of gestational diabetes mellitus.

✔ **Avoid animal protein.** Stay clear of it, specifically red meat, before and during the pregnancy and increase your intake of vegetable protein, specifically nuts to reduce the risk of gestational diabetes.

For more detailed information about what to do during pregnancy, see the section "Treating diabetes during pregnancy," later in the chapter.

Most diabetic pregnancies can be allowed to go to term at 39 weeks. However, if the mother-to-be has hypertension or a previous history of delivery problems, her doctor may advocate earlier delivery.

Taking special precautions if you've had bariatric surgery

Many more adolescents and young women are having bariatric surgery (see Chapter 9) to treat diabetes. They become pregnant at twice the rate of the general population after the surgery. These young women need to take the following precautions:

✔ Wait a year or two after surgery to conceive so that the growing fetus is not exposed to rapid weight loss in the mother.

✔ Be closely monitored for nutritional status and the fetus's growth (especially at the beginning of the pregnancy) if conception occurs earlier than a year or two after surgery.

✔ Consult with a nutritionist.

✔ If contraception is desired, use a method other than oral drugs because of malabsorption.

✔ Be tested for gestational diabetes. The surgery usually reduces the risk for high blood pressure, which makes any pregnancy more complicated, and the blood glucose often returns to normal. The usual tests can't be done in the patient with bariatric surgery because of the abnormal absorption. Monitoring the blood glucose at different times of day may be helpful (see Chapter 7).

Diagnosing gestational diabetes

The current consensus is to test all women for undiagnosed diabetes at the first prenatal visit and to screen all women for gestational diabetes because a small but significant number of patients with gestational diabetes will be missed if all women are not screened.

Everyone agrees that if your glucose tolerance is normal in weeks 27 to 31 of the pregnancy, you don't need to do more screening. If you experienced gestational diabetes during a previous pregnancy, the screening test is done much earlier — as early as the 13th week. Other reasons for earlier screening are

- ✔ Previous delivery of a large baby
- ✔ Obesity
- ✔ Glucose in the urine
- ✔ Close family members with diabetes

The screening test is done between weeks 24 and 28 of the pregnancy. No preparation is necessary. You consume 50 grams of glucose, and a blood glucose level is obtained from a vein one hour later. If the glucose level is less than 140, it's considered normal. If it's greater than 140, a further test is done before making a diagnosis of gestational diabetes, because many women who have a value greater than 140 do not necessarily have diabetes. The definitive test is a glucose tolerance test (see Chapter 2). A diagnosis of gestational diabetes is made if two or more of the samples exceed these levels:

- ✔ **Before consuming glucose:** 95 mg/dl (5.3 mmol/L)
- ✔ **One hour after consuming glucose:** 180mg/dl (10.0 mmol/L)
- ✔ **Two hours after:** 155 mg/dl (8.6 mmol/L)
- ✔ **Three hours after:** 140 mg/dl (7.8 mmol/L)

Recognizing risks to mother and baby

Whether you have diabetes before pregnancy or develop gestational diabetes, you face many considerations regarding your own health and the health of your baby.

Persistently high blood glucose left untreated has major consequences for both mother and fetus. If high glucose is present early in the pregnancy, the result may be miscarriage or *congenital malformations* (physical abnormalities that may be life threatening) in the fetus. In the third trimester, the growing fetus may exhibit *macrosomia* (abnormal largeness) that can lead to an early delivery or damage to the baby or mother during delivery. Neonatal hypoglycemia and stillbirth are also risks of high glucose.

Measuring the risks

The hemoglobin A1c (see Chapter 7) is an excellent measurement of overall glucose control and provides a good indicator for the risk of miscarriage. If a pregnant woman's hemoglobin A1c is high, it indicates that she was in poor glucose control at conception, and the likelihood of a miscarriage is greater. If overall glucose control is normal, the baby of the woman with diabetes is no more likely to be miscarried than that of a woman without diabetes.

The situation for congenital malformations is a little more complicated. The occurrence of these malformations rises with increasing glucose, but the level of *ketones* (the breakdown product of fats) also impacts their occurrence. However, measuring the ketones doesn't tell you if malformations will definitely occur.

Babies develop normally if their fathers have diabetes but their mothers don't. The environment in which the fetus is developing is responsible for the potential abnormalities. Elevated blood glucose, abnormalities of proteins and fats that result from the elevated glucose, and the loss of sensitivity to insulin explain the problems.

Early pregnancy problems

Miscarriages and congenital malformations can result from poor glucose control at conception and shortly thereafter. Both high blood glucose and low blood glucose can induce malformations. (For more on managing diabetes, see Part III.)

However, a woman in poor control of her diabetes has more trouble conceiving a baby than a woman with good glucose control, which may be the major reason that more babies aren't born with congenital malformations.

 Unlike diabetes that occurs before pregnancy, gestational diabetes mellitus does not cause congenital malformations. In gestational diabetes, blood glucose doesn't start to rise until halfway through the pregnancy, long after the baby's important body structures are formed.

Late pregnancy problems

A baby is considered large if it weighs more than 4 kilograms or 8.8 pounds at birth. Keep in mind that most large babies are the healthy offspring of mothers without diabetes. Their growth is proportional throughout the pregnancy, so their shoulders aren't out of proportion to their heads and delivery isn't complicated.

Why macrosomia occurs

Macrosomia, or abnormal largeness in a fetus, has to do with the elevated glucose, fat, and amino acid levels in the second half of pregnancy for a mother with diabetes. If these levels aren't lowered, the fetus is exposed to high levels. The high levels, especially of glucose, stimulate the fetal pancreas to begin to make insulin earlier and to store these extra nutrients. The fetus becomes large wherever fat is stored, such as in the shoulders, chest, abdomen, arms, and legs. Because they are large, macrosomic babies are delivered early in order to make the delivery easier and avoid birth trauma. However, though they are large, they are not fully mature.

However, women with pregestational diabetes or gestational diabetes need to be concerned about having a baby whose largeness is not proportional. The areas that are most responsive to insulin, where fat is stored in the baby, are the ones that enlarge the most. (See the sidebar "Why macrosomia occurs" for more information.)

Treating diabetes during pregnancy

You need to achieve a stricter level of glucose control during pregnancy than when you aren't pregnant. Your fetus is removing glucose from you at a rapid rate, so your blood glucose level is lower than usual. In addition, your body turns to fat for fuel much sooner, so you produce ketones earlier. Too many ketones can damage the fetus as well. The fact that you break down fat so early is termed *accelerated starvation.*

Monitoring your glucose and ketones

In order to maintain your blood glucose at the proper level, you must measure it more frequently. You should measure it before meals, at bedtime, and occasionally one hour after eating. Your goal is to achieve the following levels of blood glucose:

- ✔ **Fasting and premeal:** Less than 90 mg/dl (5 mmol/L)
- ✔ **One hour after eating:** Less than 140 mg/dl (7.7 mmol/L)
- ✔ **Two hours after eating:** Less than 120 mg/dl (6.7 mmol/L)

Recent studies have shown that the glucose level one hour after eating may be the most important for pregnant women with diabetes to keep under control.

You also need to check for ketones in the urine before breakfast and before supper. You can do so by placing a test strip in the stream of urine. The strip indicates whether ketones are present. If the test strip is positive, it means that you are not eating enough carbohydrates and your body is going into accelerated starvation. Too much of this condition is not good for the growing fetus.

Eating well

Your appropriate amount of weight gain depends on your weight and body mass index at the time you become pregnant. (See Chapter 3 if you're not sure how to calculate your BMI). If your BMI is normal, you should gain 20 to 25 pounds during the pregnancy. However, if you're overweight, you need to gain less weight through the pregnancy, 15 to 20 pounds. If you're obese, you should gain no more than 17 or 18 pounds. And if you're underweight, you should gain 25 to 30 pounds.

Chapter 8 tells you what you need to know about diet and diabetes, but as a pregnant woman with diabetes, you have some special requirements:

- ✔ **Your daily food intake should be 35 to 38 kilocalories per kilogram of ideal body weight.** (In this book, I use the term *kilocalories* rather than *calories,* which is typically used incorrectly.) You can use your height to determine your ideal body weight (IBW). As a woman, you should weigh 100 pounds if you are 5 feet tall, plus 5 pounds for every inch over 5 feet. For example, a 5-foot 4-inch woman should weigh 120 pounds, ideally (and *approximately,* because these numbers represent a range, not a single weight). You can change that figure to kilograms by dividing the pounds by 2.2. Then multiply that number by 35 to get the low end of the daily calorie intake and by 38 to get the high end. So if you weigh 120 pounds, you weigh 54.6 kilograms and your daily food intake should be between 1,900 and 2,100 kilocalories.

- ✔ **Your protein intake should be about 20 percent of your daily kilo-calories, or 1.5 to 2 grams per kilogram of IBW.** A woman with the IBW of 54.6 should eat about 100 grams of protein daily. Because each gram of protein contains four kilocalories, protein takes up about 400 of the 2,000 daily kilocalories.

- ✔ **Your carbohydrate intake should be 50 to 55 percent of your daily kilocalories.** If you need approximately 2,000 daily kilocalories, about 1,000 kilocalories should be carbohydrate. Because each gram of carbohydrate has 4 kilocalories, just like protein, this amounts to 250 grams of carbohydrate.

- ✔ **Your fat intake should be less than 30 percent of the total daily kilocalories.** Using 2,000 kilocalories as our target, that amounts to 630 kilocalories of fat. Because fat contains 9 kilocalories per gram, this equals 70 grams of fat a day.

Translating grams of food into amounts of specific foods would require another whole book. Because an excellent one on the subject has already been written, I refer you to the latest edition of *Nutrition For Dummies,* by Carol Ann Rinzler (John Wiley & Sons, Inc.) to get this information.

✔ **You need to eat three meals a day plus a bedtime snack.** Frequently eating helps prevent the accelerated starvation that results from the prolonged fast between supper and breakfast.

✔ **You must maintain fasting and premeal glucose levels below 90 mg/dl.** Your glucose should be less than 140 mg/dl one hour after meals.

Ask your doctor to send you to a dietician to develop a meal plan.

In addition, you can use a good multivitamin and mineral preparation. A moderate amount of exercise is also very helpful in controlling the blood glucose and keeping you in top shape during pregnancy.

Testing for fetal defects

A blood test called a *serum alpha-fetoprotein* can be done 15 weeks into the pregnancy to determine whether the fetus has neural tube defects (openings in the brain or spinal cord more common when conception occurs in a poorly controlled diabetic). At 18 weeks, an ultrasound can show any malformations of the growing fetus. An ultrasound, by directing a sound at the fetus and catching it as it bounces back to the machine, produces a picture of the fetus that shows the presence of any abnormalities. This harmless test is not painful for the mother or the fetus.

Another useful study during the diabetic pregnancy is the nonstress test. A device is placed on your abdomen that listens to the fetus's heartbeat. When the fetus moves, its heart rate normally speeds up by 15 to 20 beats per minute. This increase in heart rate should normally occur at least three times in a 20-minute period of listening.

Handling issues of gestational diabetes

If you have gestational diabetes, you don't need to worry about congenital malformations in your baby, but you need to avoid macrosomia. You need to follow the same dietary prescription as the woman with pregestational diabetes, and you need to use insulin if a careful diet does not keep your fasting blood glucose below 90, your glucose one hour after eating below 140, or your glucose two hours after eating below 120. If you can't bring yourself to use insulin shots, glyburide (see Chapter 11) has been shown to be safe for the baby because it does not pass through the placenta, although it is not approved by the FDA for this use. Your insulin regimen will probably be simpler than that of women with pregestational diabetes because your pancreas can make its own insulin. If you are taking insulin, you will stop doing so at the time of delivery.

Early ultrasound is not necessary for women with gestational diabetes unless the doctor suspects that diabetes was actually present much earlier. An ultrasound at week 38 can show whether fetal macrosomia exists. If macrosomia is present, your doctor will probably perform a cesarean section, removing the baby through·an incision made in the abdominal wall and then in the uterus.

Delivering the baby

Delivering a baby at the end of 39 weeks is best because full-term pregnancy gives the baby time to mature completely. The same is true if the mother has diabetes. If the mother doesn't go into labor spontaneously, the physician usually induces labor. The uterine contractions of pregnant women with diabetes aren't as strong as those of pregnant women without diabetes. This difference may explain the increase in rates of C-sections for these women.

If you have been taking insulin during pregnancy, nurses will monitor your blood glucose every four hours after you deliver. Your blood glucose will be maintained at 70 to 120 mg/dl with insulin, if necessary. The insulin is given in short-acting form as needed and not in large doses of long-acting insulin, which would be around in the circulation when you no longer need it.

Maintaining your health after pregnancy

If you are breastfeeding, which is always a good idea, you need to consume about 300 kilocalories *above* your usual needs. You cannot take oral agents for diabetes because they pass through the milk into the baby. For more information about breastfeeding, see *Breastfeeding For Dummies,* by Sharon Perkins and Carol Vannais (John Wiley & Sons, Inc.).

Gestational diabetes usually disappears when the pregnancy is over. However, a woman who develops gestational diabetes during pregnancy is at a much higher risk for developing diabetes later in life. If your fasting blood glucose is greater than 130 during pregnancy, the risk of developing diabetes again is as much as 75 to 90 percent in the next 10 to 15 years. Even modestly elevated blood glucose levels during a pregnancy that do not rise to the criteria for gestational diabetes are associated with a higher risk for future type 2 diabetes. You are also at much higher risk of heart disease, mainly due to the development of diabetes.

Women who don't breastfeed have a 50 percent increased risk of type 2 diabetes compared to women who never give birth. Women with gestational diabetes who breastfeed lower their risk of later diabetes.

If you had gestational diabetes, you need to have a test for glucose tolerance between 6 and 12 weeks after the pregnancy and annually after that if diabetes is not found.

Several factors predispose women with gestational diabetes to develop diabetes later on. Following are some factors that can't be changed:

- ✔ **Ethnic origin:** Certain ethnic groups, such as Mexican Americans, Native Americans, Asian Americans, and African Americans, are at a higher risk.

- ✔ **Prepregnancy weight:** Women with a higher prepregnancy weight are at a higher risk.

- ✔ **Number of pregnancies:** The more pregnancies you have, the higher your risk.

- ✔ **Family history of diabetes:** If a family history is present, you are at a higher risk.

- ✔ **Severity of blood glucose during pregnancy:** Higher blood glucose levels mean a higher risk.

On the other hand, you can reduce several risk factors:

- ✔ **Future weight gain:** Gain less weight in future pregnancies.

- ✔ **Future pregnancies:** Have fewer children.

- ✔ **Physical activity:** Increase your exercise.

- ✔ **Dietary fat:** Limit the fat in your diet.

- ✔ **Smoking and certain drugs:** Stop smoking and using drugs.

Using the drug metformin (see Chapter 11) can also help prevent future diabetes.

Women who have had gestational diabetes can use oral contraceptives with low levels of estrogen and progesterone to prevent conception. These drugs, along with hormonal replacement therapy after menopause, do not increase your risk of later diabetes. They may, in fact, decrease the risk and decrease blood glucose levels in those who have diabetes already. Women with type 1 and type 2 diabetes can use the same preparations.

Focusing on your baby's health

Increased understanding of diabetes's impact during pregnancy has resulted in a great reduction in malformations in these babies as well as the macrosomia that leads to complications at delivery. Unfortunately, many women with diabetes do not have tight glucose control at conception, so some malformations still occur. If an obvious malformation is present at birth, it is important to search for other malformations.

Also, keep in mind that the fetus was producing a lot of insulin to handle all the maternal glucose entering through the placenta. Suddenly, maternal glucose is cut off at delivery, but the high level of fetal insulin continues for a while. The danger of hypoglycemia exists in the first four to six hours after delivery. The baby may be sweaty and appear nervous or even have a seizure. It is necessary to do blood glucose tests on the baby hourly until he or she is stable and to continue testing at intervals for the first 24 hours.

Besides hypoglycemia, the baby may have several other complications right after birth:

- ✔ **Respiratory distress syndrome:** This breathing problem occurs when the baby is delivered early, but it responds to treatment. This condition is rare with good prenatal care.

- ✔ **Low calcium, with jitteriness and possible seizures:** Calcium needs to be given to the baby until its own body can take over. This condition is usually a result of prematurity.

- ✔ **Low magnesium:** This complication presents itself like low calcium and is also a result of prematurity.

- ✔ **Polycythemia:** This condition, where too many red blood cells exist, occurs for unknown reasons. Treatment requires removing blood from the baby. The amount is determined by how much extra blood is present.

- ✔ **Hyperbilirubinemia:** This condition is the product of too much breakdown of red blood cells. It is treated with light.

- ✔ **Lazy left colon:** Occurring for unknown reasons, this condition presents itself like an obstruction of the bowel but clears up on its own.

If the baby was exposed to high glucose and ketones during the pregnancy, it may show diminished intelligence. This effect is not obvious at birth but is discovered later when the baby is expected to learn something.

Large babies of poorly controlled mothers with diabetes usually lose their fat by age 1. Starting at ages 6 to 8, however, these children have a greater tendency to be obese. Controlling the blood glucose in the mother may prevent later obesity and even diabetes in her offspring.

Dealing with Polycystic Ovarian Syndrome

Polycystic ovarian syndrome (PCOS) is responsible for abnormal menstrual function in 5 to 8 percent or more of women during their reproductive years. It tends to run in families. Women with this condition often have trouble conceiving a child, and they have increased hair on their faces, arms, legs, and areas of the body that are not usually hairy in women. In addition, they often experience acne and obesity. They also have more abnormal blood fats associated with coronary artery disease.

The surprise finding in PCOS is that these women are also resistant to insulin and have increased blood levels of insulin. The greater the degree of obesity, however, the more likely the metabolic syndrome (see Chapter 5). In fact, women with PCOS who do get pregnant have a prevalence of gestational diabetes that is two to three times that of those women without PCOS. They also have higher rates of other complications of pregnancy including high blood pressure, preeclampsia, preterm delivery, and small babies.

Women with PCOS who are normal in weight do not have insulin resistance or a greater tendency to develop type 2 diabetes.

Brothers of women with PCOS who have insulin resistance also have insulin resistance, suggesting that a strong component of inheritance is present.

Another feature that women with PCOS have in common with metabolic syndrome is obstructive sleep apnea. This sleep apnea results in daytime sleepiness and high blood pressure. PCOS patients with obstructive sleep apnea tend to have insulin resistance and type 2 diabetes more often than those without.

The name of the syndrome derives from the fact that early cases of PCOS were associated with multiple ovarian cysts. More recently, the presence of ovarian cysts has not been a prominent feature of the condition, but the name has stuck.

Women with PCOS have increased levels of male-associated hormones called *androgens*. Studies have shown that androgens cause decreased insulin sensitivity when they are given to women who don't have PCOS.

The major health risks for someone with PCOS, besides infertility, are the occurrence of impaired glucose tolerance and type 2 diabetes, as well as gestational diabetes. In addition, just like patients with metabolic syndrome (see Chapter 5), these women are at greater risk for high blood pressure, abnormal blood fats, and cardiovascular disease. A group of women who had PCOS and were followed for 18 years were found to have twice the risk of diabetes compared to those without PCOS.

The most effective treatment for PCOS is lifestyle change. Weight loss and exercise often reverse the condition and prevent the development of diabetes. In very obese women with PCOS, weight-loss surgery can reverse PCOS. Oral contraceptives have been used in the past when more treatment is needed, but they don't restore fertility, which is often the main purpose of treatment. They can still be used to control the other symptoms, such as acne, irregular menses, and increased hair. Insulin sensitizing drugs, including metformin, have been very effective for treating all features of the syndrome. In a study reported in *The Journal of Clinical Endocrinology and Metabolism* in April 2005, six months of metformin was much more effective than a drug called clomiphene, a well-known inducer of ovulation, in restoring fertility. Later studies have not confirmed this.

More recently (2011), simvastatin, a cholesterol-lowering drug, has been found to be more effective than metformin in reversing PCOS and preventing complications.

Other than oral contraceptives, any treatment that is successful for reducing the acne, hairiness, and decreased insulin sensitivity in PCOS also makes the woman much more likely to get pregnant. If she doesn't want to become pregnant, she and her partner need to take the necessary precautions. For more information on polycystic ovarian syndrome, check out *PCOS For Dummies,* by Gaynor Bussell and Sharon Perkins (John Wiley & Sons, Inc.).

Part III
Managing Diabetes: The "Thriving with Diabetes" Lifestyle Plan

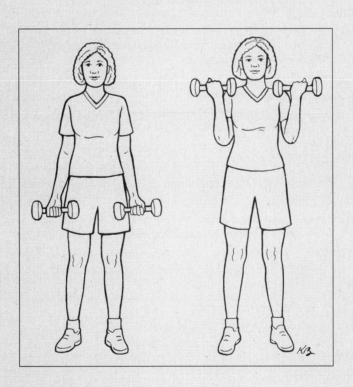

 Head to www.dummies.com/extras/diabetes for more about the effect of type 2 diabetes in parents on type 2 diabetes in their children. The interesting connection shows the importance of regarding diabetes as a family disease.

In this part . . .

✔ Get all the right tests and test your own glucose so you can discover how your food, your exercise, and your medications affect your blood glucose.

✔ Discover that you can eat food that helps to control diabetes without giving up great taste.

✔ Consider curing your diabetes with surgery, a powerful new tool that could save you years of medical treatments and a lot of money.

✔ Realize that exercise, even without weight loss, can prevent turning prediabetes into diabetes and help to control diabetes if it develops.

✔ Take the right medications at the right times and in the right amounts to maximize their ability to lower your blood glucose.

✔ Create a diabetes team made up of experts as well as family members, all of whom are dedicated to your good health.

Chapter 7

Self-Testing for Glucose and Other Key Tests

*Y*ou may wonder what you have to do to prevent the complications of diabetes that I describe in Chapters 4 through 6, and the answer is a fair amount, which I discuss in this chapter. But when you weigh the benefits that add up to a longer, better-quality life against the loss of time and money from preventive care, the benefits of preventive care win by a landslide.

With preventive care, you can take advantage of an explosion of new tests and treatments that have only been available for the last 35 years, beginning with self-testing of blood glucose in 1980 right up to new tests for overall diabetic control and multiple new hardware and software tools made possible by the latest advances in computer and Internet technology.

As Woody Allen points out, "I don't want to achieve immortality through my work; I want to achieve it through not dying." On the other hand, he says, "On the plus side, death is one of the few things that can be done just as easily lying down." Well, I don't want you to take your diabetes lying down. I want to give you the benefit of every important advance. You may not achieve immortality, but you can enjoy every day that you live.

This chapter gives you all the tools you need to detect complications in their earliest stages. And if, by chance, you are reading this section for the first time and complications have already developed, this chapter also shows you how to measure the progression or, hopefully, regression of your complications.

Testing, Testing: Tests You Need to Stay Healthy

A number of tests and measurements should be done on a regular basis. To best make sure that you get your tests done regularly, you can use the chart in Figure 7-1. This form lists the tests and you can list the results underneath. Simply copy the one in this figure and keep it up-to-date. Don't expect your doctor to keep this chart updated for you. He has too much on his mind and too many patients to get it exactly right for each one.

Date	Hemoglobin A1c	Eye Exam	Filament	TSH	Ualb	Chol	LDL	HDL	TG

Figure 7-1: A sample testing chart that you can copy to track your testing results.

© John Wiley & Sons, Inc.

Certain procedures, explained in this chapter, should be done by your doctor (and you, if feasible) according to the following schedule:

✔ **Blood glucose:** At each visit, evaluate the blood glucose measurements you've been taking. (See the section "Monitoring Blood Glucose: It's a Must," later in this chapter.)

✔ **Hemoglobin A1c:** Obtain hemoglobin A1c four times a year if you take insulin and twice a year if you don't. (See the section "Tracking Your Glucose over Time: Hemoglobin A1c," later in this chapter.)

✔ **Eye exam:** Have a dilated eye examination by an ophthalmologist or optometrist once a year or every two years if no disease is present. (See the section "Checking for Eye Problems," later in this chapter.)

✔ **Filament:** Examine your bare feet at each visit and have your doctor perform a filament test. (See the section "Examining Your Feet," later in this chapter.)

In addition to looking at the feet, you should also have an ankle-brachial index performed at least every five years.

✔ **TSH:** Your doctor should check your thyroid-stimulating hormone level when your diabetes is diagnosed and every five years thereafter if it is normal.

✔ **Ualb:** Check for microalbuminuria once a year. (See the section "Testing for Kidney Damage: Moderately Increased Albumin (MIA)," later in this chapter.)

✔ **Chol/LDL/HDL/TG:** Obtain a lipid panel once a year to monitor your total cholesterol, LDL (bad cholesterol), HDL (good cholesterol), and triglycerides. (See the section "Tracking Cholesterol and Other Fats," later in this chapter.)

In addition to the preceding tests, you should also have your doctor take your blood pressure and measure your weight at each visit. (See the sections "Measuring Blood Pressure" and "Checking Your Weight and BMI," later in this chapter.)

These tests are the *minimum* standards for proper care of diabetes. If an abnormality is found, the frequency of testing increases to check on the response to treatment.

Are doctors and patients with diabetes doing the best job of managing diabetes? Government statistics on Preventive Care Practices from the Centers for Disease Control and Prevention (CDC) suggest that they aren't. Doctors and patients are getting a little better as diabetes becomes a major health problem in the United States. The latest statistics compare the annual rates of testing for various abnormalities associated with diabetes between 1994 and 2010. They indicate some improvement, but as a whole they should be doing a lot better. Only about 60 percent of diabetic patients are doing frequent testing of blood glucose, A1C tests at least twice a year, annual eye exams, and annual foot exams.

As diabetes knowledge has grown, the guidelines for how high various tests should be in people with diabetes have changed. Unfortunately, they seem to have no effect on the results of clinical practice:

- ✔ The Joint National Committee on Prevention, Detection, Evaluation and Treatment of High Blood Pressure lowered its guidelines for blood pressure in people with diabetes in 1997 and again in 2003, but as of 2008 there was no better control, according to the CDC.

- ✔ The American Diabetes Association lowered its goal for LDL cholesterol (see later in this chapter) to less than 100 mg/dl in 1998. As late as 2010, there was no indication that patients were meeting the new goal more often than they had in 1994.

Much can be done. And that's what this chapter is all about.

Monitoring Blood Glucose: It's a Must

Insulin was extracted and used for the first time more than 90 years ago. Since that time, nothing has improved the life of the person with diabetes as much as the ability to measure his or her own blood glucose with a drop of blood.

Prior to blood glucose self-monitoring, testing the urine for glucose was the only way to determine whether your blood glucose was high, but urine testing could not tell at all whether the glucose was low. The urine test for glucose is worthless for controlling blood glucose — it actually provides misinformation. All the thousands of research papers in the medical literature before 1980, which used urine testing for glucose, are of no value and should be burned. (However, testing urine for other things, such as ketones and protein, can be of value.)

Basically, two kinds of test strips are used today. Both require that glucose in a drop of your blood reacts with an enzyme. In one strip, the reaction produces a color. A meter then reads the amount of color to give a glucose reading. In the other strip, the reaction produces electrons, and a meter converts the amount of electrons into a glucose reading.

One of the first things that was learned when frequent testing of blood glucose became feasible is that a person with diabetes, even a person who works hard to control his glucose, can experience tremendous variation in glucose levels in a relatively short time, as little as 30 minutes. This variation is especially true in association with food, but it can occur even in the fasting state before breakfast. For this reason, multiple tests are needed.

How often should you test?

How often you test is determined by the kind of diabetes you have, the kind of treatment you're using, and the level of stability of your blood glucose.

> ✔ **If you have type 1 or type 2 diabetes and you're taking before-meal insulin, you need to test before each meal and at bedtime.** The reason for this frequent testing is that you're constantly using this information to make adjustments in your insulin dose. No matter how good you think your control is, you cannot feel the level of the blood glucose without testing unless you're hypoglycemic. In fact, on numerous occasions I have had my patients try to guess their level before I test it. They are close less than 50 percent of the time. That degree of accuracy is not sufficient for good glucose control.
>
> People with type 1 diabetes should occasionally test one or two hours after a meal and in the middle of the night to see just how high their glucose goes after eating and whether it drops too low in the middle of the night. These results guide you and your physician to make the changes you need.
>
> Numerous studies have shown that increased daily frequency of blood glucose testing is significantly associated with lower levels of hemoglobin A1c and fewer complications of diabetes in patients who take insulin. There is a 0.2 percent lowering of A1c for each extra test up to a maximum of five tests.
>
> ✔ **If you have type 2 diabetes and you're on pills or just diet and exercise, testing doesn't seem to make a major difference in your glucose control.** In a large study, regular testing resulted in just a .25 percent reduction in hemoglobin A1c and even this improvement was gone by 12 months. The main reason is that patients don't use the test results to make changes in treatment.
>
> ✔ **If you're pregnant, see the testing guidelines I outline in Chapter 6.** I would guess that you're probably willing to test numerous times in a day to keep your developing fetus as healthy as possible.

The blood glucose test can be useful many other times of day in the patient on insulin:

> ✔ If you eat something off your diet and want to test its effect on your glucose, do a test.
>
> ✔ If you're about to exercise, a blood glucose test can tell you if you need to eat before starting the exercise or if you can use the exercise to bring your glucose down.

✔ If your diabetes is temporarily unstable and you're about to drive, you may want to test before getting into the car to make sure that you're not on the verge of hypoglycemia. Even if your diabetes is stable, testing at the beginning and after every couple of hours of a long drive can prevent serious hypoglycemia.

You're not being graded on your glucose test results. The human body has too much variation in it to expect that each time you take the same medication, do the same exercise, eat the same way, and feel the same emotionally, you will get the same test result. If the person who reviews your results with you sees your abnormal results as bad, he or she does not understand this point. You may want to consider finding someone who does.

Keep in mind that the occasional blood glucose test done in your doctor's office is of little or no value in understanding the big picture of your glucose control. It is like trying to visualize an entire painting by Seurat (who painted using dots of color) by looking at one dot on the canvas.

How do you use a lancet?

To get the drop of blood you need to perform a glucose test, you have to use a spring-loaded device that contains a sharp lancet. You push the button of the device, and the lancet springs out and pokes your finger. Devices that allow different depths of penetration are useful for small children.

One product that seems less painful than the others is the Accu-Chek Softclix Lancet Device. It allows you to select one of 11 depth settings so that you can penetrate your finger no deeper than necessary. Many glucose meters allow testing at other sites besides your finger, which require different depths of penetration to reach blood, so these settings can be very useful. However, the Softclix uses its own type of lancet that is a little more expensive than others on the market.

Accu-Chek also offers the Multiclix device, which holds a drum of six pre-loaded lancets. Its great advantage is that there is no handling of lancets. In most devices, you have to push the lancet into the device and pull it out to discard it. In this one, as you use one lancet it re-enters the drum and the next clean lancet drops into place. When you have used all six, you throw away the drum and put a new one in the device. It too offers 11 penetration depths. The downside is that each lancet can be used only once.

Becton Dickinson (BD) makes another lancet, called BDGenie Lancet, that works like a lancet and lancing device all in one. It is less painful and a little less expensive than other devices on the market. Becton Dickinson also makes the thinnest lancets currently available, called the BD Ultra-Fine 33 Lancets.

Although you do not have to use alcohol on your fingers, they should be reasonably clean. (My patients have done millions of finger sticks, and I've never known one of them to have an infection result.) Use the side of your finger to avoid the more sensitive tips that you don't want to hurt, especially if you use a keyboard frequently. Change fingers often so that no finger becomes very sensitive.

Remember never to use a used lancet on someone else. Each lancet lasts for a few pokes and should then be discarded in a special sharps container so it can't poke someone else accidentally. Sharps containers are available in drugstores, or you can use an empty plastic laundry detergent bottle. Check with your refuse service to make sure it is okay to leave the sealed bottle in the garbage.

Make sure you wash and dry your hands if you peel fruit just before testing yourself. Glucose in the peel can significantly modify the result.

How do you perform the test?

If you don't already own a blood glucose meter, be sure to check out the next section. All meters require a drop of blood, usually from the finger. (See the previous section, "How do you use a lancet?") You place the blood on a specific part of a test strip and allow enough time, usually between five seconds and one minute, for a reaction to occur. Some strips allow you to add more blood within 30 seconds if the quantity is insufficient. The need for a second stick of your finger is rare if you use a test strip that requires less blood. In less than a minute, the meter reads the product of that reaction, which is determined by the amount of glucose in the blood sample.

Keep the following tips in mind when you're testing your glucose:

- **If you have trouble getting blood, you can wrap a rubber band around the point where your finger joins your hand.** You will be amazed at the flow of blood. Take off the rubber band before a major hemorrhage occurs (just joking).

- **Testing blood from sites other than your fingers is generally reliable, except for an hour after eating, immediately after exercise, or if your blood glucose is low.** These other sites don't reflect the rapid changes in blood glucose that are occurring.

- **Some meters use whole blood, and some use the liquid part of the blood, called the *plasma*.** A lab glucose tests the plasma. The whole blood value is about 12 percent less than the plasma value, so you need to know which you're measuring. The various recommendations for appropriate levels of glucose are plasma values unless specifically stated otherwise. Most of the newer meters are calibrated to give a plasma reading, but check yours to be sure.

✔ **Studies have shown that the quality of test strips, which are loose in a vial, deteriorate rapidly if the vial is left open.** Be sure to cap the vial. Two hours of exposure to air may ruin the strips. Strips that are individually foil-wrapped do not have this problem.

✔ **Check the expiration date of the strips.** Expired strips won't give correct results.

✔ **Don't let other people use your meter.** Their test results will be mixed in with your tests when they are downloaded into a computer. In addition, a meter invariably gets a little blood on it and can be a source of infection.

Choosing a Blood Glucose Meter

The meter business must be a profitable one because many new meters are on the market each time I update this book. But the cost of the meter should play little part in your decision about which one to get. Most manufacturers are happy to practically give you the meter so that you're forced to buy their test strips. Each manufacturer makes a different test strip, and they're not interchangeable in other machines. Some companies even make a different strip for each different machine that they make.

Because the meters are so cheap and the science is changing so rapidly, you should get a new meter every year or two to make sure that you have state-of-the-art equipment. The cost of test strips is generally about the same from meter to meter, so the cost of strips does not have to play a big role in your meter decision, either.

The accuracy of the various machines also isn't a consideration. All are accurate to a degree acceptable for managing your diabetes. Keep in mind, though, that they do not have the accuracy of a laboratory. Meters are probably about plus or minus 10 percent compared to the lab.

Factors that may influence your purchase

Your doctor may have a meter that he or she prefers to work with because a computer program can download the test results from the meter and display them in a certain way. This analysis can be enormously helpful in deciding how to alter your therapy for the best control of your glucose.

Any meter you buy should have a memory that records the time and date so you can read that information along with the glucose result. The memory should hold at least 100 glucose values if you test four times a day, giving you 25 days' worth of readings.

Don't buy a meter without the capability to download the results to a data-management system in a computer. Bring your meter with you to your appointments so that your doctor or an assistant can download your glucose test results and evaluate them with the aid of a data-management system. Evaluating pages of glucose readings in a log book is virtually impossible.

Your insurance company also may mandate a certain meter, in which case you may have no choice.

Ask yourself the following questions when choosing a meter:

- ✔ If a small child is to use it, can the child easily use the meter and strips?
- ✔ Are the batteries common ones, or are they hard to get and expensive?
- ✔ Does the meter have a memory that I and my doctor can check?
- ✔ Is the meter downloadable to a computer program that can manipulate the data?
- ✔ Do I have to calibrate the meter every time I change to a new box of strips (an inconvenient step)?

Profiles of different meters

More than a dozen companies vie for your meter purchase. Among them, they produce more than 50 machines. Like everything in business, mergers and acquisitions have occurred and will continue to happen so that the field narrows. In the following sections, I give an overview of a number of the most common options.

In addition to these options, many other manufacturers make glucose meters including Arkay, Bionime, Fifty50 Medical, Fora Care, Infopia, Oak Tree Health, Omnis Health, U.S. Diagnostics, Walmart, and others. These companies' meters have no particular advantages not present in the meters that I describe here.

Abbott Laboratories

Abbott Laboratories purchased the MediSense Company, which first made and sold blood glucose meters. This company, which has one of the longest warranties on its meters (four years), is speedy about taking care of problems that arise. The batteries are good for 4,000 tests. They can generally be replaced by you unless otherwise noted. One clue that Abbott is really interested in customer service is that you can find the owner's guides for all their meters on the Internet.

- ✔ **FreeStyle Freedom Lite:** The FreeStyle Freedom Lite requires a tiny sample of blood, and you can add more up to a minute from the first application if you don't have enough on the strip. The Freedom Lite works with a data-management program called CoPilot Health Management System. It holds up to 400 tests, eliminating the oldest as new ones are added beyond 400, just like all the other meters described in this section. You can see a 7-, 14-, and 30-day average on the screen. No calibration is required. The meter has four programmable alarms to remind you to test. It uses CR2032 coin cell batteries available at drugstores and grocery stores. You can test away from your finger with this meter.

- ✔ **FreeStyle InsuLinx:** This meter has a touch screen that allows you to record your insulin dose. It holds 500 tests. It uses the CR2032 coin batteries and is associated with a data management program.

- ✔ **FreeStyle Lite:** This meter is identical to the Freedom Lite but is smaller, with a smaller screen and smaller buttons.

- ✔ **Precision Xtra:** This meter allows measurement of blood ketones as well as glucose. It uses its own test strips that require calibration of the meter with each new vial. The vial contains a calibration strip that is inserted into the meter before using the test strips in that vial. If you want to do a blood ketone test, you use the calibration strip that comes in that vial before inserting the ketone strip. The meter remembers the last 450 tests that you do and you can view 7-, 14-, and 30-day averages on the screen. It uses its own test strips. It has its own data-management system called Precision Xtra Advanced Diabetes Management System.

AgaMatrix

AgaMatrix was the first company to manufacture a meter that attaches to the iPhone and uses the iPhone screen to provide information. AgaMatrix also manufactures three other meters that use a CR2032 lithium coin-cell battery. They also use the Zero-Click software for data management. And they all need only a 5-microliter drop of blood.

✔ **Wave Sense Jazz:** The Jazz requires no calibration. It can remember 1,865 tests. It has seven user-settable alarms.

✔ **Wave Sense KeyNote:** The KeyNote is one of the smallest meters on the market. It remembers 300 tests. It can provide 14-, 30-, and 90-day averages on the screen. It has six alarms you can set, and it alerts you if the glucose is too low or too high. You have to calibrate the KeyNote.

✔ **Wave Sense Presto:** The Presto also remembers 300 tests and provides the same averages as the KeyNote. It also has the same alarms. You don't have to calibrate this meter.

✔ **IBGStar:** With Sanofi-Aventis, AgroMatrix developed IBGStar, the tiny meter that attaches to your iPhone, turning its screen into a meter screen. It is available for sale in Europe, and it has been approved by the FDA in the U.S. but is not yet available for sale there.

Bayer HealthCare LLC

Bayer HealthCare LLC sells five meters in the United States. The meters are accurate and carry the longest warranty in the industry (five years). You can replace the batteries at home. The meters are descendants of some of the first meters available. They allow testing away from your fingers, and no coding of the meters is required. One of them, the Contour USB, is particularly interesting.

✔ **Breeze 2:** The Breeze 2 uses a ten-test cartridge that calibrates the meter. It remembers 420 tests. It can provide 1-, 7-, 14-, and 30-day averages. The meter uses WinGlucofacts software for data management.

✔ **Contour Next:** This meter uses individual test strips that require no coding. It remembers up to 800 tests that can be downloaded and viewed with the same data-management system as the Breeze 2. It can provide a 7-, 14-, and 30-day average on the screen. It uses 3-volt lithium batteries. Contour meters use individual Contour test strips.

✔ **Contour Next USB:** The Contour Next USB is a small meter that plugs directly into the USB port of your computer and opens the Glucofacts Deluxe software, which analyzes your tests and shows you patterns, allowing you to make changes for better control, while charging your battery at the same time. The meter remembers 2,000 tests.

✔ **Didget:** Didget is a meter that plugs into the Nintendo DS and DS Lite gaming systems, rewarding your child for frequent testing, although it can be used alone. Kids who test get reward points that unlock new levels of the Nintendo games and buy in-game items. It provides 7-, 14-, and 30-day averages. It, too, uses the Contour test strips. It remembers 480 tests.

Prodigy Diabetes Care

Prodigy Diabetes Care makes three meters for the United States called Prodigy meters. The Prodigy Pocket is a small, very portable meter that comes in five colors and remembers 120 tests. The other two meters are more interesting. None of the meters require calibration. You can download them all to Prodigy's free diabetes management software.

- ✔ **Prodigy Voice:** This meter is meant for the blind. It has raised buttons. When a strip is inserted, it turns on and verbally takes the user through the setup steps and provides the reading verbally as well. It remembers 450 tests.

- ✔ **Prodigy AutoCode:** Prodigy AutoCode talks the user through the steps of testing and speaks the result. It speaks in English, Spanish, French, and Arabic. It remembers 120 tests.

LifeScan

Johnson & Johnson purchased LifeScan, one of the older meter companies. They have a number of meters in competition with one another. The company is very reliable, taking care of problems within 24 hours. You can replace the batteries in LifeScan meters at home. This company also posts its owner's manuals online in case you need to refer to them. All of their meters require user calibration, an inconvenient step.

- ✔ **OneTouch UltraMini:** This meter is small and portable. It uses a tiny blood sample. Each new vial of UltraMini test strips must be coded in the meter. It remembers 500 tests. It uses a 3-volt CR2032 coin cell battery. However, it has no way to download test results to a computer and no data-management system. Therefore, I don't recommend it.

- ✔ **OneTouch Ultra2:** This system allows testing away from the fingers. It uses a tiny sample and, therefore, can work with LifeScan's ultrafine lancets. The result is displayed in five seconds, and the blood is drawn up by capillary action. The meter has a 500-test memory that allows averaging on the screen and connects to a data port using OneTouch Diabetes Management software. You can see 7-, 14-, and 30-day averages. It uses Ultra test strips. You use buttons on the meter to set the code on the meter to the code on the bottle of test strips. You can add flags to each blood glucose test to specify whether the glucose was taken before or after a meal and whether food or exercise was involved. It uses two 3-volt CR2032 coin cell batteries, one for the meter and one for the backlight. The test is measured from whole blood but expressed in plasma-referenced units.

- ✔ **OneTouchVerio:** The Verio has a color-coded dot on the screen to tell you if your result is high, in-range, or low, which you set. It uses two included AAA batteries and comes with the OneTouch Lancing device. Only finger sticks are approved for this device. You can see 7-, 14-, 30-, and 90-day averages on the screen. It remembers 500 test results.

Nipro Diagnostics

Nipro Diagnostics makes five meters that are sold in the United States. Three of them, the TRUEtrack, TRUEbalance, and TRUEresult, have no features that differ from previous meters, but the following two are unusual:

- ✔ **TRUE2go:** The TRUE2go is claimed to be the world's smallest meter. It twists on the top of a new vial of strips. It uses a 3-volt CR2032 coin cell battery. The memory holds just 99 results. It does not work with a data-management system, so I don't recommend it.

- ✔ **Sidekick:** This meter is similar to TRUE2go in being a small meter on top of a bottle of strips, but in this case you throw away the entire meter and bottle when you use up the strips, so battery replacement is not necessary. It has a 50-test memory and no data-management system. I don't recommend it.

Roche Diagnostics

Roche Diagnostics merged with Boehringer Mannheim and now sells its meters. The batteries in these meters are replaceable at home. The meters may be used at alternate sites besides the fingers.

- ✔ **Accu-Chek Aviva:** This meter works with diabetes-management software (DMS). It has a very large memory, storing up to 500 blood glucose values, with 7-, 14-, and 30- day averages onscreen. It requires a tiny sample of blood. It comes with Spanish-language instructions and a phone number for a Spanish-speaking representative. It has a code key with each new bottle of test strips that are made just for this meter. You can set test reminders for up to four times a day with the built-in alarm. It uses a coin cell CR2032 battery.

- ✔ **Accu-Chek Compact Plus:** This meter uses a 17-test drum that requires no test-strip handling or calibration. The results are displayed in five seconds, and it has a 300-test memory that is downloadable to a DMS. You can see onscreen 7-, 24-, and 30-day averages. It uses two AAA batteries.

- ✔ **Accu-Chek Nano:** The Nano "fits in the palm of your hand." It has a downloadable 500-test memory that can be evaluated by a data management system with all the features of the other two meters.

Roche also makes a software program for people with diabetes called Accu-Chek Compass. It helps patients to better manage their diabetes by providing reports and summaries of the glucose tests.

Four noninvasive meters: Continuous glucose monitoring

Individual blood glucose measurements represent only a moment in time, and blood glucose levels can change in minutes. Potentially more useful devices that can measure blood glucose almost continuously, store the measure-ments, and download them to a computer are being developed. They may replace the meters in the preceding sections after they improve, but for now they often lag behind finger-stick measurements, especially after a meal or exercise. Each device still requires that you take blood glucose measure-ments using a finger-stick meter to calibrate these continuous meters. Many patients reject the idea of wearing the devices on their body.

Continuous monitors are most useful when the finger-stick results do not cor-relate well with the hemoglobin A1c measurements, which is especially the case in people with diabetes who take insulin, both type 1 and type 2. The doctor, knowing the direction of the blood glucose throughout 24 hours, can adjust the rapid-acting and long-acting insulin more accurately without caus-ing hypoglycemia.

Several reports in *Diabetes Care* since 2010 have shown that continuous glucose monitoring is effective in lowering the hemoglobin A1c in poorly controlled patients on insulin who have type 1 diabetes and even in well-controlled type 1 patients. It is also effective in type 2 patients on multiple insulin injections. It lowers hemoglobin A1c without increased low blood glucose and has a positive effect on quality of life. A report in January 2012 in that journal showed that even type 2 patients on pills benefited from continuous monitoring. They did significantly better during the 12 weeks they were on continuous monitoring and maintained this improvement for 40 more weeks after the continuous monitoring was stopped compared to patients who continued to use finger-stick monitoring.

These studies almost always depend on the manufacturer of the device to provide the device and to fund the study. I leave it to you to decide the effect of such support on the results of the study.

 Check with your insurance company before you purchase a continuous moni-tor. Your company may cover only a specific brand or not cover the device for type 2 diabetes. All of these continuous glucose monitors consist of a sensor under the skin connected to a transmitter that wirelessly transmits the glucose reading to a receiver. The fluid under the skin is the interstitial fluid, not the blood.

Dexcom G4 Platinum Continuous Blood Glucose Monitor

The G4 Platinum monitor by Dexcom uses a sensor that is changed after seven days. The receiver collects the information every five minutes and dis-plays it onscreen. The screen can show one-, three-, and nine-hour trends as well as alert you when the blood glucose goes above or below a set level. An alarm also sounds when the glucose is below 55 mg/dl. Software called Data

Manager 3 helps to display the data on a computer for further understanding of trends. The device is calibrated with a finger-stick glucose reading every 12 hours. It can store up to 30 days of data.

Medtronic Guardian Real-Time

The Medtronic Guardian Real-Time is a continuous glucose meter that uses a sensor that lasts three days and then must be changed. You have to calibrate the meter two hours and six hours after inserting the sensor and every 12 hours after that. You set upper and lower limits, and an alarm alerts you 30 minutes before those limits are reached. It comes in a pediatric model for children and teens. Another nice feature is that the sensor and receiver can be worn under water up to 8 feet deep for up to 30 minutes.

This monitor works with data-management software to show you trends that help you to improve your glucose control. All the results can be viewed with the CareLink Personal Therapy Software. Both the transmitter and the receiver use one AAA battery.

MiniMed Paradigm Real-Time Revel

The MiniMed Paradigm Real-Time Revel is another continuous glucose meter. Medtronic, which makes this meter and the preceding one, has a long history of working in the field of insulin pumps (see Chapter 11). This meter is combined in one apparatus with an insulin pump to accomplish the longstanding goal of creating a "closed loop" system that has been shown to be effective in controlling the blood glucose in children, adolescents, and adults with type 1 diabetes. The sensor must be changed every three days. *Closed loop* means the monitor uses the measured glucose to determine how much insulin to pump into the patient.

A report in *Diabetes Care* (December 2011) confirms the potential of the closed-loop system. In this case, the system was used in 6 of 12 pregnant women with type 1 diabetes who were well controlled (with hemoglobin A1c 6.4 percent). The other six women used conventional continuous insulin infusion without connecting to the meter. Both groups remained well controlled during their pregnancy, but the closed-loop group had less severe hypoglycemia and spent less time with low blood glucose levels.

This monitor uses the same CareLink Personal software as the Guardian Real-Time, and its features are similar.

Medtronic Minimed 530G With Enlite CGM

Just like the previous instrument, this one functions as both a glucose receiver and an insulin pump, but its sensor lasts for six days. The Enlite sensor is supposed to be more comfortable and smaller than other sensors. It isn't yet approved for use in children.

In January 2012, the FDA approved a remote continuous diabetes monitor called MySentry Remote Glucose Monitor that works with the Revel system. Now a parent sleeping in another room can monitor the glucose of her small child, as the device alerts her with an alarm if the glucose is too low or too high. If the parents of small children with diabetes can afford to shell out about $3,000 for the device, it should provide great peace of mind.

In January 2015, the FDA approved the Dexcom Share Direct Secondary Displays system that allows caregivers or other designated persons to remotely monitor the glucose levels of a diabetic with a mobile device such as a smartphone from the Internet.

How I use my patients' test results

I encourage my patients to keep their own records of their glucose levels so that they can see for themselves how they are doing. I maintain several years of records and can compare and contrast results for each patient. I use software to generate pictures of a patient's diabetic control. The figures in this sidebar show you graphics that depict test results for a typical patient before starting therapy and after insulin treatment had time to work. You can easily see how helpful the graphic information can be.

The first figure shows the patient's blood glucose levels in three different formats. The top, the Trendgraph, shows the blood glucoses each day, in this case, between 6/11 and 7/1. The shaded area represents the blood glucoses from 80 to 180 mg/dl. The line below the shaded area is the 50 mg/dl line. Each X represents a distinct blood glucose test. You can see that the glucose is often high, going up to 300, and sometimes low, going down to 50 with large excursions. This graph also shows that the mean of the tests is 159 and that 5 percent of the time, the patient is less than 80; 63.4 percent of the time, she is between 80 and 180; and 31.7 percent of the time, she is above 180.

The next figure, the Standard Day, puts all those glucose levels in a 24-hour day so that tests taken between certain hours, regardless of the day, appear close to one another. This grouping allows me to see whether the patient has a tendency to be high or low at a given time each day. The software averages out the blood glucose at different times, providing a number to compare to other time periods. This information permits me to adjust her insulin to correct for that particular time.

The bottom figure, the Pie Chart, clearly shows how much of the time this patient is high, how much of the time she is within the target of 80 to 180, and how much of the time she is below 80.

These three figures provide an excellent picture of the patient's diabetic control and permit me to easily compare it to the result of treatment.

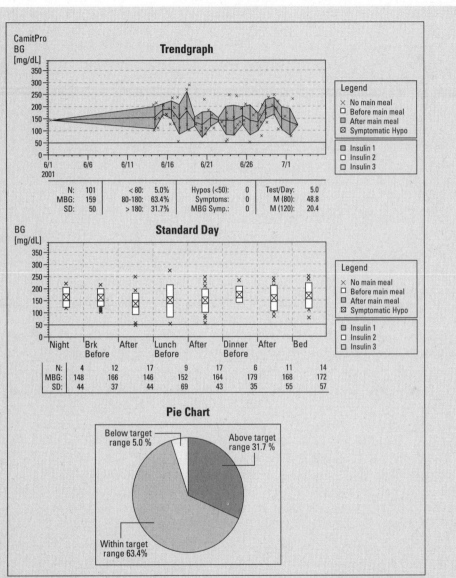

© John Wiley & Sons, Inc.

The next set of figures represents tests taken after treatment with insulin glargine (Lantus), for one week. The results are dramatic. Now almost all the glucoses are in the shaded area, and there is little excursion of the tests. A few Xs fall above 180, and a few fall below 80. The Standard Day now shows fairly low averages throughout, except perhaps after lunch. The Pie Chart shows much more in the target range and far fewer above the target range. Comparing the two graphs, the *above target range* area has dropped from 31.7 percent to 6.5 percent.

(continued)

(continued)

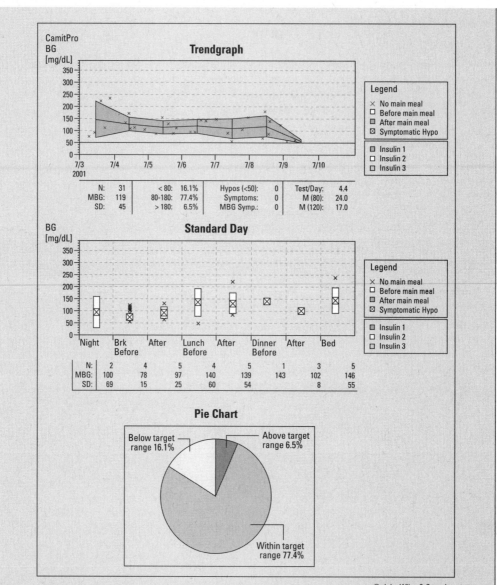

CamitPro BG [mg/dL]

Trendgraph

Legend
× No main meal
□ Before main meal
□ After main meal
⊠ Symptomatic Hypo

□ Insulin 1
□ Insulin 2
□ Insulin 3

N:	31	< 80:	16.1%	Hypos (<50):	0	Test/Day:	4.4
MBG:	119	80-180:	77.4%	Symptoms:	0	M (80):	24.0
SD:	45	> 180:	6.5%	MBG Symp.:	0	M (120):	17.0

BG [mg/dL]

Standard Day

Legend
× No main meal
□ Before main meal
□ After main meal
⊠ Symptomatic Hypo

□ Insulin 1
□ Insulin 2
□ Insulin 3

	Night	Brk Before	After	Lunch Before	After	Dinner Before	After	Bed
N:	2	4	5	4	5	1	3	5
MBG:	100	78	97	140	139	143	102	146
SD:	69	15	25	60	54		8	55

Pie Chart

Below target range 16.1%

Above target range 6.5%

Within target range 77.4%

© *John Wiley & Sons, Inc.*

I can print all these graphs and charts. In later visits, I can compare the current control with the way the patient was doing before. When patients can see so clearly how they're improving from time to time, it keeps them motivated to take their medicine and follow their diet and exercise plan.

Tracking Your Glucose over Time: Hemoglobin A1c

In order to follow your improvement with treatment, you need a test that gives you the big picture, the average blood glucose over time. As I explain in Chapter 2, the hemoglobin A1c is that test. Figure 7-2 shows you the correlation between the hemoglobin A1c and the estimated average blood glucose. By correlating the A1c with the estimated average blood glucose, you can think of the A1c in the same units as the blood glucose that you measure several times a day.

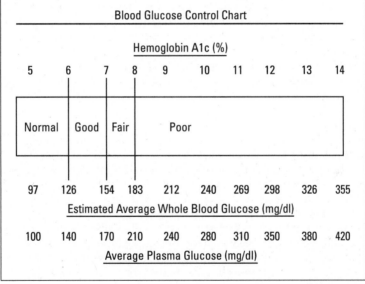

Figure 7-2: Comparison between hemoglobin A1c and blood glucose.

© John Wiley & Sons, Inc.

As you can see in the figure, a normal hemoglobin A1c of less than 6 percent corresponds to an estimated average blood glucose of less than 126, while a fair hemoglobin A1c of 7 percent reflects an average blood glucose of 155.

Large-scale studies have shown that the average hemoglobin A1c in the United States for type 2 diabetes is around 9.4 percent, which means the average blood glucose is 223. The American Diabetes Association recommends taking action to control the blood glucose if the hemoglobin A1c is 8 percent or greater, with the goal being less than 7 percent.

The American Association of Clinical Endocrinologists suggests a goal of 6.5 percent or less. Although I wish all of my patients would achieve a level of 6.5 percent, I try to get them as low as possible but still consistent with a decent quality of life, which means few to no severe hypoglycemic episodes.

Your physician should test for hemoglobin A1c as follows:

✔ Four times a year if you have type 1 or type 2 diabetes and are on insulin

✔ Two times a year if you have type 2 diabetes and are not on insulin

In my own practice, I test all patients every three months. A good hemoglobin A1c is highly motivating to keep up good self-care, whereas a poor result gives immediate feedback as to the need for tighter control.

The National Glycohemoglobin Standardization Program, created by the American Association for Clinical Chemistry, has standardized the hemoglobin A1c test so that a 6 percent result means the same thing for every patient.

A study published in *Diabetes Care* in January 2011 showed that the hemoglobin A1c changes much more frequently in gestational diabetes. The authors recommend weekly testing of the A1c to guide treatment. If you have gestational diabetes, discuss this issue with your doctor.

Bayer sells a clever home version of the hemoglobin A1c called *A1c Now*. You do a finger stick to produce a large drop of blood. The blood is mixed with a solution that is provided, and a sample of that mixture is placed in the testing device. Five minutes later, the hemoglobin A1c result appears in the device window. The device is then discarded. The device appears to be highly accurate and may save the trouble of going to a lab for this test. Because it's so quick, your doctor can have the test results while you're at his office and can act on them immediately, instead of waiting for a lab to return the test results at a later time. The test kit is available at pharmacies without a prescription, for about $30 a test. It is annually certified by the National Glycohemoglobin Standardization Program.

Another option is to collect your own blood specimen and send it to a company that runs the test and gives you and your doctor a result. Following are some companies currently doing this test:

✔ **AccuBase A1c Glycohemoglobin:** Each test costs $29.59 and includes lab analysis and reporting. It can be ordered on the Internet at Amazon. com or American Diabetes Wholesale.

• Phone: 888-872-2443

• Website: http://dtilaboratories.com/diagprod.htm

✔ **Walgreen's A1c at Home:** This testing service costs $39.99 each including lab analysis and reporting.

- Phone: 800-925-4733

- Website: `www.walgreens.com/store/c/walgreens-at-home-a1c-test-kit/ID=prod6248361-product`

The Diabetes Control and Complications Trials have shown that maintaining a hemoglobin A1c of 7 percent or less for several years early in type 1 diabetes results in diabetes complications 50 percent or lower 20 years later, even when the A1c is higher after those years.

Low thyroid function falsely raises the hemoglobin A1c. An A1c between 5.7 and 6.4 percent is an indicator of prediabetes.

Testing for Kidney Damage: Moderately Increased Albumin (MIA)

The finding of very small but abnormal amounts of protein in the urine, called moderately increased albumin (MIA) (formerly *microalbuminuria),* is the earliest sign that high glucose may be damaging your kidneys (see Chapter 5). When MIA is found, you still have time to reverse any damage.

As soon as you are diagnosed with type 2 diabetes, and within five years of being diagnosed with type 1, your doctor must order a urine test for MIA. If the test is negative, it must be repeated annually. If the test is positive, it should be done a second time to verify the result. If the second test is positive, your doctor should do the following:

✔ **Put you on a drug called an ACE inhibitor:** After you have been on this drug for some months, the test for MIA can be repeated to see whether it has turned negative. The ACE inhibitor can be stopped and restarted later if MIA appears again. If ACE inhibitors aren't tolerated, then ARBs, another class of antihypertensives, may be used. Both classes have been shown to reverse MIA and the ongoing kidney damage it reflects.

✔ **Bring your blood glucose under the tightest control possible.** Bringing it under control helps to reverse the damaging process as well.

✔ **Normalize your body fats so that your cholesterol and triglycerides are made normal.** Elevated cholesterol and triglycerides have been found to damage the kidneys. (See the section "Tracking Cholesterol and Other Fats," later in this chapter.)

✓ **Bring your blood pressure under control.** Lowering your blood pressure will help to minimize the damage to your kidneys that occurs when they are exposed to elevated blood pressure.

Doing this simple little test can protect your kidneys from damage. Ask your doctor about it if you think you've never had it done. Show him or her this page if the doctor is unclear as to why it is performed.

Up to 25 percent of patients with diabetes can have ongoing kidney damage without showing an elevated microalbumin. For this reason, the idea that all patients with diabetes should receive an ACE inhibitor may not be far-fetched.

Women who have gestational diabetes and show MIA have been found to have heart disease and kidney disease later, even if they don't develop diabetes. Persistent MIA predicts later heart disease even in the absence of gestational diabetes.

Checking for Eye Problems

All people with diabetes need to have a dilated eye exam done annually (or every two years if no eye disease is present) by an ophthalmologist or optometrist. No other physician, including the endocrinologist (yours truly excepted, of course), can do the exam properly.

For this exam, the doctor instills drops into your eyes and uses various instruments to examine the pressure, the appearance of your lens, and, most importantly, the retina of your eye.

All kinds of treatments can be done if abnormalities are found, but they must be discovered first. (See Chapter 5 for more information on eye problems.)

This test is something you must demand. Your doctor must refer you to an ophthalmologist or optometrist every year. Better yet, set up the appointment yourself with the eye doctor's nurse at the end of your first visit so that you are reminded about it each year. People who have mild type 2 diabetes and no retinopathy may be tested at two-year intervals rather than annually.

Examining Your Feet

Failing to take care of your feet leads to problems that often end in amputation. An amputation is really evidence of inadequate care. (For more on foot problems, see Chapter 5.) The doctor is not necessarily at fault here. The doctor sees you once in a while; you're with yourself much more often.

If you have any problem sensing touch with your feet, you need to take the following precautions:

✔ You must use your eyes to examine your feet every day.

✔ You must use your hand to test hot water before you step into it so that you do not get burned.

✔ You must shake out your shoes before you step into them to make sure no stone or other object is inside them.

✔ You must not go barefoot.

✔ You must keep the skin of your feet moist by soaking them in water, drying them with a towel, and applying a moisturizing lotion. (Soaking should always be accompanied by drying and moisturizing.)

Your doctor can test your ability to feel an injury by using a 10-gram filament, but, again, that is done only when you have an appointment. You can obtain one of these filaments for yourself. A couple of the places where you can get them include

✔ Lower Extremity Amputation Prevention (LEAP) Program: www.hrsa. gov/hansensdisease/leap

✔ Medical Monofilament Manufacturing, LLC: www.medicalmono filament.com, or call 508-746-7877

If you have any suggestion of a loss of sensation, at each visit to the doctor who takes care of your diabetes, you should take off your shoes and socks and have your feet inspected.

The other part of a foot examination involves checking the circulation of blood to your feet. To check the circulation, your doctor does a measurement called an *ankle-brachial index* at least once every five years. The systolic blood pressure is measured in the ankle and the arm. (See the sidebar "The meaning of your blood pressure," later in this chapter, for an explanation of systolic blood pressure.) The value for the ankle is divided by the value for the arm. An index of greater than 0.9 is considered normal. A value between 0.4 and 0.9 indicates peripheral vascular disease (see Chapter 5), and a value less than 0.4 indicates severe disease.

The ankle-brachial index should be done for any person with diabetes over age 50. Patients under 50 require the study if risk factors such as smoking, high cholesterol, and high blood pressure are present.

Tracking Cholesterol and Other Fats

Most people these days know the level of their total cholesterol, but other tests that show levels of various types of fats in the blood are needed as well.

Cholesterol is a type of fat that circulates in the blood in small packages called *lipoproteins.* These tiny round particles contain fat (*lipo,* as in liposuction) and protein. Because cholesterol does not dissolve in water, it would separate from the blood if it were not surrounded by the protein, just like oil separates from water in salad dressing. (That's why you have to shake the salad dressing each time you use it.)

A second kind of fat found in the lipoproteins is *triglyceride.* Triglyceride actually represents the form of most of the fat you eat each day. Although you may eat only a gram or less of cholesterol (an egg yolk has one-third of a gram of cholesterol), you eat up to 100 grams of triglyceride a day. (For more on the place of fats in your diet, see Chapter 8.) The fat in animal meats is mostly triglycerides.

Four types of lipoproteins exist:

- ✔ **Chylomicrons:** The largest of the fat particles, these lipoproteins contain the fat that is absorbed from the intestine after a meal. They are usually cleared from the blood rapidly. Ordinarily, chylomicrons are not a concern with respect to causing *arteriosclerosis* (hardening of the arteries).

- ✔ **Very-low-density lipoprotein (VLDL):** These particles contain mostly triglyceride as the fat. They're smaller than chylomicrons.

- ✔ **High-density lipoprotein (HDL):** Known as "good" cholesterol, this lipoprotein is the next smallest in size. This particle functions to clean the arteries, helping to prevent coronary artery disease, peripheral vascular disease, and strokes.

- ✔ **Low-density lipoprotein (LDL):** Known as "bad" cholesterol, this smallest particle is the particle that seems to carry cholesterol to the arteries, where it's deposited and causes hardening.

As you may imagine, doctors need to know which particle your cholesterol comes from in order to understand whether you have too much bad cholesterol (LDL) or a satisfactory level of good cholesterol (HDL).

You don't have to fast to test for total cholesterol and HDL cholesterol. However, you do need to fast for eight hours to find out your LDL cholesterol and triglycerides, because the blood has to be cleared of chylomicrons, which rise greatly when you eat.

TIP

You should have a *fasting lipid panel* at least each year or two. A fasting lipid panel gives you your total cholesterol, your LDL cholesterol, your HDL cholesterol, and your triglyceride levels. If your values indicate you are at low risk (LDL less than 100, HDL greater than 50), the fasting lipid panel may be done every two years.

Table 7-1 lists the current recommendations for the levels of these fats in terms of the risk for coronary artery disease.

Table 7-1	Levels of Fat and Risk for Coronary Artery Disease		
Risk	*LDL Cholesterol*	*HDL Cholesterol*	*Triglycerides*
Higher	Greater than 130	Less than 35	Greater than 400
Borderline	100 to 130	35 to 45	151 to 400
Lower	Less than 100	Greater than 45	Less than 150

You can see in Table 7-1 that the risk goes up as the LDL cholesterol goes up and the HDL cholesterol goes down. A huge study of thousands of citizens of Framingham, Massachusetts, shows that you can get a good picture of the risk by dividing the total cholesterol by the HDL cholesterol. If this result is less than 4.5, the risk is lower. If it's greater than 4.5, you're at higher risk for coronary artery disease. The higher it is, the worse the risk.

In March 2004, the story got a little more complicated. The *New England Journal of Medicine* published results of a study of more than 4,000 men who had just had heart attacks. In the study, some patients' LDL cholesterol was reduced maximally (to a mean of 62) with a large dose of a powerful drug called *atorvastatin*. The result was a major reduction, starting in just 30 days after treatment with the drug, in subsequent heart attacks, chest pain, and strokes compared to a group whose LDL was lowered only to 95. This result calls for a major reappraisal of what LDL is considered normal. Experts agree that the lowest possible LDL level is best and that this policy applies to everyone, not only people who have just had a heart attack.

Diabetes adds its own complication because of metabolic syndrome (see Chapter 5). In metabolic syndrome, the total cholesterol may not be very high, but the HDL cholesterol is low and the triglycerides are elevated. These patients also have a lot of a dangerous form of LDL cholesterol, so they are at higher risk for coronary artery disease. This increased risk must be taken into account in considering treatment for the fats.

In deciding whether and how to treat the fats, you have to consider other risk factors for coronary artery disease. You're at high risk if you have diabetes and fit any of the following conditions:

✔ You already have coronary artery disease, stroke, or peripheral vascular disease.

✔ You are a male over 45.

✔ You are a female over 55.

✔ You smoke cigarettes.

✔ You have high blood pressure.

✔ You have HDL cholesterol less than 35.

✔ You have a father or brother who had a heart attack before age 55.

✔ You have a mother or sister who had a heart attack before age 65.

✔ You have a body-mass index greater than 30.

You're at low risk if you have none of the preceding risk factors.

The treatment for abnormal fats with statins (see Chapter 11) then depends on your age and the presence of these cardiovascular disease (CVD) risk factors (see Table 7-2).

Table 7-2	Statin Treatment Based on Risk Factors	
Age	**Risk Factors**	**Statin Dose**
<40	None	None
	CVD risk factors	Moderate or high
	Overt CVD	High
40–75	None	Moderate
	CVD risk factors	High
	Overt CVD	High
>75	None	Moderate
	CVD risk factors	Moderate or high
	Overt CVD	High

All these decisions depend on obtaining a lipid (fat) panel as needed to monitor adherence.

These treatment guidelines will change as the experts have a chance to evaluate the LDL study of heart-attack victims that I discuss in this section.

After LDL cholesterol is lowered, even below 70, a higher level of HDL cholesterol has been found to be associated with fewer heart attacks than a lower level.

Measuring Blood Pressure

The United States is experiencing an epidemic of high blood pressure *(hypertension)* similar to the epidemic of diabetes. The reasons are the same:

✔ Americans are getting fatter.

✔ Americans are storing fat in the center of our bodies, the so-called *abdominal visceral fat.*

✔ Americans are getting older as a population. The fastest-growing segment of the population is over 75 years of age. Of people age 50 to 55 with diabetes, 50 percent have high blood pressure. Of people older than 75 with diabetes, 75 percent have high blood pressure.

✔ Americans are more sedentary than before.

People with diabetes have high blood pressure more often than the nondiabetic population for a lot of other reasons besides the preceding ones:

✔ People with diabetes get kidney disease.

✔ People with diabetes have increased sensitivity to salt, which raises blood pressure.

✔ People with diabetes lack the nighttime fall in blood pressure that normally occurs in people without diabetes.

Doctors generally agree that a normal blood pressure is less than 140/90. For years, the *diastolic blood pressure* (the lower reading) was considered more damaging, and an elevation in that pressure was treated with greater importance than an elevation in the *systolic blood pressure* (the higher reading). More recent studies have shown that the systolic blood pressure, not the diastolic blood pressure, may be more important. (See the sidebar "The meaning of your blood pressure" for more detailed explanations of each type of blood pressure.)

All the complications of diabetes are made worse by an elevation in blood pressure, especially diabetic kidney disease but also eye disease, heart disease, nerve disease, peripheral vascular disease, and cerebral arterial disease (see Chapter 5).

Evidence of the importance of controlling blood pressure in diabetes comes from the United Kingdom Prospective Diabetes Study, published in late 1998. This study found that a lowering of blood pressure by 10 mm systolic and 5 mm diastolic resulted in a 24 percent reduction in any diabetic complication and a 32 percent reduction in death related to diabetes.

Lowering the blood pressure to less than 120/80 is absolutely essential in diabetes. How well are doctors doing at controlling blood pressure in people with diabetes? A study in 2012 showed that only 29 percent of people with diabetes with hypertension have a blood pressure as low as 120/80.

Your doctor should measure blood pressure at every visit. Better yet, get a blood pressure device and measure it yourself. If you detect an elevation, bring it to the attention of your doctor.

The meaning of your blood pressure

What does the blood pressure measurement mean, and what is high blood pressure? When you get a reading, it usually looks something like 120/70 — it has an upper reading and a lower reading.

✔ The upper reading, called the *systolic pressure,* is the amount of force exerted by the heart when it contracts to push blood around the body. A cuff around your arm connects to a column of mercury. You, your doctor, or a machine listens for the first sound you hear on the side of the cuff away from your heart. That sound is the sound of blood finally able to overcome the pressure in the cuff and get through to the other side. The systolic blood pressure is the height of the column of mercury, read in

millimeters, just as the blood comes through. (Sometimes the cuff is not connected to a column of mercury but to a gauge that is calibrated so the reading on the gauge is in millimeters of mercury even though no mercury is present.) In our example, the systolic blood pressure reading is 120 mm of mercury.

✔ The lower reading, called the *diastolic blood pressure,* is the pressure in the artery when the heart is at rest. A valve in the heart keeps the blood from flowing backwards so that the pressure does not fall to zero (you hope). When the sound stops, the height of the mercury column gives the diastolic blood pressure, in this case 70 mm of mercury.

Pregnant women with diabetes who have high blood pressure should not take ACE inhibitors or ARBs (two classes of drugs). They're known to be harmful to the growing fetus. If you have high blood pressure and plan to become pregnant, discuss your blood pressure medication with your doctor before conceiving.

For much more information on every aspect of high blood pressure, see my book *High Blood Pressure For Dummies* (John Wiley & Sons, Inc.).

Checking Your Weight and BMI

To give you a general idea of how much you ought to weigh, you can use the following formula:

- ✔ If you're a woman, give yourself 100 pounds for being 5 feet tall and add 5 pounds for each inch over 5 feet. For example, if you're 5 feet 3 inches, your appropriate weight should be approximately 115 pounds.

- ✔ If you're a man, give yourself 106 pounds for being 5 feet tall and add 6 pounds for each inch over 5 feet. A 5-foot 6-inch male should weigh around 142 pounds.

Body-mass index (BMI) is a measurement that relates weight to height. A tall person has a lower BMI than a short person of the same weight. (See Chapter 3 for more on BMI, including instructions for calculating your own BMI.) A person with a BMI under 18.5 is considered underweight. A person with a BMI from 18.5 to 24.9 is normal. A person with a BMI from 25 to 29.9 is overweight, and a person with a BMI of 30 or over is obese. By this definition, more than 69 percent of the people in the United States are overweight or obese as of 2012.

Non-white populations like South Asians, Chinese, and blacks develop diabetes at a lower BMI. Ethnicity must be considered in developing prevention techniques and targets for ideal body weight.

You can't get a reading of your BMI by stepping on a scale, but you can get your weight. This measurement is one of the easiest in medicine. Your doctor should measure your weight at every visit.

The National Heart, Lung, and Blood Institute makes knowing your BMI easy. Using the calculator at `www.cdc.gov/healthyweight/assessing/bmi/adult_BMI/english_bmi_calculator/bmi_calculator.html`, just fill in your weight in pounds and your height in feet and inches, click "Compute BMI," and get your result.

Maintaining a BMI in the normal range makes controlling your diabetes and blood pressure easier. Also, you must eliminate obesity as a risk factor for coronary artery disease.

Testing for Ketones

When your blood glucose rises above 250 mg/dl (13.9 mmol/L), or if you are pregnant with diabetes and your blood glucose is below 60 mg/dl (3.3 mmol/L), your doctor should probably check for *ketones* — products of the breakdown of fats. Finding ketones means that your body has turned to fat for energy. If you have high glucose and find ketones, you may need more insulin. If you have low glucose and find ketones during pregnancy, you may need more carbohydrates in your diet.

Testing for ketones is done by inserting a test strip into your urine and observing a purple color. The deeper the color, the greater the ketone level. If you find a large amount of ketones, you should contact your physician. Two sources for ketone test strips are Bayer Ketostix and Nipro Trueplus Ketone Test Strips.

Testing the C-Reactive Protein

C-reactive protein (CRP) is a substance in the blood that is produced by the liver when infection or inflammation is present. It can be measured with a simple blood test. Diabetes is associated with several features that suggest that inflammation plays an important role in the disease. People who develop diabetes have higher C-reactive protein than those who don't. (Other substances associated with inflammation are also elevated in diabetes.)

Half the people with diabetes who have heart attacks have low or low-normal levels of LDL (bad) cholesterol. It is believed that inflammation plays a major role in many of these patients. Elevated CRP in the blood has been shown to directly contribute to blood-vessel damage and the formation of blood clots that cause heart attacks.

Drugs that improve diabetes lower the amount of C-reactive protein, which is also considered a marker for coronary artery disease.

Have your C-reactive protein measured with other blood tests about once a year. If the level is elevated, it may serve as a predictor of future diabetes or coronary artery disease. You need to work even harder to lower your blood glucose, improve your LDL and HDL cholesterol, and lower your blood pressure. About 90 percent of healthy individuals have CRP levels less than 3, and 99 percent have levels less than 10. This test isn't essential in diabetes.

Checking the TSH

A screening test called the *thyroid-stimulating hormone (TSH) level* is done at the time that diabetes is diagnosed and every five years thereafter if it is normal. This test is done because people with diabetes (type 1) have a higher incidence of thyroid disease than the general population, because thyroid disease is often confused with other conditions, and because hypothyroidism can lead to weight gain, which obviously isn't good for diabetes.

TSH is produced by the pituitary gland in the brain. When the thyroid gland makes the right amount of thyroid hormone, the pituitary produces the right amount of TSH to keep it working properly. The normal level in the blood is 0.5–2.5 microunits per milliliter (μU/ml).

When the thyroid makes inadequate amounts of thyroid hormone, the pituitary increases its production of TSH to stimulate the thyroid, and values of 10 or more μU/ml are not uncommon. When the thyroid makes too much thyroid hormone, it causes the pituitary to turn down its production of TSH, and values less than 0.5 μU/ml are found.

Too much thyroid hormone leads to insulin resistance, making diabetes worse than before. Too little thyroid hormone increases insulin sensitivity, so people with low thyroid function have reduced levels of blood glucose.

Low levels of thyroid hormone cause an elevation in the hemoglobin A1c in patients who don't have diabetes as well as those who do. Replacing the thyroid hormone lowers the A1c to normal if diabetes is not present.

Much more about thyroid disease and its treatment can be found in my book *Thyroid For Dummies* (Wiley).

Evaluating Testosterone in Men with Type 2 Diabetes

About one third of men in the United States over the age of 65 have low levels of testosterone, and a similar percentage of those men have diabetes. Low testosterone is associated with changes in body composition that promote diabetes like increased fat and decreased muscle. According to tests done so far, giving testosterone to these men has not resulted in persistent improvement in glucose metabolism.

Older men who have significant reduction in muscle mass and increase in fat should have their testosterone measured. If very low, treatment with testosterone may be considered by you and your doctor. Such patients should at least make a major effort to increase exercise and decrease caloric intake, which often results in a rise in testosterone.

Checking Vitamin D

Recent studies suggest a relationship between low levels of vitamin D and the development of both type 1 and type 2 diabetes. Communities that live furthest from the equator, getting less sun to make vitamin D, have the highest incidence of type 1 diabetes. Vitamin D protects the body from autoimmunity (where the body attacks itself), and type 1 diabetes is an autoimmune disease. High levels of vitamin D are associated with a lower risk of developing type 2 diabetes. In a study, people who were prediabetic were given vitamin D over three months and showed a significant improvement in glucose metabolism and reduction in hemoglobin A1c. Severe vitamin D deficiency has been shown to predict death and heart attacks in both type 1 and type 2 diabetes.

A study in the *Journal of Clinical Endocrinology and Metabolism* in September 2010 showed that blood vitamin D levels were low in obese women. The greater the degree of obesity, the lower the vitamin D. When weight was lost, the vitamin D level rose and the insulin resistance declined.

Have your vitamin D level measured with a blood test if you have prediabetes or diabetes. Take supplemental vitamin D if the level is low.

Chapter 8

Tackling What You Eat: Healthful Nutrition

*B*oy, are people big and getting bigger! The Centers for Disease Control tells everyone that more than six in ten Americans are overweight or obese. Most adults are 25 pounds heavier than people in the 1960s. And yet more than half of these overweight people think they are at a healthy weight.

The good news, according to a study in the *Journal of the American Medical Association* in January 2012, is that the prevalence of obesity and high body-mass index in the United States was the same — that is, no worse — in 2009 and 2010 as it was from 2003 to 2008. The bad news is that it's not improving.

Language specialists claim that the five sweetest phrases in the English language are

✔ I love you.

✔ Dinner is served.

✔ All is forgiven.

✔ Sleep until noon.

✔ Keep the change.

To that, most people would certainly add, "You've lost weight."

For the diabetic population, most of whom are overweight, appropriate nutrition and weight loss are not an option but a necessity. The Diabetes Control and Complications Trial clearly demonstrated that a person with diabetes who follows a careful nutrition program can reduce his or her hemoglobin A1c (see Chapter 7) by as much as 1 percent compared to the person with diabetes who is careless about diet.

In this chapter, you find out all you need to know to make your diet work for you, not only to improve your diabetes and control your blood glucose but also to feel generally that you have an improved quality of life.

Considering Total Calories First

Wanda B. Thinner, age 46, was a new type 2 diabetic patient who came to me because of high blood glucose levels, some blurring of her vision, and some numbness in her toes. She was 5 feet 5 inches tall and weighed 165 pounds. She was taking pills for the diabetes, but they weren't helping. Her doctor had told her she needed to lose weight but gave no further instructions. I started her on a diet based on the principles in this chapter. She was willing to follow the diet and lost 20 pounds, which she has kept off. Her blood glucose is now in the range of 110 most of the time. She no longer suffers from blurred vision, and her toes are beginning to improve. She isn't taking the diabetes medication and feels much better.

No matter how you slice it, your weight is determined by the number of calories you take in minus the number of calories you use up by exercise or loss of calories in the urine or bowel movements. If you have an excess of calories coming in and have insulin with which to store them, you gain weight. If you have fewer calories in than out, you lose weight. (See Chapter 7 if you're not sure how much you should weigh.) If you are overweight, you will benefit from even a small weight loss for the following reasons:

- ✔ Weight loss markedly reduces the risk of developing type 2 diabetes.
- ✔ Weight loss prevents the progression of prediabetes (see Chapter 2) into type 2 diabetes.
- ✔ Weight loss can reverse the failure to respond to drugs for diabetes that develops after responding at first (see Chapter 10).
- ✔ Weight loss reduces the risk of death from diabetes.
- ✔ Weight loss increases life expectancy in patients with type 2 diabetes.
- ✔ Weight loss has beneficial effects on high blood pressure and abnormal fats (see Chapter 7).

In an article in the *International Journal of Obesity* in June 2006, the authors from the University of Alabama and the University of Wisconsin offered ten reasons that may play a role in the obesity epidemic besides taking in excess calories:

- **Reduced length of nightly sleep:** An inverse relationship exists between weight and hours of sleep. People are sleeping less than they did before.

- **Hormones and other substances in food:** Substances like estrogens, which are put in animal feed to fatten the animals, have the same fattening effect on the humans who eat those animals.

- **Decreased exposure to high and low temperatures:** High temperatures cause sweating, and low temperatures cause shivering, both of which contribute to weight loss. Modern heat and air conditioning diminish our exposure to extremes of temperature, which is actually good for us.

- **Decreased smoking:** This phenomenon has a good side and a bad side. Cigarette smoking is the greatest public health menace that exists, but smokers do tend to be leaner than nonsmokers.

- **Use of drugs that cause weight gain:** Many of the drugs used for mental states like depression and high blood pressure cause marked weight gain and even diabetes.

- **Increases in age and ethnic groups that tend to be more overweight or obese:** Hispanic Americans, who are increasing in the population, have a much higher obesity prevalence than Caucasians. At the same time, the general population is older.

- **Increasing age of new mothers:** Older mothers tend to produce more obese children.

- **Effects in the uterus:** Maternal obesity may cause changes in the growing fetus that promote obesity.

- **Heavier women have more offspring:** These offspring, in turn, tend to be heavier.

- **Humans tend to choose heavier mates:** Heavier mates have reproductive advantages. And if your mate is heavier, you tend to become heavier.

More recently several other factors besides higher caloric intake have been suggested:

- The presence of certain bacteria in your intestine may promote increased calorie intake from food.

- Artificial sweeteners alter the population of bacteria in the digestive system, changing the metabolism of glucose, causing levels to rise higher after eating and decline more slowly.

- Excess added sugar in food even without increased total calories promotes diabetes.

Portion sizes have increased significantly both in restaurants and at home. Here are correct portion sizes for several foods:

- ✔ Three ounces of meat is the size of a deck of playing cards.

- ✔ A medium apple or peach is the size of a tennis ball.

- ✔ One ounce of cheese is the size of four dice.

- ✔ One-half cup of ice cream is the size of a tennis ball.

- ✔ A cup of mashed potatoes is the size of your fist.

- ✔ A teaspoon of butter or peanut butter is the size of the tip of your thumb.

- ✔ One-half cup of nuts is the size of a golf ball.

To have an approximate idea of how many *kcalories* (kilocalories) you need each day (not *calories,* which are much smaller, and which are incorrectly used as the common unit of food energy), you need to figure your desirable weight. Using the method described in Chapter 7, a 5-foot 6-inch male with a moderate frame should weigh around 142 pounds. Follow these steps to find the number of kcalories needed:

1. **Multiply your weight times 10.**

    This example gives a value of about 1,400 kcalories.

2. **Add kcalories for your level of exercise:**

    • A sedentary male adds 10 percent of the basal kcalories.

    • A moderately active male adds 20 percent.

    • A very active male adds 40 percent or more, depending on the length and the degree of exercise.

If the male in our example is moderately active, he needs 1,400 kcalories plus 1,400 times 20 percent (or about 300) more for a total of about 1,700 kcalories.

These formulas are true for women as well, but women usually require fewer calories to maintain the same weight as men. Be aware that this calculation is an approximation that differs not only for different people but even for the same person on different days.

Caloric needs are different for people of different ages and different levels of activity. A woman who is pregnant or breastfeeding obviously needs more kcalories (as I discuss in Chapter 6). If a person is trying to lose weight, reducing the total kcalories per day can help accomplish this goal. I say a lot more about this topic in the section on weight reduction later in this chapter.

After you determine the total kcalories you need, the question becomes how to divide the calories among various foods. Basically, three types of foods contain calories: carbohydrates, proteins, and fats. Within these foods, you have many variables, which I explain in this section.

Consuming the right amount of carbohydrates

No area in nutrition is more controversial for the diabetic person than carbohydrates. For years, the American Diabetes Association (ADA) told people with diabetes that they should eat 55 to 60 percent of their calories as carbohydrate. Other experts said that amount was too much or too little. The ADA has now modified its recommendation so that it says in the Clinical Practice Recommendations for 2012, "The recommended daily allowance for carbohydrate is 130 grams per day and is based on providing adequate glucose as the required fuel for the central nervous system without reliance on glucose production from ingested protein or fat."

Carbohydrates are the sources of energy that start with *glucose,* the sugar in your bloodstream that is one sugar molecule, and include substances containing many sugar molecules called *complex carbohydrates, starches, cellulose,* and *gums.* Some of the common sources of carbohydrate are bread, potatoes, grains, cereals, and rice.

Physicians know a lot of information about carbohydrate in the body:

- ✔ Carbohydrate is the primary source of energy for muscles.
- ✔ Glucose is the carbohydrate that causes the pancreas to release insulin.
- ✔ Carbohydrate causes the triglyceride (fat) level to rise in the blood.
- ✔ When insulin is not present or is ineffective, more carbohydrate raises the blood glucose higher.

Although the fat intake of the US population has declined because of the fear of coronary artery disease caused by cholesterol, Americans are getting fatter. In fact, 69 percent of Americans are considered overweight or obese according to the US Department of Health and Human Resources. Because Americans are not eating more protein, the culprit is most likely excess carbohydrate, such as that found in concentrated sweets, such as pastry and candy, as well as the more complex carbohydrate found in bread. Within the body, carbohydrate can be turned into fat and stored. This function was great when everyone lived in caves and got little food for prolonged periods of time, but it doesn't fit today's lifestyle, consisting as it does of abundant food (and minimal foraging for it in the supermarket).

Because carbohydrate is the food that raises the blood glucose, which is responsible for the complications of diabetes, it seems right to recommend a diet that is lower in carbohydrate than previously suggested. Furthermore, a major source of coronary artery disease in diabetes is metabolic syndrome (see Chapter 5). Because increased carbohydrate triggers increased triglyceride, which is the beginning of a number of abnormalities that lead to increased coronary artery disease, recommending less carbohydrate on this basis as well seems prudent.

My experience has been that a diet of between 40 and 50 percent carbohydrate makes controlling my patients' blood glucose much easier. It also leads to weight loss because you don't tend to substitute protein or fat for the reduced amount of carbohydrate in the diet. My patients on lower-carbohydrate diets are able to reduce the amounts of drugs they take, such as insulin, which can cause weight gain and complicate controlling their diabetes. They also have a better fat profile.

Thinking back to the example earlier in this chapter, a man on a diet of 1,700 kcalories should eat about 850 kcalories as carbohydrate. Because each gram of carbohydrate is 4 kcalories, he eats about 210 grams of carbohydrate a day. This amount, which I recommend in this case based on my experience, is higher than the recommendation by the ADA. Translating this amount into the foods you know and love, it's the same as two slices of whole-wheat bread, 1 cup of brown rice, five fruits, and a cup of baked beans a day.

Glycemic index

All carbohydrates are not alike in the degree to which they raise the blood glucose. This fact was recognized some years ago, and a measurement called the *glycemic index* was created to quantify it. The *glycemic index* (GI) uses white bread as the indicator food and assigns it a value of 100. Another carbohydrate of equal calories is compared to white bread in its ability to raise the blood glucose and is assigned a value in comparison to white bread. A food that raises glucose half as much as white bread has a GI of 50, whereas a food that raises glucose 1½ times as much has a GI of 150.

A recent study reported in the *Archives of Internal Medicine* in November 2007 showed that a group of Chinese women who tended to eat a lot of high-glycemic index rice had a significant increase in the risk of developing type 2 diabetes. Another study in the same issue showed that increasing the level of low glycemic cereal in the diet reduced the risk of type 2 diabetes in a group of black women, a group that is getting type 2 diabetes in epidemic numbers.

The point is to select carbohydrates with low GI levels to try to keep the glucose response as low as possible. A glycemic index of 70 or more is high, 56 to 69 is medium, and 55 or less is low.

Good clinical studies have shown that knowledge of the glycemic index of food sources can be very valuable. Evaluation of the diet of people who develop diabetes compared with those who don't shows that, all other things being equal, the people with the highest GI diet most often develop diabetes. After diabetes is present, patients who eat the lowest GI carbohydrates have the lowest levels of blood glucose. Patients in these studies have not had great difficulty changing to a low GI diet. The other thing that happens when low GI food is incorporated into a diet is that the levels of triglycerides and LDL (or "bad" cholesterol) fall in both type 1 and type 2 diabetes.

Switching to low GI carbohydrates can be very beneficial for controlling the glucose. You can easily make some simple substitutions in your diet, as shown in Table 8-1.

Table 8-1	Simple Diet Substitutions
High-GI Food	*Low-GI Food*
White bread	Whole-grain bread
Processed breakfast cereal	Unrefined cereals like oats and processed low-GI cereals
Plain cookies and crackers	Cookies made with dried fruits or whole grains like oats
Cakes and muffins	Cakes and muffins made with fruit or whole grains like oats
Tropical fruits like bananas	Temperate-climate fruits like apples and plums
Potatoes	Pasta and legumes
White rice	Basmati and other low-GI rice

Because bread and breakfast cereals are major daily sources of carbohydrates, these simple changes can make a major difference in lowering your glycemic index. Foods that are excellent sources of carbohydrate but have a low GI include legumes such as peas or beans, pasta, grains like barley, parboiled rice (rice that is partially boiled in the husk, making it nutritionally similar to brown rice), bulgur, and whole-grain breads.

Even though a food has a low GI, it may not be appropriate because it is too high in fat. You need to evaluate each food's fat content before assuming that all low GI foods are good for a person with diabetes.

The position of the American Diabetes Association, stated in its position paper in 2011, is that "the use of the glycemic index may provide a modest additional benefit over that observed when total carbohydrate is considered alone."

And though a food has a high GI, it may still be acceptable in your diet if it contains very little total carbohydrate. For example, cantaloupe has a GI of about 70, but the amount of total carbohydrate is so low that it doesn't raise your blood glucose significantly when you eat a normal portion. This concept is called the *glycemic load* (GL), a number that takes both glycemic index and total carbohydrates into account. A GL of 20 is high, 11 to 19 is medium, and 10 or less is low.

If you want to go into this subject in deeper detail, you can find a listing of many foods by category of food and by level of GI, portion size, and GL on the web at www.glycemicindex.com.

Fiber

Fiber is the part of the carbohydrate that is not digestible and, therefore, adds no calories. Fiber is found in most fruits, grains, and vegetables. Fiber comes in two forms:

- ✔ **Soluble fiber:** This form of fiber can dissolve in water and has a lowering effect on blood glucose and fat levels, particularly cholesterol.

- ✔ **Insoluble fiber:** This form of fiber cannot dissolve in water and remains in the intestine. It absorbs water and stimulates movement in the intestine. Insoluble fiber also helps prevent constipation and possibly colon cancer. This fiber is called *bulk* or *roughage*.

Before the current trend to refine foods, people ate many sources of carbohydrate that were high in fiber. These sources were all plant foods such as fruits, vegetables, and grains. Animal foods contain no fiber.

Because too much fiber causes diarrhea and gas, you need to increase the fiber level in your diet fairly slowly. The recommendation for daily fiber is 20 to 30 grams. Most Americans eat only about 15 grams daily.

Many of the foods listed in the previous section as having a low glycemic index contain a lot of fiber, which helps to reduce the blood glucose.

The way to eat the right amount of carbohydrate without increasing your blood glucose or triglycerides is to make it a low-glycemic, high-fiber carbohydrate. Such a diet has been shown to reduce the need for insulin in women with gestational diabetes without any negative effect on the fetus or mother. Increased dietary fiber intake has been shown to reduce the risk of death, not only from heart and blood vessel disease but also from infectious respiratory diseases.

A multinational team of researchers, publishing in the *Nutrition Journal* in December 2014 recommends dietary carbohydrate restriction as the best way to manage both type 1 and 2 diabetes. The researchers recommend replacing carbohydrate with protein.

Portioning proteins

Excluding vegetable sources of protein like soybeans, legumes, nuts, and seeds, protein in your diet is usually the muscle of other animals, such as chicken, turkey, beef, or lamb. For this reason, people used to believe that you could build your own muscle by eating lots of another animal's muscle. (The truth is that you can build up your muscle only by exercising or weight-lifting.) You need little protein to maintain your current level of muscle (or to increase it, for that matter).

Your choice of protein is very important because some is very high in fat and some is practically fat-free. The following lists can give you an idea of the fat content of various sources of protein. (In the next section, I explain how to integrate fat into your diet.)

- **Very lean:** One ounce of very lean meat, fish, or substitutes has about 7 grams of protein and 1 gram of fat. Examples include

  - Skinless white-meat chicken or turkey

  - Flounder, halibut, or tuna canned in water

  - Lobster, shrimp, or clams

  - Fat-free cheese

- **Lean:** An ounce of lean meat, fish, or substitutes has about 7 grams of protein and 3 grams of fat. Examples include

  - Lean beef, lean pork, lean lamb, or lean veal

  - Dark-meat chicken without skin or white-meat chicken with skin

  - Sardines, salmon, or tuna canned in oil

  - Other meats or cheeses with 3 grams of fat per ounce

- **Medium-fat:** An ounce of medium-fat meat, fish, or substitutes has about 7 grams of protein and 5 grams of fat. Examples include

  - Most beef products

  - Regular pork, lamb, or veal

  - Dark-meat chicken with skin or fried chicken

- Fried fish
- Cheeses with 5 grams of fat per ounce, such as feta and mozzarella

✔ **High fat:** High-fat meat, fish, or substitutes contain about 8 grams of fat and 7 grams of protein per ounce. Examples include

- Pork spareribs or pork sausage
- Bacon
- Processed sandwich meats
- Regular cheeses like cheddar or Monterey Jack

Based on the fat, you can guess that low-fat and high-fat proteins have a huge difference in kcalories. An ounce of skinless white-meat chicken contains about 40 kcalories, whereas an ounce of pork spareribs has 100 kcalories. Because most people eat a minimum of four ounces of meat at a meal, they're eating from 160 to 400 kcalories depending on the source.

My recommendation is that 20 percent of your kcalories come from protein. This would be about 350 kcalories for the gentleman who weighs 142 pounds and needs 1,700 kcalories each day. Because a gram of protein is 4 kcalories, he can eat about 90 grams of protein. Translating that into ounces of meat, because each ounce has 7 grams of protein, he can eat about 13 ounces of meat daily. For example, he can eat 6 ounces of flounder at one meal and 5 ounces of dark-meat chicken at another, with 2 cups of milk providing the rest of his protein.

Many authorities suggest less protein in the diet because protein has a damaging effect on the kidneys. Several studies have shown this to be the case, but a very large study in the *Annals of Internal Medicine* in March 2003 came to a different conclusion. It showed that high-protein diets caused increasing damage in kidneys that already had some damage but not in normal kidneys. The jury remains out on this question of lower versus higher protein diets.

Filling the fat requirement

People with type 2 diabetes have to be very aware of the fats in their diet. Fortunately, the amount of fat you need is a lot less controversial than the carbohydrate and protein in your diet. Everyone agrees that you should eat no more than 30 percent of your diet as fats. (Currently, the US population eats 36 percent of its diet as fats.)

Keep in mind that some fats are more dangerous in their tendency to promote coronary artery disease than others. These fats should make up less of the dietary fat than the safer fats.

Cholesterol is the fat everyone knows. It has been shown to be the culprit in the development of coronary artery disease, as well as peripheral vascular disease and cerebrovascular disease (see Chapter 5). The recommendation is that no more than 300 milligrams a day of fat come from cholesterol. One egg can take care of that prescription. Most other foods that you eat regularly do not contain a lot of cholesterol, but whole milk and hard cheeses like Jack and cheddar contain saturated fat, which raises the cholesterol in the body.

You also must pay attention to foods that increase triglycerides, which lead to the production of small, dense LDL particles that are connected to coronary artery disease. Abnormal fats are one component of metabolic syndrome. Triglycerides comes in several forms:

✔ **Saturated fat** is the kind of fat that usually comes from animal sources. The streaks of fat in a steak are saturated fat. Butter is made up of saturated fat. Bacon, cream, and cream cheese are other examples. Vegetable sources of saturated fat include coconut, palm, and palm-kernel oils. Eating a lot of saturated fat increases your blood cholesterol level.

✔ **Trans fatty acid** is produced when polyunsaturated fat (which I describe in the next bullet) is heated and hydrogen is bubbled through it. Fully hydrogenated, it becomes solid fat; partially hydrogenated, it has a consistency like butter and can be used in butter's place.

Trans fatty acids may contribute more to the development of heart disease than saturated fats. Keep them out of your diet! Some examples of foods high in trans fats are some cake mixes and dried soup mixes, many fast foods and frozen foods, baked goods like donuts and cookies, potato chips, crackers, breakfast cereals (even some with seemingly health-conscious names), candies, and whipped toppings. The government now requires food labels to list trans fats, so read those labels! Fortunately, food manufacturers are increasingly removing trans fats from their products.

✔ **Unsaturated fat** comes from vegetable sources. It comes in several forms:

• **Monounsaturated fat** does not raise cholesterol. Avocado, olive oil, and canola oil are examples. The oil in nuts like almonds and peanuts is monounsaturated.

• **Polyunsaturated fat** also does not raise cholesterol but causes a reduction in the good or HDL cholesterol. Examples of polyunsaturated fats are soft fats and oils such as corn oil and mayonnaise.

Eskimos eat a lot of fat (more than is recommended), and yet they have a low incidence of coronary artery disease. It has been shown that their protection comes from *essential fatty acids.* These acids are found in fish oils, which Eskimos consume in large amounts. Essential fatty acids reduce triglycerides, reduce blood pressure, and increase the time that it takes for blood to clot, which protects against a blood clot in the heart. You can have the benefits of fish oil by substituting fish for meat two or three times a week in your diet. Pills containing fish oil have not been shown to provide the same benefit. If you don't like fish (which means you have probably never tasted salmon cooked on a barbecue), you can't get this benefit.

Keeping in mind that 30 percent of your total daily calories should come from fat, less than a third of that amount should come from saturated fats. You should also keep your dietary cholesterol under 300 milligrams per day.

For the gentleman who weighs 142 pounds and needs 1,700 kcalories, who is slowly starving waiting for his dietitian to figure out how much to feed him, his final 500 kcalories can come from fat. Fat has 9 kcalories per gram, so he can eat about 56 grams of fat daily.

Remember that he has already taken in 40 grams of fat with his flounder and chicken, so he is left with only 16 grams, 8 of which come with his milk. That leaves about a teaspoon of butter from the fat sources.

Getting Enough Vitamins, Minerals, and Water

Your diet must contain sufficient vitamins and minerals, but the amount you need may be less than you think. If you eat a balanced diet that comes from the various food groups, you generally get enough vitamins for your daily needs. Table 8-2 lists the vitamins and their food sources.

Table 8-2	Vitamins You Need	
Vitamin	*Function*	*Food Source*
Vitamin A	Needed for healthy skin, bones, and eyes	Milk and green vegetables
Vitamin B_1 (thiamin)	Converts carbohydrates into energy	Meat and whole-grain cereals
Vitamin B_2 (riboflavin)	Needed to use food properly	Milk, cheese, fish, and green vegetables

Vitamin	Function	Food Source
Vitamin B$_6$ (pyridoxine), pantothenic acid, and biotin	All needed for growth	Liver, yeast, and many other foods
Vitamin B$_{12}$	Keeps the red blood cells and the nervous system healthy	Animal foods (for example, meat)
Folic acid	Keeps the red blood cells and the nervous system healthy	Green vegetables
Niacin	Helps release energy	Lean meat, fish, nuts, and legumes
Vitamin C	Helps maintain supportive tissues	Fruit and potatoes
Vitamin D	Helps with absorption of calcium	Fortified dairy products, and made in the skin when exposed to sunlight
Vitamin E	Helps maintain cells	Vegetable oils and whole-grain cereals
Vitamin K	Needed for proper clotting of the blood	Leafy vegetables, and made by bacteria in your intestine

As you look through the vitamins in Table 8-2, you can see that most of them are easily available in the foods you eat every day. In certain situations, such as if you are pregnant, you need to be sure that you are getting enough every day, so you take a vitamin supplement. Some evidence also suggests that extra vitamin C protects against colds.

As far as the other vitamins go, the proof just does not exist that large amounts of the vitamins are beneficial, and in some cases, they may be harmful. I do not recommend that you take megadoses of these vitamins.

Minerals are also key ingredients of a healthy diet. Most are needed in tiny amounts, which are easily consumed from a balanced diet. Keep the following in mind:

- ✔ **Calcium, phosphorus, and magnesium build bones and teeth.** Milk and other dairy products provide plenty of these minerals, but evidence suggests that people are not getting enough calcium. Adults should get 1,000 milligrams of calcium every day, and you should get 1,500 milligrams if you are growing up (adolescents) or out (pregnant women). Older people must be sure to eat 1,500 milligrams a day. Increased magnesium in the diet has a protective role in the development of type 2 diabetes.

✔ **Iron is essential for red blood cells and is gotten from meat and some nuts, legumes, and vegetables.** However, a menstruating woman tends to lose iron and may need a supplement.

✔ **Sodium regulates body water.** You need only about 220 milligrams a day, but you likely take in 20 to 40 times that much, which probably explains a lot of the high blood pressure in the United States. Because hypertension is so prevalent in both types of diabetes and it makes diabetic complications occur earlier, reduction of salt intake is an important consideration. Don't add salt to your food (it already has plenty in it), and you will enjoy the taste a lot more without it.

✔ **Chromium is needed in tiny amounts.** No scientific evidence shows that chromium is especially helpful to the person with diabetes in controlling blood glucose, despite reams of articles in health food magazines to the contrary.

✔ **Iodine is essential for production of thyroid hormones.** It is added to salt in order to assure that people get enough of it. In many areas of the world where iodine is not found in the soil, people suffer from very large thyroid glands known as *goiters*.

✔ **Various other minerals, like chlorine, cobalt, tin, and zinc, are found in many foods.** These minerals are rarely lacking in the human diet.

Water is the last important nutrient I discuss in this section, but it is by no means the least important. Your body is made up of 60 percent or more water. All the nutrients in the body are dissolved in water. You can live without food for some time, but you will not last long without water. Water can help to give a feeling of fullness that reduces appetite. In general, people do not drink enough water. Men need to get a minimum of 13 cups, or 104 ounces whereas women need 9 cups, or 72 ounces, of water a day from all sources (that is, from all the foods and liquids you ingest) according to the Institute of Medicine, the health arm of the National Academy of Sciences.

Counting Alcohol as Part of Your Diet

Alcohol is a chemical that has calories but no particular nutritional value; although it has been shown that a moderate amount (a glass or two of wine a day) may reduce the risk of a heart attack. Notice that I call alcohol a *chemical*. That's because alcohol is often taken to excess and does major damage to the body. It wrecks the liver and can lead to bleeding and death.

This book is not the place for a discussion of the social issues that surround the use of alcohol. Suffice it to say that excess alcohol destroys lives and families. In this section, I want to explain the part that alcohol plays in the life of the person with diabetes.

Because alcohol has calories, if you drink some, you must account for those calories in your diet. The proof of the alcohol is the percentage of alcohol in an ounce of the drink multiplied by 2. Wine that is 12.5 percent alcohol is 25 proof. Beer is around 12 proof most of the time. Liquor is often 80 proof. To determine the calories, use the following formula:

Calories = 0.8 × proof of the drink × number of ounces

For example, for a 12-ounce can of beer, you use the formula 0.8 × 12 × 12 for a total of 115 kilocalories. For a couple of 6-ounce glasses of wine, you use the formula 0.8 × 25 × 12 to come up with 240 kilocalories. You can see that the alcohol calories add up pretty quickly. You may even wonder why alcoholics are not often overweight. The answer is that alcohol becomes a staple of their diet and they develop wasting diseases associated with inadequate intake of protein, carbohydrate, fat, vitamins, and minerals.

In addition to the calories, alcohol plays other roles in diabetes. If alcohol is taken without food, it can cause low blood glucose by increasing the activity of insulin without food to compensate for it. Some alcoholics, even without diabetes, go to bed with several drinks in their systems and are unconscious the next morning because of very low blood glucose. They can have brain damage unless their bodies are able to manufacture enough glucose to wake them up.

If you're having a couple glasses of wine or other alcohol, make sure that you eat some food along with it.

A study in *Diabetes Care* in 2009 confirmed previous research findings that moderate alcohol intake (two glasses of wine daily for men and one glass for women) was protective against diabetes while more than that was harmful.

Using Sugar Substitutes

Fear of the "danger" of sugar in the diet has led to a vast effort to produce a compound that can add the pleasurable sweetness without the liabilities of sugar. Interestingly enough, despite the availability of a number of excellent sweeteners, some containing no calories at all, the incidence of diabetes continues to rise. See the section "Considering Total Calories First" earlier in this chapter for reasons why artificial sweeteners may not help diabetes. Sweeteners are divided into those that contain calories and those that do not.

Among the calorie-containing sweeteners are the following:

- **Fructose, found in fruits and berries:** Fructose is actually sweeter than table sugar *(sucrose)*. However, the body absorbs it from the intestine more slowly than glucose, so it raises the blood glucose more slowly. The liver takes it up and converts it to glucose or triglycerides.

- **Xylitol, found in strawberries and raspberries:** Xylitol is about like fructose in terms of sweetness. It is taken up slowly from the intestine so that it causes little change in blood glucose. Xylitol doesn't cause cavities of the teeth as often as the other sweeteners containing calories, so it is used in chewing gum.

- **Sorbitol and mannitol, sugar alcohols occurring in plants:** Sorbitol and mannitol are half as sweet as table sugar and have little effect on blood glucose. They change to fructose in the body. (If you read Chapter 5, you may remember sorbitol. When taken as a food, sorbitol doesn't accumulate or damage tissues.)

Sweeteners are often much sweeter than table sugar. Therefore, much less of them is required to accomplish the same level of sweetness as sugar. Following are some of the current sweeteners:

- **Saccharin:** This sweetener is 300 to 400 times sweeter than sucrose. It's rapidly excreted unchanged in the urine. Brand names include Sweet'N Low and Sugar Twin.

- **Aspartame:** This sweetener is more expensive than saccharin, but many people seem to prefer its taste. It's 150 to 200 times sweeter than sucrose. The brand name is Equal when used as a tabletop sweetener or NutraSweet when used in food and beverages.

- **Acesulfame:** This sweetener is 200 times sweeter than sucrose and does not leave an aftertaste. It can be used in cooking and is found in numerous foods and beverages. Its brand name is Sunett or Sweet One. It should not be used by people with a rare genetic disorder called phenylketonuria.

- **Sucralose:** This sweetener is obtained from sugar and is 600 times sweeter. It is very stable and can be used in place of sugar in any food. It leaves no unpleasant aftertaste. The brand name is Splenda.

- **Neotame:** Authorized by the FDA in July 2000, neotame has 7,000 to 13,000 times the sweetening power of sucrose. It isn't in commercial products yet, but food manufacturers are working with it because it can be used cooked or uncooked with no loss of sweetening. The brand name isn't yet determined.

✔ **Cyclamate:** Because it has been associated with cancer when given in huge doses, cyclamate is banned in the United States. It's 30 times as sweet as sucrose. The association with cancer has not been substantiated.

✔ **Tagatose:** Tagatose is a naturally occurring sweetener present in small amounts in fruits and dairy products. The FDA has recognized tagatose as safe. It can be purchased at most health food stores. It has about the same sweetening power as table sugar and is called Naturlose.

✔ **Stevia:** This sweetener is derived from the stevia plant, native to South America. It's marketed as SweetLeaf Stevia. It is 150 to 400 times sweeter than sugar and can be used in cooking and baking.

For people with diabetes, recommendations regarding using sugar have been changed so that some sugar is permitted. The point is to count the calories eaten as sugar and subtract that from your permissible intake. If you do this calculation, you'll have little use for either the nutritive or the non-nutritive sweeteners.

Eating Well for Type 1 Diabetes

A person with type 1 diabetes takes insulin (see Chapter 11) to control blood glucose. At this time, doctors and their patients can't match the human pancreas in the way that it releases insulin just when the food is entering the bloodstream so that the glucose remains between 80 and 120 mg/dl. Therefore, diabetic patients need to make sure that their food enters as close to the expected activity of the insulin as possible. This book is most concerned with type 2 diabetes, so I refer you to my book *Type 1 Diabetes For Dummies* (John Wiley & Sons, Inc.) for a thorough discussion of food and insulin treatment in type 1 diabetes.

Reducing Your Weight

Because most people with type 2 diabetes are overweight, weight control and reduction should be the major consideration. The benefits of weight loss are rapidly seen, even when relatively little has been lost. The blood glucose falls rapidly. The blood pressure declines. The cholesterol falls. The triglycerides drop, and the good cholesterol (HDL) rises. As I point out in Chapter 5, even a modest reduction of 10 percent of body weight has a significant positive effect on coronary artery disease.

In addition to the many other benefits, weight loss also results in significant improvement in obstructive sleep apnea.

Weight reduction is difficult for many reasons. In my experience, most patients do very well initially but tend to return to old habits. A study in *Cell Metabolism* in 2013 suggests that this tendency to regain weight is built into the human brain. When fat tissue is decreased or even increased, a central control system in the brain acts to restore the fat to the previous level by releasing a chemical called *neuropeptide,* which signals to the body that it's in starvation mode, and the body starts storing as much energy as possible. If liposuction is done, for example, the remaining cells swell up to hold more fat.

In Chapter 10, I cover the value of exercise in a weight-loss program. At this point, you need to realize that successful maintenance of weight loss requires a willingness to make exercise a part of your daily life. A recent study showed that 92 percent of people who maintain weight loss exercise regularly, while only 34 percent of those who regain their weight continue to exercise. If, for some reason, you cannot move your legs to exercise, you can get a satisfactory workout using your upper body alone.

Types of nutritional plans (NP)

The numerous methods that are available for weight loss certainly suggest that no one method is especially better than all the rest. Some are fairly drastic in the degree to which they cut calories, and weight loss is fairly rapid. But these methods are particularly prone to result in restoration of the original weight. Among the many more drastic diets are the following:

- ✔ **Very-low-calorie NP:** These plans provide 400 to 800 kcalories daily of protein and carbohydrate with supplemental vitamins and minerals. They are safe when supervised by a physician and are used when you need rapid weight loss — for example, for a heart condition. They result in rapid initial weight loss with a fall in the need for medications. Weight restoration commonly occurs, however.

- ✔ **Animal-protein NP like the Atkins:** Food is limited to animal protein sources in an effort to maintain body protein, along with vitamins and minerals. Carbohydrates are strongly discouraged. Patients often complain of hair loss. Weight is rapidly regained when the plan is discontinued. This plan isn't balanced, and I don't recommend it for more than a few weeks. Because the Atkins NP encourages foods that are high in fats, a variation called the *South Beach Diet* was developed that emphasizes decreased carbohydrates along with decreased fats.

- ✔ **LEARN NP:** The name stands for lifestyle, exercise, attitudes, relationships, and nutrition. It recommends a diet of 55 to 60 percent carbohydrate and less than 10 percent from fat.

- ✔ **Fasts:** A *fast* means giving up all food for a period of time and taking only water and vitamins and minerals. A fast is such a drastic change from normal eating habits that patients don't remain on the fast for very long, and weight is regained.

- ✔ **DASH NP:** The Dietary Approach to Stop Hypertension was designed to lower blood pressure. It consists of lean meat, poultry, and fish; whole grains; fruits and vegetables; dairy; and legumes, nuts, and seeds. High-salt foods and foods rich in saturated fats are out.

Several nutritional plans are associated with large organizations and may require that you purchase only their foods. The support given by these organizations seems to be extremely helpful in weight-loss maintenance. In addition, the slower loss of weight and the connection to more normal eating seems to result in a greater tendency to stay with the program and keep the weight off. Following are the leading contenders for this type of plan:

- ✔ **Jenny Craig:** This organization provides the food that you eat, which you must pay for. It offers some information on behavior modification and has special diets for people with diabetes. In 1997, the government required Jenny Craig to tell its customers that the weight-loss methods may be only temporary, because customers had no way to judge from its advertising that many people regain their weight.

- ✔ **Weight Watchers:** This organization emphasizes slow weight loss, exercise, and behavior modification. It charges for weekly attendance at its meetings, which are held all over the world. It doesn't require that you purchase any products, but Weight Watchers foods are available for purchase. Its point program for increasing fiber in your diet may be especially helpful to the person with diabetes.

The National Weight Control Registry, which has been running since 1993, shows that people can lose a lot of weight and keep it off. The average loss is 60 pounds and is maintained for more than five years. These "losers" do it on their own half the time. They use a combination of a low-fat diet and at least 45 minutes of exercise daily, usually walking, to keep the weight off, even though the initial weight loss was accomplished in many different ways such as a liquid diet in an organized program, other types of organized programs, or on their own. Most of them (68 percent) eat breakfast every day. The longer they kept the weight off, the easier it became to continue weight maintenance.

Vegetarian plans

Time and again vegetarian NP have been shown to reduce the risk of type 2 diabetes and to improve all aspects of the disease when diabetes is already present. Increasing the daily intake of green leafy vegetables has been especially helpful.

A report in *Diabetes Care* in 2009 looked at the diets of 60,000 men and women. The mean body-mass index was lowest in vegans (no dairy), higher in lacto-ovo vegetarians (who ate dairy and eggs), still higher in vegetarians who ate fish, and highest in nonvegetarians. The prevalence of type 2 diabetes was lowest in the vegans and rose with the mean BMI so that it was highest in the nonvegetarians. The risk of metabolic syndrome was also found to be lowest in the vegans and rose with increased meat eating. Vegans may need to add additional vitamin B12.

Consider shifting your diet in the direction of more vegetables and less animal protein. The benefits may be huge.

Mediterranean NP

Since the fourth edition of *Diabetes For Dummies* came out, a number of studies have indicated that a Mediterranean diet may be beneficial in the prevention and treatment of diabetes. In this new edition, I provide some of the rationale for that type of diet. You can also find ten new recipes from some of the finest Mediterranean restaurants in the country in the Appendix.

The first big study confirming the benefits of the Mediterranean diet was published in the *Archives of Internal Medicine* in December 2007. It showed a significant reduction in deaths from all causes. More recently, in a study published in the *Annals of Internal Medicine* in January 2014, patients who followed a Mediterranean diet supplemented with extra-virgin olive oil had a significant reduction in the onset of diabetes compared to a control group who were just given advice on a low-fat diet. Another study, published in *Diabetologica* in December 2013, confirmed the advantages of the Mediterranean diet. These are just a few of the many studies pointing to the effectiveness of the Mediterranean diet in preventing or managing diabetes.

The Mediterranean diet emphasizes the following:

- ✔ Plant-based foods such as fruits and vegetables, whole grains, legumes, and nuts
- ✔ Olive oil in place of butter or margarine

- ✔ Herbs and spices to flavor foods instead of salt

- ✔ Red meat no more often than twice a month

- ✔ Fish and/or poultry twice a week

- ✔ Alcohol in moderation (5 ounces of red wine daily for all women and men older than 65 years and 10 ounces for men younger than 65)

To start on this diet without moving to Greece, here are some suggestions:

- ✔ Make sure that most of your meal and snacks consist of fruits and vegetables, preferably unprocessed and whole. If you eat bread or cereal, make sure that it's whole grain. The same is true for rice and pasta.

- ✔ Skip butter and use olive oil on bread or pasta instead. *Tahini* (blended sesame seeds) is another great alternative to butter.

- ✔ Eat a handful of almonds, cashews, pistachios, and walnuts for a delicious snack.

- ✔ Add herbs and spices to flavor your foods.

- ✔ Grill or bake fish instead of frying or breading it. Especially good for you are tuna, salmon, trout, mackerel, and herring, fresh or in cans.

- ✔ If you eat dairy, opt for low-fat options like skim milk, fat-free yogurt, and low-fat cheese.

Refer to *Mediterranean Diet For Dummies* and *Mediterranean Diet Cookbook For Dummies* both by Meri Raffetto and Wendy Jo Peterson (John Wiley & Sons, Inc.) for more information.

The food that you find in Italian chain restaurants across the United States is not Mediterranean food. They use a lot of butter, full-fat cheese, cream sauce, meat, and white-flour pasta among other non-Mediterranean foods. So, don't think you're eating Mediterranean just because the restaurant serves pasta.

Metabolic surgery for diabetes

Metabolic surgery has been so successful in preventing and reversing diabetes that many surgeons and diabetes specialists consider diabetes a surgical disease. This surgery is so promising that I devote Chapter 9 to it.

Drugs available for weight loss

The US FDA has lately approved three oral drugs and one injectable for weight loss. They are approved for adults with a BMI of 30 or greater or a BMI of 27 or greater who have high blood pressure, type 2 diabetes, or high cholesterol.

These drugs aren't benign. If you don't accomplish some significant weight loss within 12 weeks, discontinue taking them. Make sure that your physician carefully monitors you. I have tried many different weight loss drugs in my medical practice and have never been satisfied by their effectiveness long term. I don't recommend them.

These drugs should be combined with lifestyle modification:

- **Lorcaserin (Belviq):** Approved in June 2012, it produced at least a 5 percent weight loss in 38 percent of patients with type 2 diabetes compared to 16 percent of patients given a placebo. It can cause headache, dizziness, and fatigue as well as low blood sugar.

- **Phenteramine and topiramate extended-release (Qsymia):** Approved in July 2012, it was associated with an average weight loss of 6.7 percent in 62 percent of patients (not diabetic) compared to 20 percent who received placebo after a year. It can raise the heart rate and increase the risk of birth defects (avoid taking it if you're pregnant). It also causes tingling of the hands and feet, dizziness, and constipation.

- **Naltrexone and bupropion extended release (Contrave):** Approved in September 2014, it produced a weight loss of at least 5 percent in 36 percent of patients with type 2 diabetes compared to 18 percent taking placebo. It may be associated with suicidal thoughts and behaviors as well as seizures. It raises blood pressure and heart rate. It also causes nausea, headache, and vomiting in some patients.

- **Liraglutide injection (Saxenda):** Approved in December 2014, it produced a weight loss of at least 5 percent in 49 percent of patients with type 2 diabetes compared to 16 percent of patients treated with placebo. Some serious side effects have occurred including pancreatitis, gall bladder disease, kidney disease, and suicidal thoughts. It also increases heart rate and may cause nausea, diarrhea, and vomiting as well as low blood glucose.

Behavior modification

From my years of working with obese patients, I've seen that weight loss requires more than a commitment to a sound diet and routine exercise; it requires changes in behavior with respect to food. To lose weight and keep it off, you must change your eating behavior to make your diet easier to follow. Following are some of the best techniques:

✔ Eat according to a schedule to avoid unplanned eating.

✔ Find a single place to eat all food. (Don't eat in front of the TV.)

✔ Slow down your eating to make the meal last.

✔ Put high-calorie foods away. Remove serving dishes and bread from the table.

✔ Don't dispense food to others to avoid exposure for yourself.

✔ Leave some food on your plate.

✔ Set realistic goals for weight loss. (A reasonable rate is ½ to 1 pound per week.)

✔ When eating out, be careful of salad dressing, alcohol, and bread. Share a meal.

✔ Get a ten-pound weight and carry it around for a while to appreciate the importance of losing even that little.

✔ At the market, buy from a list, carry only enough money for the food on that list, and avoid aisles containing loose foods like candy (loose fruits and vegetables are okay, though).

✔ Eat off a salad plate (a visual cue to cut portion sizes).

Incorporate one technique into your life each week (or even longer) until you feel you have mastered it and have added it to your eating style. Then go on and take up another technique.

As you go about this difficult task of losing weight and keeping it off, remember to seek the help of those around you. A loving partner provides great help through the roughest days.

In an effort to lose weight, some people with diabetes skip their insulin shots. If you do so, your body will turn to fat for fuel because glucose can't be used (see Chapter 2), and you will lose weight. However, the result is that you also lose muscle mass and your blood glucose rises very high. This situation is dangerous and not a healthy approach to weight loss.

Coping with Eating Disorders

You can't be too rich or too thin. How much damage has this statement done to society, especially the *thin* part? Young people, particularly girls, are preoccupied with their body weight. When this preoccupation becomes too great, it can result in an eating disorder.

The dangers of anorexia and bulimia

Young girls have eating disorders about ten times as often as young boys do. They either starve themselves and exercise excessively or eat a great deal and then induce vomiting and/or take laxatives and water pills. Someone who starves herself has *anorexia nervosa,* whereas someone who binges and purges has *bulimia nervosa.* By themselves, these conditions can result in severe illness and even death when carried to extremes. When combined with diabetes, the danger increases greatly.

Here are some of the clues that someone has one of these disorders:

- ✔ She eats by herself.
- ✔ She feels guilty or disgusted after overeating.
- ✔ She eats more rapidly than others do.
- ✔ She eats until uncomfortably full.
- ✔ She eats large amounts of food even when she is not hungry.

Anorexia is usually found in middle- and upper-class girls. They have a distorted body image and are fearful of weight gain. The prevalence may be as high as 1 in 200 in these girls. Their parents are usually very concerned with slimness. The girls may appear unusually thin and do not menstruate. Their malnutrition may be so severe that they die from it.

People with anorexia are in a constant state of starvation. When they have diabetes, their condition is just like that of people with type 1 diabetes before the availability of insulin. They have very low blood glucose levels, so little or no insulin is required (see Chapter 10). They develop problems with their hearts and have low blood pressure and low body temperature. They lose a lot of body musculature after the fat is gone.

People with severe anorexia may require intravenous feeding until they are stabilized a little bit, which sometimes leads to very high blood glucose levels, necessitating the use of insulin. After the life-threatening starvation is under control, good blood glucose control can be achieved with help from the patients themselves and from therapists who can help them understand their distorted body image. If the patient suffers from clinical depression, antidepressant medication may be necessary.

Bulimia involves eating large quantities of easily digested food and then purging it by vomiting and taking laxatives or water pills. These patients are usually not as severely thin as patients with anorexia. However, their backgrounds are often similar to those of anorexia patients: They may represent up to 40 percent of college-age female students. Because their weight is closer to normal, they usually menstruate normally.

Bulimia has a negative effect on diabetes because management of diabetes requires a certain amount of routine from day to day. There is no way to achieve such systematization when the amount of food coming into the body is so uncertain. However, food intake in bulimia is less severe than that in anorexia, so blood glucose levels do not fluctuate as much in this case.

However, people with bulimia are more likely to go on to adult obesity and are harder to treat psychologically. They actually do not do as well with therapy as those with anorexia, and they end up with more psychiatric problems later in life.

Sources of help

A major source of useful information is the National Eating Disorders Association. The association's website, www.nationaleatingdisorders.org, contains extensive information on this subject of eating disorders. You also call its help hotline at 800-931-2237.

The National Association of Anorexia Nervosa and Associated Disorders provides information online, including referrals to support groups, therapists, and treatment centers, at www.anad.org. You can also contact the association through the website or by calling 630-577-1330.

Chapter 9

Metabolic Surgery: A Possible Cure for Type 2 Diabetes

The first operations for obesity and diabetes were performed more than 60 years ago. In recent years more than 200,000 such operations have been performed each year with amazing results for people with type 2 diabetes. Yet most of the population with diabetes is unaware of surgery's great value. The purpose of this chapter is to begin to correct that oversight.

Metabolic surgery doesn't cure all cases of type 2 diabetes. Some people who have had diabetes for a long time and already have the complications that I describe in Chapter 5 possibly won't benefit. But many people will benefit and they should have the opportunity to decide if metabolic surgery is right for them. You can find everything you need to know to make that decision in this chapter.

Metabolic surgery that I discuss in this chapter is generally recommended for type 2 diabetes, but the patient who has type 1 diabetes with overweight or obesity may benefit as well.

Looking at the history of metabolic surgery

Viktor Henrikson, MD, performed the first operation for severe obesity in Sweden in 1952 when he recognized that some patients who had part of their small bowel removed had lost significant amounts of weight and improved other medical problems including blood pressure. He removed a large segment of the small bowel of a woman who was obese and couldn't follow a weight loss program. Unfortunately the patient didn't lose weight, but this operation opened the door.

In 1954, A. J. Kremen, MD, at the University of Minnesota performed a jejunoileal bypass in which a large segment of the small intestine was bypassed to reduce absorption of food. Others tried similar operations in the 1960s, but they were associated with serious complications. Other operations suffered from similar problems until 1966 when Edward E. Mason, MD, of the University of Iowa developed the gastric bypass, which divided the stomach into a small pouch that was connected to the small intestine and a large part of the stomach that was bypassed by food. In 1977, Ward Griffen, MD, introduced the Roux-en-Y configuration to make the gastric bypass more technically feasible. There have been many modifications since.

The next major development was the adjustable gastric band, which began as a non-adjustable band in 1978, and became an adjustable band by 1989. The FDA first approved it in 2001. The sleeve gastrectomy operation was also developed in the late 1980s. The introduction of laparoscopic procedures for metabolic surgery in this century has made the surgery almost routine.

Thus metabolic surgery has a long history, and it's surprising that more diabetic patients have not yet benefited from it.

Realizing the Benefits of Metabolic Surgery

Metabolic surgery has been so successful in preventing and reversing diabetes that many surgeons and diabetes specialists consider diabetes a surgical disease. The surgery leads to marked and long-lasting weight reduction. When the effects of metabolic surgery are compared with standard (nonsurgical) care, the results are unequivocal.

The next sections introduce you to the benefits of surgery over medical treatment for type 2 diabetes with respect to weight loss, cost, and more.

Comparing surgery versus medical weight loss

As Chapter 8 discusses, most diets don't work. When you start to diet, your brain goes into starvation mode and tries to keep you at the original weight.

A study in the *New England Journal of Medicine* in October 2011 provides the physiological basis for this. Your body begins to secrete hormones that favor weight regain. These hormones were increased not just at the tenth week when the diet ended but at 62 weeks. So you don't just regain your weight, but you actually gain more. You regain not simply because you have resumed poor eating habits but also because your body prefers to remain at the higher weight. So stop blaming yourself for regaining the weight.

A study published in *Diabetes Care* in December 2014 confirms the failure not just of diet but of the usual care of type 2 diabetes, namely diet, exercise, and drugs to promote a remission of the diabetes. In this study, 122,781 adults with type 2 diabetes were evaluated.

- A *complete remission* was defined as a year of normal blood glucose levels with a hemoglobin A1c less than 5.7 percent.
- A *partial remission* was defined as blood glucose levels less than diabetic but not normal with a hemoglobin A1c between 5.7 and 6.4 percent.
- *Prolonged remission* is complete remission for five or more years.

Only 2.8 percent of patients managed to achieve any remission, .14 percent of patients had a complete remission, and only .04 percent achieved a prolonged remission.

Considering costs

Unfortunately having diabetes is expensive. A study by the Centers for Disease Control and Prevention in the *American Journal of Preventive Medicine* in August 2013 indicated that a man diagnosed with type 2 diabetes who is between the ages of 25 and 44 will incur related costs of $124,700 over his lifetime whereas a woman will incur costs of $130,800 over her lifetime. Half of that cost results from the treatment of complications of diabetes that I describe in Chapters 4 and 5. In contrast, the average cost for metabolic surgery for diabetes is much cheaper at $22,000 in 2013.

Of course, the monetary costs represent only a small part of the cost of having diabetes. The psychological, social, and emotional costs are enormous. The reduction in the quality of life and the length of life is a major factor. The possibility of blindness, kidney failure, nerve disease with pain, and limitation of motion as well as heart attacks, strokes, and amputations are constant for a person with diabetes especially as he or she ages.

Two studies, the Diabetes Control and Complications Trial for type 1 diabetes and the Diabetes Prevention Program for type 2 diabetes, have shown that controlling the blood glucose for even a few years has major benefits 15 or 20 years later in the prevention of complications of diabetes. Even though metabolic surgery doesn't cure everyone, it's reasonable to expect that even a few years of improved glucose control can have substantial benefits in the long run. Consider the benefit for a person who had to take insulin and is now free of injections, even if he isn't cured of his diabetes.

Contemplating the other benefits

If you have always wanted to play the piano or dance the samba, don't expect metabolic surgery to bring about either one although you may feel so good and motivated by the results of surgery that you're up to doing both. You may encounter a number of healthy changes brought on by successful metabolic surgery. Here are some of them:

- Sleep apnea will improve and may disappear.
- Snoring will improve and may disappear.
- High blood pressure will disappear or greatly improve so you don't need medications.
- High abnormal blood fats will improve, and you may be able to stop medications.
- Gastroesophageal reflux with heartburn will improve or disappear.
- Metabolic syndrome, which leads to heart attacks, will improve.
- Asthma will improve.
- Arthritis will improve.
- Women who have a history of infertility due to polycystic ovarian syndrome (see Chapter 6) may become fertile after surgery. Avoid pregnancy for the first 24 months after surgery when weight loss continues.
- Abnormal liver function tests will improve.
- Early diabetes complications may reverse or at least not worsen.
- If you have little or no sexual activity before surgery, your enhanced physical and mental function after surgery as well as your increased feeling of attractiveness will probably lead to much more sexual activity after surgery if you so desire.

Considering Surgery over Traditional Diabetes Care

You may think of surgery as a radical treatment for diabetes. These sections should convince you that it isn't. In the hands of an experienced surgeon, it's no more complicated than a gallbladder operation, which has become routine. It compares favorably with what is considered both usual care and intensive care for diabetes.

Realizing that surgery is a safe option

Metabolic surgery obviously is major surgery. In the past, some deaths have been associated with it, although today deaths rarely occur. The bottom line is that it's a safe surgery.

A *meta-analysis* (a study that looks at many other studies that must incorporate strict criteria to be included) of 164 studies that was published in *JAMA Surgery* in December 2013 makes this clear. It included 161,756 patients. The conclusion was that it is both effective and safe. The mean reduction in BMI was from an initial 46 prior to the surgery to between 29 and 34 five years after the surgery. Within the first 30 days after surgery, the mortality rate was 0.22 percent and after 30 days it was 0.35 percent. This is a low rate, and when compared with the mortality rate if no surgery is done, it is relatively safe. It carries a complication and mortality rate comparable to some of the safest and most commonly performed surgeries in the United States including gallbladder surgery, appendectomy, and total knee replacement.

Comparing metabolic surgery and usual care

Medical care for diabetes can be divided into *usual care,* the kind you get from your internist or family physician and *intensive care,* the kind you get from a diabetes specialist. This section compares surgery with usual care and shows the advantage of surgery.

- A study in the *New England Journal of Medicine* in August 2012 showed that metabolic surgery can prevent type 2 diabetes. In the study, 1,658 obese patients who had metabolic surgery were matched with 1,771 obese patients who had usual care and followed for 15 years. Type 2 diabetes developed in 392 of the usual care group but only 110 in the metabolic surgery group. One point that the authors made is that the development of diabetes after the surgery was dependent on the presence of impaired fasting glucose and not the BMI before the surgery. (I discuss this point in greater depth in the later section, "Considering New Guidelines for Surgery." In other words, those individuals with prediabetes and not the heaviest individuals became diabetic.

- ✔ Another study published in November 2014 in *Lancet Diabetes and Endocrinology* followed more than 2,100 obese adults who had metabolic surgery and the same number who didn't. After up to seven years, those individuals who had surgery were 80 percent less likely to develop diabetes than those who didn't.

- ✔ A meta-analysis published in the *British Medical Journal* in October 2013 concluded that metabolic surgery leads to greater body weight loss and higher remission rates compared to usual care. They noted both improvement in quality of life and reduction in medication use.

Focusing on metabolic surgery and intensive care

Numerous studies have compared the results of metabolic surgery and intensive care for people who have diabetes. *Intensive diabetes care* is a much greater level of care than usual care. Studies that compare surgery with intensive diabetes care use a level of care that generally isn't found outside a research facility.

By the time you have a diagnosis of type 2 diabetes, you may have already had it for five years or longer. Studies that describe patients who have had diabetes for two or three years are actually describing patients who have had it for seven or eight years.

Here are a few of the results, comparing patients treated with surgery to those managed with intensive care:

- ✔ A paper in the *Annals of Surgery* in October 2013 followed 217 surgical patients for at least five years. The mean hemoglobin A1c fell to 6.5 percent from 7.5 percent whereas the fasting blood glucose went from 156 mg/dl to 114 mg/dl. Twenty-four percent of patients had a long-term complete remission whereas 26 percent had a partial remission. Thirty-four percent improved and only 16 percent remained unchanged. There was a 60 to 80 percent improvement in low high-density lipoprotein, high low-density lipoprotein, high triglycerides, and high blood pressure. Fifty-three percent showed improvement in kidney disease whereas 47 percent showed stabilization.

- ✔ Research from the Cleveland Clinic released at the 30th annual meeting of the American Society of Metabolic and Bariatric Surgery in 2013 showed a 40 percent lower risk of heart attacks and a 42 percent lower risk of strokes among 131 patients who underwent metabolic surgery and were followed for more than six years. In addition, 45 percent had a lower risk of developing kidney disease.

✔ A study of 120 patients published in the *Journal of the American Medical Association* in June 2013 compared metabolic surgery with intensive medical care. After 12 months, 28 surgical patients and 11 intensive care patients achieved a hemoglobin A1c of less than 7 percent, low-density lipoprotein levels of less than 100 mg/dl, and systolic blood pressure less than 130. Surgical patients required three fewer medications than intensive medical patients.

✔ A study published in the *New England Journal of Medicine* in March 2014 compared metabolic surgery to intensive medical care in diabetic patients who were followed for three years. The target hemoglobin A1c was 6 percent or less, which was achieved in 38 percent of the surgical group but only in 5 percent of the intensive therapy group. The best predictor for success was duration of diabetes of less than eight years.

✔ A study published in January 2015 in the *Journal of the American Medical Association* looked at 2,500 obese adults with or without diabetes. After 10 years, the death rate for those individuals who had surgery was 14 percent compared to 24 percent for those who didn't.

The evidence would seem to be overwhelming. Metabolic surgery prolongs life and causes diabetes remissions or at least a significant reduction in the severity of the diabetes. But the story isn't all gravy (pardon the pun). Some studies indicate that some patients who go into remission have a relapse after surgery.

For example, a study in *Obesity Surgery* in January 2013 showed that 68 percent of type 2 diabetic patients who were either uncontrolled or medication-controlled went into remission by five years after gastric bypass (see the "Choosing the Operation" later in this chapter for more information), but about 35 percent relapsed within five years of the initial remission. Those who relapsed were the patients with poor initial control, insulin use, and longer duration of diabetes. The authors agreed that the earlier the surgical intervention, the greater the durability of remission of the type 2 diabetes.

Getting Familiar with Guidelines for Surgical Candidates

Metabolic surgery isn't for everyone. When you have surgery for obesity, you must be committed to lifelong medical follow-up. You must be willing to give up large meals and be determined to lose weight. These sections examine the specific guidelines for you to review before talking about surgery with your doctor.

Eyeing medical determinants

In 1991 the National Institutes of Health published the indications for the appropriateness of metabolic surgery. Unfortunately these indications had very little basis in scientific evidence. Nevertheless, insurance companies have based their willingness to pay for the surgery on these criteria. The result is that many patients who should have surgery have been denied because they didn't fit these criteria:

- ✔ Any patient with a body mass index (BMI) greater than 40 (see Chapter 3 for an explanation of BMI).

- ✔ Patients with a BMI of 35 or greater who have another medical condition such as type 2 diabetes, high blood pressure, heart disease, severe joint disease, or obesity-related severe psychological problems when less invasive methods of weight loss have failed.

- ✔ Metabolic surgery can result in substantial weight loss and is an available option for well-informed and motivated patients so the surgery is limited to patients who are acceptable operative risks.

- ✔ Patients opting for surgery should be followed by a multidisciplinary team so patients should find such a team.

- ✔ Lifelong medical surveillance after surgery is a necessity so patients who don't recognize the need for this should be excluded.

Noting psychological determinants

Most surgical programs also insist on a number of psychological determinants in addition to the physical determinants. They include the following:

- ✔ The individual needs to demonstrate adherence to recommendations by attending appointments, practicing self-monitoring with recordkeeping, making time for healthy eating and activity, taking medication, and completing blood work.

- ✔ The individual must have an understanding of the benefits and limitations of a surgical procedure to assist with management of his obesity.

- ✔ The risks of surgical intervention must not be excessive and must be lower than the risks of not providing the treatment.

- ✔ If psychological disorders such as depression are present, they won't necessarily prevent surgery, but they need to be treated.

Knowing who shouldn't have surgery

Not every person who needs the surgery can have it. These are some of the current criteria that exclude the operation:

- ✔ BMI less than 35
- ✔ Age less than 18 or greater than 65
- ✔ A medical condition that makes surgery too risky
- ✔ Clinically significant or unstable mental health concerns
- ✔ Unrealistic expectations for surgery
- ✔ A history of poor compliance with lifestyle, medical, or mental health interventions
- ✔ Pregnant, breast-feeding, or planning a pregnancy within two years of surgery
- ✔ Smokers (must quit at least eight weeks before surgery) — all smokers must participate in smoking-cessation programs after surgery.

I discuss the validity of these criteria in the later "Considering New Guidelines for Surgery" section.

Choosing the Operation

A number of operation choices are available, all of which are considered safe. Some are more effective than others. The following sections describe a few of the most common.

They're divided into restrictive operations and malabsorptive operations. The *restrictive operations* reduce the food you can eat but don't interfere with your absorption of food. The *malabsorptive operations* interfere with the absorption of food by your intestines. All the operations are done *laparascopically,* which means the surgeon makes very small incisions in your abdomen and inserts long, slender operating instruments through these incisions.

As a result, you have much less postoperative discomfort and recover faster compared to an operation where your abdomen is opened. An even newer type of operation is single incision laparoscopic surgery. The surgeon makes a single incision through the belly button, avoiding the four to five incisions of traditional laparoscopic surgery. There is a better cosmetic result, faster recovery, and less pain.

The three operations that I discuss in the following sections tend to be the most commonly performed at the Bariatric Centers of Excellence. A number of other types of metabolic surgery have been developed including bilio-pancreatic diversion with or without duodenal switch, vertical banded gas-troplasty, jejunoileal bypass, and others. These other operations have been associated with short-term and long-term complications, particularly lack of absorption of key vitamins and minerals. However, if the more common oper-ations aren't successful for one reason or another, these other operations may be considered as a next step.

Adjustable gastric banding (AGB)

The adjustable gastric banding (AGB) is a restrictive operation. An adjust-able band is placed close to the top of your stomach, creating a small upper pouch and a much larger lower pouch. The normal stomach is about the size of a football. The small upper pouch is the size of a golf ball. The upper pouch can hold very little food. You get full quickly, and your feelings of hunger disappear when the pouch is full. In addition, a nerve called the *vagus* nerve runs along the stomach. The band squeezes the nerve when the pouch is full, sending a signal to your brain to stop eating.

The band is connected via a tube to an injection port under the skin. A salt solution inflates the band to the extent needed to promote sufficient weight loss.

Patients who have AGB tend to lose less weight than those who have a mal-absorptive procedure. However, to lose weight, you must follow a strict diet. Christine Ren-Fielding, MD, of the New York University Langone Weight Management Program has published a study of 100 people with diabetes who have had AGB. Forty percent had complete remission of their diabetes, 40 percent had improvement, and 20 percent had no change or worsened after five years. Improvement correlated with the amount of weight lost.

Advantages of AGB include the following:

- ✔ It induces excess weight loss of 40–50 percent.
- ✔ It involves no cutting of the stomach or rerouting of the intestines.
- ✔ It requires a shorter hospital stay, usually less than 24 hours.
- ✔ It's reversible and adjustable.

✔ It has the lowest rate of postoperative complications.

✔ It has the lowest rate of vitamin and mineral deficiencies.

Here are the disadvantages:

✔ The patient experiences slower weight loss.

✔ More patients fail to lose 50 percent of excess weight.

✔ It leaves a foreign object in the body.

✔ It has the highest rate of reoperation.

Roux-en-Y gastric bypass (RYGB)

The Roux-en-Y gastric bypass (RYGB) is mostly a restrictive procedure but has some malabsorption associated with it. The stomach is stapled to create a small upper pouch totally closed off from the larger lower pouch. The upper pouch is attached to the small intestine so that the upper third of the intestine is bypassed, resulting in some malabsorption. The larger lower part of the stomach empties into the intestine, but no food can get to it so only digestive juices flow through it.

Anita Courcoulas, MD, of the University of Pittsburgh Medical Center reported that patients who had a RYGB operation had a 27 percent weight loss compared to 17 percent for those who had AGB. In the later section, "How the surgery works," I show the benefit of RYGB compared to vertical sleeve gastrectomy (VSG) and AGB. RYGB may be the operation of choice for the person with type 2 diabetes who has had it longer and it isn't well controlled.

RYGB has these advantages:

✔ Long-term weight loss is significant, up to 60 percent.

✔ Favorable changes in intestinal hormones occur.

The disadvantages include

✔ It's the most complicated of the surgeries.

✔ It may result in vitamin and mineral deficiencies.

✔ It has a longer hospital stay.

Vertical sleeve gastrectomy (VSG)

VSG is another restrictive operation. The stomach is divided so that the part left in the patient is a tube that isn't much wider than the intestine into which it empties, about 25 percent of the size of the original stomach. The operation results in an early feeling of fullness similar to the AGB that I describe previously. The other part of the stomach is removed, and absorption isn't affected.

A study published in the *Journal of Visceral Surgery* in April 2013 compared the effects of AGB, RYGB, and VSG in terms of weight loss and postoperative complications and death with 26,558 operations evaluated. The conclusion was that VSG is midway between AGB and RYGB. The weight loss is less than RYGB but more than AGB. Complications and death are less than RYGB but more than AGB. Despite the fact that VSG doesn't cause as much weight loss as RYGB, sleeve gastrectomy has become the most popular method of weight loss surgery in the United States, surpassing laparoscopic gastric bypass, which had been the most common procedure for decades, as of November 2014. In 2013 in the United States, VSG accounted for 42.1 percent of the bariatric procedures performed, followed by gastric bypass (34.2 percent), gastric band (14 percent), and others (1 percent).

VSG may be best in the earlier stages of diabetes. Five years after VSG only 10 percent of patients with more severe diabetes taking insulin were still in remission, whereas 59 percent of those taking oral antidiabetic drugs were in remission and 81 percent of those who were about to develop diabetes but not yet on drugs hadn't developed the disease. This was the case even though the severe diabetics lost as much weight from the operation as the less severe cases.

Advantages of this surgery include

- There is rapid and significant weight loss.
- There is no foreign body or rerouting of the intestine.
- It has a brief hospital stay of two days.
- Favorable changes in intestinal hormones reduce hunger.

Some of the disadvantages are

- It's not reversible.
- Long-term vitamin deficiencies may occur.

The longer an individual has type 2 diabetes, the more resistant he or she is to remission.

How the surgery works

The restrictive operations, AGB and VSG, work by simply reducing your food intake so that you lose weight over time. In addition, your vagus nerve is compressed earlier than usual. There is no change in the way food travels through your stomach and intestines. With the combined restrictive and malabsorptive operation, RYGB is different. After RYGB, patients rapidly lower their glucose and require less or no medications, even before the large weight loss occurs.

A study published in *Diabetes Care* in August 2013 helps to explain the different effect of RYGB. Sixty patients with uncontrolled type 2 diabetes (a mean hemoglobin A1c 9.7) were divided into three groups of 20. One group had intensive medical therapy (IMT). A second group had IMT plus RYGB. A third group had IMT plus VSG. They were tested at the beginning of the study and at 12 and 24 months. At 24 months, the mean hemoglobin A1c was 6.7 for RYGB, 7.1 for VSG, and 8.4 for IMT. BMI fell 0.2 for IMT, 8.7 for RYGB, and 8.2 for VSG. Although the weight loss was about the same for the two surgeries, loss of *truncal fat,* the fat that is believed to cause insulin resistance, which can lead to diabetes, was much greater for the RYGB group. Insulin sensitivity increased by 2.7 fold for the RYGB, but only 1.2 for the VSG, and it didn't improve after IMT. RYGB restored normal beta-cell function (see Chapter 3), but VSG and IMT didn't.

The explanation for the better effect of RYGB is probably because this operation, unlike VSG or IMT, causes dramatic changes in hormones that promote normal pancreatic function. These changes are greater for RYGB than they are for VSG. It's also possible that the food restriction after surgery explains the improvement although you would expect it to be the same for both surgeries.

Preparing for Surgery

Prior to having surgery, you need to do a number of things. These sections tell you all you need to know and do.

Finding the right surgeon

The key to a successful outcome is to find the right surgeon and the right surgical program. You can find both in an accredited Bariatric Center of Excellence (COE). *Bariatrics* is the branch of medicine that treats obesity.

To become a COE certified hospital, a hospital must go through a rigorous reporting process and inspection and perform a minimum of 140 bariatric surgical procedures each year. Two institutions do the inspections, collect data, and accredit hospitals: The American Society of Metabolic Surgeons and the Surgical Review Corporation. To find a COE, check out www. surgicalreview.org/locate/.

COE must go through rigorous training including the following courses and others:

✔ Obesity sensitivity training

✔ Proper moving of an obese patient

✔ Recognizing the signs and symptoms of bariatric surgery complications

✔ Post-op care of the bariatric patient

✔ Bariatric surgery post-op nutrition

Getting ready for surgery

After your surgeon has determined that surgery is right for you, you must take a number of steps to get ready. Most COE have you do the following:

✔ Attend an information session.

✔ Organize your medical records for your physical and nutrition assessment.

✔ Meet with a psychologist.

✔ Obtain a nutritional assessment with a dietitian.

✔ Schedule a consultation with one of the surgeons.

Furthermore, you have a bunch of blood tests taken, both as a baseline to see the changes that surgery brings and screening to make sure that your tests are what they are expected to be. The tests will probably not be normal, but shouldn't be too abnormal. Your doctor will review the tests with you to clarify your condition before surgery.

In addition to the usual tests such as a hemoglobin A1c, cholesterol, and triglyceride panel, electrolytes (sodium, potassium, chloride, and CO_2), and a serum chemistry profile (glucose, calcium, liver function, and kidney function), you should have a vitamin D test, a vitamin B12 test, a folate test, a total iron, and iron binding capacity. These latter tests represent the nutrients that you may need to take after the surgery if you don't absorb enough of them. These tests should be repeated at every three to six months for the first year and annually after the surgery throughout your life.

Identifying Short-Term and Long-Term Complications of Surgery

If you have metabolic surgery, you need to know what to expect if a problem should occur. Although the instances of problems are low, they still do occur occasionally, both just after surgery and long after surgery. The latter problems are mostly due to failure to take in enough of the vitamins and minerals that are essential to health and tend to occur more after malabsorption procedures than restrictive procedures. These sections examine the short-term and long-term problems associated with metabolic surgery.

Managing your medications after surgery

You have probably been on some potent medications for your diabetes and other medical problems prior to surgery. The rapid fall in weight requires that you adjust or discontinue your medications immediately after surgery. Obviously you do so with the help of your physician, but you need to make sure that the correct changes are made. See Chapter 11 for more information concerning these medications. Here are some of the recommended changes based on the medication you are taking:

✔ Stop taking sulphonylureas. If not, you'll probably develop hypoglycemia.

✔ Discontinue metformin, but your physician may add it back if your fasting blood glucose continues to be elevated after surgery.

✔ Stop drugs in the class DPP-4 inhibitors, drugs with names like Januvia, Onglyza, Tradjenta, and Nesina.

✔ Discontinue drugs in the class GLP-1 analogs such as Byetta, Bydureon, Victoza, Tanzeum, and Trulicity.

✔ Stop rapid-acting insulin.

✔ Reduce the dose of long-term insulin (Levimir and Lantus) by half and discontinue it if your blood glucose drops into the hypoglycemic range.

✔ Check your blood pressure and reduce or eliminate blood pressure drugs if your blood pressure is low or you're dizzy. Check with your doctor before doing so. Blood pressure usually drops within a month of surgery.

✔ Have your cholesterol checked and reduce or eliminate drugs that you're taking for it in consultation with your doctor.

Make sure that you monitor your blood glucose after surgery. You should probably do it every four hours until it stabilizes at a normal level of less than 100 mg/dl in the fasting state or 140 mg/dl after eating.

Listing short-term problems

Short-term complications can arise from any metabolic surgery and include the following:

- Internal bleeding that mostly stops spontaneously but occasionally requires reoperation
- Infection
- Blood clots in the legs that can travel to the heart and lungs
- Leaks after surgery, where tissue has been sewed together, which are suggested by a sustained rapid heart rate, rapid breathing, and fever
- Partial collapse of the lungs

Noting long-term problems

Certain long-term complications are common to all three types of metabolic operations. Complications that are common to all include

- Nausea or vomiting
- Excess or loose skin
- Small bowel obstruction with symptoms that include abdominal bloating, cramping, pain, nausea, and vomiting
- Stomach ulcers with pain, nausea, or vomiting and intolerance to foods

Each surgery also has its own long-term complications.

- With AGB, the band can slip or cause erosions. Although the average rate of band slippage is only 5 percent, if it slips, it can result in obstruction so no food can pass, resulting in nausea, vomiting, heartburn, and excessive weight loss.
- You may also experience leakage of the fluid in the band, causing the band to loosen so you have an initial feeling of fullness as the stomach is filled but rapid tolerance of more solid food and weight gain.

✔ You may also suffer from a nighttime cough after AGB.

✔ RYGB has complications peculiar to it. There can be closure of the opening through which food passes as a result of scar formation. Loss of tolerance to both solid and liquid food will follow. There can be an enlargement of the small opening between the two stomach parts so the patient tolerates more solid food and no longer loses weight. Also there is a condition called *dumping syndrome* when food and fluid pass into the small intestine too fast. Early symptoms include nausea, vomiting, stomach pain, diarrhea, and a feeling of fullness. Late symptoms due to low blood sugar include sweating, weakness or dizziness, nervousness, and the other symptoms of low blood sugar described in Chapter 4.

Other rare but possible complications can include instances of inadequate intake of key vitamins and minerals that can occur much later after surgery in months or years. You can experience a deficiency in any of the following, along with their expected symptoms:

✔ **Iron:** These symptoms due to anemia begin with feeling weak or tired and problems concentrating. Later the patient experiences brittle nails, pale skin, shortness of breath, and sore tongue. Iron deficiency is prevented by taking iron supplements as suggested by your doctor along with extra vitamin C, which promotes iron absorption.

✔ **Vitamin D and calcium:** Your doctor can discover this deficiency through a bone densitometry study, which may show bone loss. To avoid bone loss, take 2,000 international units of vitamin D daily plus 1,500 mg of calcium.

✔ **Vitamin B12:** This deficiency can cause symptoms of anemia similar to iron deficiency, but if present for a long time, you can get nerve damage including confusion, dementia, depression, poor balance, and numbness and tingling of the hands and feet

✔ **Folic acid:** This deficiency can cause fatigue, gray hair, ulcers in the mouth, and a swollen tongue.

✔ **Vitamin A:** This deficiency can cause loss of tearing of the eyes, loss of nocturnal vision, and decreased immunity.

Adhering to the recommendations of the COE is essential for your follow-up to surgery. Blood tests can detect them. With the exception of vitamin D and calcium, you can usually prevent vitamin deficiencies by taking two multivitamins daily.

Eating Properly and Exercising after Surgery

Success after surgery depends on your willingness to eat and exercise appropriately. The surgery can help you a great deal, but it's up to you to follow the recommendations of the nutrition counselor and an exercise trainer. These sections discuss eating and exercising after your surgery.

Focusing on nutrition after surgery

You can do a lot to help the weight loss when it comes to what you eat. Here are suggestions that can make the process much easier for you:

- Drink only fluids for the first few weeks after surgery. A *fluid* is anything you can drink through a straw.
- After you're eating solid foods, eat three small meals plus two small snacks daily. Check with a dietitian for an understanding of small meals.
- Choose mostly solid foods.
- Take no more than one cup of solid food at a meal.
- Chew food well and eat slowly so you feel full.
- Don't eat textures that are hard to chew like tough meats, stringy vegetables, and soft and doughy breads.
- Avoid fluids within 30 minutes of solid foods.
- Consume beverages between meals and snacks.
- Avoid carbonated beverages.
- Avoid foods with lots of added sugar.

Comprehending why you may gain weight

It's possible to gain weight despite these surgeries. Some reasons may be an indication of surgical failure, inappropriate eating behaviors, or psychological complications. As a result, you need to continue with nutrition and activity counseling as well as long-term medical management. If you believe that you're doing everything right, you may need to see the surgeon to verify that the operation is still working. Some of the reasons you may gain weight include the following:

✔ Increased intake of calories

- Due to consuming liquids within 30 minutes of solid food

- Due to a slow rate of eating so you don't feel full

- Adaptation to feeling full over time

- Consuming carbonated beverages that stretch the pouch

✔ Eating high calorie foods

✔ Eating larger meals five times or more daily

✔ Consuming high caloric beverages

✔ Decreasing activity

✔ Decreased metabolic rate due to age, decreased muscle mass, or medication

✔ Changes in mental health that affect your lifestyle

Exercising before and after surgery

Exercise is an essential part of success after metabolic surgery. Patients who exercise sufficiently not only lose more weight but also show greater improvement in blood glucose and hemoglobin A1c. Exercise must be measured objectively and developed with your doctor so that both of you are in full agreement. These sections can help you start on the right foot.

What the patient records

Part of the initial evaluation prior to surgery is taking a history of exercise. Most patients report that they do exercise before surgery and report a substantial increase after surgery. However, when exercise is measured objectively, what the patient reports isn't nearly often accurate. When patients are given a pedometer (which counts steps) prior to surgery, most are found to do less than 5,000 steps daily, a level that is considered sedentary. Sufficient physical activity is 10,000 steps daily. Using another device called the SenseWear armband, researchers found that patients spent 80 percent of their time sedentary prior to surgery while the general population spends only 65 percent sedentary.

When patients are asked to record their exercise after metabolic surgery, researchers note the same discord between reported and actual exercise. Patients report an increase of 100 to 500 percent in their exercise. If the patient wears an objective-measuring device, no increase in physical activity or even a decrease is found in patients who aren't given an exercise program after surgery. Postoperative patients were found to accumulate only 23 minutes per week of moderate-to-vigorous physical exercise.

What exercise accomplishes

A program called Bari-Active showed that preoperative face-to-face counseling with a personal trainer for 45 minutes three times a week resulted in better weight loss and decreased percentage of body fat compared to usual care alone.

Another study of RYGB and AGB patients after surgery compared patients treated with dietary counseling to those with dietary counseling plus an exercise program. After 12 weeks, the exercise group showed improved objectively measured fitness and better blood glucose levels after meals even though the two groups didn't differ in weight reduction or food intake. The briefness of the study may be the reason the exercise group didn't show more weight loss.

Even though Bariatric Center Network requirements state that all patients should receive exercise counseling after surgery, only 22 percent of patients of accredited programs report that they have been counseled.

Some physicians may be reluctant to recommend physical activity prior to surgery. However, the Department of Health and Human Services activity guidelines state "adults with chronic conditions obtain important health benefits from regular physical activity; when adults with chronic conditions do activity according to their abilities, physical activity is safe."

Based on the evidence, most sports and health organizations recommend that healthy and overweight or obese individuals do at least 60 minutes of moderate-intensity physical activity per day (refer to Chapter 10 for more information).

These are some of the reasons to begin physical activity before metabolic surgery:

- ✔ Better aerobic fitness may help reduce surgical complications, improve healing, and expedite postoperative recovery.

- ✔ Preoperative counseling teaches the patient that metabolic surgery is associated with positive behavior changes.

- ✔ If addressed early, barriers to physical activity after surgery are diminished.

- ✔ Success in preoperative physical activity leads to success in postoperative physical activity.

Developing your exercise plan

You need to work with your metabolic surgery team to develop a program that you're willing to do and the team believes is beneficial.

The American College of Sports Medicine recommends that patients with current symptoms or history of metabolic, cardiac, or pulmonary disease be referred to a cardiologist for an evaluation including a graded exercise test to minimize the risk of injury, stroke, and/or heart attack before starting a moderate to vigorous intensity exercise program.

Feeling dull aches at the beginning of an exercise program means that increased blood is flowing into muscles causing swelling or microtears in the muscle or connective tissue. This generally resolves with time.

There are many different types of exercise (see Chapter 10), including aerobic exercise, strength training, and flexibility exercises. All are important, but the greatest benefit comes from aerobic exercise, which improves heart and lung function after metabolic surgery.

For aerobic exercise to be productive, do at least 10 minutes if possible, six times a day, or 60 minutes, which is optimal for daily exercise. Guidelines recommend that you exercise every day, so make it part of your daily life. The more time you're moving and the less time you spend in front of the TV or the computer, the better for your health.

Choosing the right activity for you is very important because it encourages you to stick with it. Walking may be the best choice, but if you have pain or a physical limitation, cycling or an elliptical trainer may be better. Swimming or water aerobics may be even better for the person with joint pain.

There may be many barriers that prevent you from exercising. Here are some of them and how you may overcome them:

- **Lack of confidence in your ability:** You may overcome it by working with a trainer to whom you explain your limitations.

- **Excessive fatigue:** You may address it by beginning with low-level exercises and shorter exercise periods as you work your way up to longer exercise periods.

- **Pain with activity:** The pain diminishes if you choose classes that are designed for people with limitations or exercise in the pool.

- **Fear of injury:** Start at low activity levels or in a swimming pool.

- **Lack of belief in your ability to meet exercise guidelines:** Start slow and build up slowly as you improve.

Discuss with your doctor the type, duration, frequency, and intensity of physical activity. Set up a timeframe for achieving more vigorous levels of activity and also determine a level at which you can comfortably remain so that you're physically fit without injury. You need to use an objective measure such as a pedometer to check your accomplishments. If you're going to do strength training, work with a trainer to set goals and use the equipment properly. Make sure that you follow up in person or on the phone with your clinician at regular intervals both to show that you're improving your fitness and to set new goals.

If you do weight training, don't lift more than 5 to 10 pounds for the first four weeks after surgery.

Along with your new weight, becoming physically fit by exercising before and after metabolic surgery makes a huge difference in your health, your self-esteem, and your appearance.

Hearing from Real Patients

The patients in this section are all real. Their names and any identifying features have been changed to protect their privacy. They have willingly and generously offered their stories in order to provide you with the experiences of people who have gone through it so you can see for yourself what to expect.

Patient GM

GM is a 47-year-old teacher whose type 2 diabetes was diagnosed in 1996. He remembers being overweight as a child and as a teenager. His parents and grandparents were all normal in weight. He is an only child. Although his parents didn't encourage him to eat excessively, his grandparents did. He feels that he made many bad food choices as he grew up. He did some running, biking, and climbing as a child.

In 1996, he suffered through a serious of setbacks and life changes when his father died, he married, and he started his career. At that time, he started eating much more food than before and his weight increased significantly. His exercise declined after he fell on some ice and ruptured two discs in his back.

Over the years he has made many attempts to lose weight, but the weight never stayed off. In 1991, he tried an all-liquid diet, for six months and lost 60 pounds, but rapidly regained the weight when he returned to regular eating patterns. He weighed 230 pounds on his six-foot-two frame even after the weight loss. He tried portion control and a modified Atkins diet without success. He never took diet pills because he had sleep apnea and was taking pills to help him sleep. The diet pills would have worked against sleep.

In 2004 he heard about the gastric band and actually had the surgery. At the time there was only one size and it was not right for him. It didn't allow the passage of any food through his stomach. The band was removed a few weeks after it had been put in place.

He took multiple pills for his diabetes including metformin, glyburide, and sitagliptin. In addition, he took simvastatin for his cholesterol. He didn't have to take medication for his blood pressure. He also suffered from sleep apnea and used a CPAP machine to treat this.

In 2013, he discovered that the gastric band was now adjustable and decided to try to have the surgery again. By that time his weight was up to 358 pounds. His hemoglobin A1c ran between 9.8 and 10.1 for the previous five years although the addition of sitagliptin reduced it to 7.7. After speaking to several surgeons, he decided that the gastric sleeve operation, which would be permanent, would be a better choice. He had the surgery at New York University in April 2014. At the time, he was completely confident that this operation would work for him.

The surgery went well although at first he had difficulty swallowing. He remained in the hospital for two days. For the first four to six months after the operation, he suffered from nausea and vomiting about three times a week. He was told that this would improve as the sleeve stretched, and it did. It now occurs two to three times a month depending on what he eats.

In the year after the surgery, he lost 158 pounds and now weighs 200 pounds. He has stopped all medications for diabetes and for his cholesterol. His hemoglobin A1c is 5.1. He has continued to use the CPAP machine, but is getting a sleep study to see if he needs it anymore. He is an avid scuba diver, does yoga, and rides bicycles.

GM says he doesn't think about food, although he never did. He doesn't eat between meals. He has chosen not to make use of support groups. He is now investigating plastic surgery to remove some of the stretched skin from his heavier days. He is delighted with the results of surgery.

Patient MS

MS is now 32 years old. She believes that she began to gain weight when she was in the third grade when a cousin died. At 18, she had no menstrual periods and lost hair. Her doctor diagnosed her with polycystic ovarian syndrome (refer to Chapter 6). She was found to be prediabetic with insulin resistance and placed on metformin and birth control pills. She was extremely anxious and depressed.

In 2006 at the age of 23, when she was 292 pounds at five-feet-five, she began to try to lose weight, accompanying her diet with a great deal of exercise. She had a personal trainer, attended a weight loss program, and worked out seven days a week, including spin classes, boxing classes, jogging, and boot camp. She was able to lose 120 pounds in a year, but put it back on in 18 months.

At age 28 she was put on Byetta followed by Victoza, both injections to promote weight loss, but she had side effects and came off them. She was never on pills for blood pressure or cholesterol. She took Meridia, a pill for weight loss, but didn't lose weight.

She didn't date, thinking that it wasn't an option for her. At age 29 she had a terrible experience related to her weight loss that convinced her to do something. She is an elementary school teacher. One of the students, not in her class, was having trouble. Just at that time she went to lunch with several of the teachers and the principal. The mother of the student happened to be at the restaurant and took a picture of the group, thinking they were discussing her child. She published the picture on Facebook. Others added their comments, one of which was "the teacher on the left (MS) probably eats her students." This comment convinced MS to do something that she considered radical at the time — surgery for her obesity — although now she considers it conservative.

MS had a friend who had been successful with metabolic surgery three years earlier. MS tried to find a surgical program and discovered the New York University program through a friend's co-worker.

She went to the introductory program at NYU and discovered that it probably has the world's most experience with metabolic surgery. She was able to relate to the chief surgeon, who, himself, had the surgery years before. She went thinking the gastric sleeve surgery was right for her, but later came away believing that the adjustable gastric band (AGB) was better for her needs.

About 18 months ago she had the AGB surgery. It took a total of about an hour. She was discharged the next day because her surgery was postponed until 7 p.m. After surgery, she had nausea that responded to medications.

Since the surgery, she has lost half of her weight and now fluctuates around 150 pounds. She had a problem with kidney stones a year after surgery and was found to be anemic. She hadn't been taking her vitamins. The anemia corrected when she did take them.

She now dates frequently and has lost most of the anxiety that she had since age 18. She has come off the metformin and the birth control pills. Two months ago, when she stopped the birth control pills, she had her first menstrual period since age 18, which suggests that her polycystic ovarian syndrome along with her insulin resistance and prediabetes is under control without medications.

Her opinion of metabolic surgery has radically altered. She encouraged her mother to undergo the surgery and wants others to know the surgery is life altering and life enhancing.

Patient MP

Patient MP is a 68-year-old physician who has had type 2 diabetes since 2000. He was slim until he started medical school at age 22 and then began to gain weight. He reached his maximum weight of 350 pounds in 2004. He is 6 feet tall. MP loses weight when he is depressed. One of his children died at a year old in 1975, and he lost a great deal of weight then. Three others of his children developed cancer at age 5 and he lost weight each time but regained all of it thereafter. Those three children and three others are fine now.

His parents were never obese, and his father is living and well at age 94. He has one brother and two sisters, none of whom are obese or have had diabetes.

MP has tried all kinds of weight loss programs including starvation, Weight Watchers, a medically supervised dietary supplement, and diet pills with little result. He has never significantly exercised. He never experienced any single traumatic incident that convinced him to have surgery.

He hasn't had complications of diabetes, such as eye disease, kidney disease, nerve disease, or heart disease. Prior to surgery, he required insulin injections to control his diabetes. Since surgery, he is off insulin, but he must take diabetes pills for control. His last hemoglobin A1c was 5.8. Prior to surgery he took two pills for his blood pressure, but now needs only one. He took a pill (a statin) for his cholesterol before surgery and continues to take it, although he is uncertain he needs it.

Before his surgery he had sleep apnea. He required removal of the uvula in his mouth to reduce his snoring, but the apnea continued. The surgery cured his sleep apnea.

In the course of his medical practice he met a bariatric surgeon and was impressed by the results of metabolic surgery. This surgeon recommended the NYU Bariatric program to him. He had his surgery, an adjustable gastric band, in 2002. The surgery went well, and he was discharged the next day. Over the next two years, his weight dropped to 180 pounds and has stabilized between 190 and 210.

Since the surgery, MP has had a single kidney stone, but he's unsure if it was related to the surgery. He also had low blood iron but no anemia, and supplements of iron made the iron level normal.

He finds that he can't eat much meat because it's too dense and gets stuck in his small stomach pouch when he does eat it. He must chew his food very well.

MP makes full use of the adjustable feature of the gastric band. When he is about to go on vacation, he has it loosened so that he can eat more normally. When he returns, he has it tightened. He refers to this as a band break. He did the same thing recently when he had to have a total knee replacement. Rather than bother the nurses and the hospital with his special needs, he had his band loosened, ate normally in the hospital, and had it tightened when the surgery was finished.

He is convinced that he should have had the surgery much earlier. It might have made it possible to stop all or at least more of the pills that he still takes.

Considering New Guidelines for Surgery

Until some medication becomes available that can cure type 2 diabetes, surgery is the only treatment that can cure diabetes at this time. Unfortunately, the criteria for selecting patients, developed in 1991, and still used by insurance companies for authorizing surgery (see the section "Getting familiar with guidelines for surgical candidates" earlier in this chapter) weren't based on scientific evidence and haven't been brought up-to-date. Doctors know a lot more about who should have the operation, who can benefit most, when the operation should be done, and which operation will work best for which patient.

Researchers and doctors still have a lot to learn, but here are some of the factors that should be considered:

- Medical management is unlikely to cause a remission of type 2 diabetes.
- The earlier the surgery is done in the course of diabetes, the more likely there will be a persistent cure. In the Swedish Obese Subjects study, 47 percent of newly diagnosed patients treated with surgery remained in remission after 15 years but only 9 percent of patients who had diabetes more than three years remained in remission after 15 years.

✔ The severity of glucose intolerance, not the BMI, should determine the need for surgery. A group of patients with poorly controlled type 2 diabetes underwent RYGB. Eighty-eight percent had a complete remission and the diabetes didn't return during a six-year follow-up. BMI may be elevated by large amounts of muscle. The distribution of the excess fat determines whether it will cause medical problems.

✔ Some patients with advanced diabetes don't do well with surgery. If complications are present and established, surgery may not help.

✔ The best operation for early diabetes is probably VSG. The AGB may also be used.

✔ The best operation for more advanced diabetes is probably RYGB.

Recognizing these facts, in 2012 Interdisciplinary European Guidelines were published that stated, "Patients with type 2 diabetes with BMI greater than or equal to 30 and less than 35 may be considered for bariatric surgery on an individual basis, as there is evidence-based data supporting bariatric surgery benefits in regards to type 2 remission or improvement."

Two studies in the *Journal of the American Medical Association* in 2014 showed that people with a BMI between 30 and 35 lost far more weight (as much as 50 pounds) and achieved greater improvement in hemoglobin A1c compared to patients treated intensively without surgery, and that people with a BMI between 30 and 40 who had RYGB were five times more likely to reach their metabolic treatment goals than lifestyle patients.

A study of patients treated with AGB surgery reported at the International Diabetes Federation world congress in December 2013 from Australia confirms the value of surgery at lower BMIs. Type 2 diabetes patients with a BMI of 25 to 30 who received a laparoscopic gastric band achieved significantly greater weight loss (11 kilogram versus 1 kg) and significantly higher rates of remission (52 percent versus 8 percent) than did those treated with standard medical care. The surgical patients who didn't have a complete remission also required much less medication to reduce their hemoglobin A1c. All surgical patients on insulin were able to stop it while many standard care patients had to intensify treatment. In addition, the quality of life was greatly improved in the surgical patients. All patients had their diabetes for less than five years.

Given the high cost of lifelong type 2 diabetes and the fact that early surgical treatment leads to many more lifelong remissions than standard care or later treatment, it's in the interest of insurance companies to spend a little more up front to save thousands later on, not to mention the advantages to the patient.

Therefore, I offer the following recommendations for metabolic surgery:

✔ All patients with type 2 diabetes who are acceptable candidates for metabolic surgery and have a BMI of 25 or greater should be offered metabolic surgery, which should be paid for by insurance if the patient has insurance. Because the Asian population develops diabetes at a lower BMI, their cutoff should be a BMI of 23.

✔ Patients who have had diabetes for three years or less (really eight years because most patients have the diagnosis made after five years) should be offered VSG or AGB. This recommendation is subject to change if research shows that patients do just as well with this surgery if they have had it for four years or if three years is too long to wait. It is also subject to change if one or the other of these surgeries is clearly found to be superior.

✔ Patients who have had diabetes for more than three years should be offered RYGB.

✔ All surgeries should be done at a Bariatric Center of Excellence by a surgeon who has extensive experience with the recommended surgery.

✔ The US government or one of its subsidiaries should launch a major program to establish many more Bariatric Centers of Excellence and train many more surgeons to begin to get this epidemic under control.

My recommendations are based on the best currently available research and may change as new information is presented or published.

Chapter 10

Creating Your Exercise Plan

In This Chapter

▶ Understanding the importance of exercise

▶ Tailoring exercise for type 1 and type 2 patients

▶ Determining how long and how hard to exercise

▶ Picking an activity you like

*I*n the Standards of Medical Care in Diabetes 2015, the American Diabetes Association makes the following recommendations:

✔ Adults with diabetes should perform at least 150 minutes each week of moderate-intensity aerobic physical activity (50 to 70 percent of maximum heart rate), spread over at least three days per week, with no more than two consecutive days without exercise.

✔ In the absence of a medical reason not to, adults with diabetes should perform resistance training that involves all muscle groups at least twice per week.

✔ Adults older than 65 should follow the physical guidelines if possible and if not possible, be as physically active as able.

✔ All individuals, including those with diabetes, should limit the amount of time being sedentary by breaking up extended amounts of time (greater than 90 minutes) sitting.

If your time is limited, you don't have to set aside an hour daily to do your physical activity, although that amount would be best. Since the last edition of this book, numerous studies have suggested that many other approaches to exercise can greatly improve control of type 2 diabetes and prevent prediabetes from turning into diabetes. Here are some of the best approaches:

✔ Doing just two 20-second sprints (high intensity) on an exercise bike three times a week has been shown to prevent type 2 diabetes and to lower the blood glucose if diabetes is present.

✔ Doing one minute of high-intensity exercise followed by one minute of rest, performed for 20 minutes (for a total of 10 minutes of intense exercise), three times a week, dropped average blood glucose levels from 137 mg/dl to 119 mg/dl.

✔ Using a pedometer to ensure a minimum amount of daily walking may reduce your chance of getting diabetes by half.

In this chapter, you discover why exercise is important, how much and what kinds you need to do to make a difference, and which specific exercises are best for you.

Getting Off the Couch: Why Exercise Is Essential

More than 80 years ago, the great leaders in diabetes care declared that diabetes management has three major aspects:

✔ Proper diet

✔ Appropriate medication

✔ Sufficient exercise

When the diabetes experts wrote their recommendations for proper care, the isolation and administration of insulin had just recently begun, and they were focusing specifically on how to control type 1 diabetes. Since that time, many studies have shown that exercise doesn't normalize the blood glucose or reduce the hemoglobin A1c (see Chapter 7) in type 1 diabetes. Many other studies have shown that exercise *does* normalize blood glucose and reduce hemoglobin A1c in type 2 diabetes. A study published in *Diabetes Care* in March 2012 showed that resistance exercise is associated with more prolonged reductions in blood glucose than aerobic exercise in type 1 diabetes.

Although exercise can't replace medication for the type 1 diabetic, its benefits are crucial for patients with both types of diabetes. Even modest physical activity may cancel out the adverse impact of diabetes on the heart and blood vessels.

The major aspects for diabetes management described here came before the advent of surgery for diabetes beginning in the 1950s as I describe in Chapter 9.

Recent evidence has shown that it isn't just necessary to exercise but that spending too much time in sedentary activities is detrimental to your health. That is the reason for the new recommendation to limit sedentary time. Get up every 90 minutes and move around. Or get yourself one of those new standing desks.

Preventing macrovascular disease

The major benefit of exercise for both types of diabetes is to prevent *macrovascular disease* (heart attack, stroke, or diminished blood flow to the legs). Macrovascular disease affects everyone, whether they have diabetes or not, but it's particularly severe in people with diabetes. Exercise prevents macrovascular disease in numerous ways:

- Exercise helps with weight loss, which is especially important in type 2 diabetes.
- Exercise lowers bad cholesterol and triglycerides, and it raises good cholesterol.
- Exercise lowers blood pressure.
- Exercise lowers stress levels.
- Exercise reduces the need for insulin or drugs.
- Exercise reduces C-reactive protein, a cause of heart and blood vessel disease in diabetes (see Chapter 7).

Providing other benefits

In addition to its major benefits in the prevention of macrovascular disease, exercise provides a number of other very important benefits:

- Exercise has been shown to improve pancreatic beta-cell function, the very cells that produce insulin.
- Exercise is medicine for the brain. It stimulates the production of nerve cells, which prevent loss of memory, improve thinking, and enhance judgment.
- Higher levels of physical activity at midlife are associated with exceptional health among women at age 70 or older.
- Increased physical activity prevents weight gain as you age and weight regain if you diet.

✔ Exercise, even without weight loss, reduces the risk of diabetes.

✔ Higher levels of physical activity before pregnancy or in early pregnancy significantly lower the risk of gestational diabetes.

Taking charge of your health

John Plant is a 46-year-old male who has had type 1 diabetes for 23 years. He takes insulin shots four times daily and measures his blood glucose multiple times a day. He follows a careful diet.

Prior to developing diabetes, he was a very active person, participating in vigorous sports and doing major hiking and mountain climbing. At the time of his diagnosis, his doctor warned him that he would have to give up many of the most strenuous activities because he would never know his blood glucose level and it might drop precipitously during heavy exercise. He ignored this advice and continued his active way of life. He found that he could do with much less insulin than his doctor prescribed and rarely became hypoglycemic. He has been able to continue these activities without limitation. His blood glucose level is generally between 75 and 140. His last hemoglobin A1c was slightly elevated at 5.7 (see Chapter 7). A recent eye examination showed no diabetic retinopathy (see Chapter 5). He has no significant microalbuminuria in his urine and no tingling in his feet (see Chapter 5).

Is John lucky? You bet he is. But like most "luck," his is based on a self-realization that the human body is made up of both a mind and a body. If humans were meant to spend their lives munching potato chips in front of a TV set, why would they have all these muscles?

When a new diabetic patient enters my office, I give him a bottle of 50 pills. I instruct him not to swallow the pills but to drop them on the floor three times daily and pick them up one at a time. The condition a person is in can be judged by which thing he or she takes two at a time: pills or stairs.

To take charge of your own health, check out the many health resources that I have gathered at www.dummies.com/extras/diabetes.

Understanding your body mechanics during exercise

The feeling of fatigue that occurs with exercise is probably due to the loss of stored muscle glucose.

With exercise, insulin levels in nondiabetics and people with type 2 diabetes decline because insulin acts to store and not release glucose and fat. Levels of glucagon, epinephrine, cortisol, and growth hormone increase to provide more glucose. Studies show that glucagon is responsible for 60 percent of the glucose, and epinephrine and cortisol are responsible for the other 40 percent. If insulin did not fall, glucagon could not stimulate the liver to make glucose.

You may wonder how insulin can open the cell to the entry of glucose when insulin levels are falling. In fact, two things are at work here. Glucose is getting into muscle cells without the need for insulin, and the rapid circulation that comes with exercise is delivering the smaller amount of insulin more frequently to the muscle. The muscle seems to be more sensitive to the insulin as well, which is exactly what the person with type 2 diabetes hopes to accomplish when insulin resistance is the major block to insulin action.

One way to preserve glucose stores is to provide calories from an external source. Any marathoner knows that additional calories can delay the feeling of exhaustion. The timing is important. If the glucose is given an hour before exercise, it will be metabolized during the exercise and increase endurance. However, if it's given 30 minutes before exercise, it may decrease stamina by stimulating insulin, which blocks liver production of glucose.

Fructose can replenish you when you're doing prolonged exercise. This sweetener can replace glucose because it is sweeter but is absorbed more slowly and does not provoke the insulin secretion that glucose provokes. Fructose is rapidly converted into glucose inside the body. (See Chapter 8 for more on fructose.)

Reaping the benefits

As your body becomes trained with regular exercise, the benefits for your diabetes are very significant. Your body starts to turn to fat for energy earlier in the course of your exercise. At the same time, the hormones that tend to raise the blood glucose during exercise are not produced at the same high rate because they aren't needed. Because you don't require as much insulin, your insulin doses can be reduced, and avoiding hypoglycemia during exercise becomes much easier.

Exercising When You Have Diabetes

If you have diabetes and have not exercised previously, you should check with a doctor prior to beginning a new exercise program, especially if you're over the age of 35 or if you've had diabetes for ten years or longer. You should also check with a doctor if you have any of the following risk factors:

- The presence of any diabetic complications like retinopathy, nephropathy, or neuropathy (see Chapter 5)
- Obesity
- A physical limitation
- A history of coronary artery disease or elevated blood pressure
- Use of medications

You need to discuss these issues with your doctor in order to choose the appropriate exercises. I say more about the choice of exercise in the section "Is Golf a Sport? Choosing Your Activity" later in this chapter.

When you begin to exercise, whether you have type 1 or type 2 diabetes, you can take many steps to make your experience safe and healthful. Following are some important steps to take:

- Wear a bracelet identifying your first and last name, type of diabetes, food or drug allergies, and emergency contact numbers for your doctor and a family member or close friend.
- Test your blood glucose very often.
- Choose proper socks and shoes.
- Drink plenty of water.
- Carry treatment for hypoglycemia.
- Exercise with a friend.

And here are some things to avoid when you exercise:

- Don't assume that you have to buy lots of special clothing to exercise. The right shoes and socks are essential, but other than that, you need special clothing only if your sport demands it (such as soft pants for cycling).
- Don't expect to lose weight in certain spots by repetitively exercising them.
- Don't exercise to the point of pain.
- Don't get too focused on using exercise gadgets like belts or other objects that don't require you to move.

Working out with type 1 diabetes

People with type 1 diabetes or type 2 on insulin depend on insulin injections to manage blood glucose. They don't have the luxury of a "thermostat" that automatically shuts off during exercise and turns back on when exercise is finished. After an insulin shot is taken, it is active until it's used up.

If you have type 1 diabetes, you have to avoid overdosing on insulin before exercise, which can lead to hypoglycemia, or underdosing, which can lead to hyperglycemia. If your body doesn't have enough insulin, it turns to fat for energy. Glucose rises because it is not being metabolized but its production is continuing. If exercise is particularly vigorous in a situation of not enough insulin, the blood glucose can rise extremely high.

Reducing your insulin dosage prior to exercise helps prevent hypoglycemia. One study showed that an 80 percent reduction of the dose allowed the person with diabetes to exercise for three hours, whereas a 50 percent reduction forced the person with diabetes to stop after 90 minutes due to hypoglycemia. Each person with diabetes varies, and you must determine for yourself how much to reduce insulin by measuring the blood glucose before, during, and after exercise.

Another way to prevent hypoglycemia, of course, is to eat some carbohydrate (see Chapter 8). You need to have some carbohydrate (which quickly raises blood glucose) available during exercise.

In addition, the site of the insulin injection is important because it determines how fast the insulin becomes active. If you are running and inject insulin into your leg, it will be taken up more quickly than an injection into the arm would be.

You can exercise whenever you will do it faithfully. If you like to sleep late and you schedule your exercise at 5:30 a.m., you probably won't consistently do it. Your best time to exercise is probably about 60 to 90 minutes after eating because the glucose is peaking at this time, providing the calories you need; if you exercise then, you avoid the usual post-eating high in your blood glucose, and you burn up those food calories. If you take insulin and prefer early-morning exercise, check your blood glucose and eat a snack if you are below 150 mg/dl. Don't exercise just before bedtime; it may cause hypoglycemia while you are sleeping.

Working out with type 2 diabetes

Other than the insulin discussion, many of the suggestions for type 1 patients in the previous section apply to type 2 patients as well.

What are aerobic and anaerobic exercise?

Aerobic exercise is exercise that can be sustained for more than a few minutes, uses major groups of muscles, and gets your heart to pump faster during the exercise, thus training the heart. I give you many examples of aerobic exercise throughout this chapter.

Anaerobic exercise, on the other hand, is brief (sometimes a few seconds) and intense and usually cannot be sustained. Lifting large weights is an example of an anaerobic exercise. A 100-yard dash is another example.

With sufficient exercise and diet, some people with type 2 diabetes can revert to a nondiabetic state. This state doesn't mean that they no longer have diabetes, but it certainly means that they will not develop the long-term complications that can make them so miserable later in life (see Chapter 5).

Determining How Much Exercise to Do

Unless you have a physical abnormality, you have no limitation on what kind of exercise or how much you can do. You should select one or more activities that you enjoy and will continue to perform.

Exerting enough effort

In the recent past, exercise physiologists said that you needed to make sure that you monitored your exercise intensity by periodically checking your heart rate. Your exercise heart rate was supposed to be based on your age. The usual formula to figure this out is to take the number 220, subtract your age, and multiply that number by 60 to 75 percent to get the recommended exercise heart rate for aerobic exercise. (See the sidebar "What are aerobic and anaerobic exercise?" if you're not sure what aerobic exercise is.)

Now studies have shown that people can sustain aerobic exercise at higher heart rates. Perhaps the best way to know whether you're meeting your exercise goals is to use the perceived exertion scale described in the sidebar "Checking the value of your exercise."

The younger you are, the faster your exercise heart rate may be. Like everything in this book, your exercise heart rate is an individual number. If you are a world-class athlete training for your ninth marathon, your exercise heart rate may be higher. If you have some heart disease, your exercise heart rate may be significantly lower.

Checking the value of your exercise

Measuring your pulse during exercise (or even at rest) may be hard for you. Instead, you can use the perceived exertion scale. Exercise is given a descriptive value from *extremely light* to *extremely hard* with *very light, light, somewhat hard,* and *very hard* in between. You want to exercise to a level of *somewhat hard,* and you will be at your target heart rate in most cases. As you get into shape, the amount of exertion that corresponds to *somewhat hard* will increase.

Here is a description of these various levels of exercise:

✔ **Extremely light exercise** is very easy to do and requires little or no exertion.

✔ **Very light exercise** is like walking slowly for several minutes.

✔ **Light exercise** is like walking faster but at a pace you can continue without effort.

✔ **Somewhat hard exercise** is getting a little difficult but still feels okay to continue.

✔ **Very hard exercise** is difficult to continue. You have to push yourself, and you're very tired. At this level, you have trouble talking. The very hard level of exercise is most beneficial.

✔ **Extremely hard exercise** is the most difficult exercise you've ever done.

Do not continue exercising if you have tightness in your chest, chest pain, severe shortness of breath, or dizziness.

Devoting an hour a day

When you know your maximal exercise heart rate, you can choose your activity and use the perceived exertion scale to be sure that you achieve that level during exercise. I must repeat that the best choice of exercise for you is an exercise you enjoy and will continue to perform.

The choices are really limitless. The number of kilocalories you use for any exercise is determined by your weight, the strenuousness of the activity, and the time you spend actually doing it. In the past it was suggested that in order to have a positive effect on your heart, you need to do a moderate level of exercise for 20 to 45 minutes at least three times a week. In 2002, the Institute of Medicine (the medical division of the National Academies) recommended that in order to maintain health and a normal body weight, you need to do one hour of exercise a day.

An hour (not an apple) a day keeps the doctor away! Moderate aerobic exercise done for an hour every day provides enormous physical, mental, and emotional benefits. Exercise cancels out the changes induced by overfeeding and reduced activity.

You need to warm up and cool down for about five minutes before and after you exercise. Stretching is one possibility for both warm-up and cool-down. I am not going to discuss stretching in detail because the importance of stretching for the healthy exerciser is not clear. One study showed that a group of runners who did not stretch did better than a group who did. Most doctors agree that stretching after an injury is appropriate, but whether all the advice about stretching before exercise for an uninjured person is much ado about nothing is yet to be determined. If you do stretch, do not stretch to the point that it hurts, or you risk tearing muscle. See the excellent book *Fitness For Dummies,* by Suzanne Schlosberg and Liz Neporent (John Wiley & Sons, Inc.), for more about stretching.

Making moderate exercise your goal

Moderate exercise has a moving definition. If you're out of shape, moderate exercise for you may be slow walking. If you're in good shape, moderate exercise may be jogging or cross-country skiing. Moderate exercise is simply something you can do and not get out of breath. For ideas on the types of exercise you can do, see the following section.

How long can you stop exercise before you start to decondition? It takes only about two to three weeks to lose some of the fitness your exercise has provided. Then it takes up to six weeks to get back to your current level, assuming that your holiday from exercise does not go on too long.

Is Golf a Sport? Choosing Your Activity

The following factors can help you determine your choice of activity:

✔ Do you like to exercise alone or with company? Pick a competitive or team sport if you prefer company.

✔ Do you like to compete against others or just yourself? Running or walking are activities you can do alone.

✔ Do you prefer vigorous or less-vigorous activity? Less-vigorous activity over a longer period is just as effective as more-vigorous activity.

✔ Do you live where you can do activities outside year-round, or do you need to go inside a lot of the year? Find a sports club if weather prevents year-round outside activity.

✔ Do you need special equipment or just a pair of running shoes?

✔ What benefits are you looking for in your exercise: Cardiovascular, strength, endurance, flexibility, or body fat control? You should probably look for all these benefits, but you may have to combine activities to get them all in.

✔ Do you have any balance problems? Swimming and water aerobics are great choices for you.

Perhaps a good starting point in your activity selection is to focus on the benefits. Table 10-1 gives you some ideas.

Table 10-1	Match Your Activity to the Results You Want
If You Want to . . .	*Then Consider . . .*
Build up cardiovascular condition	Vigorous basketball, racquetball, squash, cross-country skiing, handball, swimming
Strengthen your body	Low-weight, high-repetition weight lifting; gymnastics; mountain climbing; cross-country skiing
Build up muscular endurance	Gymnastics, rowing, cross-country skiing, vigorous basketball
Increase flexibility	Gymnastics, yoga, judo, karate, soccer, surfing
Control body fat	Handball, racquetball, squash, cross-country skiing, vigorous basketball, singles tennis

You can tell from this table that living in places with plenty of snow is helpful because cross-country skiing is on almost every list. On the other hand, so is vigorous basketball, so you don't have to give up exercise if you live in a warm climate like Florida.

The special needs of many of these sports may turn you off to exercise. The curious thing is that the best exercise that you can sustain for life is right at your feet. A brisk daily walk improves heart function, adds to muscular endurance, and helps control body fat. So many people drive their cars to the gym and try to park as close as possible so that they can get to the building with as little effort as possible. Seems a little strange, doesn't it?

Of course, the social benefits of exercise are very important. You are together with people who are concerned with health and appearance. These people usually share many of your interests. People who like to jog often like to hike and climb and camp, too. Many lifetime partnerships begin on one side of a tennis court (and some end there as well).

Cross-training, where you do several different activities throughout the week, is a good idea. Cross-training reduces the boredom that may accompany doing one thing day after day. It also permits you to exercise regardless of the weather because you can do some things indoors and some outside.

Table 10-2 lists a variety of activities, including some that don't exactly fit into the category of *exercise* but offer some interesting comparisons. Next to each activity, I include the amount of kilocalories that a 125-pound person and a 175-pound person burn in 20 minutes.

Table 10-2	Calories Burned in 20 Minutes at Different Body Weights	
Activity	*Kilocalories Burned (125 pounds)*	*Kilocalories Burned (175 pounds)*
Standing	24	32
Walking, 4 mph	104	144
Running, 7 mph	236	328
Gardening	60	84
Writing	30	42
Typing	38	54
Carpentry	64	88
House painting	58	80
Playing baseball	78	108
Dancing	70	96
Playing football	138	192
Golfing	66	96
Swimming	80	112
Skiing, downhill	160	224
Skiing, cross-country	196	276
Playing tennis	112	160

Everything you do burns calories. Even sleeping and watching television use 20 kilocalories in 20 minutes if you weigh 125 pounds.

A study published in the *European Journal of Preventive Cardiology* in December 2014 looked at 2,768 people to measure the benefits of yoga compared to exercise or no physical activity. The authors found that yoga is as beneficial as aerobic exercise and much more beneficial than no exercise in the prevention of heart and blood vessel disease. Yoga was found to reduce blood pressure, cholesterol, and weight.

Your choice of an activity must take into account your physical condition. If you have diabetic neuropathy (see Chapter 5) and can't feel your feet, you don't want to do pounding exercises that may damage them without your awareness. You can swim, bike, row, or do armchair exercises where you move your upper body vigorously. One of my favorite machines that give you a good workout without trauma to your joints is the elliptical trainer, but you may have to join a club to get at one unless you buy one for home.

A study published in the *Journal of the American College of Cardiology* in February 2015, which followed joggers for a total of 12 years, showed that 1 to 2.4 hours of light jogging per week is the healthiest form of running. Over the 12-year period, strenuous joggers were as likely to die as sedentary non-joggers.

If you have diabetic retinopathy (see Chapter 5), you won't want to do exercises that raise your blood pressure (like weight lifting), cause jerky motions in your eyes (like bouncing on a trampoline), or change the pressure in your eyes significantly (like scuba diving or high mountain climbing). You also should not do exercises that place your eyes below the level of your heart, such as when you touch your toes.

Patients with nephropathy (see Chapter 5) should avoid exercises that raise the blood pressure for prolonged periods. These exercises are extremely intense activities that you do for a long time, like marathon running.

Some people have pain in the legs after they walk a certain distance. It may be due to diminished blood supply to the legs so that the needs of the muscles in the legs cannot be met. Although you need to discuss this problem with your doctor, you do not need to give up walking. Instead, determine the distance you can walk up to the point of pain. Then walk about three-quarters of that distance and stop to give the circulation a chance to catch up. After you rest, you can go about the same distance again without pain. By stringing several of these walks together, you can get a good, pain-free workout. You may even find that you are able to increase the distance after a while because this kind of training tends to create new blood vessels.

Is there a medical condition that should absolutely prevent you from doing exercise? Short of chest pain at rest, which must be addressed by your doctor, the answer is no. If you can't figure out an exercise that you're able to do, get together with an exercise therapist. You will be amazed at how many muscles you can move that you never knew you had.

Walking 10K Steps a Day

The idea of walking 10,000 steps a day may seem like a huge, unattainable goal to you, but you may be surprised. This goal is certainly worth striving toward because, as I discuss previously in this chapter, walking is one of the most beneficial exercises you can do. All of your steps count, and 10,000 steps can be all the daily exercise you need to do in addition to resistance training (weight lifting, for example).

The first step toward reaching this goal is to buy a *pedometer,* a device that you wear on your belt or wrist that counts each step you take. Don't buy a fancy one with a lot of bells and whistles. All you need is to be able to count your steps and, if you want, to convert the steps into miles. To do this, you need to know how far you walk each time you take a step. Walk ten steps, measure the distance, and divide by ten to get your stride length. Input this number in the appropriate place in the pedometer, and it will give you the miles that correspond with the steps you walk.

Accusplit pedometers work very well. The model I like is the Accusplit Accelerometer Pedometer, which records your steps and the time you spend walking. You can find it at www.accusplit.com. If you want to be more fancy and technical, get yourself a pedometer that you can synchronize with a site on the Internet, like the Fitbit. You and your friends and relatives can sync to the same page on the Internet, and you can see how you're doing compared to them. I find it to be a great motivator. It also acts as an alarm to wake you without disturbing others; it can count your sleep and has other functions.

Begin by doing your usual amount of exercise each day. Remember to record the steps at the end of the day and reset the button on the pedometer to zero. After seven days, add up the steps and divide by seven to get your daily count. You'll probably find that you're doing between 3,000 and 5,000 steps a day. This level of steps is considered a sedentary level.

Next, you want to build up your daily number. Use the catchy phrase *10k a day* to remind you to do extra walking to reach 10,000 steps. Here are some tips to help:

✔ Get a good pair of walking shoes or sneakers and replace them when they begin to wear out.

✔ Leave your car parked. If you can make a trip in an hour or less by foot, save your gas money and add substantially to your daily step count.

✔ Try to add a few hundred steps a week. Begin by identifying a baseline day in your first week when you did the most steps, and make every day like that one. Each week, add a few hundred more.

✔ Find an exercise buddy to walk with you. It's much more fun.

✔ Keep a record of the number of steps involved in various walks you take so you can easily get the steps you are missing on any given day.

✔ Use stairs instead of the elevator, whether you're going up or down.

✔ Take a walk at lunchtime daily.

✔ Stop if you feel pain, and check with your doctor before continuing.

If you don't have a pedometer, or if you want to count other types of exercise toward your walking goal, use the following conversions:

✔ 1 mile = 2,100 average steps

✔ 1 block = 100 average steps

✔ 10 minutes walking = 1,200 steps on average

✔ Biking or swimming = 150 steps per minute

✔ Weight lifting = 100 steps per minute

✔ Roller skating = 200 steps per minute

If you like tangible rewards for what you do (besides the reward of a lower blood glucose, a lower cholesterol, a lower blood pressure, and possibly a lower weight), join the President's Challenge at `www.presidentschallenge.org`. It provides a place to record your activity, and it offers all kinds of information on activities for every age. You choose what you like to do, and every time you do it you record your progress. It gives you points toward awards.

If you prefer to follow an actual trail, take a virtual walk on the American Discovery Trail, a 5,048-mile walk across America from Delaware to California. You can find it at `www.discoverytrail.org`. Every time you walk, convert your steps into miles and see how far they take you along that trail. The website has links to all the sights you would see.

A study in the *Archives of Internal Medicine* in June 2003 provides the best evidence for the benefits of walking. Diabetics who walked at least two hours a week had a 40 percent lower death rate than inactive diabetics.

Another study in *Diabetes Care* in June 2005 entitled "Make Your Diabetic Patients Walk" followed for two years 179 patients with type 2 diabetes who were divided into six groups. The groups differed in the amount of increased exercise they did. For example, the first group did a little more exercise by the end of the study, whereas the last group did much more exercise by the end of the study. The other groups fell in between those extremes.

The results were that the highest exercisers had the lowest blood pressure, greatest weight loss, greatest reduction in total cholesterol and bad cholesterol, greatest increase in good cholesterol, greatest reduction in blood glucose, and greatest reduction in money spent on drugs. Although the people who did the least exercise had no change in the cost of their annual medications, the highest exercisers had a reduction of $660 per year. What are you waiting for? Take the first steps!

Lifting Weights

Weight lifting is a form of anaerobic exercise. (See the sidebar earlier in this chapter if you're not sure what anaerobic exercise is.) It involves the movement of heavy weights, which can be moved only for brief periods of time. It results in significant muscle strengthening and increased endurance.

Doctors are looking for drugs that can increase insulin sensitivity (see Chapter 11). You need look no further. Lifting weights has been shown in several studies to accomplish this. Writing in *Diabetes Care* in September 2007, a group of investigators from the Centers for Disease Control showed that muscle-strengthening activity significantly increased insulin sensitivity, thereby lowering the blood glucose and the hemoglobin A1c in 4,500 adults between the ages of 20 and 70.

Older adults from age 50 and above who were given only eight weeks of flexibility and resistance training had substantial improvement in strength and flexibility while their glucose levels improved as well.

Because weight lifting causes a significant rise in blood pressure as it is being done, people with severe diabetic eye disease should not do it unless your blood pressure is under very good control. Check with your doctor.

Weight training, which uses lighter weights, can be a form of aerobic exercise. Because the weights are light, they can be moved for prolonged periods of time. The result is improved cardiovascular fitness along with strengthening of muscles, tendons, ligaments, and bones. Weight training is an excellent way to protect and strengthen a joint that is beginning to develop some discomfort.

I recommend that you do seven different exercises with light weights every other day, or daily if possible. Choose weights that permit you to do each exercise ten times in a row, for three sets of ten with a rest in between each set. You should need only five to ten minutes to complete all seven, and the benefits will be huge. These exercises are the bicep curl, shoulder press, lateral raise, bent-over rowing, good mornings, flys, and pullovers. You may want to do them initially with a trainer to make sure you do them correctly.

Figure 10-1 shows the bicep curl. To do this exercise:

1. **Hold the dumbbells along the sides of your body, palms facing forward.**

2. **Raise the dumbbells until your elbows are fully bent.**

3. **Slowly lower the dumbbells to the original position.**

Figure 10-2 shows the shoulder press. To do this exercise:

1. **Hold the dumbbells with your palms facing each other and your elbows bent.**

2. **Raise the dumbbells over your head, turning your palms to face forward.**

3. **Lower the dumbbells to the original position.**

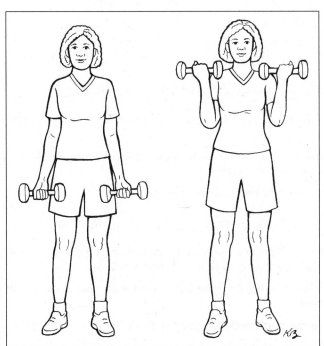

Figure 10-1:
Bicep curl.

Illustration by Kathryn Born

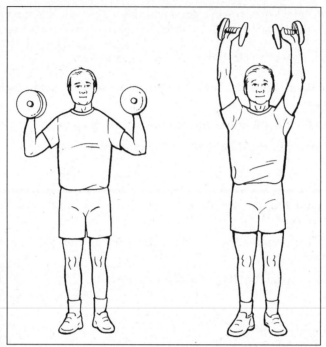

Illustration by Kathryn Born

Figure 10-2:
Shoulder
press.

Figure 10-3 shows the lateral raise. To do this exercise:

1. **Hold the dumbbells along the sides of your body, palms facing each other.**

2. **Lift the dumbbells out to the sides, palms facing the floor, until they are above your head.**

3. **Lower the dumbbells down to your sides.**

Figure 10-4 shows bent-over rowing. To do this exercise:

1. **Hold a dumbbell in each hand, arms hanging down, legs straight, and back bent as necessary toward the floor.**

2. **Raise the dumbbells up to your chest with your back parallel to the floor.**

3. **Lower the dumbbells toward the floor.**

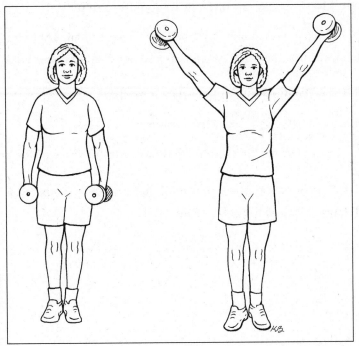

Figure 10-3:
Lateral
raise.

Illustration by Kathryn Born

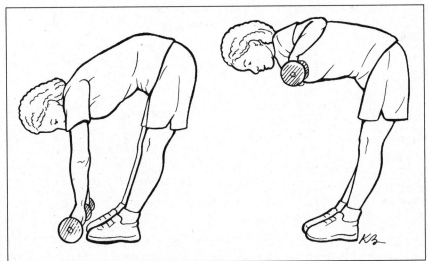

Figure 10-4:
Bent-over
rowing.

Illustration by Kathryn Born

Figure 10-5 shows good mornings. To do this exercise:

1. **Hold the ends of one dumbbell above your head, arms straight.**

2. **Lower the dumbbell forward as you bend so that your back is parallel to the floor.**

3. **Raise the dumbbell to the original position.**

Figure 10-6 shows flys. To do this exercise:

1. **Lie on your back and hold the dumbbells out to each side at the shoulder.**

2. **Lift the dumbbells together until they are above your head.**

3. **Lower them to the sides again.**

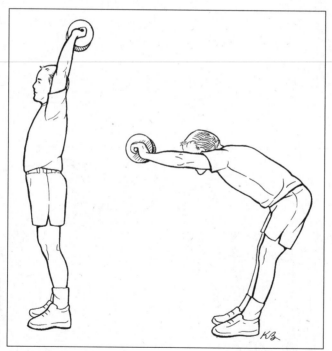

Figure 10-5:
Good
mornings.

Illustration by Kathryn Born

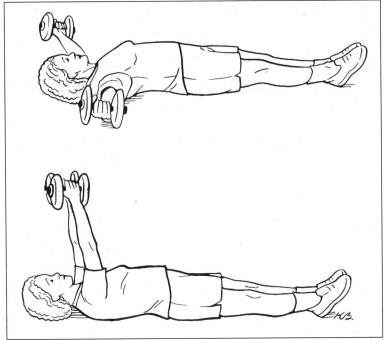

Illustration by Kathryn Born

Figure 10-6:
Flys.

Figure 10-7 shows pullovers. To do this exercise:

1. **Lie on your back holding one dumbbell with both hands straight up above your head.**

2. **Lower the dumbbell with your arms straight to the floor behind your head.**

3. **Raise the dumbbell back above your head.**

Older people in nursing homes who are given weights of just a few pounds have shown excellent return of strength to what appeared to be atrophied muscles. The benefits for you will be that much greater.

Weight training may be good for the days that you do not do your aerobic exercise, or you can add it for a few minutes after you finish your activity. Weight training is also good for working on a particular group of muscles that you feel is weak. Very often, these muscles are in the back. Weight-training exercises can isolate and strengthen each muscle.

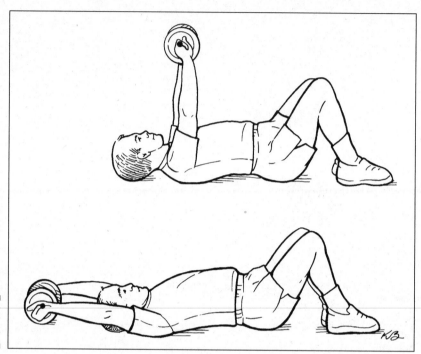

Figure 10-7:
Pullovers.

Illustration by Kathryn Born

If you do a lot of aerobic exercise that involves the legs, you may want to use upper-body weight training only. I can tell you from personal experience that you gain both a stronger upper body and an enhanced ability to do your usual exercise.

Chapter 11

Medications: What You Should Know

In This Chapter

▶ Taking pills to control blood glucose

▶ Using insulin injections

▶ Combining insulin and oral agents in type 2 diabetes

▶ Avoiding drug interactions

Chapter 9 discusses some excellent surgical options available to help you address your diabetes. You may wonder why even bother with pills or shots when the surgery can take care of the problem. A few different answers may apply to you:

✔ You may not want surgery.

✔ If you do, it may be some time before you can have surgery.

✔ Millions of people with type 2 diabetes need the surgery, and not that many surgeons are available.

✔ You may not be the right candidate for surgery.

Meanwhile, keeping your blood glucose, your blood pressure, and your cholesterol under control with medications if necessary are critical to prevent complications from developing.

You don't know how lucky you are (but I'm about to tell you). You are the beneficiary of the greatest advances in diabetes medications in the history of the disease. From 1921, when insulin was isolated and used for the first time, to 1955, when a class of glucose-lowering drugs called *sulfonylureas* became available, insulin was the only option for treating diabetes. For another 40 years, nothing new showed up in the United States — until 1995. Now many newer classes of drugs, each in its own way, lower blood glucose.

Since the last edition of this book, new medications have been introduced and older medications have run into trouble. You find the latest information on all those changes in this chapter.

If you have diabetes and diet and exercise aren't keeping your blood glucose under control, you need to see your doctor about taking medication. In this chapter, you find out all you need to know to use diabetes medications effectively and safely.

This chapter helps you become an educated consumer. Not only can you find out about the medication you're taking and how it works, but you also discover when to take it, how it interacts with other medications, what side effects it may cause, and how to use several medications together, if necessary, to normalize your glucose. Right now, today, you have all the tools needed to control your diabetes, and there are more to come. In the immortal words of the great entertainer Al Jolson, "You ain't seen nothin' yet."

Taking Drugs by Mouth: Oral Agents

For years, insulin shots were the only treatment available for diabetes. Most people do not care for shots. You may be an exception, but I doubt it. Fortunately, drugs that can be taken by mouth have been available for some time. One thing you should know about these pills: You can take them or leave them, but they work much better if you take them.

Sulfonylureas

Scientists discovered sulfonylureas accidentally when they noticed that soldiers who were given certain sulfur-containing antibiotics developed symptoms of low blood glucose. When scientists began to search for the most potent examples of this effect, they came up with several different versions of this drug. Sulfonylureas all have the following characteristics:

- They work by making the pancreas release more insulin.

- They are not effective in type 1 diabetes where the pancreas is not capable of releasing any insulin.

- Sometimes they don't work when first given (primary failure), but they almost always stop working within a few years after you start them (secondary failure). Sulfonylureas continue to be used because, for most people, they improve glucose control for at least those first few years.

✔ They are all capable of causing hypoglycemia.

✔ When you use any of a class of antibiotics called *sulfonamides,* the glucose-lowering action of the sulfonylureas is prolonged.

✔ They should not be taken by pregnant women or nursing mothers, with the exception of glyburide, which has been shown to be safe. Check with your doctor.

✔ They can be fairly potent when given in combination with one of the other classes of oral agents.

Following are the sulfonylureas that are currently in use:

✔ **Glyburide (brand names Micronase, Diabeta, and Glynase):** Among the foreign brand names for glyburide are Antibet, Azuglucon, Betanase, Gliban, Glibil, Gluben, and Orabetic. Pretty confusing, huh? Glyburide comes in 1.25, 2.5, and 5 mg. The usual starting dose is 2.5 to 5 mg with breakfast, and the maintenance dose is 1.25 to 20 mg. Glyburide leaves the body equally in the bowel movement and the urine, so patients with either liver or kidney disease are at greater risk for low blood glucose. Glyburide is carried around the bloodstream bound to proteins, so if you take other drugs that bind to proteins, such as aspirin, the activity of glyburide may increase. When these drugs are withdrawn, the activity of glyburide may decrease. Other than hypoglycemia, the incidence of negative effects is very low.

Glynase is a form of glyburide that is slightly more active because it is absorbed better, so less is required for the same effect. The starting dose is 1.5 mg, and it's available in 1.5-mg, 3-mg, or 6-mg tablets with a maximum dose of 12 mg.

You can take either form of glyburide once a day in the morning, but sometimes it works better when given twice a day.

A French study published in the *Journal of Clinical Endocrinology and Metabolism* in November 2010 showed that the death rate due to heart attacks in people taking glyburide was three times greater than those taking glipizide or glimepiride (see the following bullets). If you are on glyburide, discuss switching to one of the others with your doctor.

✔ **Glipizide (brand names Glucotrol and Glucotrol XL):** Among the foreign brand names are Digrin, Glibenase, Glican, Glyco, Glynase (which is the same name as glyburide in the United States), Mindiab, Napizide, and Sucrazide. Glipizide is similar to glyburide but slightly less potent, so pills come in 5 and 10 mg. You take it 30 minutes before food. The starting dose is 5 mg. Up to 40 mg can be given daily in several doses. Because it's less potent, glipizide is preferred for elderly patients.

Glucotrol XL is an extended release form of glipizide that lasts for 24 hours, so it usually is given as 5 or 10 mg once a day.

✔ **Glimepiride (brand name Amaryl):** This drug also lasts a longer time and is fairly potent, so it is given once a day. It comes in 1-, 2-, and 4-mg sizes with a maximum daily dose of 8 mg.

Amaryl is combined with rosiglitazone (trade name Avandia, discussed in the later section "Rosiglitazone") to form a medication called Avandaryl. It's also combined with pioglitazone (trade name Actos, discussed in "Pioglitazone") as the drug Duetact.

Choosing among the second-generation sulfonylureas, I generally select glimepiride because of its long duration of action. All three of the drugs are available as generic preparations.

A study published in *Diabetes Care* in November 2014 showed that a longer duration of sulphonylurea use (six years or greater) was associated with a significantly higher risk of developing coronary heart disease but not strokes. Discuss changing treatment after five years with your doctor.

Metformin

Metformin, brand names Glucophage, Fortamet, and Glumetza, is an entirely different kind of glucose-lowering medication. Outside the United States, it's called Benoformin, Dextin, Diabex, Diaformin, Fornidd, Glucoform, Gluformin, Metforal, Metomin, and Orabet.

More than 30 years ago, the United States banned a sister medication called *phenformin* because of an association with a fatal complication. Metformin has been used in Europe for years without much trouble and was finally approved in the U.S. in 1995. Metformin is rarely, and perhaps never, associated with the fatal complication *lactic acidosis* that caused phenformin to be banned. A study reported in the *Archives of Internal Medicine* in November 2003 stated that no evidence exists to date that metformin therapy leads to lactic acidosis.

Metformin has the following characteristics:

✔ It lowers the blood glucose mainly by reducing the production of glucose from the liver (the *hepatic* glucose output).

✔ It works for both type 1 and type 2 diabetes because (unlike the sulfonylureas) it does not depend on stimulating insulin to work.

✔ It may increase the sensitivity of the muscle cells to insulin and slow the uptake of glucose from the intestine.

✔ It's available in 500-, 850-, and 1,000-mg tablets. It is also available as a liquid containing 500 mg per 5 milliliters called Riomet and as an extended release form containing 750 mg.

✔ The maximum dose is 2,500 mg taken in divided doses with each meal.

✔ A relatively inexpensive generic form is available, which is just as good as any of the brand name forms.

✔ Used by itself (a treatment called *monotherapy*), it does not cause hypoglycemia. However, when given in combination with the sulfonylureas, hypoglycemia can occur. If low blood glucose is persistent, the dose of sulfonylurea is reduced.

✔ It must be taken with food because it causes gastrointestinal irritation, but this side effect declines with time.

✔ It's often associated with weight loss, possibly from the gastrointestinal irritation or because of a loss of taste for food.

✔ It's not recommended if you have significant liver disease, kidney disease, or heart failure.

✔ It's usually stopped for a day or two before surgery or an X-ray study using a dye and restarted two days later.

✔ It's not recommended for use by alcoholics.

✔ It's not recommended for use in pregnancy or by nursing mothers except for women with polycystic ovarian syndrome in the first trimester and gestational diabetes.

✔ Metformin reduces the occurrence of heart and blood-vessel disease as well as cancer in diabetes and should probably be continued if insulin is added in type 2 diabetes. It significantly reduces major heart and blood vessel damage compared to sulphonylureas.

✔ After gastric bypass, uptake of metformin in the intestine is increased, so a reduction in dosage may be necessary.

✔ A study in *Diabetes Care* in October 2013 noted that metformin use is associated with reduced mental function that may be reversed by vitamin B12 and calcium.

Metformin was previously stopped when kidney disease occurred. The drug is considered to be so useful that experts now recommend continuing to use it and perhaps lowering the dose except in very severe kidney disease, when it must be stopped. Recent evidence (*JAMA Internal Medicine*, December 2014) supports the use of metformin in patients with mild to moderate kidney disease. Discuss continuing it with your doctor if you have kidney disease and diabetes.

Metformin can be a very useful drug, especially when *fasting hyperglycemia* (high blood glucose upon awakening) is present. Metformin has some positive effects on the blood fats, causing a decrease in triglycerides and LDL cholesterol and an increase in HDL cholesterol. About 10 percent of patients fail to respond to it when it is first used, and the secondary failure rate is 5 to 10 percent a year. It occasionally causes a decrease in the absorption of vitamin B12, a vitamin that is important for the blood and the nervous system.

Bristol-Myers Squibb, the maker of Glucophage (one of the trade names of metformin), and other drug makers have come up with new preparations of metformin, which, they believe, have some advantages over the original drug:

- **Glucophage XR:** The original preparation of metformin has to be taken at each meal. However, Glucophage XR lasts for 24 hours and comes in a 500-mg strength. Its longer-lasting effects help overcome the problem of patients not taking their medication the required multiple times a day as well as reducing gastrointestinal side effects. Glumetza is the same drug by Biovail Pharmaceuticals.

- **Glucovance:** This pill combines glyburide (a sulfonylurea described in the previous section) with metformin at a dose of 250 or 500 mg. The various combinations are 1.25 mg of glyburide with 250 mg metformin, 2.5 mg glyburide with 500 mg metformin, and 5 mg glyburide with 500 mg metformin. The advantage is the convenience of having to take only one pill instead of two. Glyburide/metformin is the generic form. But note the warning about glyburide in the previous section.

- **Metaglip:** Made by Bristol-Myers Squibb, this drug combines metformin 250 mg and glipizide 2.5 mg. Glipizide/metformin is the generic form that also comes in 500 mg/5 mg.

- **Avandamet:** This drug is a combination of 4 mg of rosiglitazone (Avandia; which I describe in the section "Rosiglitazone," later in this chapter) and 500 mg of metformin. It's a potent combination of two drugs that act differently to improve insulin sensitivity.

- **ACTOplus Met:** This pill combines 500 or 850 mg metformin with 15 mg pioglitazone (Actos), which I discuss in the later section "Pioglitazone." Takeda makes it.

- **Janumet:** Janumet combines 500 or 1,000 mg metformin with 50 mg sitagliptin, a member of a new class of drugs called DPP-4 inhibitors (which I address in a later section). It is made by Merck.

In my experience, the combination drugs work better than giving two drugs separately. This effect may reflect the greater compliance that results when a single pill is given compared to two separate pills. If you are already taking both of the drugs separately that are available in a combination pill, ask your doctor about getting the single pill that contains both.

Alpha-glucosidase inhibitors

Alpha-glucosidase inhibitors are drugs that block the action of an enzyme in the intestine that breaks down complex carbohydrates into simple sugars that can be absorbed. Taking alpha-glucosidase inhibitors results in a slowing of the rise in glucose after meals. The carbohydrates are eventually broken down by bacteria lower down in the intestine, producing a lot of gas, abdominal pain, and diarrhea — the main drawbacks of these drugs.

The following two alpha-glucosidase inhibitors are currently being used:

✔ **Acarbose (brand name Precose):** This drug seems to have much greater popularity in Europe than it does in the United States. It was the first alpha-glucosidase inhibitor on the market. Following are its main characteristics:

- It's supplied in 25-, 50-, and 100-mg strengths.

- The recommended starting dose is 25 mg at the beginning of each meal. This dose can be increased to 50 or 100 mg three times daily, depending on the blood glucose. The highest dose is not given unless the patient weighs more than 130 pounds.

- It does not require insulin for its activity, so it works for both type 1 and type 2 diabetes.

- It does not cause hypoglycemia when used alone but does in combination with sulfonylureas. If hypoglycemia is persistent, the dose of sulfonylurea is decreased.

- It should not be used by people with intestinal disease.

- Many people do not like it because of the gastrointestinal effects.

- The lowering of glucose and hemoglobin A1c is modest at most.

✔ **Miglitol (brand name Glyset):** This medication was the second alpha-glucosidase inhibitor introduced. Its characteristics are identical to acarbose. It comes in 25, 50, and 100 mg. Curiously Bayer is the manufacturer of both drugs.

Because these drugs block the breakdown of complex carbohydrates, hypoglycemia occurring with acarbose or miglitol and sulfonylurea combinations must be treated with a preparation of glucose, not more complex carbohydrates.

In my own practice, I haven't found a use for either of the drugs in this section. I tried acarbose on a number of patients, and even though they started at a low dose and gradually built up to a more effective level, they complained about the gas and abdominal pain and asked me to take them off the drug. Because I was not seeing much change in the blood glucose, I did not object. I see no reason to expect that miglitol would be any different.

Thiazolidinediones (The glitazones)

This group of drugs for diabetes is the first type of medication that directly reverses insulin resistance.

Troglitazone

Troglitazone, brand name Rezulin (called Prelay outside the United States), was the first oral agent for type 2 diabetes that actually reversed the basic lesion in this disease, namely the insulin resistance. It does so by causing changes within the muscle and fat cells where the insulin resistance resides. These changes take several weeks to occur, and if the patient stops taking troglitazone, they take several weeks to subside.

In March 2000, because of continuing occurrences of severe liver disease sometimes leading to death in a small number of patients taking troglitazone, the FDA removed troglitazone from the market. The other glitazone drugs currently on the market have not had this problem, although the FDA requires monitoring the patient's liver function when these drugs are first used.

Rosiglitazone

Rosiglitazone was the second thiazolidinedione to be approved by the FDA. GlaxoSmithKline markets it as Avandia. Rosiglitazone has the following properties:

- It's available as 2-, 4-, and 8-mg tablets.

- Tablets are taken with or without food once a day.

- The recommended starting dose is 4 mg, and 8 mg is the maximum starting dose. Increases in the dose are made no more often than every two to four weeks. Rosiglitazone may take three months or longer to have its maximum effect.

- Because it improves insulin resistance, this drug has its greatest effect on the blood glucose after eating, rather than the first morning glucose.

- By itself, rosiglitazone doesn't cause hypoglycemia. It results in hypoglycemia only when combined with insulin or sulphonylurea.

- If rosiglitazone is given to a patient on sulphonylurea or metformin, those drugs must not be stopped when rosiglitazone is started because it takes so long to work.

- Rosiglitazone is *insulin sparing*, meaning the body doesn't have to make as much insulin to control the blood glucose. It and pioglitazone, which I discuss in the next section, may have their best use in the most insulin-resistant patients, identified by increased waist circumference, low HDL cholesterol, and fatty liver.

✔ The drug is eliminated from the body through the bowels, so no adjustment of the dose is needed when the kidneys are poorly functioning.

The following problems are associated with the drug:

✔ It causes water retention and swelling of the ankles, especially in the older population. The water retention may also be responsible for a mild decrease in red blood cells. People with heart failure shouldn't take it.

✔ Some infertile women find they become more fertile on rosiglitazone. It may cause unintended pregnancies.

✔ It's associated with an increased risk of fractures in women, especially older than age 65.

Pioglitazone

Pioglitazone, manufactured by Eli Lilly and Takeda in the United States, was the third thiazolidinedione to come to market. The brand name is Actos, and it has the following properties:

✔ The initial dose is 15 mg once a day with or without food, but most patients require 30 or even 45 mg. It comes in all three sizes.

✔ In addition to restoring fertility in some women who are infertile due to insulin resistance, pioglitazone reduces estrogen levels in women taking estrogen and may result in making hormone-based contraception, such as birth-control pills or Depo-Provera, less effective.

✔ Pioglitazone has been shown to reduce bad (LDL) cholesterol particles in people with or without diabetes (as reported in *Diabetes Care,* September 2003).

✔ Pioglitazone has been shown to be associated with increased osteoporosis in women.

✔ Pioglitazone has not been shown to be associated with a higher incidence of heart attacks.

✔ It is authorized for use alone, with insulin, with metformin, or with a sulfonylurea.

Pioglitazone, like rosiglitazone, has been associated with decreased bone mineral density and increased fractures in older women. After 18 months of treatment with pioglitazone, patients have a two or three times greater risk of a fracture than people who never used the drug. The fractures occur especially in the hip or wrist. Pioglitazone has also been found to cause or worsen heart failure (which is why it is contraindicated for use in patients with heart failure) and has been associated with increased bladder cancer

Pioglitazone 30 mg has been combined with glimepiride 2 or 4 mg in a pill called Duetact made by Takeda.

Meglitinides

Each of the drugs in the meglitinides group has about the same activity, although they are chemically somewhat different. They are chemically unrelated to the sulfonylureas but work by squeezing more insulin out of the pancreas just like the sulfonylureas do. They are taken just before meals to stimulate insulin for only that meal.

Following are the two drugs in this class:

- **Repaglinide (brand name Prandin):** This medication was the first meglitinide. Here are the characteristics of repaglinide:

  - It is available as 0.5-, 1-, and 2-mg tablets and is taken just before or up to 30 minutes before meals.

  - The starting dose is 0.5 mg with a mild elevation of blood glucose or 1 or 2 mg if the initial blood glucose is higher. The dose may be doubled once a week to a maximum of 4 mg before meals.

  - Because it acts through insulin, repaglinide can cause hypoglycemia.

  - It's not recommended during pregnancy or for nursing mothers.

  - It's not used with the sulfonylureas but can be combined with metformin.

  - Repaglinide lowers the blood glucose and the hemoglobin A1c effectively when used in combination with metformin.

  - It's mostly broken down in the liver and leaves the body in the bowel movement. Therefore, if liver disease is present, the dose has to be adjusted downward.

  - Despite the lack of excretion through the kidneys, increases in the dose have to be made more carefully when kidney impairment is present.

Experience with repaglinide has shown that it causes no problems when given with nondiabetes medications. It's bound to protein in the blood, so medications like aspirin (which also bind to protein) may, theoretically, increase its activity. I have not seen this as a problem with my patients who are on this medication.

A combination of repaglinide and metformin is called PrandiMet, and it has two strengths, 1 mg or 2 mg of repaglinide plus 500 mg of metformin. It is taken two or three times daily, 15 to 30 minutes before meals.

✓ **Nateglinide (brand name Starlix):** This drug is very similar to repaglinide in its activity. However, it comes in 60 and 120 mg. The starting dose is usually 120 mg before each meal; if a meal is skipped, no dose is taken. If hypoglycemia occurs, the dose is lowered to 60 mg. The features of repaglinide also apply to nateglinide, other than the dosage. A report in *Diabetes Care* in July 2003 showed that repaglinide combined with metformin is a more potent combination than nateglinide with metformin.

Nateglinide is available as a generic, but repaglinide is not, so the less expensive choice is nateglinide.

DPP-4 inhibitors

This class of drugs has a different mechanism from any of the previous classes of oral agents. They affect a hormone called *glucagon-like peptide-1* (GLP-1), which is made in the small intestine and has a number of positive effects for people with diabetes:

✓ It slows the movement of food in the intestine.

✓ It reduces the production of glucagon from the pancreas. Glucagon raises the blood glucose.

✓ It increases insulin levels.

✓ It decreases food intake (by decreasing appetite), leading to weight loss.

✓ It normalizes the blood glucose in many patients.

The only problem with GLP-1 is that an enzyme called *dipepdipyl peptidase-4 (DPP-4)* rapidly breaks it down. Therefore, under usual circumstances, GLP-1 isn't around long enough to have these effects in a major way.

The class of drugs called DPP-4 inhibitors blocks the rapid breakdown of GLP-1 and prolongs its actions. They cause hypoglycemia when used with sulfonylureas, so the dose of the latter drug is usually reduced. They reduce the hemoglobin A1c about the same as the sulfonylureas but less than metformin. Over the long term, they have been found to reduce atherosclerosis and inflammation, a deterrent to heart disease. The kidneys excrete them, so their dosage has to be reduced when kidney disease is present, with the exception of linagliptin (see later in this section).

Currently, five DPP-4 inhibitors are on the market:

✔ **Sitagliptin (brand name Januvia):** Approved in 2006, this Merck drug comes in 25, 50 and 100 mg. The dose is 100 mg daily. Because the kidneys excrete this drug, people with kidney disease must take lower doses. It can cause stomach discomfort. It can be taken in combination with a sulfonylurea, metformin, or insulin

The problem with sitagliptin is that the amount of lowering of the hemoglobin A1c is less than 1 percent. In addition, it does not result in weight loss, which, I believe, is the major advantage of GLP-1.

Sitagliptin is available in combinations as the following drugs:

  • Janumet, containing 50 mg of sitagliptin and 1,000 mg of metformin or 50/500

  • Juvisync, containing 100 mg of sitagliptin and 10 mg of simvastatin or 100/20 or 100/40

✔ **Saxagliptin (brand name Onglyza):** Saxagliptin was approved in 2009. It comes as 2.5- and 5-mg tablets. The recommended dose is 2.5 or 5.0 mg once daily. It may be given with a sulfonylurea, metformin, or insulin.

Saxagliptin is available in combination with extended-release (XR) metformin as Kombiglyze XR, containing 2.5 mg saxagliptin and 1,000 mg metformin or 5 mg saxagliptin and 500 or 1,000 mg metformin.

✔ **Linagliptin (brand name Tradjenta):** This drug was approved in 2011. It comes as 5-mg tablets, and the recommended dosage is 5 mg once daily. It may be used in the same combinations as the other DPP-4 inhibitors. At the end of January 2012, the FDA approved a combination of linagliptin 2.5 mg and metformin, either 500 mg or 1,000 mg, which is called Jentadueto.

✔ **Vildagliptin (brand name Galvus):** Vildagliptin comes in 50-mg tablets, and the recommended dose is 50 mg twice daily. It isn't recommended for pregnant or breast-feeding women. Eucreas is a mixture of vildagliptin and metformin.

✔ **Alogliptin (brand name Nesina):** Nesina comes in 6.25, 12.5, and 25 mg. The recommended dose is 25 mg once daily. The smaller tablets are for people with kidney problems. It shouldn't be used in pregnant or nursing women. Alogliptin is available as Kazano with metformin and as Oseni with pioglitazone.

Only one head-to-head trial of the DPP-4 inhibitors — saxagliptin versus sitagliptin — has been done. The two drugs were found to have the same potency.

Bile acid sequestrants

Bile acid sequestrants are drugs that are used to reduce the total cholesterol and the LDL cholesterol. When they were being used for that purpose, it was noted that they also lowered the blood glucose and the hemoglobin A1c. Although the lowering of hemoglobin A1c is modest, about 0.5 percent, these drugs may have a place in prediabetes or mild type 2 diabetes. They do not cause hypoglycemia.

The FDA has authorized the use of colesevelam (brand name Welchol) for this treatment. It can be used for both type 1 and type 2 diabetes. Side effects include constipation and nausea. Colesevelam comes as 625-mg tablets as well as 1,875- and 3,750-mg powder packets. The dose is 3,750 mg once daily. It may be used alone or with other oral hypoglycemic agents and does not cause weight gain.

Bromocriptine

Bromocriptine is another drug long used for a different illness that has been found to have glucose-lowering effects. It has been used to treat Parkinson's and to treat brain tumors that produce too much growth hormone or prolactin. It was discovered to lower the blood glucose and the hemoglobin A1c to a slightly greater extent (hemoglobin A1c reduced 0.6 to 0.7 percent) than the bile acid sequestrants but by a different mechanism. It also reduces triglycerides and free fatty acids without causing hypoglycemia or weight gain.

Side effects include nausea, dizziness, and headache in less than 15 percent of patients. The dose of bromocriptine (called Cycloset) is one 0.8-mg tablet increased by one tablet per week up to a maximum of 4.8 mg. It may be used by itself or with other oral agents. The generic version of bromocriptine does not work for people with diabetes.

SGLT2 inhibitors

This new group of drugs called *sodium glucose co-transporter 2 (SGLT2)* inhibitors works by preventing glucose from being reabsorbed by the kidneys so it's excreted in the urine, thereby lowering the blood glucose. These drugs don't cause hypoglycemia, but may result in some weight loss and decreased blood pressure. They can reduce the A1c by 0.7–0.9 percent. Don't use them during pregnancy or when breast-feeding.

Currently three different ones are on the market, and I'm sure there will be more. Their dosage must be decreased if you have kidney damage. Because they cause a lot of glucose to spill in the urine, they may cause urinary tract infections, increased urination, and yeast infections of the genital areas, especially in women. They can also cause some dehydration and low blood pressure with possible dizziness or fainting. The three drugs are

- **Canagliflozin (brand name Invokana):** Canagliflozin was the first in this group approved by the FDA in 2013. It comes in 100 and 300 mg. The starting dose is 100 mg before the first meal. It is also available with metformin as Invokamet.

- **Dapagliflozin (brand name Farxiga):** Released by the FDA in January 2014, dapagliflozin comes in 5 and 10 mg, and treatment starts at 5 mg. There is little clinical difference between dapagliflozin and canagliflozin. It also comes with metformin as Xigduo XR.

- **Empagliflozin (brand name Jardiance):** This is the latest "me too" drug (a drug made by a different company that has no advantages over previous drugs) in this class, released by the FDA in August 2014. It comes as 10- and 25-mg tablets, and the starting dose is 10 mg. Its actions appear to be identical to the other two SGLT2 inhibitors.

Combining oral agents

Taking one oral agent alone often does not control the blood glucose sufficiently to prevent complications of diabetes. (A hemoglobin A1c of less than 7 percent is the goal; see Chapter 7.) In this section, I explain how you can use two or more of these drugs together.

You should never take a drug, or a combination of drugs, as a convenient way of avoiding the basic diet and exercise that are the keys to diabetic control. (See Chapters 8 and 10 for more information on these crucial points.)

I currently start all new type 2 patients who are mildly out of control on metformin. I give this medication at least two weeks to work. Many patients need no more treatment than this in addition to their diet and exercise. I usually begin with a dose of 500 mg twice daily and raise it to 1,000 mg twice daily if the blood glucose is still elevated after two weeks.

If 2,000 mg of metformin does not control the patient's blood glucose, sitagliptin or another DPP-4 inhibitor is an excellent second drug to add at this point, usually at a dose of 100 mg once daily.

When a patient is taking these two drugs but still has slightly elevated blood glucose, I add a sulfonylurea. I like to use a longer-acting form, such as glimepiride, because I always prefer a drug that can be taken only once a day over drugs that require multiple dosing. I have found that 2 to 4 mg of glimepiride combined with the other drugs is all the treatment needed to achieve the goal.

A few patients still have elevated blood glucose and hemoglobin A1c levels, even with the preceding treatments. For them, repaglinide in place of the sulfonylurea usually does the trick. Starting with a dosage of 1 mg before each meal, those patients have found this medication to be very helpful.

If low blood glucose starts to be a problem, the dose of the sulfonylurea or repaglinide is lowered because the other medications are not responsible for hypoglycemia.

If there is still a little way to go to get the hemoglobin A1c down to 7 percent, colesevelam or bromocriptine may do the trick.

Many diabetes specialists believe that the pancreas gradually fails to make insulin in type 2 diabetes and that most patients need to take insulin sooner or later (see the sidebar "Combining insulin and oral agents in type 2 diabetes"). My experience is that giving insulin early on is not necessarily needed and that the modern medications, particularly metformin, can delay or eliminate the need for insulin. Certainly, numerous people with diabetes are well controlled with only a small dose of an oral medication. And I have seen many others who used insulin when nothing else was available but have since stopped taking it and do not appear as though they will ever need it again. Some people need no drugs at all. Several of my patients with long-standing, poorly controlled type 2 diabetes, who have been able to change their lifestyle and lose weight with diet and exercise, have been able to stop all medications as well.

Some patients still don't lower their hemoglobin A1c to 7 or below despite all the above medications, or do so initially but not later. These patients are given insulin or the injectable drugs described in the next section.

New injectable drugs

In the earlier discussion of DPP-4 inhibitors, I mention that those drugs work by blocking the breakdown of the natural hormone GLP-1. The effects of GLP-1, such as increasing the secretion of insulin and decreasing the uptake of glucose, have been called the *incretin effect*. The incretin effect includes slow emptying of the stomach with an early sensation of fullness. They often cause weight loss. Recent studies suggest that the incretin effect is lost early in type 2 diabetes. Because incretins have been shown to preserve beta-cell function, some experts believe they should be used early in the treatment of type 2 diabetes, but they aren't yet recommended for initial treatment. The following sections introduce you to several forms of GLP-1 that are in use.

All of the drugs in this group shouldn't be given to anyone with medullary thyroid cancer and shouldn't be given to pregnant or nursing women. They can't be used in type 1 diabetes because insulin production is mostly gone with that condition. The kidneys don't excrete them, so their dose doesn't have to be changed with kidney disease.

Exenatide

Amylin Pharmaceuticals and Eli Lilly have been able to extract a substance from the venom of a lizard called the Gila monster that acts like GLP-1 but does not break down nearly as fast. This substance is used in the medication exenatide (trade name Byetta). The pharmaceutical companies have also been able to produce a second injectable substance called *pramlintide* with many similar properties.

Exenatide is a powerful form of GLP-1 that lasts for several hours. It is taken within an hour before breakfast and supper. It may only be used in type 2 diabetes and comes in pens containing either 5 or 10 micrograms per dose. It may be used with metformin or a sulfonylurea or combinations of those drugs. It can sometimes cause substantial weight loss and eliminate the need for all of those drugs. It is associated with nausea, and in rare cases it can't be used because the nausea is so severe. Hypoglycemia is frequent when it is used with a sulfonylurea. The dosage of the sulfonylurea is then reduced. At present it may be used with long-acting insulin but not short-acting or rapid-acting insulin.

Exenatide has been found to be linked to pancreatitis (true for all GLP-agonists), an inflammation of the pancreas that causes abdominal pain, nausea, and vomiting and can be fatal. Whether and how exenatide may cause pancreatitis is not clear.

This drug has proved to be very valuable in the treatment of type 2 diabetes. It is sometimes necessary to use more than the maximum recommended dose of 20 micrograms a day.

Liraglutide

Liraglutide (brand name Victoza) is another form of GLP-1. Liraglutide can be injected once a day without relation to meals. It has been shown to lower the hemoglobin A1c to a greater extent than twice-daily exenatide. It also causes more weight loss, increased reduction in fasting plasma glucose, and more blood pressure lowering. Nausea is a minor side effect.

Liraglutide is started at a dose of 0.6 mg by injection and raised to 1.8 mg daily over two weeks.

Liraglutide has been associated with tumors of the thyroid gland in animals but not humans.

Extended-release exenatide

In January 2012, the FDA approved once-weekly extended-release exenatide (brand name Bydureon). It's more effective than twice-daily exenatide but has about the same potency as daily liraglutide. The obvious advantage is one shot a week instead of 14. The FDA had previously rejected it twice in 2010 until the manufacturer, Amylin Pharmaceuticals, satisfied the FDA's objections. It is a new formulation, and time will tell its place in the management of type 2 diabetes.

Pramlintide

Pramlintide (brand name Symlin) is an extract from the same beta cells of the pancreas that produce insulin. The hormone in its natural state in the body is called *amylin*. It has a number of valuable properties for type 1 and type 2 diabetes, including the following:

- ✔ It blocks the secretion of glucagon, a major hormone that tends to raise blood glucose (see Chapter 2 for details).
- ✔ It slows the emptying of the stomach so that glucose is absorbed more slowly.
- ✔ It causes loss of appetite and weight loss.

Pramlintide, therefore, has an important effect on the rate at which glucose appears in the blood after eating. These effects occur when pramlintide reaches certain centers in the brain.

Because amylin comes from the same cells that make insulin, it's absent in type 1 diabetes just as insulin is absent in type 1 diabetes. It was thought that providing amylin to a patient with T1DM might improve the blood glucose. However, naturally occurring amylin has chemical properties that make it unusable as a pill or an injection. Mainly, it couldn't be made to dissolve in any liquid. A small change in the chemical structure made it possible to dissolve the new chemical while retaining all the properties of amylin.

Pramlintide is taken before meals that contain at least 30 grams of carbohydrate or 250 kilocalories. It doesn't mix with insulin. Because pramlintide is so potent, the insulin dose must be reduced by half. It can cause nausea and hypoglycemia.

The starting dose of pramlintide for type 1 diabetes is 15 micrograms before meals, and it's increased by 15 micrograms every three days. The maximum daily total dose is 180 micrograms. For type 2 diabetes, the starting dose is 60 micrograms before major meals, and it can be increased to 120 mcg if necessary.

Pramlintide hasn't been studied in pregnancy or while breast-feeding, so it shouldn't be used during these conditions. Children may use it.

You should probably not use pramlintide if you have hypoglycemia unaware-ness (see Chapter 4) or a form of diabetic neuropathy called gastroparesis (see Chapter 5), which makes the stomach empty slowly.

Other new injectable drugs

Here are a few other new injectable drugs available on the market.

- **Albiglutide (brand name Tanzeum):** Albiglutide is injected once a week under the skin, without regard to meals. The starting dose is 30 mg, but it can be raised to 50 mg. It comes in a single dose pen. It differs little from liraglutide.

- **Dulaglutide (brand name Trulicity):** This is yet another once weekly GLP-1. It's available as 0.75 and 1.75 mg single dose injection pen or a single dose prefilled syringe. I find nothing that differentiates this drug from the others.

  In February 2015 the FDA authorized the sale of Glyxambi, which is a combination of linagliptin and empagliflozin. Just what the world desper-ately needed (just joking).

Taking Insulin

If you have type 1 diabetes, insulin is your savior. If you have type 2 diabetes, you may need insulin at some point in the course of your disease. Insulin is a great drug, but most people take it through a needle, and that's the rub (or the pain). Inventors have come up with many different ways to administer insulin, but using a syringe and a needle has been the standard for so long that most patients continue to do so. In this section, I tell you about the newer methods, which you should at least consider because they are easier and possibly more accurate than the old method. However, the new syringes and needles are just about painless.

Until a few years ago, insulin could be obtained only by extracting it from the pancreas of a cow, pig, salmon, or some other animal. This wasn't entirely satisfactory because those insulins are slightly different from human insulin.

Using them resulted in an immune reaction in the blood and certain skin reactions. The preparation was purified, but tiny amounts of impurities always remained. In 1978, researchers were able to trick bacteria called *E. coli* into making human insulin. Almost all insulin is now perfectly pure human insulin. Soon, no insulin besides human insulin will be available.

Previously, insulin came in two different strengths, U40 and U80, which meant 40 units per milliliter or 80 units per milliliter. This system was confusing, especially if the wrong syringe was used — you had to use a U40 syringe for U40 insulin. To eliminate confusion, all insulin commonly used in the United States is now U100, or 100 units per milliliter (there is a U500 form for severe insulin resistance), and all syringes are U100 syringes. This standardization does not necessarily apply in Europe or elsewhere, so check the insulin strength and the markings on the syringe.

Considering insulin options

In the human body, insulin is constantly responding to ups and downs in the blood glucose. In order to avoid having to take many shots a day, forms of insulin were invented to work at different times. The following list explains the various forms of insulin:

- ✔ **Rapid-acting lispro insulin:** Lispro insulin (called *Humalog insulin* by its manufacturer, Eli Lilly) begins to lower the glucose within five minutes after its administration, peaks at about one hour, and is no longer active by about three hours. Lispro is a great advance because it frees the person with diabetes to take a shot just when he or she eats. With the previous short-acting insulin (regular insulin), a person had to take a shot 30 minutes prior to eating. Because its activity begins and ends so quickly, lispro does not cause hypoglycemia as often as the older preparations.

  Novo Nordisk has come out with *insulin aspart* (called NovoLog), which has characteristics indistinguishable from lispro insulin.

  Sanofi-Aventis produces insulin glulisine (trade name Apidra), which is similar in its properties to the other two rapid-acting insulins.

- ✔ **Short-acting regular insulin:** Regular insulin takes 30 minutes to start to lower the glucose, peaks at three hours, and is gone by six to eight hours. Until Humalog, NovoLog, and Apidra came along, patients used this preparation before meals to keep their glucose low until the next meal.

- ✔ **Intermediate-acting NPH:** This drug begins to lower the glucose within 2 hours of administration and continues its activity for 10 to 12 hours. It can be active for up to 24 hours. The purpose of this kind of insulin is to provide a smooth level of control over half the day so that a low level of active insulin is always in the body, an attempt to parallel the situation that exists in the human body.

✔ **Long-acting insulin glargine and detemir:** Aventis sells an insulin called *insulin glargine,* which goes by the trade name Lantus. Studies have shown that insulin glargine has its onset in 1 to 2 hours after injection, and its activity lasts for 24 hours without a specific peak time of activity, which is exactly what is needed to control the blood glucose over an entire day. Insulin glargine is released in a smooth fashion from the site of injection, and it doesn't matter if you inject the abdomen, the thigh, or the deltoid. Because of its smooth and predictable activity, insulin glargine does not tend to cause low blood glucose at night, which often happens with NPH insulin. However, one disadvantage of insulin glargine is that it can't be mixed with other insulins in one syringe.

I have used this insulin in a number of my patients with type 1 diabetes and have been extremely pleased with the results. I now use it with all new type 1 diabetes patients.

Insulin detemir or Levemir has similar properties to glargine but does not last quite as long. It is a product of Novo Nordisk.

If you do not have good diabetic control (defined as hemoglobin A1c of 7 percent or less) with NPH insulin, ask your doctor to consider using insulin glargine or detemir.

✔ **Premixed insulins:** Several mixtures are available: one with 70 percent NPH insulin and 30 percent regular; one with a 50–50 mix of NPH and regular; one with a 75–25 mix of NPH-like insulin and lispro insulin; and one with a 70–30 mix of NPH-like insulin and insulin aspart. These insulins are helpful for people who have trouble mixing insulins in one syringe, have poor eyesight, or are stable on a preparation that does not change. Insulins that are not premixed are better for young, fairly stable type 2 diabetics.

Whichever type of insulin you take, you need to know a few basic things about its use:

✔ Insulin may be kept at room temperature for four weeks or in the refrigerator until the expiration date printed on the label. After four weeks at room temperature, the insulin should be discarded.

✔ Insulin does not take too well to excessive heat, such as direct sunlight, or to excessive cold. Protect your insulin against these conditions.

✔ You can safely give an insulin shot through clothing.

✔ If you take less than 50 units in a shot, you can use $\frac{1}{2}$-cc syringes that make it easy to measure up to 50 units. If you take less than 30 units, you can use $\frac{3}{10}$-cc syringes.

✔ Shorter needles may be more comfortable, especially for children, but the depth of the injection helps to determine how fast the insulin works.

> ✔ You can reuse disposable syringes a couple of times.
>
> ✔ Used syringes and needles must be disposed of in a puncture-proof container that is sealed shut before being placed in the trash.

As of February 2015, a new option is available that you should know about. The FDA approved inhaled insulin called Afrezza from Sanofi and MannKind Corporation. Both type 1 and type 2 diabetes patients can use it. It's a dry powder that is placed in a small, portable inhaler and taken just before meals. It can't be used in acute situations like diabetic ketoacidosis (see Chapter 4) or in people with chronic lung disease. If you really hate those needles, ask your doctor if you can give it a try.

Shooting yourself

Whatever type of insulin you use, you may be taking it by syringe and needle. (I discuss other delivery options later in the chapter, in the sections "Delivering insulin with a pen," and "Delivering insulin with an external pump.")

Combining insulin and oral agents in type 2 diabetes

Sometimes the characteristics of the currently available oral agents do not provide the tight control needed to avoid complications. This problem is particularly common after many years of type 2 diabetes. In such cases, insulin may be required. Insulin may be added in a number of ways, but often a shot of glargine insulin at bedtime is all that is needed to start the day under control and continue it with oral agents. For example, metformin may control the daytime glucose very well after eating, but the first morning glucose may need the overnight shot of glargine insulin. By gradually increasing the dose of glargine, most patients with type 2 diabetes on oral agents can be controlled so that their hemoglobin A1c is 7 or below.

As type 2 diabetes progresses, the oral agents may be less effective, and insulin is taken more often. Two shots a day of intermediate and short-acting insulin may do the trick. Usually you take two-thirds of the dose in the morning and one-third before supper because you need short-acting insulin to control the supper carbohydrates. In this situation, 75 percent protamine lispro (like NPH) and 25 percent lispro insulin may be useful, allowing the patient to measure from only one bottle. This combination is especially valuable in the older person with diabetes, where the tightest level of control is not being sought because the expected lifespan of the patient is shorter than the time necessary to develop complications. In this patient, doctors want to prevent problems like frequent urination leading to loss of sleep or vaginal infections, so they give enough to treat this but not so much that a frail, elderly patient is having hypoglycemia on a frequent basis.

Drawing insulin up is done in the same way no matter which type of insulin is involved. If you look at the syringe in Figure 11-1, you see that it's lined. Starting at the needle end of the syringe, you'll find nine small lines above the needle, followed by a tenth longer line where the number 10 may be found. Each line is one unit of insulin. Above the 10-unit line, you'll find a succession of four small lines followed by a larger line representing 15, 20, 25, and so on.

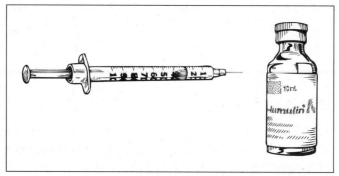

Figure 11-1:
The insulin syringe and bottle.

Illustration by Kathryn Born

If the insulin is short-acting, long-acting, or regular, the bottle should be clear, and you do not have to shake the bottle. The other kinds of insulin are cloudy, and you need to roll the bottle a few times to suspend the tiny particles in the liquid. A new bottle has a cap on the top, which you break off and discard. When you're ready to take insulin, wipe the rubber stopper in the top of the bottle with alcohol.

Pull up the number of units of air that corresponds to the number of units of insulin you need to take. Turn the insulin bottle upside down and penetrate the rubber stopper with the needle of the syringe. Push all the air inside and pull out the insulin dose you need. Because air replaces the insulin, the pressure inside the bottle is unchanged and no vacuum is created. Check to make sure that you have the right amount of the right insulin and no air bubbles in the syringe.

To give the injection, use alcohol to wipe off an area of skin on your arm, chest, stomach, or wherever you're injecting it. Insert the needle at a right angle to the skin and push it in. When the needle has penetrated the skin, push the plunger of the syringe down to zero to administer the insulin.

If you're taking two kinds of insulin at the same time (but not insulin glargine), you can mix them in one syringe, thus avoiding two shots. Here's how you do that:

1. **Wipe both bottles with alcohol.**

2. **Draw up the total units of air corresponding to the total insulin you need.**

3. **Push the units of air into the longer-acting insulin bottle that corresponds to the number of units of longer-acting insulin you need, and withdraw the needle without drawing any insulin.**

4. **Push the rest of the units of air into the shorter-acting insulin bottle, and withdraw the correct units of insulin.**

5. **Go back to the longer-acting bottle and withdraw the correct units of insulin from there.**

   By doing this, you do not contaminate the shorter-acting insulin with the additive in the longer-acting insulin.

Where you inject the insulin helps determine how fast it works. The site that most rapidly absorbs insulin injections is the abdomen, followed by the arms and legs and then the buttocks. You may use these differing rates of uptake of the insulin to get faster action when your blood glucose is high. If the body part that gets the insulin is exercised, the insulin enters more quickly. If you use the same injection site repeatedly, the absorption rate slows down, so rotate the sites.

The timing of your insulin injections helps to determine the smoothness of your glucose control. The more regular you are in your injections, your eating, and your exercise, the smoother your glucose level.

Conducting intensive insulin treatment

Intensive insulin treatment is essential in type 1 diabetes if you hope to prevent the complications of the disease. This treatment means measuring your blood glucose at least before each meal and at bedtime, plus using both short-acting and longer-acting insulin to keep the blood glucose between 80 and 100 before meals and less than 140 after eating. How you do this is the subject of this section.

In a person who doesn't have type 1 diabetes, a small amount of circulating insulin is always present in the bloodstream, and after eating, insulin increases temporarily to control the glucose in the meal. Intensive insulin treatment attempts to mirror the activity of the normal human pancreas as much as possible.

In intensive insulin treatment, you usually take a certain amount of longer-acting insulin at bedtime. I prefer insulin glargine because it produces a smooth basal level of glucose control over 24 hours. In addition, you take a dose of rapid-acting insulin before each meal. I prefer lispro because I have the most experience with it. The dose of lispro is determined by the expected grams of carbohydrates in the meal you're about to eat, as well as by your blood glucose at that moment. Your doctor should provide you with a list of how much insulin to take for a given situation. Each patient is different, and the dosage must be individualized.

Using the carbohydrates in a meal to determine your insulin dose is called *carbohydrate counting.* The key to this system is to know the carbohydrates in your food. Here is where you make use of your friendly dietitian, who can go over your food preferences and show you how many carbohydrates are in them. The dietitian can also show you where to find carbohydrate counts for any other foods that you may eat.

You also need to know how many grams of carbohydrate are controlled by each unit of insulin you take. This number is determined by checking your blood glucose an hour after eating a known amount of carbohydrate. For example, one person may need 1 unit to control 20 grams of carbohydrate, while another person needs 1 unit to control 15 grams of carbohydrate. If both of them eat a breakfast of 75 grams of carbohydrate, the first person might take 4 units of lispro, whereas the second person takes 5 units of lispro. Then additional units are added for the amount that the blood glucose needs to be lowered. A typical schedule is to take 1 unit for every 50 mg/dl that the blood glucose is above 100 mg/dl. Insulin can also be subtracted if the blood glucose is too low. For every 50 mg/dl that the glucose is below 100, subtract 1 unit. (To see how carbohydrate counting works in practice, see the sidebar "Carbohydrate counting to maximum health.")

By measuring your blood glucose frequently, you can find out how different carbohydrates affect your blood glucose. By using the carbohydrate sources that have a low glycemic index, you need less insulin to control them. (See Chapter 8 for more on carbohydrates.)

As you attempt to help your body mirror normal insulin and glucose dynamics, you often have to deal with a greater frequency of hypoglycemia. The best way to handle hypoglycemia is by eating slightly smaller meals and using the unused calories as between-meal snacks. This technique smoothes the ups and downs.

At what point do you adjust your insulin glargine? If you find that several mornings in a row your fasting blood glucose is too high, you might add a unit or two to your bedtime glargine. If it's too low, you might reduce your insulin glargine by a unit or two or try eating a small bedtime snack. A high blood glucose level throughout the day is an indication to raise the glargine. Getting a lot of hypoglycemia at different times of day is a reason to lower the glargine. These adjustments are best done in consultation with your doctor. If, however, you're unable to see your doctor, you can put your knowledge to use and make these adjustments on your own.

ANECDOTE

Carbohydrate counting to maximum health

To find out how you can accomplish carbohydrate counting in everyday life, take a typical type 1 patient. Salvatore Law is a 41-year-old who has had type 1 diabetes for 31 years. He has been well controlled because he follows a good diet, does lots of exercise, and takes his insulin appropriately. He takes 30 units of insulin glargine at bedtime.

Law has a list of dosages of lispro insulin that tells him to take 1 unit of insulin for each 20 grams of carbohydrate he eats. He is about to have breakfast and knows that it will contain 80 grams of carbohydrate. Therefore, he needs four units of lispro insulin. He measures his blood glucose before breakfast and finds that it is 202 mg/dl. His doctor has told him to take an extra unit of lispro insulin for each 50 mg/dl above 100 mg/dl. He adds two more units for a total of six units of insulin taken just before breakfast.

At lunch, his blood glucose measures 58. He is about to have a lunch of 120 grams of carbohydrate, so he needs 6 units for that. However, he reduces it by 1 unit for the glucose measurement that is approximately 50 mg/dl lower than 100, so his final dose is 5 units.

Before supper, Law's blood glucose measures 120. His supper contains only 60 grams of carbohydrate, so he needs 3 units for that. He does not have to adjust the dose because the glucose is close to 100, so he takes only 3 units.

At bedtime, his blood glucose is 108, so he is doing very well. Unless the blood glucose is 200 or greater, he does not need to take any bedtime lispro because he is taking insulin glargine to control his glucose overnight.

Adjusting insulin when you travel

If you're traveling between time zones, you may wonder if you need to change your insulin routine while you're gone. Time changes of less than three hours require no modifications, but changes above three hours require progressively more. You should probably discuss these changes with your physician before you go.

Say that you're taking the red-eye flight at 10 p.m. from San Francisco, arriving at 6 a.m. at Kennedy Airport in New York. If you are taking insulin glargine or detemir, you don't have to change your dose. Just start using lispro (or any other rapid-acting insulin) at the beginning of your meals (which you'll be eating three hours earlier than usual because of the time change).

When you return to California, you add three hours to your day. In this case, you need to take an extra measurement of your blood glucose. If it's around 150, you need do nothing, but if it's 200 or more, take a couple of units of lispro insulin to bring it down. If your blood glucose is much below 100, eat a small snack. Again, you do not have to adjust your insulin glargine.

Delivering insulin with a pen

Several manufacturers, including Eli Lilly, Owen Mumford, Diesetronic, Novo Nordisk, Sanofi-Aventis, and Becton Dickinson, have sought ways to make delivering insulin easier. The insulin pen, shown in Figure 11-2, is one useful tool. The pen doesn't eliminate the need for needles, but it does change the way you measure your insulin. Either the pen comes with an insulin cartridge already inserted, or the cartridge is placed inside the pen just like an ink cartridge used to be put in a pen and replaced when it runs out.

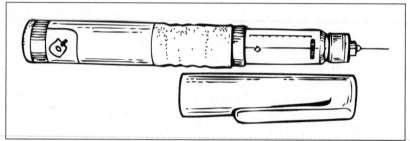

Figure 11-2:
The insulin
pen.

Illustration by Kathryn Born

Each cartridge contains 1.5 or 3.0 milliliters of insulin — either NPH, regular, lispro, aspart, glargine, detemir, a mixture of NPH and lispro (such as 75 percent NPH-like lispro and 25 percent lispro), or a mixture of NPH plus aspart. You can then dial the amount of insulin that you need to take. Each unit (sometimes 2 units) is accompanied by a clicking sound so the visually impaired can hear the number of units. The units also appear in a window on the pen. If you draw up too many units, one of the pens forces you to waste the insulin by pushing it out of the needle, while others allow you to reset the pen and start again. Depending on the pen, you can deliver from ½ to 80 units of insulin. You screw on a new needle as needed.

A number of different companies make pens for their own insulin. Available pens include the following options:

- **Autopen:** This pen is available in four different models. Two contain a 1.5-ml cartridge, and two contain a 3-ml cartridge. Within each size, one pen delivers Humalog insulin in 1-unit increments, and the other pen delivers Humalog insulin in 2-unit increments.

- **Humalog Mix 75/25, Humalog Mix 50/50, Humalog KwikPen, Humulin Mix 70/30, and Humulin N:** All these prefilled, disposable pens contain 3 ml of the particular kind of insulin you use.

- **HumaPen Luxura HD:** This pen is used for Humalog insulin when half-unit doses are needed, particularly in children.

✔ **Levemir FlexTouch Pen:** This prefilled disposable pen contains 3 ml of Levemir insulin.

✔ **NovoLog FlexPen and NovoLog 70/30 FlexPen:** These prefilled, disposable insulin syringes contain 3 ml of insulin.

✔ **NovoPen Junior:** This pen takes NovoLog cartridges containing 3 ml of insulin, and they can be measured in half-unit doses.

✔ **NovoPen 3:** This pen holds NovoLog 3-ml cartridges.

✔ **SoloStar:** This disposable pen contains 3 ml of Lantus insulin.

Insulin pens require needles, and you must match the pen with the proper needle in order for the pen to work properly. If the needles don't come with the pen, the instructions with the pen tell you which needle to use.

Should you shift from your syringe and needle to a pen? If you're comfortable with the syringe and needle and feel your technique is accurate, you probably have no reason to do so. If you're new to insulin, have some visual impairment, or feel that you're not getting an accurate measurement of the insulin, a pen may be the solution for you.

In February 2015, the FDA issued a warning against allowing others to use your pen. Even if needles are changed, there may be blood in the pen cartridge that could cause infection of the other user.

Delivering insulin with a jet-injection device

Jet-injection devices (see Figure 11-3) are for people who just can't stick a needle into their skin. At around $1,000 or more, they're expensive, but they last a long time and replace the syringe and needle.

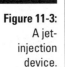

Figure 11-3: A jet-injection device.

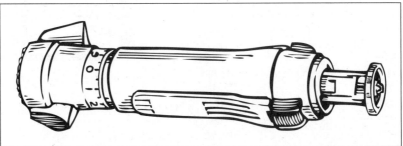

Illustration by Kathryn Born

The only jet injection device that I could verify is still on the market is the Insujet, a device that is made in the Netherlands by the European Pharma Group at www.insujet.com. To contact the company for information about the device, you can e-mail info@insujet.com.

A large quantity of insulin is taken into the injection device, enough for multiple treatments. The amount of insulin to be delivered is measured, usually by rotating one part of the device while the number of units to be delivered appears in a window. The device is held against the skin. With the press of a button, a powerful jet of air forces the insulin through the skin into the subcutaneous tissue, usually with no pain perceived by the patient. The devices come in a lower power form for smaller children. These devices can deliver up to 50 units at one time.

Should you try an insulin jet injector? If you have no trouble with the syringe and needle or find the pen to be an easy substitute, you don't need a jet injector. If you hate needles or need to give frequent shots to a small child who is very resistant to them, a jet injector may solve your problems.

Delivering insulin with an external pump

For some people — and you may be one of them — the external insulin pump (see Figure 11-4) is the answer to their prayers. These devices are as close as you currently can come to the gradual administration of rapid-acting insulin that is normally taking place in the body. They're expensive, costing more than $4,000, but the insulin pump may be the answer for patients who simply cannot achieve good glucose control with syringes, pens, or jet injectors.

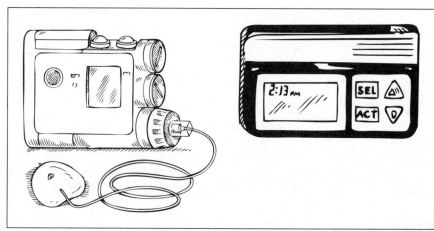

Figure 11-4: The insulin pump with its infusion set.

Illustration by Kathryn Born

Currently, six companies — Animas, Insulet, Medtronic MiniMed, Roche, Sooil Development, and Tandem — sell these pumps, which are the size of a pager. Inside the pump is a motor. A syringe filled with short-acting insulin is placed within the pump, with the plunger against a screw that slowly pushes it down to push insulin out of the syringe. The end of the syringe is attached to a short tube, which ends in a needle pushed into the skin of the abdomen. Insulin is slowly pushed under the skin. The Insulet device, called the OmniPod, has the infusion set built in and doesn't require tubing.

The rate at which insulin slowly enters under the skin is called the *basal rate*. It can be set, by way of computer chips, to vary as often as every half hour to an hour. For example, from 8 a.m. to 9 a.m., the pump may deliver 0.8 units, while from 9 a.m. to 10 a.m., the pump may deliver 1.0 unit, depending on the needs of the patient. This amount is determined, of course, by measuring the blood glucose with a meter (see Chapter 7).

When the patient is about to eat a meal, he or she can push a button to deliver extra insulin, called a *bolus* of insulin. (The amount is determined by carbohydrate counting, which I explain earlier in this chapter.) You can get extra insulin if the blood glucose is too high at any time.

Pump usage has its advantages:

✔ It's flexible because the bolus is taken just before meals.

✔ It often smoothes out the swings of glucose during the day because the insulin is administered slowly and in small variable doses, depending on insulin requirements at different times of day.

✔ It can be rapidly disconnected and reconnected to take a shower or swim. (However, it can take a little getting used to when worn to bed.) Or insulin delivery can be suspended during exercise to prevent hypoglycemia after exercise.

✔ It's safe from overdosage because it has built-in protective devices.

However, pump usage has definite disadvantages besides the high cost:

✔ Infections of the skin are frequent because the infusion set is left in place for several days. These infections are usually mild, however.

✔ Overall diabetic control is not necessarily better with the pump than with other ways of delivering insulin, especially with the new insulin glargine. The latest proof of this was an article published in *Journal of Diabetes and Its Complications* in November 2010.

✔ Because the patient receives only short-acting insulin, if insulin stops entering, ketoacidosis may come on rapidly (see Chapter 4).

✔ Some patients are allergic to the tape that holds the infusion set onto the skin.

✔ Blood glucose must be measured often to adjust the pump for optimal control.

Pump usage is definitely not treatment to be done on your own at the beginning. You need a diabetologist to help with dosages, a dietitian to help you calculate amounts of boluses based on carbohydrate intake, and someone from the manufacturer to teach you how to set the pump and to be available to fix any malfunctions.

If you use a pump and your blood glucose rises above 250 mg/dl, take the following steps:

1. **Take a bolus of insulin with the pump to bring it down. (The amount is determined by your sensitivity to insulin.)**

2. **Recheck your glucose in an hour.**

3. **If the glucose is still above 250 mg/dl, use a syringe to take more insulin.**

4. **Check your infusion set.**

5. **Check the ketones in your urine and report to a doctor if the amount is moderate to large.**

6. **Recheck your glucose every two hours and use more insulin as needed.**

Is an insulin pump for you? If you're willing to invest the time and effort at first, if your schedule is very uncertain, particularly with respect to meals, and if your glucose control has not been good with other means, you should look into this option.

My patients who use the pump have generally had positive experiences. Now that they have it, none of them are willing to give up the pump. Occasionally, they disconnect the pump to allow their skin to heal. They have generally shown improved glucose control and a better hemoglobin A1c.

Do I recommend using an insulin pump? With insulin glargine, you can accomplish a continuous basal control of the blood glucose much like the pump does. The pump proponents say that you need to be able to alter the basal dose for different conditions throughout the day, and you can't do that with a single shot of insulin. However, I am not sure that it makes a great difference in the course of controlling the blood glucose.

Is one pump better than another? All seem to have excellent mechanical features, and all provide you with the ability to adjust your insulin in several ways. They all have alarms for any eventuality like blockage of the tube, an electrical failure, and so forth. They try to differentiate themselves by offering different options for how the insulin is delivered, but you may find that you need the help of a rocket scientist to figure out those differences.

One pump that does deserve special mention, because it is the wave of the future, is the Medtronic MiniMed Paradigm Real Time Revel. This pump is sold with the OneTouch UltraLink Blood Glucose Monitor. Readings taken by the monitor are wirelessly sent to the pump, which uses a software program to calculate the bolus of insulin to be given, taking into account the carbohydrates about to be eaten, which you must enter into the pump. The wearer must accept the bolus before it is delivered. This product is just short of the so-called *closed loop system,* where the blood glucose determines the amount of insulin to be given, just as the normal pancreas is constantly doing. The pump chooses the boluses, but it does not constantly alter the basal level of insulin, because no continuing information about the current blood glucose level is given. The wearer must test the blood glucose with the meter in order for the pump to know glucose levels.

For an extensive discussion of the various types of insulin pumps that are available, their pros and cons and much more about using a pump to deliver insulin, see my book *Type 1 Diabetes For Dummies* (Wiley).

Utilizing aids to insulin delivery

For those of you still using the old needle-and-syringe method, I want you to be aware of numerous aids that can make taking insulin easier for you:

- ✔ **Spring-loaded syringe holders:** You place your syringe in the holder, hold it against the skin, and press a button. The needle enters and administers the insulin. Examples are Inject-Ease and Autoject 2.

- ✔ **Syringe magnifiers:** These magnifiers help visually impaired people administer insulin. Examples are Insul-eze, BD Magniguide, and Syringe Magnifier by Apothecary.

- ✔ **Syringe-filling devices:** You can feel and hear a click as you take up insulin. An example is Count-A-Dose.

- ✔ **Subcutaneous infusion sets:** A catheter is placed under the skin, and injections are made into the catheter instead of the skin to reduce punctures. Many units are available.

- ✔ **Needle guides:** You can use these guides when you can't see the rubber part of the insulin bottle to insert the needle to take up the insulin. An example is Safe Shot.

Call your local American Diabetes Association branch or look in the back of the ADA's *Diabetes Forecast* magazine to find sources for these products.

If you take a drug that makes you prone to hypoglycemia, you need to wear a medical bracelet or necklace that identifies you as a person with diabetes who may be hypoglycemic. Numerous companies make these products.

Using Other Medications

Most of this chapter is devoted to medications that lower the blood glucose, but diabetes involves more than elevated blood glucose levels. People with diabetes often have high blood pressure and high cholesterol, and they suffer more sickness when exposed to influenza or pneumonia. You need to consider this fact in the overall management of your disease.

If you have high blood pressure (see Chapter 7), then lifestyle changes, including weight loss and physical activity, may be all you need to control the condition. However, if lifestyle changes alone don't work, numerous medications are available that control blood pressure. See my book *High Blood Pressure For Dummies* (John Wiley & Sons, Inc.) for a complete discussion of this subject. Controlling blood pressure is as important as controlling blood glucose in preventing diabetic complications.

Most people with diabetes also have elevated levels of LDL (bad) cholesterol (see Chapter 7). Excellent drugs are available to manage this problem if lifestyle changes don't suffice. See *Controlling Cholesterol For Dummies* (John Wiley & Sons, Inc.) by Carol Ann Rinzler and Martin W. Graf, MD, for the answers to your questions on this topic. Cholesterol control is another cornerstone of excellent diabetic care. A study published in the *New England Journal of Medicine* in March 2004 indicates that when it comes to LDL cholesterol, the lower, the better. Talk to your doctor about this topic.

Statin drugs are the most frequently used for lowering LDL cholesterol. However, statin use in postmenopausal women is associated with an increased risk for type 2 diabetes, so discuss it with your doctor.

People with diabetes, especially those whose glucose is poorly controlled, are prone to become sicker when they develop influenza or pneumonia. Excellent vaccinations for these illnesses are available. Flu vaccine is given annually, and pneumonia vaccine is given once if you are older than 65 and received a previous vaccination more than five years ago. In 2011, the Advisory Committee on Immunization Practices at the Centers for Disease Control recommended that all unvaccinated adults with diabetes aged 19 to 60 be vaccinated against hepatitis B virus as soon as a diagnosis of diabetes is made. Those individuals 60 and older should be vaccinated if they're expected to have a satisfactory immune response.

Finally, aspirin has been shown to reduce sickness and death due to coronary artery disease (which I discuss in Chapter 5). Because coronary artery disease is such a prominent feature of diabetes, many doctors recommend that all patients with diabetes take a daily aspirin tablet. However, the American Diabetes Association doesn't recommend it for diabetics at low risk of a heart attack. Diabetics may need more than the usual dose of a baby aspirin to reduce their risk of heart attacks; a full adult pill may be necessary.

Avoiding Drug Interactions

Studies have shown that some patients with diabetes are taking as many as four to five drugs, including their diabetes medications. These drugs often interact, and the results can be harmful. Sometimes (believe it or not) even your doctor is not aware of the interactions of common drugs. You need to know the names of all the drugs you take and whether they affect one another.

Many common medications used for the treatment of high blood pressure also raise the blood glucose, sometimes bringing out a diabetic tendency that may otherwise not have been recognized:

- ✔ **Thiazide diuretics** often raise the glucose by causing a loss of potassium. Among these drugs are chlorothiazide (Diuril) and metolazone (Zaroxolyn), which are similar to hydrochlorothiazide.

- ✔ **Beta blockers** reduce the release of insulin and include such drugs as propranolol (Inderal), metoprolol (Lopressor), and atenolol (Tenormin).

- ✔ **Calcium channel blockers** also reduce insulin secretion. They include nifedipine (Adalat), verapamil (Calan), diltiazem (Cardizem), verapamil (Isoptin), amlodipine (Norvasc), and nifedipine (Procardia).

- ✔ **Minoxidil** can raise blood glucose.

Drugs used for other purposes can also raise blood glucose:

- ✔ **Corticosteroids,** even in topical use, can raise blood glucose.

- ✔ **Cyclosporine,** used to prevent organ rejection, can raise the blood glucose by poisoning the insulin-producing beta cell.

- ✔ **Diphenylhydantoin,** known as Dilantin, is a drug for seizures and blocks insulin release.

- ✔ **Nicotinic acid and niacin,** used to raise HDL and lower cholesterol, can bring out a hyperglycemic tendency.

✔ **Phenothiazines,** such as prochlorperazine (Compazine), mesoridazine (Serentil), trifluoperazine (Stelazine), and chlorpromazine (Thorazine), can block insulin secretion and cause hyperglycemia. Many of the newer antipsychotic drugs also cause insulin resistance.

✔ **Thyroid hormone,** in elevated levels, raises the blood glucose by reducing insulin from the pancreas and increasing the breakdown of insulin.

Oral contraceptives were previously accused of causing hyperglycemia when the dose of estrogen was very high, but current preparations are not a problem.

Many common medications, either on their own or by doing something to make the oral drugs that lower blood glucose more potent, also lower the blood glucose. The most important of these include the following:

✔ **Salicylates and acetaminophen,** known as aspirin and Tylenol, can lower the blood glucose, especially when given in large doses.

✔ **Ethanol,** in any form of alcohol, can lower the blood glucose, particularly when taken without food.

✔ **Angiotensin-converting enzyme inhibitors,** used for high blood pressure, such as quinapril (Accupril), captopril (Capoten), benazepril (Lotensin), fosinopril (Monopril), lisinopril (Zestril and Prinivil), and enalapril (Vasotec), can lower the blood glucose, though the mechanism is unclear.

✔ **Alpha-blockers,** another group of antihypertensives that includes prazosin, lower the glucose as well.

✔ **Fibric-acid derivatives** like clofibrate (Atromid-S), used to treat disorders of fat, cause a lowering of blood glucose.

If you start a new medication and suddenly find that your blood glucose is significantly higher or lower than usual, ask your doctor to check for the possibility that the new medication has a definite glucose-lowering or glucose-raising effect.

Finding Assistance Obtaining Drugs

Diabetes can be expensive, especially if you need several drugs to control your blood glucose. The pharmaceutical companies understand, and several offer programs to provide medication for a period of time. Table 11-1 tells you what you need to know about these companies.

All these programs require you to get a prescription from your doctor. The doctor usually fills out forms that state that the patient meets the financial requirements and needs the drug. Not all companies give away free drugs for life. But if you cannot afford to buy a drug that you're taking, do not hesitate to call the company and ask whether it has a patient-assistance program.

Table 11-1	How You Can Get Drug Supplies		
Company	**Primary Medication**	**Program Name**	**Phone Number**
Xubex Pharmacy	Metformin	Free Medication Program	866-699-8239
Eli Lilly	All insulin preparations	Lilly TruAssist	855-559-8783
RxOutreach	Glyburide	Rx Outreach	800-769-3880
Novo Nordisk	Insulin preparations	Patient Assistance Program	866-310-7549
Pfizer	Glipizide, glipizide extended release, chlorpropamide	Pfizer RxPathways	866-706-2400
Sanofi-Aventis	Insulin glargine	Patient Assistance Program	800-981-2491

Chapter 12

Assembling Your Diabetes Team

....

....

Shakespeare said it: "All the world's a stage." That quote applies to diabetes beautifully. You have many roles in life, and one of them is the role of a person with diabetes. But as with any production, you're not expected to do it all alone. You have a large cast and crew who are eager to help you, but you must be willing to ask for their help and know how to use them so that they can give you their best. Believe me, as a member of that crew, everyone wants to give you their best.

The question is, do you want your play to be a comedy or a tragedy? You hold all the major positions, so the choice is entirely up to you. And remember, as with all plays, life goes on offstage. You may also be a brother or sister, mother or father, boss or employee, and so on. Fortunately, the life skills that you discover as someone with diabetes are applicable to all your other roles.

The Internet is a goldmine of information. The resources it offers deserve mention in this chapter on using all the tools available to manage your diabetes.

Your Role as Author, Producer, Director, and Star

Being the author, the producer, the director, and the star may seem like a lot of responsibility — and it is. Unlike many short-term illnesses where the doctor knows what has to be done, instructs you to do it, writes a prescription, and cures you, diabetes is your daily companion for life. No one, not even your mother or spouse, can be with you all of the time. Therefore, you're the one who writes the script and the action. You decide whether you'll take your medication or exercise regularly. You determine whether you'll follow a diet that will control your weight and your blood glucose.

You're the one who needs to gather the resources needed to play the role properly. In this sense, you're the producer. You need your props and your theater, the equipment, the medications, and the environment in which to manage your diabetes. Your environment may be a comfortable home where you can eat the proper diet and a good exercise facility where you can burn up calories while you strengthen your heart. Or it may be the sidewalk where you can safely walk or jog.

After you have the resources, you need to direct your cast and crew to make your play come out the way you envision it. You're the one who sees to it that the primary physician obtains a hemoglobin A1c (see Chapter 7) every three or four months and that you visit the eye doctor at least once a year. The physician is dealing with many patients each day and can easily forget your specific needs, so you must let the doctor know what they are and not expect him or her to read your mind. You may be dealing with other doctors who treat your heart, your lungs, and other parts of you. Each doctor needs to know all the medications you take.

Finally, you're the star of the show. That role is both an honor and a responsibility. Although you may wish that you had never been chosen for this particular role, you have it. You can make of it what you will. You can learn all your lines (understand your disease) and speak them fluently (take your medications, follow your diet, and so on), or not. Obviously, not studying your lines is a lot easier, but in that case, the result can be a tragedy. Take proper care of yourself, and the smile on your face and that of all your fellow cast members and crew will clearly indicate that you have written, produced, directed, and starred in a comedy.

The Primary Physician: Your Assistant Director

In the United States, where you can find numerous specialists, only 8 percent of people with diabetes are regularly seen by a specialist. Because of the large size of the diabetic population and the requirements of a healthcare system with limited resources, the other 92 percent are in the hands of more general doctors, primary physicians, who have to deal with many other illnesses besides diabetes.

Although using a primary physician instead of a specialist may seem not conducive to the best care, I can say many good things about it. Besides diabetes complications, you may have other things go wrong, and the primary physician can handle them as well. After all, if you had only mild heart disease, you might not require a cardiologist, and your primary physician could also manage your bronchitis very well.

You should expect your primary physician to have a decent working knowledge of diabetes. Chapter 7 describes the proper way to follow a person with diabetes. The various tests are essential to your health, and the primary physician must know which ones to order and when to send you to a specialist because your needs are beyond his or her expertise.

The Diabetologist or Endocrinologist: Your Technical Consultant

One type of specialist, an endocrinologist, should have the most in-depth knowledge of the management of diabetes. She has several years of advanced training (on top of the years of training in general internal medicine) and devotes her practice to taking care of people with diabetes, plus patients with problems of the thyroid, adrenals, or other glands. A *diabetologist* is an endocrinologist who takes care of only diabetic patients.

If you have type 1 diabetes, you will certainly see an endocrinologist sooner or later. If you have type 2 diabetes and get into trouble with complications or control, you'll be sent to an endocrinologist for consultation. You have the right to expect that this physician will be able to answer most questions that arise during the care of diabetes.

This doctor will be up on the newest treatments for diabetes, so if you have questions about the future of diabetes care, ask her. This doctor should also have the best understanding of all the drugs currently used for diabetes, how they interact with each other, their side effects, and other drugs that interact with them.

If you're not satisfied with the answers you're getting from your primary physician, ask for a referral to a specialist. Many health plans today try to steer you away from the specialist because this doctor orders more expensive tests and costs more to see by virtue of the extra years of specialty training. But do not take no for an answer. If your primary doctor will not refer you, find one who will.

If your endocrinologist or diabetologist makes any changes to your treatment, report those changes to your primary physician. One of the big problems in medicine is the lack of communication between medical-care providers of all types, not just doctors.

For your own sake, make sure that all your medical-care providers know what the others are doing for you. Carry a list of your medications and show it each time you have a doctor visit. You may even want to carry the actual medications so the doctor can verify that you are getting the medications in the strengths that she thinks you are getting.

The Eye Doctor: Your Lighting Designer

The eye doctor (*ophthalmologist* or *optometrist*) ensures that your diabetes does not damage your vision. This doctor has had advanced training in diseases of the eye. Your primary-care physician must see to it (no pun intended) that you have an examination by this specialist at least once a year and more often if necessary.

The eye doctor examines you for the conditions I outline in Chapter 5. He must send a report to your primary physician. He should also take the opportunity to educate you about diabetic eye disease.

An ophthalmologist or optometrist must dilate the pupils of the eyes in order to do a proper examination.

Sometimes the good deed of restoring vision leads to unexpected, negative consequences. One ophthalmologist I talked to told me that he restored the vision of a diabetic patient, only to have the patient buy a gun and nearly shoot someone with whom he had a grievance.

The Foot Doctor: Your Dance Instructor

The foot doctor, or *podiatrist,* is your best source of help with the minor (and some of the major) foot problems that all people suffer. You should go to her if you have such problems as toenails that are hard to cut, corns and calluses, and certainly any ulcer or infection of your foot. It's especially important to visit the podiatrist if you have any neuropathy (see Chapter 5). In that case, you're better off not trying to cut your toenails by yourself.

Foot doctors I spoke with emphasized that the earlier you see a podiatrist, the less likely you are to have a minor problem turn into a major disaster. For example, an infected toe that would respond to soaking by the person without diabetes may need antibiotics, special shoes, and surgical removal of dead tissue in the person with diabetes.

The doctor can tell you which preparations you should not use on your skin. She can show you how important it is that you give lesions time to heal and not rush to put weight on your injured feet. Many podiatrists also give you a list of do's and don'ts for the proper care of your feet, such as conducting daily inspections, avoiding extreme heat, and so on. Chapter 5 details all the things you need to do to preserve good foot health.

The Dietitian: Your Food-Services Provider

This person serves one of the most important roles in your care. Because most diabetes is type 2, and type 2 is greatly worsened by obesity, a good dietitian can really help you to control your blood glucose both by eating the right foods and amounts and helping you to lose weight. The dietitian can also show you which foods belong to which energy source — carbohydrate, protein, and fat. (See Chapter 8 for more on your diet.)

People with type 1 diabetes need to know how food interacts with mandatory insulin injections. The dietitian can teach you to count carbohydrates so that you know how much insulin to take for your meals. (See Chapter 11 for more on carbohydrate counting.)

A good dietitian usually holds up a mirror to you, showing you not only what you eat but how you eat as well. When do you consume most of your calories, and where do they come from? All ethnic foods can be adjusted so that you enjoy the foods you have always eaten while you stay within the bounds of a diabetic diet. A good dietitian is the best source for this kind of information.

The dietitian can also show you what a portion of food really means. This demonstration is an eye-opener in most cases. You usually find that you have been eating portions much larger than necessary. Unfortunately, when it comes to a diabetic diet, you can't have your cake and eat it, too. But you can see in the Appendix, which offers gourmet recipes for people with diabetes, that every culture makes delicious food that is actually good for the person with diabetes. For even more information on this important topic, see the latest edition of my book *Diabetes Cookbook For Dummies* (John Wiley & Sons, Inc.).

One thing you want to be sure of is that the dietitian is flexible in her approach to food. You may have to follow a few rules about where your calories come from, but you should have plenty of room for variation within those rules. The diet you are ultimately given should take into account your preferences as well as the fact that the amount of carbohydrate, protein, and fat is different for different individuals. Any dietitian who simply hands you a printed diet and says "Go follow it" is doing you no favor.

The Diabetes Educator: Your Researcher

Every person in your play is actually an educator in addition to his other role, but an actual diabetes educator is specially trained to teach you what you need to know about every aspect of diabetes so that you properly take care of yourself. He should have *CDE* (Certified Diabetes Educator) after his name. A CDE has taken extensive courses in diabetes and has passed an examination.

A diabetes educator teaches you how to take your insulin or pills, how to test your blood glucose, and how to acquire any of the other skills you need. You can find many diabetes educators in a diabetes education program. After you have gotten over the shock of having diabetes, asking your primary physician to refer you to such a program is a good idea. After you have gone through the program, go back and update yourself every few years. New drugs and new procedures are constantly being discovered. A diabetes educator can be a wonderful source of information about these advancements while making sure that you continue in your good diabetic habits.

Although individual education classes may be hard to find and be more expensive than group classes, studies suggest that individual education of people with diabetes is more effective than group education. Glucose control was better and patients' behavior and psychological adjustment were more improved.

The Pharmacist: Your Usher

The role of the usher may not sound important, but how will you enjoy the play if you can't find your seat? The pharmacist is your guide to all the medications and tools required to control your blood glucose and manage any complications that you develop. She ushers you into the use of all these strange and new products. You may see your pharmacist more often than you see any other of your crew who are actually in the medical field.

Each time you start a new medication, a good pharmacist checks to make sure that it does not conflict with other medicines you are taking. The pharmacist tells you about side effects and makes sure that your doctor is checking you for adverse drug reactions or interactions. The pharmacist may give you a printout that you can take home and refer to, telling you all you need to know about your new medication.

Many pharmacists also prepare a list of medications that you take, telling you each drug's strengths and dosage frequency. You can carry this list around in case any doctor ever needs to know what you take.

Modern pharmacists also do a lot of educating. Posters in the pharmacy explain diseases and drugs. Pharmacists can tell you about helpful over-the-counter drugs that your doctor doesn't prescribe. They are also often aware of new drugs and treatments before they become well known. Some pharmacies have blood-pressure devices that you can use for free, as well as glucose meters.

The Mental-Health Worker: Your Supporting Actor

Your mental-health worker may be a psychiatrist, a psychologist, or a social worker, or your primary physician may play this role. This person comes in handy whenever you have days when you feel you just can't cope. (See Chapter 1 for more about dealing with the emotional aspects of diabetes.) The mental-health worker supports you and gets you going again. Diabetes certainly proves the fact that all diseases are both physical and emotional.

Your Family and Friends: Your Captivated and Caring Audience

Your audience is the people you live with, eat with, and play with. Your family and friends can be a tremendous source of help, but you must clue them in to the fact that you have diabetes. If you have type 1 diabetes, you can teach them how to recognize when your glucose is too low, in case you're ever too ill to take care of yourself. If you have type 2, ask them to moderate their diet so that you can follow yours. A diabetic diet is good for anyone. Complying with your diet is difficult enough, and you don't need your family exposing you to high-calorie foods.

A family member or friend can also become your exercise partner. Sticking to a program is a lot easier when a partner is counting on you to show up to work out. Your family and friends can also accompany you when you visit the doctor and remind you to ask the doctor a question or to follow the instructions you received.

Let these people know about your diabetes and buy them a copy of this book so that they better understand what you are going through and how they can best help you.

The Internet: Your Potential Partner in Lifestyle Change

Type 2 diabetes is a lifestyle disease. Some harmful choices for your lifestyle contributed to your development of type 2 diabetes and some helpful choices will help you control it or prevent it if you don't have it yet. Unlike the people in your life, who can hardly be there with you 24 hours a day, the Internet is only a mouse click away at any time. On the Internet you can find help for the two key aspects of your lifestyle that affect diabetes, diet and exercise.

Because weight loss is the main preoccupation of millions of Americans, numerous websites promise incredible results. Probably the single most important feature of a site that will truly help you to succeed is continued feedback. If you get regular new advice (at least weekly) and peer support in the form of message boards where you can interact with others, you will lose three times as much weight as with sites that only provide diet and exercise information on a noninteractive web page.

For additional resources, go to www.dummies.com/extras/diabetes.

Sites for diet and weight loss

Following are some of the better sites for diet and weight loss:

✔ **www.ediets.com:** This site gives you a choice of many different diets and provides the food as well as weekly updates and suggestions. You can choose from more than 22 diet plans, and eDiets.com prides itself on the tastiness of its foods, so one of the plans is sure to appeal to you. You can consult with their nutritionists to develop a diet that meets your needs. If, for example, you have a heart issue, the company will tailor your diet for you. Fitness is an important component of their diets.

✔ www.diet.webmd.com: This site uses a questionnaire to develop a "diet just for you." The diet, which is called a nutritional plan, is personalized and nutritionally sound. You fill out a daily nutritional journal that the people at WebMD comment on. They analyze your progress and nutritional needs each week. WebMD is filled with useful information for people who must lose weight for any reason. It also emphasizes fitness, as any good diet program should.

✔ http://shapeup.org: This is the web address of Shape Up America!, a nonprofit organization founded by former surgeon general C. Everett Koop, MD. It offers lots of free information about nutrition and also advocates for your health. For example, it is working to get the federal government to label beer, wine, and spirits with nutritional information and to classify obesity counseling and treatment as essential health benefits so your insurance has to pay for it.

Sites for exercise programs

Here are some of the better websites for exercise programs:

✔ www.freetrainers.com: This site offers individualized fitness programs with individual advice and message boards for reading the experiences of others and offering your own. They have something for everyone from beginning exercisers to established fitness devotees. You can even find a training partner at this site.

✔ workoutsforyou.com: At this site, you can get a personalized fitness program, weekly e-mail tips, and unlimited e-mail consultations. There are lots of member testimonials in case you want to read the experience of others. You have to pay for information and a program at this site.

✔ www.global-fitness.com: This website for Global Health and Fitness offers a large amount of information on fitness with lots of feedback from trainers. It touts itself as the first weight-loss and fitness program on the Internet, starting in 1996. It is another site where you pay for information and training.

None of these sites tell you about the people who did not do so well or even the ratio of successful to unsuccessful clients. Don't spend a lot of money up front until you are sure the program is what you need and what works for you. Good luck!

Finding reputable websites

Not everything that you find on the Internet is true, let alone reputable. The Health on the Net Foundation has established a set of principles that any site on the Internet can adhere to. From its website at www.hon.ch, you can search for medical sites that follow these HONcode principles:

- **Principle 1:** Any medical or health advice provided and hosted on this site is only given by medically trained and qualified professionals unless a clear statement is made that a piece of advice offered is from a non-medically qualified individual or organization.

- **Principle 2:** The information provided on this site is designed to support, not replace, the relationship that exists between a patient/site visitor and his or her existing physician.

- **Principle 3:** Confidentiality of data relating to individual patients and visitors to a medical/health website, including their identity, is respected by this site. The website owners undertake to honor or exceed the legal requirements of medical/health information privacy that apply in the country and state where the website and mirror sites are located.

- **Principle 4:** Where appropriate, information contained on this site is supported by clear references to source data and, where possible, have specific HTML links to that data. The date when a clinical page was last modified is clearly displayed (typically at the bottom of the page).

- **Principle 5:** Any claims relating to the benefits/performance of a specific treatment, commercial product, or service is supported by appropriate, balanced evidence in the manner outlined in Principle 4.

- **Principle 6:** The designers of this website seek to provide information in the clearest possible manner and provide contact addresses for visitors that seek further information or support. The webmaster displays his or her e-mail address clearly throughout the site.

- **Principle 7:** Support for this website is clearly identified, including the identities of commercial and noncommercial organizations that have contributed funding, services, or material for the site.

- **Principle 8:** If advertising is a source of funding, the site clearly says so. A brief description of the advertising policy is displayed on the site. Advertising and other promotional material is presented to viewers in a manner and context that facilitates differentiation between it and the original material created by the institution operating the site.

If a site agrees with these principles, you can bet the information on it is very reliable.

Part IV

Special Considerations for Living with Diabetes

Seven tips to making a restaurant dinner a healthful experience

- Drink a large glass of water 10 minutes before you have your meal so you feel more full.

- Check the menu before you go to make sure there are entrées that work for your diabetes.

- If there is a delay in getting your table, ask for some carrot sticks and celery until you can be seated.

- Don't drink any wine until you can have some food with it.

- Consider splitting your entrée with another guest to reduce the number of calories and carbohydrates.

- You can have dessert, but share it with others at the table and try to be satisfied with a bite or two.

- If you take insulin, wait until you get food containing carbohydrates, protein, or fat before taking your injection.

The Patient Protection and Affordable Care Act (PPACA) provides a unique opportunity to compare how often diabetes is discovered when people have medical insurance and when they don't. Go to www.dummies.com/extras/diabetes for more information that describes the difference and the consequences.

In this part . . .

✔ Know how to help your child manage his or her diabetes and avoid possible problems.

✔ Regulate diabetes in the elderly and handle any challenges before they become more serious.

✔ Identify any potential occupational and insurance problems so you can overcome them.

✔ Be up-to-date on what's new in diabetes and work closely with your doctor on cutting-edge treatments and care.

✔ Recognize and ignore what doesn't work in diabetes care and treatment.

Chapter 13

Managing Diabetes in Children

*W*hen I wrote the first edition of this book, in 1998, almost all diabetes in children was type 1 diabetes. Since then, a vast change in this situation has taken place. The incidence of type 2 diabetes is rapidly approaching the incidence of type 1 diabetes in children, and the culprits to blame for this huge increase are obesity and lack of exercise. I have a lot more to say about this problem in the section on type 2 diabetes in children later in this chapter.

There are still plenty of new cases of type 1 diabetes in children. This chapter contains basic information about the care for those children; for a full discussion of type 1 diabetes, see my book *Type 1 Diabetes For Dummies* (John Wiley & Sons, Inc.).

Children with diabetes present special problems that adults with diabetes do not have. Not only are they growing and developing from babies to adults, but they have problems of psychological and social adjustment. Diabetes can add complications to a period of time that is not exactly smooth, even without it.

Many doctors believe that if a child has diabetes, the whole family really has the disease because everyone must adjust to it. And because diabetes is the second most common chronic disease in children after asthma, it is no small problem.

In this chapter, you find out how to manage diabetes in your child at each stage of growth and development. You need to remember that your child is first a child and then a child with diabetes. And you also need to remember that no one is to blame for your child's diabetes. Although diabetes is a serious problem, it's nothing you and your child can't handle.

Dealing with Diabetes in Your Baby or Preschooler

If your infant or preschooler is diagnosed with diabetes, you may feel overwhelmed. The information in this section can help you understand that this diagnosis isn't the end of the world — it's the beginning of many years of special care for your child.

Nurturing a diabetic infant

Although type 1 diabetes doesn't usually show up in babies, it can, and you should know what to expect when it does. Obviously, your baby is not verbal and cannot tell you what is bothering him or her. And you may miss the fact that the baby is urinating excessively in his or her diaper. The baby will lose weight and have vomiting and diarrhea, but these symptoms may be ascribed to a stomach disorder rather than diabetes. When the diagnosis is finally made, the baby may be very sick and require a stay in a pediatric intensive care unit. Do not blame yourself for not realizing that your baby was sick with diabetes.

Type 2 diabetes is almost never seen in babies. The current epidemic of type 2 diabetes in children is the result of excessive weight gain, which is rare in babies and toddlers. The treatments described below are for type 1 diabetes.

After the diagnosis of T1DM is made, the hard work begins. You must learn to give insulin injections and to test the blood glucose in a child who will be reluctant to have either one done. You have to learn when and what to feed the baby, both to encourage growth and development and to prevent low blood glucose.

At this stage, you don't need to be as worried about tight glucose control as you will be later on. There are several reasons why not. First, the baby's developing neurological system can be damaged by frequent, severe low blood glucose, so the glucose is permitted to be higher now than later on. Second, studies show that changes associated with high blood glucose leading to diabetic complications do not begin to add up until the prepubertal years, so you have a grace period during which you can allow less tight control.

According to a study in *Diabetes Care* in June 2011, vitamin D deficiency is associated with increased prevalence of diabetic eye disease in children and adolescents. Make sure your child has sufficient vitamin D. It's available as drops that you can add to your baby's food.

On the other hand, a small baby is very fragile. He or she has less of every-thing, so small losses of water, sodium, potassium, and other substances lead more rapidly to a very sick baby. If you keep the baby's blood glucose around 150 to 200 mg/dl (8.3 to 11.1 mmol/L), you are doing very well.

Taking care of a toddler with diabetes

Diagnosing diabetes in your preschooler may be just as difficult as it is in the baby. The child may still be preverbal and running around in diapers.

A preschooler is beginning the process of separating from his parents and starting to learn to control the environment (by becoming toilet-trained, for example). This separation process makes it more difficult for you, the parent, to give insulin injections and test the glucose. You must be firm in insisting that these things be done. You'll need to do them yourself because a small child neither knows how to do them nor understands what to do with the information generated by the glucose meter.

Because a toddler's eating habits may not be very regular, the use of very short-acting insulin like lispro is especially helpful (see Chapter 11). Very soon, people with diabetes should have a way of measuring the blood glucose in a painless fashion, which will be of great assistance in monitor-ing children.

Becoming an educated caregiver

For a time of variable duration in the child with type 1 diabetes — a so-called "honeymoon period" — your child will have seemingly regained the ability to control his or her blood glucose with little or no insulin. This period always ends, and it isn't your fault that it does. When it ends, you have to work with your child's doctor, dietitian, and diabetes educator to find out how to con-trol diabetes with insulin.

To give your child appropriate care, you need to know how to do the follow-ing things:

- ✔ **Identify the signs and symptoms of hyperglycemia, hypoglycemia, and diabetic ketoacidosis (see Chapters 4 and 5).** Each child has a particu-lar way of expressing low or high blood glucose, for example, by becom-ing quiet or loud. Learn the signs for your child, and let anyone else who cares for the child know them.

- ✔ **Administer insulin (see Chapter 11).** Thanks to rapid-acting insulin, you can wait to see how much the baby is eating before you decide on the amount of insulin.

✔ **Measure the blood glucose and urine ketones (see Chapter 7).** Very frequent blood glucose measurements are essential. The more information you have, the better the control and the less frequent the hypoglycemia. Most children need between four and seven blood glucose measurements a day to achieve excellent control.

Toddlers who are toilet-trained may have accidents when their glucose is high, because high glucose causes a large quantity of urine.

✔ **Treat hypoglycemia with food or glucagon (see Chapter 4).** Young children require half the adult dose of glucagon. Glucagon may cause a toddler to vomit, but it still raises the blood glucose.

✔ **Feed your diabetic child (see Chapter 8).**

✔ **Set an example for lifelong exercise for your child by exercising with her.**

✔ **Know what to do when your child is sick with another childhood illness.** If your child must go to the hospital, approach it as a positive experience — a chance to get a tune-up.

Your responsibilities as the parent of a diabetic baby or preschooler are extensive and time-consuming. Training your usual helpers to take over, even for a short time, is especially difficult. Unless you hire a professional to take over for a while, you may not get very much time away from your diabetic infant.

Placing your child in preschool is a difficult decision. You can do so only if you are sure that the adult supervisors are fully aware of your child's needs and willing to provide for them.

Your other children may resent the attention that you pay to this one child. If your other children start to misbehave, this may be the reason.

Helping Your Primary-School Child with Diabetes

Around age 10, some children are found to have type 2 diabetes. Important differences exist in the way type 1 and type 2 are recognized and treated. Therefore, I discuss each type separately in this section. In 1990, less than 4 percent of children diagnosed with diabetes had type 2. In 2003, the figure had risen to more than 30 percent. In 2007, almost one of every two children with diabetes had type 2 diabetes. For a discussion of why that number has grown so rapidly, see the section "Preventing and Treating Obesity and Type 2 Diabetes in Children," later in this chapter.

Coping with type 1 diabetes

In some ways, type 1 diabetes care gets a little easier with a primary-school child, but in other ways, it gets more difficult. Your child can finally tell you when he or she has symptoms of hypoglycemia, so that part is easier to recognize and treat. But you must begin to control the blood glucose more carefully because your child is reaching the stage where control really counts.

You still have a child who is growing and developing, so nutrition remains critical. You must provide enough of the right kinds of calories to fuel the growth process. A snack such as 4 ounces of apple juice and a graham cracker between breakfast and lunch, between lunch and supper, and at bedtime can help smooth out glucose control and avoid hypoglycemia.

With age, your child is going to do more to separate from you. He or she may insist on giving insulin shots and doing blood tests. Studies indicate that primary-school years are not a good time for you to give up these tasks, certainly not completely. Your child may not be physically capable of performing them and, in an attempt to hide the disease from peers, may not perform them at all during school. Diet may also suffer at school as the child tries to fit in and not stand out by eating the things that diabetes requires.

Managing hypoglycemia

Because you are beginning to tighten the level of glucose control, hypoglycemia is more of a risk, especially at night. At this stage (and from now on), you can avoid hypoglycemia by taking any or all of the following steps:

- ✔ Give a bedtime snack regularly.
- ✔ Give cornstarch at bedtime. Cornstarch is slowly broken down, so it provides glucose over a longer period of time. One to two tablespoons of uncooked cornstarch can be added to milk (shake well), yogurt, or pudding, or you can try a commercial product such as NiteBite, which can be given before bedtime.
- ✔ Measure and treat low blood glucose before bedtime.
- ✔ Occasionally check the blood glucose at 3 a.m.
- ✔ Ask your child about symptoms of nighttime low blood glucose, such as nightmares and headaches.
- ✔ Be sure your child does not skip meals.
- ✔ Have your child eat carbohydrates before exercising.

At least one member of your family must be able to administer glucagon by injection to treat hypoglycemia should you be unable to get your child to eat or drink.

Handling school issues

When your child goes to school or a daycare setting, you need to address new problems. One issue is that he interacts with other children, wants their approval, and wants to fit in. Your child may consider diabetes a stigma and be very reluctant to share it with other children. A plan of treatment that interferes with school and friendships may be very unwelcome.

Other issues may arise regarding the school's willingness to participate in your child's care. To best handle these issues, you must be aware of your rights.

Federal laws, especially the Diabetes Education Act of 1991, specify that diabetes is a disability and that it's unlawful to discriminate against children with diabetes. If a school receives federal funding or is open to the public, it has to reasonably accommodate the special needs of the diabetic child.

Any school receiving federal funds must develop a *Section 504 plan* to meet the needs of the disabled child. This plan refers to Section 504 of the Rehabilitation Act of 1973, and it takes every need of the child into account from the moment she is picked up in the morning by a bus driver (who must know how to help the child with a diabetic problem) until she arrives back home at the end of the day. The plan includes the child's self-care abilities, and it lists trained personnel by name and responsibility.

If you plan to send your child to a private school that receives no federal funds, before enrolling, insist on a plan of care for your child identical to a 504 plan.

The law requires that a diabetic child be able to participate fully in all school and after-school activities. Therefore, provisions must be made for blood glucose testing, for treatment with insulin, and for taking snacks or going to the bathroom as needed.

The written Section 504 treatment plan is developed by your doctor, you, and the school nurse, and relevant people in the school have assigned roles. The plan must include

- Blood glucose monitoring
- Insulin administration
- Meals and snacks
- Recognition and treatment of hypoglycemia
- Recognition and treatment of hyperglycemia
- Testing of urine ketones as indicated

As the parent, you are responsible for providing all supplies for testing and treatment. The school provider has a responsibility to understand and treat hypoglycemia, to test the blood glucose and treat it when the level is outside certain parameters, to coordinate meals and snacks, and to permit excused appointments to the doctor as well as restroom use. There is no reason that your child should not participate fully in school.

You have to provide a kit every day for school that contains everything the child needs to test the blood glucose and, if necessary, the urine for ketones. The kit must also include any necessary insulin and syringes. A list of signs and symptoms of high and low blood glucose is another useful addition to this kit. A source of food must be available to the child throughout the school day, both for snacks and prevention of hypoglycemia during exercise. The teachers need to know to remind the child to eat. The child must be free to eat when necessary and not have to request food from the teacher.

These kits and food sources also have to go with the child whenever the child leaves school — for example, for a fire drill or a field trip.

Recognizing and treating type 2 diabetes

A number of clues point to a child having type 2 diabetes rather than type 1:

- ✔ The child is overweight rather than underweight at diagnosis.

- ✔ Symptoms, such as thirst and increased urination, are mild or not present at all; if they are present, they have been going on for a long time (often months).

- ✔ The child has a strong family history of type 2 diabetes.

- ✔ The child's glucose level at diagnosis is usually lower than the glucose of a patient with type 1.

- ✔ The child belongs to an ethnic group at increased risk for type 2, such as African American, Hispanic, Asian, or Native American.

- ✔ The child has *acanathosis nigricans,* dark or thickened patches on the skin between the fingers and toes, on the back of the neck, and on the underarms. These patches are present in 90 percent of type 2 patients.

- ✔ An older girl may have irregular menses caused by polycystic ovarian syndrome (see Chapter 6).

Despite these clues pointing to type 2, the two types of diabetes can be confused for several reasons. Type 1 diabetic children may be overweight. Type 2 children may have ketones in their urine, just as type 1 patients do. The glucose level at diagnosis in some type 1 children is not very elevated. And the overall occurrence of type 2 is still low enough that the doctor may not think of the possibility.

Some children actually have "double diabetes." These children have type 1 diabetes but were overweight or obese at the time the diagnosis was made. In these children, lifestyle modification plays an important role in the treatment. Weight loss and exercise will help to bring the glucose under control, even though insulin is the primary treatment.

An important thing to remember is that type 2 diabetes responds to treatment with insulin much more rapidly than type 1, and the child may not need insulin at all after a proper diet and exercise are established. No child with type 1 diabetes can live without insulin except possibly.

If you have an overweight child — one who is more than 120 percent of his or her ideal weight for height — you should request that your doctor screen him or her for diabetes every two years by using a fasting blood glucose test.

The treatment of type 2 diabetes, both in children and adults, starts with lifestyle change. You, the parent, must make the commitment to exercise with your child every day. You should meet with a dietitian and discuss a diet for the whole family that provides sufficient nutrition for the growing child while allowing for weight loss. If these two things are accomplished, no more steps will be necessary. That means limiting TV and computer time so the child is active rather than passive. You might consider getting a pedometer for your child and encouraging him or her to build up the number of steps taken each day, with prizes for reaching goals.

Shifting responsibility to the child

As your child grows and matures, you will constantly be concerned with the question of when to let him or her take over. Tim Wysocki, PhD, looked at 648 children to see when they were able to take over key skills. He found that 50 percent of children had mastered the following tasks at the younger age in the ranges below, whereas 75 percent had mastered the tasks at the older age. You can use these results as a general guide for your child.

- ✔ Pricking finger with lancet: 5–6

- ✔ Performing blood glucose test with a meter: 6–7

- ✔ Stating symptoms of high blood glucose: 7–9

- ✔ Giving injections to self: 8–10

- ✔ Drawing up mixture of two types of insulin: 10–11

- ✔ Stating reasons for need to change insulin dose: 8–12

- ✔ Testing urine for ketones: 8–14

- ✔ Adjusting food intake according to blood glucose: 9–14

- ✔ Adjusting insulin dose according to blood glucose: 13–18

If diet and exercise do not return the blood glucose to normal, oral hypogly-cemic agents (see Chapter 11) are used. Currently, metformin is the only oral drug approved by the FDA for children. If oral agents fail, insulin is given.

Managing Your Adolescent's Diabetes

Until 10 years ago, only 3 percent of cases of diabetes in adolescents were due to type 2 diabetes. Presently 45 percent of new cases of diabetes in adolescents are due to type 2 diabetes. In non-Hispanic blacks, it represents 58 percent of new cases, in Asian/Pacific Islanders 70 percent, and in American Indians 86 percent.

If an adolescent or young adult has type 2 diabetes, the information in the previous section applies, because the goal remains the same no matter what the age: Normalize the child's weight and increase exercise in order to achieve normal blood glucose levels. Therefore, I focus my attention in this and the next section on type 1 diabetes roughly corresponding to the teenage years.

Your adolescent or teenager with type 1 diabetes will provide some of your biggest challenges. This is the time period when most childhood diabe-tes begins. The Diabetes Control and Complications Trial (see Chapter 3) showed that tight glucose control can be accomplished beginning at age 13 and that this control can prevent complications. The higher frequency of severe hypoglycemia that accompanies tighter control was not found to be damaging to the brain of a child at this age. However, children at this age do not think in terms of long-term blood glucose control and prevention of com-plications. So they're not willing to do many of the tasks required to control their diabetes on a regular basis.

The goal of treatment at this stage is a hemoglobin A1c between 7 and 9 percent (see Chapter 7). A value above 11 percent indicates poor control. (This isn't true for smaller children, who are allowed to have a higher hemoglobin A1c.)

The outlook for children with type 1 diabetes has improved dramatically in the last few years. Up to 2000 their life expectancy was 19 years less than the general population. Between 2000 and 2011 life expectancy increased to just 4 years less than the general population.

This stage is when your child is most eager to become independent. You don't want to give up all control at this time for several reasons:

  ✔ Your child actually does better if he or she has limits that are clearly stated and enforced.

✔ The "shame" of diabetes may cause the child to skip shots and food, especially around friends.

✔ The problem of eating disorders (see Chapter 8) may pop up at this time, especially among girls trying to maintain a slim body image. Girls with diabetes know that if they skip their injections, they lose weight. They may ignore the high blood glucose that results.

✔ Teenagers with diabetes may still be unable to translate levels of blood glucose into appropriate action.

The hormonal changes that occur in puberty are often associated with insulin resistance. These physical changes may be a source of loss of control rather than any failure of your child to follow the diabetic treatment plan. Upward adjustment of the insulin may overcome this problem.

Strenuous exercise may play an even greater role in the life of your child at this age, and type 1 diabetes is no reason to prohibit exercise. The result will be a significant reduction in the amount of insulin required after exercise. The blood glucose measurements will help you to define your child's need for insulin. If your child plays a team sport, the coach and teammates must be aware of the diabetes and permit your child to eat, go to the bathroom, and take insulin as required.

Make sure that your child snacks regularly; keep snacks readily available no matter where your child may be.

Handing Over the Reins to Your Young Adult Child with Diabetes

When your child becomes a young adult, you definitely want to give up the control that has helped her to thrive up to this point. Your child should be doing her own testing. She is ready to leave the pediatric level and begin to work with doctors who care for adults, so you will probably be out of the loop. Your child should now have the skill to choose appropriate insulin treatment based on blood glucose levels and calories of carbohydrate consumed (see Chapter 11).

Your child now has new challenges, including finding work, going to college, finding a future mate, and finding a place to live independently. At the same time, the reluctance to admit to diabetes and the desire for a thin body continue to complicate care.

Off to college

When your child leaves for college, he or she has all the responsibility for the diabetes. Your job is simply to make sure that all the equipment for testing the blood glucose and administering insulin is available to your child. You should also make the college aware of your child's medical condition. Encourage your child to find one or more people at the college, such as a roommate or sports teammate, who are prepared to help when necessary.

Two issues are particularly important to discuss before the student leaves for school: alcohol use and sexual activity. Alcohol use may significantly increase in college, which means that your child may consume many empty calories and run the risk of severe hypoglycemia if he or she fails to eat properly. If you have a diabetic daughter, discuss with her the risk of pregnancy when diabetes is not in control. (See Chapter 6 for information.) Young adults of both sexes should know how to prevent sexually transmitted diseases.

College, like the rest of your child's life, can be experienced just as it would be if diabetes were not present. The key is planning.

Diabetes care must be intensive at this point (see Chapter 11). Multiple shots of intermediate and short-acting insulin are taken. Your child must follow a diabetic diet (see Chapter 8), and an exercise program is essential (see Chapter 10). The rest of this book really has to do with the tasks that your young adult child with diabetes faces.

Preventing and Treating Obesity and Type 2 Diabetes in Children

The epidemic of obesity, which has spread to children in the United States in the past few decades, has led to a much higher prevalence of type 2 diabetes in children than was ever seen before. As many as one-third of all US children are overweight or obese. However, only a fraction of these children go on to develop diabetes.

A number of medical conditions can cause obesity in children, but they represent probably 1 percent of the causes. Most of them can be diagnosed during the course of a good physical examination by your child's pediatrician. By far, the major reason for obesity in children is too many calories in and too few burned up by exercise.

Even without diabetes, obesity is a burden for children. The obese child faces severe psychological and social consequences:

✔ Lower respect from peers than other disabled children get

✔ Less comfortable family interactions

✔ Poor body image

✔ Low self-esteem

Defining obesity in children

The definition of obesity in children age 2 to 19 is based on the body-mass index, BMI (see Chapter 7). A child is obese or overweight if his BMI is at the 95th percentile or greater for his age and sex. He is overweight if the BMI is between the 85th and 95th percentile. You can find the growth charts that indicate the percentiles for BMI at www.brightfutures.org/bf2/pdf/pdf/GrowthCharts.pdf.

Obesity is not just responsible for type 2 diabetes. It can also provoke a number of other dangerous medical conditions in children. These include

✔ Metabolic syndrome, discussed in Chapter 5, leading to an increased tendency for heart attacks and strokes

✔ Polycystic ovarian syndrome, discussed in Chapter 6, leading to infertility, abnormal menstrual periods, and hairiness in girls

✔ Heart disease due to the increased work of the heart

✔ High blood pressure, which can damage the heart and the kidneys

✔ Sleep disorders like obstructive sleep apnea with snoring and increased blood pressure

✔ Fatty liver with abnormal liver enzymes in the blood

✔ Gallbladder disease

✔ Bone and joint diseases due to the weight on the bones

✔ Skin abnormalities like acanthosis nigricans, black velvety patches on the joints and under the arms

✔ Nervous-system diseases such as increased pressure in the brain with headache and visual disturbances

Preventing obesity in children

Prevention of obesity is much preferred over treating the damage that it does. You can do the following things to prevent obesity in your child:

- ✔ Try to have a normal weight before you become pregnant.

- ✔ Exercise throughout your pregnancy.

- ✔ Breastfeed for at least six months. A study in *Diabetes Care* in March 2011 showed that it reduces the occurrence of obesity in your child and reduces the increased obesity in your child associated with exposure to your diabetes while in the uterus.

- ✔ Eat meals together as a family.

- ✔ Avoid sugary drinks and fatty foods.

- ✔ Restrict time for sedentary activities like TV or computers. Adolescent boys with screen time of two hours or more daily have twice the risk of insulin resistance compared to boys with less than two hours.

- ✔ Don't allow your child to participate in fundraisers that sell candy and cookies.

- ✔ Insist on exercise daily and do it with your child.

Changes are coming in schools. New federal guidelines set calorie caps on meals in school, gradually reduce the amount of salt in school foods, eliminate trans fats from school food, and reduce the amount of fat in milk and other foods. Food companies are reformulating foods that they sell to schools to meet these guidelines.

The outlook for children with type 2 diabetes is much worse than type 1 diabetes with much earlier death due to heart disease, on average just 27 years after the diagnosis is made. The incidence of high blood pressure and kidney disease including kidney failure also rises rapidly. Treatment must be improved.

Dealing with type 2 diabetes

Adding type 2 diabetes to obesity can be devastating. The consequences of the preceding problems may lead to failure to manage the diabetes because the child wants to avoid any activity that makes him or her even more different from his or her peers.

You must help your obese child to lose weight because most obese children become obese adults. With the assistance of a dietitian, you can figure out the food that your child can eat to maintain growth and development without gaining more weight. One of the most helpful techniques is to take the child into the supermarket and point out the difference between empty calories and nourishing calories. Another is never to make high-calorie food, such as cake and candy, a reward. Finally, if you keep problem foods out of the house, there is much less likelihood that your child will eat them.

When type 2 diabetes develops, treatment should begin as early as possible to minimize the development of complications. Depending on the severity of the diabetes, the treatment can utilize any or all of the following approaches:

- **Lifestyle changes:** Parents must set an example of good dietary and exercise habits. Some studies suggest that if parents go first, children will follow. The best diet is one that emphasizes a variety of vegetables, some fruits, and small amounts of protein with minimal processed carbohydrates like candy and pastries. The best exercise is what you will continue to do regularly.

- **Drugs:** The currently available drugs, with the exception of metformin, are either not recommended for children under 16 years of age or not useful for long-term treatment. A study in the *New England Journal of Medicine* in June 2012 showed that adding rosiglitazone to metformin increased the number of children in control of their diabetes, so the addition of other drugs may be changing.

- **Surgery:** All of the information about metabolic surgery for diabetes in adults in Chapter 9 pertains to children, although it's important that they have attained maturity of their skeleton, which is usually age 13 for girls and 15 for boys. The presence of depression or an eating disorder doesn't preclude surgery. Weight-loss surgery is safe for adolescents, but they tend to have low adherence to vitamin supplementation after surgery, which must be addressed.

Because it's reversible, adjustable gastric banding is probably the operation of choice in children. Experience with 110 teenagers who had this surgery at the New York University Program for Surgical Weight Loss showed an average 55 percent weight loss with no complications or deaths.

The International Pediatric Endosurgery Group has published bariatric surgery recommendations for children and adolescents. Essentially, the recommendations exclude children who have not attained final or near-final adult height. The BMI must be greater than 40 kg/m^2 or greater than 35 kg/m^2 if other diseases such as diabetes or heart disease are present. A trial of lifestyle change has been unsuccessful. The family unit should have a psychological evaluation and be stable. The surgeon should be experienced and have a team that can do long-term follow-up. The adolescent will adhere to healthy dietary and exercise habits after surgery.

Surgery in preadolescents or in people planning to become pregnant within two years isn't recommended.

Taking Special Care of Sick Children

The comments in this section apply primarily to a child with type 1 diabetes, because children with type 2 diabetes do not lose diabetic control to nearly the same extent.

Any child is susceptible to all the usual childhood illnesses, but diabetes complicates your child's care during these times. An illness can affect diabetes in opposite ways. An infection may increase the level of insulin resistance so that the usual dose of insulin is not adequate. Or it may cause nausea and vomiting so that no food or drink can stay down, and the insulin may cause hypoglycemia. For this reason, you need to measure the blood glucose in your sick child every two to four hours. If the glucose is over 250 mg/dl (13.9 mmol/l), you need to give extra short-acting insulin (see Chapter 11). If it's under 250, you give more carbohydrate-containing nutrients.

You also need to test ketones in your child's urine or blood once or twice a day (see Chapter 7) while he or she is sick, especially if the glucose is over 300 mg/dl. If the ketones become elevated, you need to discuss the situation with your doctor.

You should probably feed your child with clear liquids like tea and soda during the sick days. Don't offer your child milk, because it upsets the stomach. As long as your child can hold down clear liquids, you can continue to take care of him or her. If clear liquids cannot be held down, you must contact your doctor and bring your child to the hospital.

While the blood glucose remains over 250 mg/dl, use tea, water, and diet soda so as not to add calories of carbohydrate. When the blood glucose is less than 250 mg/dl, you can use regular soda or glucose drinks.

Checking for Thyroid Disease in Type 1 Children

Because type 1 diabetes is an autoimmune disease (see Chapter 2), it is not surprising that children with type 1 have other autoimmune diseases more commonly than unaffected children. The disease that is found most commonly in association with type 1 diabetes is *autoimmune thyroiditis*. This condition is discovered by obtaining a blood test that shows an abnormal increase in proteins in the blood called *thyroid autoantibodies.* In a study of 58 patients with type 1 diabetes *(Diabetes Care,* April 2003), 19 were found to have autoimmune thyroiditis.

Autoimmune thyroiditis usually results in no symptoms, but occasionally it causes low thyroid function *(hypothyroidism),* and even more rarely it causes high thyroid function *(hyperthyroidism).* Autoimmune thyroiditis is found mostly in girls between 10 and 20 years of age. This condition is easily treated, as I explain in my book *Thyroid For Dummies* (Wiley).

Autoimmune thyroiditis is so common in type 1 diabetes that patients are recommended to be screened yearly for thyroid disease with a simple blood test that checks the level of thyroid-stimulating hormone (TSH).

Appreciating the Value of Team Care

When your child is first diagnosed with diabetes, the stress can be overwhelming. The guilt that comes with this diagnosis may leave you unable to help your child much at first and certainly unable to learn all that you need to know to master the areas of importance to the health of your child. Therefore, you must depend on the help of a diabetes care team throughout the duration of his or her childhood, and especially when the diagnosis is first made.

Another resource that can be tremendously valuable for you and your child is a diabetes summer camp. These camps are located all over the country and provide a safe, well-managed place where your child can go and be in the majority. He or she can learn a great deal about diabetes while enjoying all the pleasures of a summer camp environment. (Certainly not a minor benefit is the opportunity for you to have time off for perhaps the first time in years.)

You can find an extensive list of camps for diabetic children throughout the United States by going to www.childrenwithdiabetes.com/camps/index.htm. It's one of the many services of the website "Children with Diabetes."

In Chapter 12, I compare diabetes to a stage play. There, the person with diabetes was the author, the producer, the director, and the star. When you have a child with diabetes, he or she is the star, but you take on the roles of author, producer, and director. You obviously have a great responsibility, but it's one that I feel certain you can handle. Just don't try to do it alone. Use your medical experts as well as your family and friends to make it manageable.

Chapter 14

Diabetes and the Elderly

*E*veryone wants to live a long time, but no one wants to get old. Nevertheless, getting old is better than the alternative. Woody Allen says the one advantage of dying is that you don't have to do jury duty. I think I would rather do jury duty.

The first issue I have to tackle in this chapter is defining *elderly*. Every year my definition seems to change, but I think it's fair to talk about the age of 70 as the beginning of being elderly. Using that definition, by the year 2020, more than 20 percent of the United States population will be elderly. As much as one-fifth of that elderly population will have diabetes.

Elderly people with diabetes have special problems. Because of those special problems, they're hospitalized at a rate that is 70 percent higher than the general elderly population. In this chapter, you find out about those problems and the way to handle them.

For additional resources, check out www.dummies.com/extras/diabetes.

Diagnosing Diabetes in the Elderly

The incidence of diabetes in the elderly (which is almost always type 2 diabetes) is higher for many reasons, but the main culprit seems to be increasing insulin resistance with aging. Half of the elderly population has prediabetes.

A study in *Diabetes Care* in August 2008 suggests that the increased insulin resistance associated with aging is due to exactly the same causes as that found in younger people, namely physical inactivity and obesity. However, as a result of decreasing height with age, the body mass index (BMI) isn't a good indicator of obesity in the elderly. The waist circumference is better. A BMI of 30 may not indicate the same level of increased risk of a heart attack in an elderly person as it does in a younger person. A BMI of 30–35 is associated with only a slight increase in risk. The pancreas seems to be able to make insulin at the usual rate. The fasting blood glucose actually rises very slowly as you get older. The glucose after meals, however, rises much quicker and leads to the diagnosis.

Because the fasting blood glucose is usually normal, the hemoglobin A1c (see Chapter 2) is used to make the diagnosis in the elderly population. A hemoglobin A1c that is above 6.5 percent is considered diagnostic of diabetes. Results that fall between normal and that value are in a gray zone that probably indicates prediabetes (see Chapter 2).

The Diabetes and Aging Study (*Diabetes Care,* June 2011) showed that a hemoglobin A1c of 8 percent was associated with the lowest rates of complications and death in older diabetic patients while a level of less than 6 percent was associated with higher death rates.

Elderly people with diabetes often don't complain of any symptoms. When they do, the symptoms may not be the ones usually associated with type 2 diabetes, or they may be confusing. Elderly people with diabetes may complain of loss of appetite or weakness, and they may lose weight rather than become obese. They may have incontinence of urine, which is usually thought of as a prostate problem in elderly men or a urinary-tract infection in older women. Elderly people with diabetes may not complain of thirst because their ability to feel thirst is altered.

Evaluating Intellectual Functioning

You need to evaluate the intellectual function of an elderly person with diabetes because managing the disease requires a fairly high level of mental functioning. The patient has to follow a diabetic diet, administer medications properly, and test the blood glucose. Studies have shown that elderly people with diabetes have a higher incidence of *dementia* (loss of mental functioning) and Alzheimer's disease than nondiabetics, making it much harder for them to perform these tasks.

A study in *Diabetes Care* in October 2010 indicated that some loss of intellectual function in the elderly was due to large changes in blood glucose during each day. Treatment that moderates these changes may be helpful. Another study in *Diabetes Care,* in November 2008, showed that microalbuminuria (see Chapter 7) was predictive of loss of intellectual function and drugs that reversed microalbuminuria (ACE inhibitors or angiotensin receptor blockers) were protective.

The patient can take *cognitive screening tests* to determine his or her level of function. Testing helps determine whether the patient can be self-sufficient or will need help. Many older people who are living alone with no assistance really require an assisted-living situation or even a nursing home.

Considering Heart Disease

The major cause of death in elderly people with diabetes is a heart attack. Strokes and loss of blood flow in the feet are also much more common in diabetics than nondiabetics. Usually, elderly diabetics not only suffer from diabetes but also have high blood pressure and high cholesterol, are overweight or obese, and do little exercise.

After the diagnosis of diabetes is made, it is too late for prevention, but a major effort should be made to control the glucose, the blood pressure, and the cholesterol in order to postpone the onset of vascular disease.

If you have been smoking for decades, although you can't do much about cancer or emphysema, you can prevent sudden death associated with cigarette smoking. That complication of smoking disappears in a few days of no cigarettes.

Preparing a Proper Diet

Diet and exercise are the foundations of good diabetic care for the elderly just as they are in the younger population. Elderly diabetic patients do disproportionately better with lifestyle change than the younger population. Even light physical activity significantly reduces the incidence of diabetes, especially among the overweight or obese. Fifteen minutes of moderate walking after meals improved the glucose intolerance of older people with prediabetes. The information I provide in Chapter 8 (on diet) and in Chapter 10 (on exercise) should be used to create a wellness plan to manage diabetes as well as to help the elderly patient feel good and ward off any other health issues.

Diminishing intellectual function can have a negative effect on the diet of elderly people with diabetes, because they may not understand or be able to prepare a proper diabetic diet. The elderly have other problems when it comes to proper nutrition:

✔ They may have poor vision and be unable to see to read or cook.

✔ They may have low income and be unable to purchase the foods that they require.

✔ Their taste and smell may be decreased, so they lose interest in food.

✔ They often have a loss of appetite.

✔ They may have arthritis or a tremor that prevents cooking.

✔ They may have unhealthy teeth or a dry mouth.

Any one of these problems may be enough to prevent proper eating by the elderly person, with the result that the diabetes is poorly controlled.

Anyone over the age of 65 who has Medicare Part B insurance coverage is covered for the services of a dietitian for *medical nutrition therapy*. Be sure to take advantage of this benefit. The dietitian can analyze the elderly person's current intake and make recommendations to insure a balanced diet that will help with control of the blood glucose.

Avoiding Hypoglycemia

The elderly, who are already somewhat frail, are especially hard-hit by the consequences of hypoglycemia and are especially prone to it because of several factors:

✔ Their food intake may be uncertain.

✔ They may be taking multiple medications.

✔ They may sometimes skip medications.

✔ They often live alone.

✔ Their mental state may not permit them to recognize when they are becoming hypoglycemic.

✔ Their kidney function is often impaired, causing many diabetic medications to last longer than in a younger person.

The hemoglobin A1c goal for healthy elderly adults is 7 percent. However, if the life expectancy is less than five years, the elderly person is frail, or the risks of intensive therapy outweigh the benefits, the goal is 8 percent. This decreased level of control will help to avoid hypoglycemia. Refer to Chapter 4 for more information on hypoglycemia.

Using Medications

Medications that may lower blood glucose to abnormally low levels, such as the sulfonylureas and insulin, are not the drugs of first choice in the elderly. As I explain in the previous section, hypoglycemia hits elderly patients particularly hard and should be avoided if at all possible. With that goal in mind, I explain the proper order of drug usage for elderly diabetics in this section. Each of these medications is discussed in detail in Chapter 11.

Elderly people are often on several medications, and the monthly expense for drugs may be great enough to cause them to skip doses or not buy the drug. As I explain many times in this book, compliance with your treatment routine is essential to good health. If you are not taking your diabetes medication(s) as prescribed, you must let your doctor know.

- ✔ Metformin is probably the first drug to try because it doesn't increase insulin secretion (which can lead to hypoglycemia) and because it's inexpensive. Kidney function, which is decreased in the elderly, must be checked when using this drug. The doctor should measure the level of creatinine in the blood. Previously the drug was stopped if evidence suggested kidney disease. Recent evidence (December 2014 *JAMA Internal Medicine*) supports the use of metformin in patients with mild to moderate kidney disease. The drug should be started at a low dose of 500 mg and gradually increased over several weeks to avoid stomach and intestinal problems. A study in *Diabetes Care* in October 2013 noted that metformin use is associated with reduced mental function that may be reversed by vitamin B12 and calcium.

- ✔ Sulfonylureas are added when a second drug is needed. However, sulfonylureas can cause hypoglycemia — especially the older drug chlorpropamide. The newer drugs in this category, such as glyburide and glipizide, are preferred; glipizide may not cause hypoglycemia as often. Your doctor should start you on half the usual dose and raise it slowly over a number of weeks.

The sulfonylurea-like drugs called the *meglitinides* (repaglinide and nateglinide) may have an advantage in the elderly because they do not last as long. Nateglinide is also available in a generic form.

Drugs like acarbose (Precose), in the class called alpha-glucosidase inhibitors (see Chapter 11), have a very limited effect on the blood glucose and a lot of intestinal side effects. I do not recommend their use in the elderly.

If pills fail to provide reasonable control of the blood glucose so that the hemoglobin A1c is lower than 9, the patient must use insulin. A shot of glargine at bedtime, combined with taking a pill during the day, often accomplishes the desired level of control. Two drug classes that are beginning to have a greater role in diabetes in the elderly are the GLP-1 agonists and the DPP-4 inhibitors (see Chapter 11). Two daily injections of exenatide (Byetta) or the new once-a-week preparation may be very helpful in achieving some weight loss and lowering of the blood glucose. Sitagliptin (Januvia) or the other DPP-4 inhibitors may provide all the extra glucose control needed by the patient.

There is a 20 percent decrease in deaths due to heart attacks in elderly diabetics who take statins, so these drugs are recommended for all elderly diabetics unless there is a medical reason not to give them. Lowering the blood pressure with drugs also lowers heart attack risk, but no benefit exists in lowering the systolic blood pressure below 140. The evidence for a beneficial effect of low dose aspirin in the elderly is uncertain.

Dealing with Eye Problems

Elderly people with diabetes are at risk for the eye problems brought on by the disease, and these problems can affect all aspects of proper diabetes care. Older patients often get cataracts, macular degeneration, and open-angle glaucoma in addition to diabetic retinopathy.

Fortunately, the risk of developing eye diseases associated with diabetes has been found to decrease as people age, at every level of hemoglobin A1c. For example, a 70-year-old with a hemoglobin A1c of 11 is at much lower risk than a 60-year-old with the same hemoglobin A1c.

An eye examination is recommended every two years if it remains negative for diabetic eye disease. One of the biggest failures in diabetes care is that as many as one-third of the elderly never have an eye examination at all. If no examination is done, how can disease be found when it is early enough to treat? When problems are detected, they can be treated, and the patient's vision can be saved.

Coping with Urinary and Sexual Problems

Urinary and sexual problems are common in elderly people with diabetes and greatly affect quality of life. An older person with diabetes may experience paralysis of the bladder muscle so that urine is retained; when the bladder fills, overflow incontinence is the result. Also, an older person may be unable to get to the bathroom fast enough. Or, spasms in the bladder muscle may lead to incontinence. The result may be frequent urinary-tract infections. A urologist may be able to help.

Almost 60 percent of all men over the age of 70 are impotent, and 50 percent have no *libido* (the desire to have sex). The percentages are even higher for diabetic men. These problems can have many causes (see Chapter 6), but older men are especially likely to have blockage of blood vessels with poor flow into the penis. The elderly take an average of seven medications daily, many of which affect sexual function.

To have sex at any age, you need sexual desire and the physical ability to perform, you need a willing partner, and you need a safe, private place. Any or all of these factors may be missing for the elderly.

Treating sexual dysfunction may not be necessary if the male and his partner are okay with the situation. If they aren't, Chapter 6 points out a number of treatments for potency problems.

Monitoring Foot Problems

The risk of foot problems is much higher in elderly patients because they have diminished circulation. It is essential that you examine your feet with your eyes to check for foot problems, or if your parent or loved one has diminished intellectual function, that you examine his feet daily. Make sure the doctor checks his feet at every visit. Almost half of elderly patients can't see or reach their feet, so it must be done by someone else.

Most foot problems are reversible if found early. Regular foot doctor visits may be as routine as visits to the dentist. See Chapter 5 for more information on prevention and treatment of foot problems.

Considering Treatment Approaches

When deciding on treatment for an elderly patient with diabetes, you first have to consider the individual. Does this person have a low life expectancy? Or is this person physiologically young, with the possibility of living for 15 or 20 more years? If the patient is only 65 years old and in relatively good health, he or she has a life expectancy of at least 18 more years — plenty of time to develop complications of diabetes, especially macrovascular disease, eye disease, kidney disease, and nervous system disease. That person may require more intensive diabetes care than someone who is older and has worse overall health.

A study of a large representative population of elderly people with diabetes published in *JAMA Internal Medicine* in January 2015 showed that 51 percent were relatively healthy, 28 percent had intermediate health, and 21 percent had poor health, although the average hemoglobin A1c for the group was 7 percent. This level suggests that many elderly people with complex or poor health are being overtreated and suffering from hypoglycemia. Diabetics in patients older than age 75 have double the rate of emergency department visits for hypoglycemia than the general population.

The level of care provided to an elderly patient may be basic or intensive:

- ✔ **Basic care** is meant to prevent the acute problems of diabetes like excessive urination and thirst. You can accomplish this goal by keeping the blood glucose under 200 mg/dl (11.1 mmol/L). Basic care is used for an elderly person with diabetes who is not expected to live very long, either because of the diabetes or other illnesses.

- ✔ **Intensive care** is meant to prevent diabetic complications in an elderly person expected to live long enough to have them. The goal here is to keep the blood glucose under 140 mg/dl (7.7 mmol/L) and the hemoglobin A1c as close to normal as possible while avoiding frequent hypoglycemia. Elderly patients who have had diabetes for 20 or more years have a higher death rate when treated intensively.

The benefits in terms of preventing complications of diabetes are much greater when the hemoglobin A1c is lowered from 11 to 9 than when it is lowered from 9 to 7. The goal of treatment for many elderly people can be set higher in order to avoid hypoglycemia.

Treatment always starts with diet and exercise. Education about both can be of great value, especially if the patient's spouse is also involved. I discuss diet in the section "Preparing a Proper Diet," earlier in this chapter, and in Chapter 8.

Exercise may be limited in the elderly person with diabetes. Recent studies have shown that exercise is helpful even in the very old because it reduces the blood glucose and the hemoglobin A1c. However, because elderly patients have more coronary artery disease, arthritis, eye disease, neuropathy, and peripheral vascular disease, exercise just may not be possible. (See Chapter 10 for more on exercise.)

If an elderly patient can't walk at all, he or she may still be able to do resistance exercises sitting in a chair. These exercises increase strength and lower the blood glucose.

When diet and exercise are inadequate to control an elderly patient's diabetes, medications must be added. I discuss medications in the section "Using Medications," earlier in this chapter, and in Chapter 11.

Understanding the Medicare Law

In 1998, the federal government began to offer benefits for the 4.2 million people with diabetes who are eligible for Medicare (over age 65). Under the policy, all people with diabetes enrolled in Medicare Part B or Medicare Managed Care are eligible to receive coverage of glucose monitors, test strips, and lancets. It does not matter which method they use to control their disease.

If you're enrolled in Medicare, you can get these benefits by having your physician prescribe the supplies and document how often you use them.

The Health Care Financing Administration, which administers Medicare, has also passed regulations that permit people with diabetes to get reimbursed for education programs. In addition, if you have Medicare insurance and have type 1 diabetes, you are eligible for Medicare to pay for your insulin pump.

To find out more about Medicare, call the Medicare Hotline at 800-633-4227. The government provides a hotline for the hearing-impaired at 877-486-2048. For a complete rundown of Medicare coverage of diabetes supplies and services, go to www.medicare.gov/publications/pubs/pdf/11022.pdf.

Chapter 15

Dealing With Occupational and Insurance Problems

*A*fter we got his diabetes under control, one of my patients wrote to his mother, "Dear Mom, I'm not working, but my pancreas is." Most people need to work, and some people even want to work. People need to work for the same reason that a certain man didn't turn in his brother-in-law who thought he was a chicken: We need the eggs.

As a person with diabetes, when you try to get a job, you may run into various forms of discrimination. Part of the problem is the fear that the company will have to pay higher insurance premiums if it hires a person with a chronic illness. Part of the problem is a lack of understanding of the great strides that have been made in diabetes care so that a person with diabetes often has a better record of coming to work than a nondiabetic.

In this chapter, you find out what you need to know when you apply for work, health insurance, and life insurance. You discover how to work the healthcare system so that you derive the greatest benefits possible at the lowest cost.

Traveling with Diabetes

Whether you travel for your job or for pleasure, if you need insulin injections and must carry syringes and needles, you have to follow the rules of the Transportation Security Administration (TSA) if you fly within the United States. Airlines outside the United States may have different rules; check with your airline before you travel overseas.

The TSA instructs that you should "make sure injectable medications are properly labeled (professionally printed label identifying the medication or a manufacturer's name or pharmaceutical label). Notify the screener if you are carrying a hazardous waste container, refuse container, or a sharps disposable container in your carry-on baggage used to transport used syringes, lancets, etc." Updated information is available at the TSA website: www.tsa.gov/traveler-information/travelers-disabilities-and-medical-conditions. You can also call the TSA call center at 855-787-2227.

The TSA permits prescription liquid medications and other liquids needed by persons with disabilities and medical conditions. These items include

- All prescription and over-the-counter medications (liquids, gels, and aerosols) including K-Y jelly, eye drops, and saline solution for medical purposes

- Liquids including water, juice, or liquid nutrition or gels for passengers with a disability or medical condition

- Life-support and life-sustaining liquids such as bone marrow, blood products, and transplant organs

- Items used to augment the body for medical or cosmetic reasons, such as mastectomy products, prosthetic breasts, bras or shells containing gels, saline solution, or other liquids

- Gels or frozen liquids needed to cool disability or medically related items used by persons with disabilities or medical conditions

If the liquid medications are in volumes larger than 3 ounces each, they may not be placed in the quart-size bag used for personal liquids of less than 3 ounces. They must be declared to the Transportation Security Officer.

Specifically with respect to medications for diabetes, notify the Security Officer that you have diabetes and are carrying your supplies with you. (Medication and supplies you are going to use should be in your carry-on luggage.) The following diabetes-related supplies and equipment are allowed through the checkpoint after they have been screened:

- Insulin and insulin-loaded dispensing products (vials or box of individual vials, jet injectors, biojectors, EpiPens, infusers, and preloaded syringes)

- Unlimited number of unused syringes when accompanied by insulin or other injectable medication

- Lancets, blood glucose meters, blood glucose meter test strips, alcohol swabs, meter-testing solutions

- Insulin pump and insulin-pump supplies (cleaning agents, batteries, plastic tubing, infusion kit, catheter, and needle; insulin pumps and supplies must be accompanied by insulin)

- Glucagon emergency kit

- Urine ketone test strips

- Unlimited number of used syringes when transported in sharps disposal container or other similar hard-surface container

- Sharps disposal containers or similar hard-surface disposal container for storing used syringes and test strips

Here are some suggestions for managing your diabetes if you're changing time zones:

- Obtain a list of doctors in the countries you will visit who speak your language. To find English-speaking doctors, you can contact the US embassy in each country or go to the website of the International Association for Medical Assistance to Travelers, `http://iamat.org/ doctors_clinics.cfm`.

- If using an insulin pump, change the basal hourly rate to the same dose every hour so that whether it's 8 a.m. or 8 p.m., the same dose is given. When you arrive in the new time zone, you can adjust the basal rate back to your usual doses.

- If you use long-acting insulin, change a single dose to two half doses 12 hours apart.

- Stick to your regular schedule using local time for any oral medications.

Wherever you go, make sure you wear a bracelet or necklace that identifies you as a person with diabetes.

Knowing Where You Can't Work

You may have grown up watching Eliot Ness on television and had your heart set on being a member of the Federal Bureau of Investigation. If you require insulin, forget it. The FBI has a policy called a *blanket ban* on hiring certain groups of people, including people with diabetes who take insulin. A blanket ban does not take into account the condition of the individual, the past employment history, the way the person manages his or her diabetes, or the responsibilities of the position. It simply says, in effect, "You've got the disease, so you can't work here." This policy is a throwback to the days before 1980, when a person with diabetes could never be sure what his blood glucose was doing.

Another important institution that has a blanket ban in place is the United States military. If you have any kind of diabetes, you are not eligible to serve. If you develop diabetes after you've been in the military, you will probably be discharged. This policy doesn't make a lot of sense because many countries have people with diabetes in their military forces and have no difficulty with them, but so it goes.

Fortunately, blanket bans in the United States are falling faster than Babe Ruth home runs. For example, the Department of the Treasury lifted a blanket ban on becoming a member of the Bureau of Alcohol, Tobacco, and Firearms if you have insulin-requiring diabetes. Recently, several states lifted a ban on hiring people with diabetes to be school-bus drivers. This action resulted from lawsuits against several school districts that fired drivers with spotless driving records just because they had diabetes. (This reversal doesn't mean that no safeguards against risky drivers exist. Drivers are being evaluated on a case-by-case basis before they are accepted to drive children, which is fair.)

Previously, commercial drivers with diabetes could drive within a state but could not cross state lines. Now the Department of Transportation (DOT) looks at people with diabetes on a case-by-case basis to determine if they're fully able to drive commercially from state to state. As long as the person has no history of hypoglycemia with unconsciousness, the DOT grants an exemption that permits the individual to drive between states, with reconsideration taking place every two years.

At one time, people with diabetes who took insulin were banned from becoming firefighters. Now they are permitted to serve in this work, too, on a case-by-case basis. However, the rule says they must have a hemoglobin A1c of less than 8 percent. I believe this policy needs to be changed because people function perfectly well at higher levels of hemoglobin A1c, even at 10 or 11 percent.

Another blanket ban that is falling is the ban on piloting airplanes. For 37 years, a person who took insulin could not fly a plane. In 1996, the Federal Aviation Administration (FAA) reconsidered its ban based on the great advances in controlling diabetes. The FAA decided to permit people to fly privately but not for commercial airlines. Even if they have a private license, however, they can't use it outside the airspace of the United States. Applications for a pilot's license are evaluated on a case-by-case basis.

Flying a plane: It's not easy, but it's worth it

Getting a pilot's license is not easy but is well worth the effort for the person who loves to fly. To be successful, you must have no other disqualifying conditions, such as arteriosclerotic disease of the heart or brain, diabetic eye disease, or severe kidney disease (see Chapter 5). You must have had no more than one hypoglycemic reaction with loss of consciousness in the last five years and have had at least a year of stability after that. You must be evaluated by a specialist every three months after you get the license and measure your blood glucose multiple times a day. You must carry a glucose meter and meter supplies in flight, along with supplies for rapid treatment of hypoglycemia. Your blood glucose must be between 100 and 300 mg/dl (5.5 to 16.6 mmol/L) a half hour before takeoff, every hour of the flight, and a half hour before landing. However, you're not expected to measure your blood glucose in flight if doing so interferes with properly flying the plane. Phew! If Lindbergh were diabetic, he never would have made it to Paris.

Is there ever a justification for a blanket ban? The answer is no, and it has been proved in a number of studies. In one study of accidents of all kinds, people with diabetes actually had fewer accidents, including automobile accidents, than groups of people without diabetes. In another study of people over age 65 with diabetes, the rate of automobile accidents was no greater than that of the nondiabetic groups.

Becoming Familiar with Workplace Law

A number of laws protect you in the workplace if you work in the United States, but the most important is probably the Americans with Disabilities Act (ADA) of 1990. This act states,

> *The determination that an individual poses a "direct threat" shall be based on an individualized assessment of the individual's present ability to safely perform the essential functions of the job.*

In 1998, the US Court of Appeals ruled that the ADA protects Americans with diabetes. The act applies to employers with 15 or more employees. What the ADA means is that you are qualified for a particular job if you can perform the essential functions of the job as determined by the employer, with or without reasonable accommodation. Therefore, you can't be discriminated against in hiring, firing, promotion, training, pay, or any other aspect of employment because you have diabetes. Your boss cannot ask whether you have diabetes but can expect you to pass a physical examination to verify that you are well enough to do the job.

The Federal Rehabilitation Act of 1973 is an important law that protects you when you apply for a federal job or a job in a company that receives federal assistance. A person with diabetes is specifically protected under this law. The most important provision states,

> *No otherwise qualified handicapped individual in the United States shall, solely by reason of his handicap, be excluded from the participation in, be denied the benefits of, or be subjected to discrimination under any program or activity conducted by the Executive agency. . . .*

To exclude you, federal agencies have to prove that you will not be able to perform safely if given the job. That proof is hard to come by and puts the burden on them, not you. They must decide on a case-by-case basis. As I note earlier in the chapter, the FBI and the military are exempt from this law.

Curiously, a problem arose in the Americans with Disabilities Act when diabetes began to respond so well to treatment. Only a person with a disability could sue under this act. In a perfect example of a Catch-22 (where you can't avoid a problem because of contradictory rules), people with diabetes were no longer considered disabled, so even though they were discriminated against, they couldn't sue. In 2008, President George Bush signed the Americans with Disabilities Act Amendments Act, bringing diabetics again under the act.

What can you do if you run into discrimination on the job due to your diabetes? You can contact the US Equal Employment Opportunity Commission (EEOC). You can find your nearest EEOC office on the web at www.eeoc.gov/field/index.cfm or call 202-663-4900. You may have only 180 days from the alleged discriminatory act to file the charge. Another alternative is to call the American Diabetes Association at 800-DIABETES (800-342-2383) to request a free packet of information, plus assistance from a legal advocate.

Navigating the Health-Insurance System

You can get insurance for your medical care several ways. The Patient Protection and Affordable Care Act (PPACA or Obamacare) has made it possible for many people who didn't have health insurance to have some coverage. The following sections explain how the PPACA works together with private insurance, Medicare, and Medicaid.

Employer insurance

Half of the US population has insurance through its employer. Any employer with 50 or more employees must provide health insurance under PPACA. Employers with less than 50 employees have marketplaces set up by the government where they can buy less expensive insurance and may get tax breaks if they do. These marketplaces can't charge more if the employee is sick or for a preexisting condition.

Government insurance

A third of the population has government insurance. Under the PPACA, Medicare (elderly) insurance is similar to what it was before the act, but Medicaid has expanded to cover more poor people. However, the governor of each state must decide whether to allow Medicaid expansion in that state. In states that agree to expand Medicaid, the government covers most of the costs. In those that don't, no more poor people are covered than before.

Private insurance

A tenth of the population (30 million people) buys insurance. Currently, there are two major forms of payment for medical care — fee-for-service and capitated payment — with a lot of hybrids in between. The old *fee-for-service* method pays the medical provider — whether a physician, a lab, or a hospital — based on the number of services provided. More services and procedures mean more profit for the provider. So the incentive is to do more in order to make more money (not that providers would ever do more than is necessary for the money).

The other main method of reimbursement is *capitation*. Here the provider gets a fixed amount of money for each patient. The risk is divided among many patients so that if one costs more, ideally another will cost less. This system is the basis of the health maintenance organization (HMO), which hires physicians to provide the care. HMOs look to enroll people who cost as little as possible for their medical care.

Because they seem to end up costing less money overall, capitation plans are growing while fee-for-service plans are declining. The government is even encouraging HMOs to enroll Medicare recipients in order to reduce costs. At the same time, the government requires HMOs to enroll people who cost more, like most people with diabetes.

Each state has a health insurance marketplace where insurance companies compete for your business by offering plans with more or less coverage that vary in cost from expensive to cheap. These plans can't charge more for people who are sick or have preexisting conditions. The federal government gives tax credits to those individuals with incomes below a certain level. Regardless of cost, all plans cover doctor visits, hospital visits, maternity visits, and mental health visits. Children can remain on their parents' plan until age 26 and can buy low-cost catastrophic coverage until age 30.

If you don't know what your state marketplace is, start with www. healthcare.gov.

As a healthcare consumer, you want to look for a large group containing many patients because such a group can spread out your extra expenses among many people who don't consume as much medical care. Before you sign up, ask several questions:

✔ What is your total annual cost, and how often is a payment required?

✔ Will you have a *deductible,* meaning that you have to pay the first so-many dollars before the insurance starts paying?

✔ Will you have a *copayment,* meaning that every time you use a provider, you have to pay some dollars?

✔ Does your plan pay for durable medical equipment, like an insulin pump (see Chapter 11), which can be very expensive? (You want to ask this even if, when you sign up, you may not foresee a need for it.)

✔ Will your plan pay for your diabetes medication and diabetes supplies, and to what extent?

✔ Can your physician order any medications you need, or is he or she restricted to certain medications?

✔ How often will you need to travel to the pharmacy to pick up medications? (Some plans make you go back every 30 days.)

✔ Are you covered for specialists, particularly eye doctors and foot doctors?

✔ Are you limited to certain hospitals, certain physicians, and certain laboratories? (If so, this restriction may be much more inconvenient for you, not to mention possibly requiring you to change from a physician with whom you are very comfortable.)

✔ Is home healthcare included in the plan, and to what extent?

After you sign up for a plan, you need to be vigilant to be sure you are getting what you paid for. You and your physician may need to make many phone calls to get what you need, but if you persist you can often come away with a "Yes." The insurance company may provide goods and services that are excluded in your original contract if you're persistent.

Important changes for people with diabetes

The Patient Protection and Affordable Care Act signed by President Obama in March 2010 has had profound effects on the ability of the person with diabetes to get affordable medical care. Beginning in 2010, insurers could no longer deny insurance coverage to children because of preexisting conditions. Since 2014, adults have the same right. Also beginning in 2010, insurers could no longer drop people who are diagnosed with a new condition such as diabetes or its complications.

Here are some other important provisions of the new law:

✔ Creating the Cures Acceleration Network to finance research into cures for diseases

✔ Creating a new National Diabetes Prevention Program to fund grants for community efforts to help people with diabetes

✔ Requiring restaurant chains with 20 or more locations to post calorie counts for every item they sell

✔ Allowing employers to use workplace wellness programs to reward employees

✔ Permitting no annual limit on benefits after January 1, 2014

✔ Allowing no coverage waiting periods greater than 90 days after January 1, 2014

✔ Reducing and eventually eliminating the amount that Medicare patients have to pay for their medications (the doughnut hole) by 2020

✔ Providing more payment for preventive medical care

No insurance

Another tenth of the population doesn't have any insurance, even under PPACA. PPACA mandates a fine if you have no insurance, but the government waves the fine if you absolutely can't afford to buy insurance. For more information on the Affordable Care Act and its provisions in your state, go to http://obamacarefacts.com/obamacare-facts/.

Changing or Losing a Job

One of the major reasons why people with diabetes used to stay in jobs they didn't care for was their fear of losing their health insurance. These days, this worry doesn't have to stop you, because several laws protect you from the loss of health insurance if you change or lose your job.

The Consolidated Omnibus Budget Reconciliation Act (COBRA) stipulates that your employer must keep you on your current health insurance for as long as 18 months after your job ends and longer if you are disabled. If your child is at the age when he or she is no longer covered under your policy, the child's coverage can continue for up to three years. You, rather than your employer, have to pay the premiums for this continued insurance. The other way to continue health insurance if you lose your job is to buy it from your state's insurance marketplace.

If you are leaving work because of retirement at age 65, sign up for Medicare without fail. It is a generous program (which you supported while you were working) that recognizes the specific needs of people with diabetes. Since 1998, Medicare has expanded its coverage to include blood glucose monitors and test strips after your physician certifies the need. It also offers payment for specific types of outpatient diabetes education programs, as long as they are considered necessary by your physician. And recently it has begun to pay for nutrition counseling and eye examinations. Most plans pay for an insulin pump, insulin, and syringes. To find out more about Medicare, call the Medicare Hotline at 800-633-4227. The government provides a hotline for the hearing-impaired at 877-486-2048.

Considering Long-Term Care Insurance

People with diabetes are living longer and longer, and you're going to need a way to pay for your care when you can no longer pay health-insurance premiums. When you're 90, your 88-year-old wife will most likely not be in a position to pay for your insurance, nor will your 65-year-old daughter. Medicare doesn't cover most of your long-term care expenses. Medicaid does cover some long-term care, but not everything you may need. This is where long-term insurance may help, if you can afford it. Obama's Healthcare Act steps in here by allowing payment of monthly premiums through payroll deduction to buy long-term care as of January 2011.

If you have plenty of money and want to protect it from the financial hit of a long-term illness, long-term insurance is for you. If you have little money, then the years of premiums are going to wipe out your savings, and you may end up needing to drop the policy before you even use it.

One big problem is that many companies that sell long-term insurance don't cover people with diabetes. If you can get this type of insurance coverage while you're still working, you may be able to get into a large group where your particular illness is not considered and the premiums may be relatively low. However, you'll obviously be paying those premiums for a longer time than if you start coverage when you are older.

Before you buy, you should check several important features of a long-term care insurance policy:

- What are the *benefit triggers,* the physical limitations that trigger coverage? To make this determination, generally insurance companies look at activities of daily living, such as the ability to bathe yourself, dress yourself, eat without help, go to the bathroom, and get out of bed. When you can't perform one or more of these tasks, benefits begin.

- How much of the cost of care does the insurance pay, some or all?

- What levels of care does the policy provide? Your policy may offer coverage only for adult day-care services or may cover anything up to and including living in a nursing facility.

- Is a waiver of premiums built in so that you don't have to pay premiums when you are disabled?

- Is the policy guaranteed renewable so you can renew no matter whether you use it, although the premiums will be higher?

Whatever you do, if you buy long-term care insurance, make sure you take good care of yourself so you live long enough to get some benefit from it.

Shopping for Life Insurance

As you may expect, the situation with life insurance and people with diabetes is in a state of flux. Insurance companies like to calculate your chance of dying and charge you (or turn you down) based on those calculations. Many companies are using calculations based on the life span of people with diabetes in 1980 or before. Using those statistics, diabetics clearly died earlier than their nondiabetic friends. Thus, the cost of life insurance is greater for people with diabetes than nondiabetics.

As new studies are done, they should indicate that the life spans of people with diabetes and nondiabetics are approaching equality. In some cases, people with diabetes, who take better care of themselves than people without a chronic illness, are living even longer. So the situation is improving, and insurance companies will catch up sooner or later. Can you imagine the surprise if insurance companies were ever to charge people with diabetes less than others because of their good habits?

Insurance companies look at levels of blood glucose and the hemoglobin A1c. Try to get yourself in excellent control before you apply. You may be able to save a bundle or get your insurance much more easily.

With the Internet, you can quickly find and compare the cost of insurance at numerous companies based on your age; your habits (warning: If you smoke, you pay through the nose); and the presence of conditions such as diabetes, high blood pressure, and high cholesterol. Many companies take a standard rate for a healthy person with no diseases and add 50 percent more if you have diabetes. Of course, your actual cost depends on your specific circumstances, including your age when you first buy the insurance.

Chapter 16

Eyeing What's New in Diabetes Care

*I*n previous editions of *Diabetes For Dummies,* I have enthusiastically spoken about the great efforts of pharmaceutical companies to provide you with the best drugs to lower your glucose, reduce your blood pressure, and lower your cholesterol. In this edition I have the sad responsibility to warn you about these same pharmaceutical companies.

As a consequence of my skepticism, I'm not going to talk about new drugs in this chapter but rather about how to make informed choices about medications and new products that may make managing your disease easier. In addition, you find out about major efforts to get cells that don't usually make insulin to turn into the insulin-producing beta cells. I also tell you about some possible links between diabetes and other medical conditions.

Protecting Yourself from the Dangers of New Drugs

In an effort to instantly gratify their stockholders and find the next "billion dollar drug," drug companies seem to have lost sight of their major goal, which is to find drugs that are both effective and safe for the treatment of diabetes.

Although some drug companies continue to pursue this goal, many of them are guilty of the following misconduct:

✔ Withholding studies that they have paid for that show that their drugs are not as effective as they claim. A study in the *New England Journal of Medicine* in January 2008 showed that the companies that make antidepressants allowed 94 percent of positive studies to be printed but only 14 percent of negative studies. Even the positive studies, if carefully evaluated, weren't nearly as positive as the companies claimed. This behavior isn't limited to companies that make antidepressants.

✔ Strongly advertising the one study that shows positive effects when many others show negative effects.

✔ Withholding studies that indicate their drugs may have dangerous side effects.

✔ Promoting their drugs for purposes that are not permitted by the FDA.

✔ Advertising their drugs as though they are the best or only treatment when older and better treatments exist.

✔ Providing catered lunches and samples to doctors to convince them to use their drugs. A basic conflict of interest exists in the relationship between doctors and pharmaceutical companies.

✔ Paying large sums of money to private doctors to do "studies" of their drugs that rarely find negative things about the drugs.

✔ Paying rebates to private doctors to use their drugs, whether or not they are the best choice for the patient.

These problems are not limited to doctors and the pharmaceutical industry. Any time "advisors" are also salespeople, they advise the purchase of what they sell. But just because this practice takes place in every industry doesn't make it right. And in the medical industry, it's often a matter of life or death.

What steps can you take to avoid the dangers I outline above? Here are a few suggestions:

✔ **Don't ask your doctor to prescribe new drugs that are heavily promoted by advertising.** Too few people have used them and too little time has passed to truly know the potential of these new drugs.

✔ **Don't take samples from your doctor.** Drug companies use samples to get you and your doctor hooked on their drug.

✔ **Don't ask for a drug just because a key organization like the American Heart Association, the American Diabetes Association, the Endocrine Society, or others promotes the drug.** These organizations have become big and fat from the money provided by those drug companies.

> ✔ **Do wait several years before trying a new drug.** The drugs that are currently available are more than adequate to control your blood glucose, your blood pressure, and your cholesterol *if you take them as prescribed.*

Checking the Role of Intestinal Organisms in Type 2 Diabetes

Obesity has been found to change the composition of the bacteria in the human intestine. These bacteria increase the absorption of food from the intestine, resulting in more obesity. When bacteria from lean men are transplanted into the intestine of men with metabolic syndrome, the recipients show increased insulin sensitivity — an improvement in their condition. By examining the intestinal bacteria of people at high risk for diabetes, researchers may be able to predict the future development of diabetes.

Transplantation of intestinal bacteria has been successful in treating a highly pathological organism called *Clostridium difficile,* which causes severe inflammation of the colon. More recently, it has successfully treated other chronic gastrointestinal infections. Changing the intestinal bacteria in a person with type 2 diabetes may prove to be another weapon in the arsenal of the diabetes specialist.

Eating One Meal a Day to Control Diabetes

Diabetes doctors have been looking for the best way for type 2 diabetics to eat in order to control their diabetes. A group in Sweden published its study in *PLoS ONE* in November 2013 comparing three different diets: a low-fat diet, a low-carbohydrate diet, and the Mediterranean diet. The first two were spread over three meals, whereas the Mediterranean diet was a single large lunch with red wine. The researchers looked at the effects of these diets on blood glucose, blood fats, and other hormones.

Although the low-carbohydrate diet reduced glucose more than the low-fat diet, the low-carbohydrate diet resulted in a higher level of a fat called *triglyceride.* The Mediterranean diet induced the least increase in glucose. The traditional Mediterranean diet didn't include breakfast. Thus, the authors of this study suggest that the person with type 2 diabetes should reconsider his meal arrangements and perhaps limit meals to one a day.

Losing Weight with Gastric Artery Embolization

Left gastric artery embolization, which means closing off the left gastric artery, the artery to the stomach, with some obstructive agent, results in a significant loss of weight. Patients who had this procedure lost 8 percent of their body weight compared to patients who had other arteries to the stomach shut off. The explanation may be that the left gastric artery supplies the part of the stomach that makes *ghrelin,* a hormone that stimulates appetite. Embolization probably suppresses ghrelin.

The study at Harvard Medical School was presented at the meeting of the Radiological Society of North America in November 2013. Fifteen patients underwent left gastric artery embolization for the treatment of bleeding from the stomach. Researchers then reviewed the patients' records after the procedure. They found that the patients who had gastric artery embolization lost a mean of 7.9 percent of their body weight within three months. The authors suggested that the study needed to be repeated with a larger group where the patients were randomly assigned to one procedure or another.

Blocking the Vagus Nerve for Weight Loss

Cutting of the vagus nerve was once used for the treatment of stomach ulcers. These patients commonly lost weight after the procedure.

In January 2015 the Food and Drug Administration approved an implanted device for the treatment of obesity called the Maestro System. Implantation takes 60 to 90 minutes and is done on an outpatient basis. The rechargeable device is implanted along the left side of the chest with electric leads that surround the *vagus nerve,* a nerve that runs along the stomach. It may be used for people with a BMI of 40 or greater, or those with a BMI of 35 to 40 plus another cardiac risk such as high blood pressure, high blood fats, or diabetes. The Maestro System doesn't sever the vagus nerve but blocks it on a daily schedule to reduce hunger.

The device was shown to work in a study of 239 people, with 162 receiving the active device and 77 receiving a sham operation. Those who had the active operation lost 24.4 percent of their excess body weight whereas those who had the sham operation lost 15.9 percent of their excess body weight.

People who had the active procedure had a 3.7 percent adverse reaction rate consisting of mild or moderate heartburn or abdominal pain.

Lowering Blood Glucose in Pregnancy

As explained in Chapter 6, prevention of gestational diabetes is important in preserving the health of the growing fetus and the mother and avoiding complications of birth. Controversy has been continuing as to whether higher-than-normal blood glucose levels that did not reach the level of diabetes posed a danger to mother and child.

A large number of medical centers combined to form the Hyperglycemia and Adverse Pregnancy Outcomes Study Cooperative Research Group to answer this question, among others. They published their results in the *New England Journal of Medicine* in May 2008.

The group evaluated blood glucose levels in 23,316 pregnant women. They looked at the birth weight of the newborns and their levels of C-peptide. Higher levels of C-peptide indicate that the fetuses were exposed to higher levels of glucose and had to make more insulin, which tends to cause fat accumulation in the babies.

The study found that birth weight and C-peptide levels have a continuous association in the babies even though the mothers' glucose level didn't reach that diagnostic of diabetes. Even at these lower levels of maternal blood glucose, the rate of necessary cesarean sections at delivery (because of a large baby) was higher, and newborns had a higher rate of low blood glucose (a consequence of too much insulin production in the newborn when the maternal supply of glucose is cut off at birth).

A later study from the same group (in *Diabetes Care* in March 2012) showed that the hemoglobin A1c was not a useful alternative to an oral glucose tolerance test in predicting complications in the pregnancy.

If you have been tested for gestational diabetes and don't reach the criteria for that diagnosis, the outcome of your pregnancy will still be improved by careful diet and regular exercise.

Using an Endoscopic Duodenal-Jejunal Bypass Liner for Weight Loss

In Chapter 9, I discuss metabolic surgery as a cure for diabetes. Specialists have been trying to find a substitute for surgery that will accomplish the weight loss without the cutting. The duodenal-jejunal bypass liner may be one solution.

The duodenal-jejunal bypass liner is a sleeve that doesn't allow food to pass through to be absorbed. It's delivered to the beginning of the small intestine using an *endoscope,* a tube that goes through the mouth, through the stomach, and into the small intestine.

It was shown to be effective in a study involving 77 obese patients. Thirty-eight had the sleeve inserted and were placed on a diet whereas 39 followed the diet but didn't have the sleeve inserted. After six months, those patients with the sleeve had lost 32 percent of their excess weight whereas those patients without the sleeve lost 6.4 percent of their excess weight. The hemoglobin A1c improved to 7 percent in the sleeve group but only 7.9 in the other group.

Adverse reactions included upper abdominal pain, back pain, nausea, and vomiting, none of which were severe. However the device had to be removed in one patient due to gastro-intestinal bleeding and two patients due to migration of the liner down the intestine.

The duodenal-jejunal bypass liner has the added advantage of being reversible. It may be removed at any time in the same way it was inserted.

Placing a Gastric Balloon

The gastric balloon is yet another attempt to accomplish the benefits of surgery without the cutting. A balloon is placed in the stomach and filled with a salt solution to keep it in place. The result is similar to the adjustable gastric band that I discuss in Chapter 9. The capacity of the stomach is greatly diminished so that the patient eats much less and loses weight.

Past problems with the balloon occurred when the balloon burst and passed into the intestine, blocking the bowels. A new version called the ReShape Duo overcomes this problem by using two connected balloons. If one bursts, the other prevents the other balloon from entering the intestine. The liquid in the balloon contains a dye that is absorbed and turns the person's urine blue, alerting the patient to the rupture and allowing the physician to remove the balloon and replace it.

The balloons are removed after six months to reduce the risk of stomach ulcers that result from friction with the stomach. They may be particularly useful in people who need quick weight loss for heart surgery or cancer treatment but are too sick to have real metabolic surgery.

People who used the balloons plus lifestyle change lost 28.5 percent of their excess weight compared to an 11.3 excess weight loss for people who did lifestyle change only.

On August 5, 2015 the FDA approved the ORBERA Intragastric Balloon System after studies showed that although the balloon must be removed after six months, significant weight loss continues for a year or longer. Some people with diabetes may benefit from this treatment.

Understanding the Importance of the ACCORD Trial

The ACCORD (Action to Control Cardiovascular Risk in Diabetes) trial is a study of 10,250 people who have had T2DM and are at high risk to have a heart attack. The average hemoglobin A1c was 8.2 percent, which is higher than the average patient with T2DM. The patients were randomized into two treatment arms, a standard treatment arm that had a goal of an A1c target between 7 and 7.9 percent and an intensive treatment arm that had a goal of an A1c target less than 6 percent.

All patients already had known heart disease, diabetes, and at least two of the following additional risk factors:

- ✔ High blood pressure
- ✔ High cholesterol
- ✔ Obesity
- ✔ Smoking habit

When patients with these characteristics are allowed to maintain their usual A1c of 8.2 percent, their death rate is 50 per 1,000 patients per year.

The study was due to be completed in 2010, but in early February 2008, the researchers announced that they were closing the part of the study that attempted to get the A1c down to 6 percent because there was a higher death rate among the intensively treated patients than the other group. Here were the results up to that point:

- ✔ The intensive group had an average A1c of 6.4 percent.
- ✔ The standard group had an average A1c of 7.5 percent.
- ✔ The standard group had a death rate of 11 per 1,000 patients per year.
- ✔ The intensive group had a death rate of 14 per 1,000 patients per year.

Therefore, although the death rate for both groups was far below the level for these people with an A1c of 8.2 percent initially (11 or 14 versus 50 per 1,000), the intensively treated group that reached their goal had a slightly greater death rate than the standard group that reached their goal.

Subsequent papers from this study published in the *New England Journal of Medicine* in April 2010 have shown the following information:

- ✔ The use of combination therapy with a statin drug and a fibrate (see Chapter 11) didn't reduce the rate of fatal heart or nonfatal heart attacks or strokes compared with a statin alone in these high-risk patients.

- ✔ Targeting a blood pressure of less than 120 mmHg didn't reduce the risk of fatal and nonfatal major heart attacks compared to a blood pressure target of 140 mmHg in these high-risk patients.

The moral of this story isn't that intensive treatment is dangerous in T2DM, but that intensive treatment is dangerous in this population of high-risk patients with heart disease and other risk factors.

Note that the death rate for both groups is much lower than that of the poorly treated patients. These patients are so sick that the difficulties associated with trying to keep their blood glucose at a level of 100 mg/dl all the time may be too great.

The more you control your blood glucose early in diabetes, the less chance that you will get to the point of the patients in this study.

Taking Advantage of Metabolic Memory

The Diabetes Control and Complications Trial, the results of which were published in 1993, showed that tight control of the blood glucose in type 1 diabetes substantially reduces the occurrence of complications of diabetes. Although the formal study ended in 1993, researchers continued to follow 90 percent of the participants. They called the follow-up the Epidemiology of Diabetes Interventions and Complications. Their results were published in the *New England Journal of Medicine* in December 2005 and December 2011.

Although the intensively treated group had only 6.5 years of intensive treatment, the long-term risk of complications, particularly kidney disease, was significantly reduced, even after 18 years during which the two groups had essentially the same level of treatment. This phenomenon is called *metabolic memory,* the tendency of the body to remember the very good treatment, resulting in a decrease of complications over time compared with the group not treated intensively.

Very good control of the blood glucose early in the disease has benefits that last for decades. Maintain that level of control, and you reduce the chance of complications enormously.

Chapter 17

Discovering What Doesn't Work When You Treat Diabetes

In This Chapter
▶ Recognizing the signs that a treatment won't work
▶ Identifying drugs, diets, and other treatments that don't help

*E*veryone wants a quick and easy solution to their problems. For every problem, five people offer a quick and easy answer. Just send in the money. These cheats have got what it takes to take what you've got.

Being fooled by these claims may be a lot more serious for you than for the person who walked up to the man dressed as a polar bear who was promoting soft drinks in a shopping center. The first man said: "Don't you feel foolish, dressed like a bear?" The "bear" replied: "Me, foolish? You're the one talking to a bear."

This chapter tells you as much as I know about diabetes tests and treatments that don't work. Don't expect to find every "wonder cure" for diabetes that you've read or heard about. As soon as this book is published, new, more seductive claims will be made. I hope that you will remain skeptical, use the information in this chapter to test claims out, and check with your doctor before you try something that may do more harm than good.

If you want additional resources to figure out your options for what works with diabetes treatment and care, check out www.dummies.com/extras/diabetes.

Developing a Critical Eye

Many clues can alert you that a treatment may not work. Here are a few:

✔ **If a treatment is endorsed by a Hollywood star or a sports figure, be highly skeptical.** Always consider the source and make sure that it's reputable. In this case, the fame of the star is being used to convince you, not any special knowledge that he or she possesses.

✔ **If the treatment has been around for a long time but is not generally used, don't trust it.** If a treatment has been around for a while and really works, it will have been tried in an experimental study where some people take it and some don't. Doctors and medical texts recommend drugs that pass that test.

✔ **If it sounds too good to be true, it usually is.** An example would be the claims about chromium improving blood glucose levels. The study that "proved" it was done on chromium-deficient people, a situation that does not exist in the United States.

✔ **Anecdotes are not proof of the value of a treatment or test.** The favorable experiences of one or a few people are not a substitute for a scientific study. Perhaps those people did respond to the drug (or supplement or miracle cure), but it may have been for entirely different reasons.

A lot of information about diabetes is available on the web. I provide the best resources currently available for diabetes at www.dummies.com/extras/diabetes. The same rules apply when you consider the validity of claims made on the web, with a few extra rules thrown in:

✔ **Don't rely on search engines for validity.** Search engines do not check claims for validity.

✔ **Go to the site of the claim and see whether most of the information there makes sense.** If you find a lot of silly information, that should be a red flag. If you still feel the treatment might work, ask the webmaster (the person who develops the site) for references. If none are forthcoming, forget about the idea.

✔ **Go to sites that you know are reliable to see whether you can find the same recommendations.** The treatments discussed on sites like the American Diabetes Association (ADA) and the Diabetes Monitor (Appendix A) can be relied on. When a treatment's value is uncertain, these sites can usually tell you the truth.

✔ **Go to medical conferences put on by reputable experts.** You will be given web addresses that are reliable.

Identifying Drugs and Supplements That Don't Work

In the past decade, so many drugs have been touted as the cure for diabetes that you would think everyone would be cured by now. The fact is, as I say again and again, you *do* have the tools right now to control diabetes, but the solution is not as simple as taking a pill. If it were, this book would not be necessary. In this section, I tell you about some drugs that have received unwarranted hype because they "worked" in a few people.

The Federal Trade Commission is concerned with all the phony "cures" for diabetes. They have set up a phony website called "Glucobate" that promises to be a cure for diabetes. When you click on "Order Now" they tell you about the hoax and offer tips to avoid being scammed, most of which you will find in this chapter.

Here are just a few of the false claims found in several websites that illustrate the available false information. You must be very wary before you change your treatment.

- Diabetes drugs offer few benefits and simply don't live up to their claims.

- Practically all anti-diabetic drugs result in weight gain and eventual total dependency upon insulin injections.

- Anyone can reverse type 2 diabetes and stop type 1 diabetes in its tracks in less than four weeks with the right plan.

- These treatments can improve diabetes: bitter gourd, curry leaves, aloe vera, guava, fenugreek, black plum or Indian blackberry, mango leaves, okra, holy basil, flax seeds, psyllium husk, and ginger.

If you participate in a clinical research study of a new drug, a system is in place to protect you. Make sure that a review board in an institution that has been approved to do the research has approved the study. Such institutions are usually accredited by an established organization like the Association for the Accreditation of Human Research.

How the ADA labels new drugs

The American Diabetes Association evaluates new therapies and places them in one of four categories:

- Clearly effective

- Somewhat/sometimes effective or effective for certain categories of patients

- Unknown/unproven but possibly promising

- Clearly ineffective

If you're about to try a new therapy that has not been recommended by your doctor and is not discussed in this book, you may want to contact the ADA and find out its position on the treatment. Of course, if you're involved in a clinical trial that is trying to determine the effectiveness of a therapy, no one will know whether it works or not.

See the sidebar "How the ADA labels new drugs" for information on how the American Diabetes Association evaluates new treatments.

Chromium

You can find articles singing the praises of chromium for controlling the symptoms of diabetes in all kinds of magazines and newspapers and on the Internet. Should you take supplements of chromium?

The strongest case for chromium comes from a study of people with type 2 diabetes in China. They were given high doses of chromium and were found to improve their hemoglobin A1c, blood glucose, and cholesterol while reducing the amount of insulin they had to take. However, these people were chromium deficient in the first place. People in the United States and other countries where the diet is sufficient in chromium do not have this deficiency and do not show improvement in glucose tolerance when they take chromium. In addition, chromium is present in such small amounts normally that it is hard to measure even in people without chromium deficiency.

The exact amount of chromium you need in your diet is uncertain but is estimated to be 15 to 50 micrograms daily. People who take much more than that tend to accumulate it in their livers, where it can be toxic. Some studies suggest that chromium can cause cancer in high doses.

For now, the evidence does not support the use of chromium in diabetes except for people who are known to be chromium deficient.

Aspirin

People who take the sulfonylurea drugs (see Chapter 11) sometimes have a greater drop in blood glucose when they take aspirin. This drop is because aspirin competes with the other drug for binding sites on the proteins that carry sulfonylureas in the blood. When they're bound to protein, the sulfonylureas are not active; when they're free, they are. Aspirin knocks the sulfonylureas off so that they're free. As a result, aspirin has been recommended as a drug to lower blood glucose.

By itself, aspirin has little effect on blood glucose. Its effect with sulfonylureas is so inconsistent that it can't be reliably depended on to lower the blood glucose.

Cinnamon

A number of articles in the medical literature since 2001 have suggested that cinnamon lowers the blood glucose in type 2 diabetes and improves fat levels as well. To verify these claims, a study called a meta-analysis was done and published in *Diabetes Care* in January 2008. In a meta-analysis, an analysis is done of all studies that are randomized so that the subjects don't know if they are getting the drug or a placebo. In this case, none of five studies showed that cinnamon had a positive effect either on the blood glucose or blood fats. You may have noticed the same thing if you were taking a daily dose of a teaspoon of cinnamon. You can cease and desist!

Pancreas formula

Pancreas formula is sold on the Internet as a mixture of herbs, vitamins, and minerals that help diabetes. No clinical or experimental evidence shows that pancreas formula does anything of value in the human body. The claims that are made for this "treatment" are not supported by factual evidence.

Fat Burner

You may hear and read a lot of advertising for the Fat Burner product in reputable newspapers and on reputable radio stations. Advertisements claim that you can "burn fat without diet or exercise," and they will even throw in, ABSOLUTELY FREE, a bottle of Spirulina to enhance your Fat Burner weight-control program. If you believe this is possible, I have a bridge I would like to sell you, *cheap.* In order to burn fat, you must exercise and stop taking in large amounts of carbohydrates or other sources of calories.

Ki-Sweet

The literature for Ki-Sweet offers another lesson in being skeptical. The creators of this "miracle" sweetener claim that it has a "special designation from the American Diabetes Association." The ADA denies the claim, but how many people will buy something when they see ADA approval and not bother to see whether it's true? No evidence exists that Ki-Sweet, made by squeezing the juice of kiwi, has any advantages over other sweeteners (which I discuss in Chapter 8).

The facts about aspartame

Many news sources report that aspartame (see Chapter 8) causes cancer. Because so many people eat and drink products that contain aspartame, I want to clarify the facts.

Aspartame is an acceptable artificial sweetener with no known dangers to human beings. No evidence shows that aspartame causes cancer when used in normal amounts. The Food and Drug Administration has an acceptable daily intake for food additives, including a 100-fold safety factor. It is inconceivable that anyone would use more aspartame than that.

Gymnema sylvestre

Gymnema sylvestre is a plant found in India and Africa that is promoted as a glucose-lowering agent as part of an alternative medical treatment called _Ayurvedic medicine._ _Gymnema sylvestre_ has never been tested in a controlled study in humans. One statement in its advertising is, "For most people, blood sugar lowers to normal levels." No evidence exists that this is the case.

Avoiding Illegal Drugs

Drugs like cocaine, heroin, speed, and marijuana aren't just illegal; they're especially harmful for the person with diabetes for several reasons:

- ✔ Some make you excessively hungry, and you take in too many calories.
- ✔ All cause you to lose your awareness of hypoglycemia, so you don't treat it.
- ✔ All cause a loss of judgment that results in the failure to take medications, eat properly, and exercise.
- ✔ Some cause a reduced insulin response to food, so you become hyperglycemic.
- ✔ Some cause you to lose your appetite, so you become hypoglycemic and malnourished with vitamin deficiencies.

Not a lot of valid information is available about each illegal drug's impact on diabetes, because we cannot do studies where these drugs are given to one group of diabetics while a control group takes a placebo. But we do know the following:

- ✔ Marijuana (grass, weed, bud, cannabis) causes increased appetite, which results in taking in too many calories.

✔ Amphetamine (speed, Dex, crank) and ecstasy (derived from amphetamine and also called MDMA, E, X, adam, bean, and roll) increase the body's metabolic rate, resulting in hypoglycemia because the user often does not eat properly and is unaware of the onset of low blood glucose.

✔ Cocaine (coke, snow, nose candy, dust, toot) and freebase cocaine (crack, rock) lead to food deprivation, increased metabolism and caloric needs, and vitamin deficiency.

✔ Heroin (dope, junk, smack) is similar to cocaine but has additional risks associated with injections, such as infection.

Do you need any more reason to get high on exercise rather than drugs?

Knowing the Dangers of Some Legal Drugs for Other Purposes

Just because a drug is legal does not mean it has no undesirable side effects. Several classes of drugs need to be used with caution. They may cause weight gain, prevent normal metabolism, and have many other effects that negatively affect your diabetes. This list is not exhaustive. One of the first places to look if you are doing everything right but still have poor control of your blood glucose is among the medications you take for other reasons.

Antipsychotics

In an issue of *Diabetes Care* (February 2004), four major medical associations warned that second-generation antipsychotic drugs, used to treat a variety of severe mental illnesses, can cause rapid weight gain, most of which is fat, leading to prediabetes, diabetes, insulin resistance, and abnormal blood fats.

The drugs differ in their risks, but clozapine (Clozaril, made by Novartis) and olanzapine (Zyprexa, made by Eli Lilly) appear to be the worst offenders. Other drugs named include risperidone (Risperdol, made by Johnson & Johnson), quetiapine (Seroquel, made by AstraZeneca), ziprasidone (Geodon, made by Pfizer), and aripiprazole (Abilify, made by Bristol-Myers Squibb).

If you are taking one of these drugs, ask your doctor to screen and monitor you for evidence of weight gain and insulin resistance. The benefits of taking the drug may outweigh the risks. In the article, the panel suggests that baseline screening consisting of a medical history and physical examination along with fasting glucose and blood fats be done before using the drug.

If you are overweight or obese, you should receive nutritional and physical activity counseling if you take one of these drugs. If you are at risk of developing diabetes, your doctor should use the drug that is least associated with this problem.

AIDS medications

Certain drugs that control AIDS, called *protease inhibitors,* block the body's ability to store glucose, so people who use them may develop diabetes. More than 80 percent of the people who use them develop excess stomach fat, and half develop glucose intolerance. More than 10 percent develop diabetes. Table 17-1 shows the specific drugs with their brand names and manufacturers.

Table 17-1	Protease Inhibitors That Affect Glucose Metabolism	
Generic Name	*Brand Name*	*Manufacturer*
Saquinavir (hard gel)	Invirase	Hoffman–La Roche
Saquinavir (soft gel)	Fortovase	Hoffman–La Roche
Ritonavir	Norvir	Abbott Laboratories
Indinavir	Crixivan	Merck
Nelfinavir	Viracept	Pfizer
Amprenavir	Agenerase	GlaxoSmithKline
Lopinavir and ritonavir	Keletra	Abbott Laboratories
Atazanavir	Reyataz	Bristol-Myers Squibb
Fosamprenavir	Levixa	GlaxoSmithKline

You should be screened before starting these drugs, and your doctor should monitor you carefully for weight gain and glucose intolerance. If diabetes does develop, the protease inhibitors are continued and the diabetes is treated. So far, none of the protease inhibitors stands out as more likely to cause diabetes.

Recognizing Diets That Don't Work

For the overweight person with type 2 diabetes, any diet that causes some weight loss helps for a time. But you have to ask yourself these questions:

✔ Am I prepared to stay on this diet indefinitely?

✔ Is this diet healthy for me in the long run?

✔ Does it combine all the features I need — namely weight loss, reduction of blood glucose, and reduction of blood fat levels — with palatability and reasonable cost?

If you can say yes to all these questions, the diet will probably work for you.

So how do you know which diets are healthy and effective, and which aren't? First, take a close look at Chapter 8, where I discuss diet in much more detail. Next, develop a discerning eye for defects in the latest diet fads.

When you walk into a reasonably large bookstore, you may be overwhelmed by the number of diet books. But the more books that are written about this subject, the less we seem to know for certain. Why would authors bother to write dozens of new books on dieting each year if the solution rested in some older book? You can bet that word of mouth would have made that book the all-time bestseller in any category.

The diet books in print these days are way too numerous to list here, but they can be grouped into a few categories:

✔ **Diets that promote a lot of protein with little carbohydrate:** The trouble with these diets is that they're not a healthy and balanced approach. Unless you use tofu as your source of protein, you will be getting a lot of fat in your diet, much of it saturated fat, which is not good for you. The diet is lacking in vitamins that a supplemental vitamin pill may or may not provide. Few people stay on such a diet for long. How many people can eat chicken for breakfast, lunch, and supper? The diet is also lacking in potassium, an essential mineral.

People who do follow this kind of diet for a long time also find that they have problems with hair loss, cracking nails, and dry skin. Their breath and their urine smell of acetone because of all the fat breakdown. They become very dry and need to drink large quantities of beverages.

I see a place for this diet as a starter. Some people with type 2 diabetes who have high blood glucose levels show rapid improvement when started on a diet like this. As the glucose comes under control, the diet can be changed to a more balanced one.

✔ **Diets that promote little or no fat:** The people who can follow a diet that is less than 20 percent fat deserve a new designation — *fatnatics*. This kind of diet is extremely difficult to prepare and perhaps even more difficult to eat unless you're a rabbit. In order to make up the calories, people on this diet eat large amounts of carbohydrates. Chapter 8 makes it clear why this is not a good idea for people with diabetes.

Like the protein diet, this diet may be lacking in essential vitamins and minerals, especially the fat-soluble vitamins. Rarely do people stay on such a diet after they leave the confines of a spa or other sanctuary where the diet is promoted. However, this approach may also be a good way to start a dietary program for a person with type 2 diabetes, as long as the total calories are not greater than the daily needs of that individual.

✔ **Very-low-calorie diets:** These diets require taking in food and drinks that contain less than 800 kilocalories daily (and generally do not taste very good). They are lacking in many essential nutrients and must be supplemented by vitamins and minerals. This approach cannot form the basis of a permanent diet because the dieter would eventually become emaciated. Most dieters who start this kind of program do not last on it and regain every ounce they have lost and then some. (There are always exceptions, of course.)

I do not like this kind of diet even as a starter diet because it is so unlike usual eating habits that people rapidly find it to be intolerable. Eating is a basic part of human existence, and it's a source of great pleasure for people and other animals. A diet that takes away this fundamental activity cannot be tolerated for very long.

The transition from a very-low-calorie diet to a balanced diet is very difficult and rarely succeeds.

What about hypnosis?

The National Institutes of Health, a very respected source, has listed hypnosis as a treatment for "stabilization of blood sugar in diabetes." Although it has a disclaimer that says that publishing this statement does not imply endorsement of the treatment, the fact that the statement comes from the NIH gives this treatment credibility. The only trouble is that no experimental evidence exists that proves the usefulness of hypnosis. So you have to be wary, even when the advice comes from the most respected of sources.

Part V
The Part of Tens

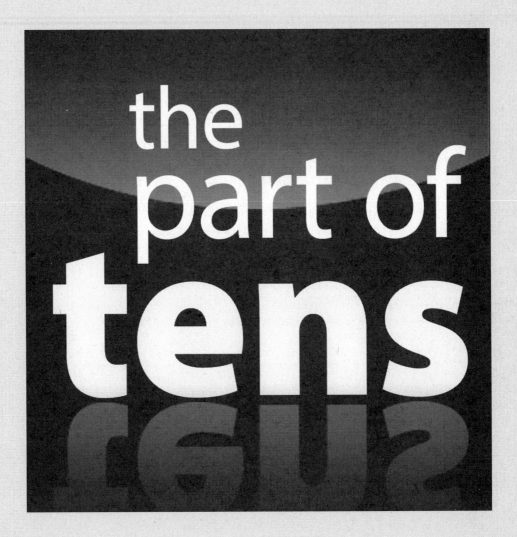

Refer to www.dummies.com/extras/diabetes for ten ways to prevent type 2 diabetes. They represent just a small sample of what you can do.

In this part . . .

- ✔ Observe ten important commandments for great diabetes care to help manage your condition and lead a normal life.

- ✔ Debunk common myths about diabetes so that you aren't confused about them.

- ✔ Get the experts and your family and friends to help you in your journey with diabetes.

- ✔ Know how to tell the difference between truth and fiction in diabetes care.

Chapter 18

Ten Commandments for Excellent Diabetes Care

In This Chapter

▶ Understanding the importance of monitoring, dieting, testing, and exercising

▶ Solidifying prevention with medication, the right attitude, and planning

*W*hen I originally wrote this chapter, I came up with 20 things you had to do in order to prevent or reverse the effects of diabetes. I decided that was too much to ask of you, so I reduced the list to ten essentials. Surely you can do everything in this chapter when you consider that it is only half as difficult!

Can you pick and choose what you will do? No. Everything here is essential to living a long and high quality life with diabetes. You wouldn't want to save your sight and lose your kidneys. So read this chapter very carefully and practice every recommendation. And if you think I should have left any of the other ten behaviors in, let me know.

Major Monitoring

You have this incredibly compact and accurate glucose meter. Now you want to use it to find out how your blood glucose is doing at any time of day or night under any circumstances. You don't feel well. Is it low blood glucose or the beginning of a cold? Test! You just ate a large portion of pasta. Did it raise your blood glucose too much? Test! You can monitor your glucose in so many ways, almost without pain, that you have no excuse for not doing so. And you don't have to do it with a finger stick every time. Most meters allow you to do it in other parts of your body — your arm, leg, or abdomen for example — especially when the blood glucose would not be expected to change rapidly as it would during or after exercise or after a meal. At those times, you should only use your finger.

People with type 1 diabetes need to test at least before meals and at bedtime because their blood glucose level determines their dose of insulin. People who have stable type 2 diabetes may test once a day at different times or twice a day. If you're sick or about to start a long drive, you may want to test more often because you don't want to become hypoglycemic — or hyperglycemic for that matter. The beauty of the meter is that you can check your blood glucose in less than ten seconds any time you feel it's necessary.

Devout Dieting

If you are what you eat, then you have the choice of being controlled or uncontrolled depending on what you put into your mouth. If you gain weight, you gain insulin resistance, but a small amount of weight loss can reverse the situation. The main point you should understand about a "diabetic diet" is that it's a healthy diet for everyone, whether they have diabetes or not. You should not feel like a social outcast because you're eating the right foods. You don't need special supplements; the diet is balanced and contains all the vitamins and minerals you require (although you want to be sure you're getting enough calcium and vitamin D).

You can follow a diabetic diet wherever you are, not just at home. Every menu has something on it that's appropriate for you. If you're invited to someone's home, let them know you have diabetes and that the amount of carbohydrate and fat that you can eat is limited. If that fails, limit the amount that you eat. (See Chapter 8 for more on your diet.)

A person with T2DM who follows a careful diet can reduce his hemoglobin A1c by 1 percent or more. This translates into a reduction in the occurrence of complications like eye disease, kidney disease, and nerve disease of more than 25 percent. Is that benefit worth your effort?

Tenacious Testing

The people who make smoke detectors recommend that you change the battery without fail each time you have a birthday. You should use the same simple device to remember your "complication detectors." Make sure that your doctor checks your urine for tiny amounts of protein and your feet for loss of sensation every year around the time of your birthday. It takes five to ten years to develop complications of diabetes. When you know the problem is present, you can do a lot to slow it down or even reverse it. Never has it been truer that "an ounce of prevention is worth a pound of cure." (For more on complications that may develop, see Chapters 4 and 5.)

I make it very easy for you to get the tests you need at the time you need them. The online cheat sheet for this book at www.dummies.com/ cheatsheet/diabetes gives you the current testing recommendations. Make a copy for your doctor if he or she does not already have such a list. Demand that you get the tests when they are due. A doctor with a busy medical practice may forget whether you have had the tests you need, but you don't have an excuse for forgetting. Make sure she tests your hemoglobin A1c, your blood pressure, and your cholesterol among other things.

Enthusiastic Exercising

When you take insulin (as opposed to pills), controlling your diabetes is a little harder because you have to coordinate your food intake and the activity of the insulin. But I have patients who have had diabetes for decades and have little trouble balancing their food and insulin. They are the enthusiastic exercisers. They use exercise to burn up glucose in place of insulin. The result is a much more narrow range of blood glucose levels than is true of the insulin takers who do not exercise. They also have more leeway in their diet because the exercise makes up for slight excesses.

I am not talking about an hour of running each day or 50 miles on the bike. Moderate exercise like brisk walking can accomplish the same thing. The key is to exercise faithfully. (For more on exercise, see Chapter 10.) Thirty minutes of moderate exercise every day will not just improve your diabetes. It will also reduce the possibility of a stroke, a heart attack, and many cancers, and just keep you feeling generally good. Exercise can reduce your hemoglobin A1c by 1 percent or more, just like diet.

Lifelong Learning

When I see a patient new to me who has had diabetes for some time, I am amazed at the lack of knowledge of many fundamental areas of their disease. You would think that they would want to know anything that might help them to live more comfortably and avoid complications.

So much is going on in the field of diabetes that I have trouble keeping up with it, and it's my specialty. How can you expect to know when doctors come up with the major advances that will cure your diabetes? The answer is lifelong learning. After you get past the shock of the diagnosis, you are ready to learn. This book contains a lot of basic stuff that you need to know. You can even take a good course in diabetes. Then you need to keep learning. Go to meetings of the local diabetes association. Become a member of the

American Diabetes Association and get its terrific magazine called *Diabetes Forecast,* which usually contains the state-of-the-art developments.

Remember that a lot of misinformation is available on the web, so you must be careful to check out a recommendation before you start to follow it. Even information on reliable sites may not be right for your particular problem.

Above all, never stop learning! The next thing you learn may be the one that will cure you.

Meticulous Medicating

Compliance, which means treating your disease in accordance with your doctor's instructions, is a term that has special relevance for the patient with a chronic disease like diabetes who must take medications day in and day out. Sure, it's a pain (even if you could take insulin by mouth and not by injection). But the basic assumption is that you're taking your medication. Your doctor bases all his or her decisions on that assumption. Some very serious mistakes can be made if that assumption is false.

Check with your pharmacist to make sure that your pills don't interfere with one another. Some pills are taken with food; others are taken with no food for a period before and after that medication. Taking them correctly is just as important as taking them at all.

Every time a study is done on why patients' health conditions do not improve, compliance is high up or leads the list of reasons. Do you make a conscious decision to skip your pills, or do you forget? Whatever the reason, the best thing to do is to set up a system so that you're forced to remember. Keeping your pills in a dated container quickly shows you if you have taken them or not. You can even divide the pills by time of day.

Appropriate Attitude

Your approach to your disease can go a long way toward determining whether you will live in diabetes heaven or diabetes hell. If you have a positive attitude, treating diabetes as a challenge and an opportunity, managing your disease is easier and your body actually produces chemicals that make it happen. A negative attitude, on the other hand, results in the kind of pessimism that leads to failure to diet, failure to exercise, and failure to take your medications. Plus, your body makes chemicals that are bad for you when you are depressed.

Diabetes is a challenge because you have to think about doing certain things that others never have to worry about. It brings out the quality of organization, which can then be transferred to other parts of your life. When you're organized, you accomplish much more in less time.

Diabetes is an opportunity because it forces you to make healthy choices for your diet as well as your exercise. You may end up a lot healthier than your neighbor without diabetes. As you make more and more healthy choices, you feel and test less and less like a person with diabetes.

Preventive Planning

Life is full of surprises (like the sign on a display of "I Love You Only" Valentine cards: Available in Multipacks). You never know when you will get more than you bargained for. That is why having a plan to deal with the unexpected is so important. Say you're invited to someone's home, and she serves something that you know will raise your blood glucose significantly. What do you do? Or you go out to eat and are given a menu of incredible choices, many of which are just not for you. How do you handle that? You run into great stress at work or at home. Do you allow it to throw off your diet, your exercise, and your compliance with your doctor's orders?

A little advance planning can overcome any eating challenge. Discuss good foods with the people who regularly cook for you. Check out the calorie breakdown of the foods you eat at fast food places, usually available on the Internet. Many restaurants provide the nutritional breakdown on their websites. Make a diet for yourself and follow it.

The key to these situations is the realization that it's not possible for everything to go right all the time. In the case of the friend who cooked the wrong thing for you, you can at least eat a small portion to limit the damage. At the restaurant, you should come prepared with the food choices you know will keep you on your diet. It may be better not to look at the menu and simply discuss with your waiter what is available from your list of correct foods.

Fastidious Foot Care

A recent headline read: "Hospital sued by seven foot doctors." I would certainly not like to treat any doctor with seven feet or even a doctor who is seven feet tall. Whether you have two feet or seven feet, you must take good care of them. The problem occurs when you can't feel with your feet because of neuropathy (see Chapter 5). You can easily know when this problem exists just by checking with a 10-gram filament. If your feet cannot feel the filament, they will not feel burning hot water, a stone, a nail in your shoe, or an infected ulcer of your foot.

When you lose sensation in your feet, your eyes must replace the pain fibers that would otherwise tell you there is a problem. You need to carefully examine your feet every day, keep your toenails trimmed, and wear comfortable shoes. Your doctor should inspect your feet at every visit.

Diabetes is the primary cause of foot amputations, but this drastic situation is entirely preventable if you pay attention to your feet. Test bath water by hand, shake your shoes out before you put them on, wear new shoes only a short while before checking for pressure spots, and get a 10-gram filament and see whether you can feel it. If you smoke, you are especially at a high risk for an amputation of your toes or foot. The future of your feet is in your hands.

The other aspect of fastidious foot care is making sure the circulation in the blood vessels of your feet remains open. This test is done by your doctor performing an ankle-brachial index on all patients with diabetes older than age 50 and younger patients who have risk factors for arterial disease such as smoking and high blood pressure (see Chapter 5). It quickly tells you and your doctor if you're experiencing a problem with your circulation.

Essential Eye Care

You're reading this book, which means you are seeing this book. So far, there are no plans to put out a Braille edition, so you had better take care of your eyes or you will miss out on the wonderful gems of information that brighten every page.

Caring for your eyes starts with a careful examination by an ophthalmologist or optometrist. You need to have an exam at least once every two years (or more often if necessary). If you have controlled your diabetes meticulously, the doctor will find two normal eyes. If not, signs of diabetic eye disease may show up (see Chapter 5). At that point, you need to control your diabetes, which means controlling your blood glucose. You also want to control your blood pressure because high blood pressure contributes to worsening eye disease, as does high cholesterol.

Although the final word is not in on the effects of excess alcohol on eye disease in diabetes, is it worth risking your sight for another glass of wine? Smoking has definitely been shown to raise the blood glucose in diabetes. Even at a late stage, you can stop the progression of the eye disease or reverse some of the damage if you stop smoking now.

Chapter 19

Ten Myths about Diabetes That You Can Forget

● ●

In This Chapter

▶ Separating diabetes fact from fiction

▶ Being wise about your medical care

● ●

Myths are a lot of fun. They're never completely true, but you can usually find a tiny bit of truth in a myth. The trouble is that some myths can hurt you if you allow them to determine your medical care. This chapter is about those kinds of myths — the ones that lead you to fail to take your medication or stay on your diet, or even lead you to take things that may not be good for you.

Perfect Treatment Yields Perfect Glucoses

Doctors are probably as responsible as their patients are for the myth that perfect treatment results in perfect glucose levels. For decades, doctors measured the urine glucose and told their patients that if they would just stay on their diet, take their medication, and get their exercise, the urine would be negative for glucose. Doctors failed to account for the many variables that could result in a positive test for glucose in the urine, plus the fact that even if the urine was negative, the patient could still be suffering diabetic damage. (The urine becomes negative at a blood glucose of 180 mg/dl [10 mmol/L] in most people, a level that still causes damage.)

The same thing is true for the blood glucose. Although you can achieve normal blood glucose levels most of the time if you treat your diabetes properly, you can still have times when, for no apparent reason, the glucose is not normal. So many factors determine the blood glucose level at any given time that this should hardly be a surprise.

Type 2 Diabetes Occurs in All Overweight People and Not in Normal Weight People

Type 2 diabetes has a strong genetic influence. If you have a parent or sibling with diabetes, you're more likely to develop it. Obesity is a major risk factor for diabetes, but not everyone who is obese develops diabetes, and just because you're slim doesn't mean that you won't develop type 2 diabetes.

A look at the statistics makes this point clearly. More than 200 million overweight adults older than 20 live in the United States of whom more than 100 million are obese (a BMI greater than 30). Yet the total number of adults with diabetes is just 30 million. Ninety million Americans have prediabetes. A study in the *Journal of the American Medical Association* in August 2012 showed that about 12 percent of newly diagnosed people with type 2 diabetes were normal in weight at the time of diagnosis. Furthermore, those who were normal in weight had a higher *morbidity rate* (tended to die) earlier than those individuals who were obese. ***Note:*** Don't take this as a recommendation to become obese. Obesity has plenty of other risks associated with it.

You Can't Enjoy Your Food

I hope you will not become a victim of this myth after reading this book. I provide recipes from great restaurants and chefs that clearly deserve the designation "gourmet" throughout Appendix A. If you want more info on the great food you can enjoy, see the latest edition of my book *Diabetes Cookbook For Dummies* (John Wiley & Sons, Inc.). Chapter 8 discusses that no food is forbidden to the person with diabetes. The key is moderation and not allowing yourself to gain weight.

Diabetes is not caused by sugar or fat or any other specific food. Type 2 diabetes typically occurs when the total food consumption leads to weight gain (weight gain is not always present) in a person who is genetically inclined to develop diabetes. Even then, regular exercise may postpone or prevent diabetes. Eating together is one of the most common social events, and by using the information in Chapter 8, you can continue to enjoy food despite diabetes.

You Can Tell the Level of Your Blood Glucose by How You Feel

Many of my patients have claimed that they can tell their blood glucose level by how they feel, and I have challenged them to prove it. Guess who wins every time, with the exception of significant hypoglycemia? Sure, if your blood glucose is below 50 mg/dl and you are sweaty and have palpitations and a headache, you know that you are low — but even then, you don't know how low. Therefore, you don't know how much treatment to give yourself to bring it back up but not too high.

Patients with high blood glucose rarely can tell within 50 mg/dl what their level is. Less than half of patients who guess come close to the correct answer. People who don't test but who instead rely on the way they feel will suffer one or several of the short-term and long-term complications described in Chapters 4, 5, and 6.

People With Diabetes Get More Colds and Other Illnesses

One problem that people with diabetes don't have is a tendency to develop colds and other minor illnesses. A number of risk factors for the development of colds include some of the following:

✔ Being a child, especially if your parent(s) smokes

✔ Being exposed to secondhand smoke as an adult

✔ Taking medication that suppresses the immune system

People with type 2 diabetes do develop high blood pressure and high cholesterol more often. A number of other diseases including some cancers, arthritis, and bone fractures are more common in diabetics. Refer to Chapter 5 for more about this topic.

If You Need Insulin, You're Doomed

Many people with type 2 diabetes believe that once they have to take insulin, they're on a rapid downhill course to death. This is not so. If you're using insulin, it probably means that your pancreas has pooped out and cannot produce enough insulin to control your blood glucose, even when stimulated by oral drugs. But taking insulin is no more a death sentence for you than it is for the person with type 1 diabetes.

Some people believe that insulin itself causes complications like impotence or other damage. No evidence supports this theory. One study suggested that using insulin to lower the blood glucose so the hemoglobin A1c was less than 6 percent caused more deaths than lowering it to a more modest level like 7 percent.

This study examined patients who had already had a heart attack and were quite sick when the study began. Even so, the doctors could not get the patients' hemoglobin A1c to the level they wanted with insulin. The goal was set too low. It does not take lowering to 6 percent to prevent complications in new patients with diabetes; 6.5 percent will accomplish this. First of all, using insulin is often a temporary measure for when you're very sick with some other illness that makes your oral drugs ineffective. When the illness is over, your insulin needs end.

Secondly, you may be on insulin because oral agents you tried failed to control your glucose. I see many people in this situation who can be taken off the insulin and given one of the newer oral agents, which actually control their glucose better than the insulin.

One typical patient came to me on 60 units of insulin weighing 180 pounds with a hemoglobin A1c of 7.4. I gradually lowered his insulin as I added rosiglitazone to his treatment. He lost 22 pounds, came off insulin entirely, and now has a hemoglobin A1c of 6.

Thirdly, elderly people with diabetes may need insulin to keep their blood glucose at a reasonable level but do not need very tight control because their probable life span is shorter than the time it takes to develop complications. Their treatment can be kept very simple. The insulin is being used to keep them out of immediate trouble, not to prevent complications.

Finally, people with type 2 diabetes who truly need to be on insulin intensively need to check their blood glucose more often and live more like a person with type 1 diabetes. I hope you realize that with today's methods, this level of intensive treatment means a much higher quality of life than it used to.

People with Diabetes Shouldn't Exercise

If any myth is really damaging to people with diabetes, it is this one: People with diabetes shouldn't exercise. The truth is exactly the opposite. Exercise is a major component of good diabetes management — one that, unfortunately, all too often gets the least time and effort on the part of the patient as well as his or her care providers.

And I'm not just talking about aerobic exercise where your heart is beating faster. Some form of muscle strengthening needs to be a part of your lifestyle. (See Chapter 10 to find out the benefits of muscle strengthening.) If you have a muscle that you can move, move it!

You Can't Give Blood Because You Have Diabetes

Having diabetes doesn't preclude giving blood. However the person with diabetes must fulfill the following criteria:

- ✔ Your blood glucose should be under control.
- ✔ You should be in good health.
- ✔ Your blood pressure should be under 180/100.
- ✔ You shouldn't be anemic.

If you're going to give blood, make sure you have a good meal without fatty foods before the donation and drink extra fluids to make up for the blood loss. Eat some extra fish, raisins, and spinach to replenish your iron.

If You're Sick and Can't Eat, You Can Skip Your Diabetes Medications

When you get sick, you make more of the hormones that tend to raise the blood glucose. So even though you don't feel like eating, you probably need to take your medications, and maybe even more than usual, particularly if you are on insulin.

How can you know what to do? Test your blood glucose! That handy meter will help you decide if things are okay, if your control is a little off, or if you need to contact your doctor for advice. Even if you don't do much testing because your blood glucose is generally so good, you may want to test every four to six hours during illness if you find that your glucose is high, low, or unstable.

Diabetes Wrecks Your Sense of Humor

After the initial stages of accepting diabetes, your sense of humor should return. (See Chapter 1 for more on dealing with diabetes.) If your humor doesn't return, it's no laughing matter.

Dr. Joel Goodman, director of The HUMOR Project, pointed out in a lecture I attended that you "jest for the health of it." Numerous scientific studies have shown the health benefits of laughter.

The comedian Steve Allen pointed out in an interview (performed by Dr. Goodman) that there is humor in every aspect of life — you just have to look for it. The saying goes, "Someday we'll laugh about this." The question is, "Why wait?"

My diabetic patients have been the source of many funny stories, some of which I tell in this book. I want to give you the assignment of coming up with *at least* one funny story from your diabetic past. Send me an e-mail at drrubin@drrubin.com or write me a note about it. Of course, what you think is funny may not be funny to someone else. This is clearly shown by our individual preferences in comedians. Ask ten of your friends who their favorite comedian is and see if you don't come back with 12 answers.

Soak Your Feet Daily if You Have Diabetes

Here's an eleventh myth since you just gave me a standing ovation for writing this book. A standing ovation deserves a brief encore.

This myth causes more damage than it prevents. Soaking the feet tends to dry them. The skin can crack and infection can occur, which is, of course, the opposite of what you are trying to accomplish. Protect your skin by using a moisturizing lotion on a regular basis.

Make sure you inspect your feet every day, particularly if there is any question about your ability to feel abnormalities in your feet. Washing your feet with a good soap containing a moisturizing lotion is a good time to do that inspection.

Follow that up by applying a thick (not a thin or watery) moisturizing lotion to your feet. They will continue to give you good service for many years to come.

Chapter 20

Ten Ways to Get Others to Help You

In This Chapter

▶ Teaching friends and loved ones about hypoglycemia

▶ Making sure your primary physician is following the standards of care

▶ Finding an exercise partner

▶ Enlisting other types of help

Diabetes is a social disease. No, I don't mean that you catch it like herpes. I mean that you can't continue very long with diabetes without calling on the help and expertise of others. Asking for help is not such a bad thing. People who regularly interact with others seem to live longer and have a higher quality of life.

Diabetes has become so pervasive in the United States that practically everyone either knows someone who has diabetes or has it himself. There is a huge, growing body of knowledge about all aspects of diabetes, but you have to be willing to share your diagnosis with others so they can help you. These days I even get new patients when people who know they have diabetes share their diagnosis and symptoms with someone else and that person realizes that he has diabetes as well.

In this chapter, you discover how to make use of the great resources that are available to people with diabetes. So many knowledgeable people are out there — it would be a shame not to utilize their information. (Why, even I use my colleagues' knowledge on very rare occasions!)

Explain Hypoglycemia

If you take either insulin or one of the sulfonylurea medications (see Chapter 11), you may become hypoglycemic. Occasionally, hypoglycemia can be so severe that you're unaware of the problem. At that point, someone in your environment needs to know the symptoms of hypoglycemia and how to treat it. Chapter 4 contains all that information.

You may want to make a list of the signs and symptoms of hypoglycemia and pass it around to your family and friends. You should keep that list and an emergency kit to treat hypoglycemia at home and at work. You may even want to wear a medical alert bracelet so someone can identify your problem when none of these people are around.

Follow the Standards of Care

Decades of following diabetes patients, along with increasing scientific knowledge, has led to the establishment of "standards of care" for people with diabetes. These recommendations usually appear in a supplement to the January issue of *Diabetes Care,* a journal of the American Diabetes Association. I outline these standards in Chapter 7 and on the cheat sheet for this book, which you can find online. By following the standards of care, you have a good chance of avoiding the short- and long-term complications of diabetes. If these complications have already occurred, you have a good chance of having them diagnosed while they are still treatable.

You are the one who needs to make sure that you get an annual eye examination, get your urine tested for microalbumin and your nerves tested for sensation, and get all the other tests that must be done regularly and routinely. (See Chapter 7 for more on these tests.) You can't do these tests alone, however. You need your physician to order the tests and send you to the eye doctor. Don't expect your physician to remember all these details. Just as you have trouble keeping to a program of care over a lifetime, your physician does much better with acute illnesses than chronic ones.

Find an Exercise Partner

Few people continue a regular exercise program completely on their own; I also have trouble doing so. However, when you know that someone is waiting for you, you tend to perform the exercise much more regularly. I have many patients who are regular exercisers because I emphasize exercise so much. All of them exercise with a partner.

If you belong to a club, finding an exercise partner is easy. First, you select the sport, and then you hang out in the place where the sport is played. If the sport is a racket sport, you will soon find others at about your level. If the sport is something like running, you have to be a little forward and ask whether you can join someone or a group about to run. The people you can keep up with are your natural exercise partners.

If you're not a member of a club, finding an exercise partner is a little more difficult. You may have to approach people with whom you work, or you may need your significant other to commit to exercising with you. Most people are happy to walk with you, and some will run and bike with you. Cyclists seem to like group activity, and you can check out listings at a local bike shop or the Sunday newspaper in the activities section to find a group. If you can't seem to find an exercise partner, try a personal trainer.

Use Your Foot Doctor

Your foot doctor is your first line of defense against lesions of the foot. He or she knows what the foot should look like and will notice problems very early, when they're still reversible. Your doctor probably has a foot doctor that he likes to work with.

One of the most useful things the foot doctor can do is to cut your nails. It is too easy to accidentally cut your skin when you try to cut your own nails. If you have diabetes, the consequences can be serious.

Should you notice an abnormality, you must get to the foot doctor immediately. In this situation, you are much better off erring on the side of too much rather than too little medical care. In my practice, I ask the patients about their feet at every visit and examine the feet of those who have been found to have neuropathy (see Chapter 5) in the past. If I discover a foot problem, the foot doctor sees it that day.

Doctors have performed the first hand transplantation, which seems to be going well, but as far as I know, no plans exist to do a foot transplantation. Take good care of your feet because they have to last a lifetime. Your foot doctor can be your major ally in this endeavor.

Enlist Help to Fight Food Temptation

Ever since Adam and Eve, the problem of temptation has been on the front burner. For a diabetic, the constant temptation is to eat foods that do not further your major diabetic goal, which is to control your blood glucose. The opportunities for screwing up your diet are boundless. Just like your exercise partner, your "food partner" — your significant other — can make staying on your diet a lot easier for you.

If your partner cooks most of the meals in your household, he or she has a responsibility to prepare the right kinds of foods. To do so, your partner must know what to make and what to avoid (see Chapter 8). If you go to the dietitian, take your partner along.

Numerous books of recipes and meals are written specifically for people with diabetes. The first cookbook you should look at is *Diabetes Cookbook For Dummies* (John Wiley & Sons, Inc.), which I wrote with Cait James. That book would not have been written if it didn't offer a special feature — the recipes of some of the finest chefs in the United States and Canada. I include a number of good recipes in Appendix A of this book. You can also go to www. dummies.com/extras/diabetes for a list of great websites.

I believe that one big problem in diabetes (as well as the nondiabetic obese population) is large portions of food. One of the simplest of diets is to eat the same foods but half as much. As I worked with the chefs in the various restaurants represented in Appendix A, again and again they remarked to me that Americans eat much more food in a portion than Europeans. Americans have learned to avoid fat, but they eat too much carbohydrate.

When it comes to eating out, your loved one can steer you to restaurants where you can choose foods that work for you. When you're in the restaurant, he or she can point out the healthy choices. The best way to direct you is to set an example of appropriate eating for you.

If you're asked to dinner in someone's home, your partner can help by telling your host in advance that you have diabetes and need to avoid eating certain foods. It is unwise, however, to turn your loved one into a nag. Asking to be reminded each time you stray from your diet will lead to hostility.

Expand Your Diabetes Knowledge

The person who serves as your diabetes educator is the source of a huge amount of necessary and sometimes critical information. Every person with diabetes ought to go through a program of education after the initial shock of the diagnosis is past (see Chapter 1). Never hesitate to ask a question, no matter how basic you think it may be. You will be surprised by how many others want the same information. Insurance will generally pay for yearly education, but check your insurance to be sure.

Of course, every caregiver should be a diabetes educator as well. When you are past the formal diabetes education program, don't hesitate to ask questions of your physician, your dietitian, or any of the other people in your team (see Chapter 12).

Knowledge about diabetes is expanding so fast that great advances are arriving almost daily. Some of these advances may be just what you need.

Fit Your Favorite Foods into Your Diet with a Dietitian

Years ago, a diagnosis of diabetes meant that you had to make enormous changes in your diet. This adjustment was hard enough for people who ate the usual American diet but much harder for people who came from another culture and had an entirely different diet. Fortunately, this situation has changed dramatically.

The dietitian's job is to come up with a diabetic diet plan based on *your* food choices, not those of the dietitian. If you have special dietary needs because of your culture, a dietitian must be able to accommodate those needs if they are reasonable.

Members of your culture ate the foods that you like for generations without developing diabetes in large numbers. The main reasons they didn't develop diabetes in large numbers are that they did not eat the large portions you eat and they were much more physically active than you are. If you want to keep enjoying "your" foods, eat and exercise like your great-grandparents.

Don't be satisfied with a printed sheet of paper with the heading "Diabetic Diet." The key word in diabetic diets is *individualization*. You probably won't stay on a diet that you do not enjoy.

Seek Out Appropriate Specialists

The specialist who knows the most about diabetes is the *diabetologist* (or endocrinologist), a physician with advanced training in diabetes care who maintains his or her edge by attending diabetes meetings regularly and keeping up with the literature by reading the most important clinical diabetes journals. In addition, these days an up-to-date specialist has to be aware of what is on the Internet and how to differentiate reality from hype. This person can explain the latest advances in diabetes to you.

Not only do you want to find a diabetes specialist, but should you develop a complication of diabetes, you also want to use a specialist in that area. At the first sign of kidney disease associated with diabetes, ask your doctor to refer you to a nephrologist. Have an eye doctor examine your eyes every two years or more often if necessary. If there is any question of loss of sensation or abnormal muscle movements, see a neurologist. If there is any indication of heart trouble, get a referral to a cardiologist.

The pace of advances in diabetes is amazing. A general physician cannot keep up with it. The diabetes specialist concentrates on diabetes and the other specialists concentrate on their fields, and that is to your benefit.

Discuss Your Meds with the Pharmacist

One of your most valuable and least utilized resources is your pharmacist. He or she is loaded with information about drug actions, interactions, side effects, proper dosage and administration, and contraindications, as well as what to do in case of an overdose. Every time you get a new medication, you can have your pharmacist run it against the medications you're already taking and see whether any problems might occur. Thanks to computers, this comparison should take only a few minutes. If you work with one drug store, you should be able to get a printout of your entire list of medications, which you can carry with you in case you ever need medical care.

The pharmacist can also save you money by recommending generic equivalents to the brands that your doctor prescribes. The doctor may have good reason to prescribe them, so the pharmacist will check with him before giving you a different medication.

The information in the computer tends to be all-inclusive. If a drug has ever had a side effect, no matter how rare, it will probably be in the computer. The drug manufacturer wants to be able to say that it warned you about every possibility. If a side effect or drug interaction is serious, discuss it with your physician before you start the new medication.

Share This Book with Everyone

If you really want your friends and loved ones to understand what you're going through, why not give them a copy of this book and ask them to read it? You can select the chapters that are most important to you. Your family and friends will probably be delighted to have a resource they can understand, and you can expect a lot more help from them.

When I began writing this book, I did so because I saw a need for information that could be understood by most people without the benefit of a medical-school education. At the same time, I wanted you to have a little fun because "a spoonful of sugar helps the medicine go down." But I did not want to trivialize diabetes, and hope I have not done so. If you believe I have succeeded in what I set out to do, share this book with others.

Appendix

Mini-Cookbook

· ·

*T*his appendix should make it clear to you that you can have great food from every ethnic corner of the world and still stay within the requirements of a diabetic diet. In a short appendix like this, I could not include every possible type of food, but I tried to select foods that most people enjoy either at home or in a restaurant. This edition includes several recipes featuring Mediterranean food. I chose the restaurants from among the best in the country, with an emphasis on San Francisco because that is where I reside and (happily) get to try them. I've also included a sampling of delicious salad recipes from my book *Diabetes Cookbook For Dummies* (John Wiley & Sons, Inc.). If you like what you see, pick up a copy for even more delectable diabetic-friendly recipes.

Getting to Know the Contributing Restaurants and Chefs

The chefs and restaurants who contributed recipes were a pleasure to work with and deserve great praise for their willingness to accommodate the needs of diabetic diners. Some restaurant recipes were altered slightly to keep them appropriate for a diabetic diet, but changes were never done without the approval of the chefs who created them. Some of their recipes may take a little longer than others to prepare, but all are worth the time and the effort. In any case, you can go to the restaurant that provided the recipe, order that meal, and know that you are on your diabetic diet.

Avra Estiatorio

The flavors of the Mediterranean have been cultivated and coveted for more than two thousand years. Avra Estiatorio gives you the best of what this ancient tradition has to offer — classic Mediterranean specialties and the freshest fish available. From the moment you walk in, you're surrounded by

Mediterranean charm, with exposed wood-beamed ceilings, soft arched walls, and tapestries you feel like you've been transported to a Greek isle. The open kitchen, with its magnificent fish display, prepares the freshest selections from the sea, including Mediterranean specialties such as barbounia, lithrini, and fagri.

Avra Estiatorio, 141 East 48th Street, New York, NY. 212-759-8550
`www.avrany.com`

Border Grill

Situated in Santa Monica, California, the critically acclaimed Border Grill restaurant features the bold foods of Mexico. The original restaurant is joined by Border Grill Downtown LA and Border Grill Las Vegas, as well as the Border Grill Truck, a gourmet taco truck on the cutting edge of the street-food scene in Los Angeles.

The restaurants and truck are the inspiration of two women who are chefs, restaurateurs, cookbook authors, and television personalities: Mary Sue Milliken and Susan Feniger. They are well known from Bravo's *Top Chef Masters* and Food Network's *Two Hot Tamales* and are natural teachers who enjoy sharing their passion for bold flavors and strong statements through many media. If you find, as I did, that their recipes make you hunger for more, look for their book *Mexican Cooking For Dummies* (John Wiley & Sons, Inc.).

Border Grill, 1445 Fourth St., Santa Monica, California. 310-451-1655.
`www.bordergrill.com/`

Greens

When residents of the San Francisco Bay area think of great vegetarian food, Greens is the first name that comes to mind. Greens uses the freshest ingredients, many of which come from the Zen Center's Green Gulch Farm, across the Golden Gate Bridge in Marin County. This brief trip results in no loss of freshness for the fine seasonal organic produce.

Chef Annie Somerville came to Greens in 1981 and became executive chef in 1985. She continues to create outstanding dishes with a balance of colors and flavors and contrast of textures. In addition to the Green Gulch and Start Route Farms in Marin County, she uses artisan cheeses from west Marin and Sonoma counties. She has authored the award-winning book *Field of Greens: New Vegetarian Recipes from the Celebrated Greens Restaurant* (Bantam).

Greens, Fort Mason, Building A, San Francisco, California. 415-771-6222.
www.greensrestaurant.com.

Gerald Hirigoyen

Gerald Hirigoyen is the chef and owner of several San Francisco restaurants, including Piperade and Lauburu. By whatever designation, his food is straightforward and flavorful, and the social atmosphere is full of character and energy. The high quality of the food is in contrast to the moderate prices of everything on the menu. Much of the menu can be enjoyed not only for taste but also for the healthful qualities of the food.

Gerald Hirigoyen trained in the Basque region of France and in Paris with some of the great names in French cuisine. He came to San Francisco in 1980 and ran the kitchens of several fine restaurants, but in 1991, he decided to go out on his own and start his restaurant. He has received numerous awards and much recognition for the quality of his food. *Food and Wine* magazine called him one of 1994's "Best New Chefs in America."

Luna Blu

Chef Renzo Azzarello is from a seaside resort Taormina Sicily and began his chef training at a young age, learning how to cook as a child in his family's bed and breakfast kitchen. He has worked in, managed, and owned several restaurants in the Bay Area, mainly in San Francisco. During this time he increased his knowledge of California resources and infused his Italian cuisine background with local ingredients. Azzarello knows that the only way to create fantastic food is to have the right ingredients, fresh natural sustainable produce, a happy team who are eager to learn, and people who enjoy nourishing artisanal food. He is environmentally conscious due to his strong connection with the ocean; he believes we should live life sustainably and leave our blue planet healthy for future generations of all creatures. He and his wife Crystal established their restaurant, Luna Blu in 2013. The food you eat at Luna Blu is rare and special, something you find once in a blue moon.

Luna Blu, 35 Main Street, Tiburon, CA. 415-789-5844

Paulette Mitchell

Paulette Mitchell, the author of 13 cookbooks, is known for her quick-to-prepare recipes with gourmet flair. She is the author of the award-winning *15-Minute Gourmet* cookbook series. She also is a video producer of Telly

Award–winning travel and culinary videos as well as a media spokesperson, freelance writer, culinary speaker, cooking instructor, and television personality. As an avid world traveler, Paulette is most inspired by flavors from diverse cultures both near and far.

Paulette's most recently published cookbook is *The Complete 15-Minute Gourmet: Creative Cuisine Made Fast and Fresh* (Thomas Nelson), which features 350 delicious recipes from around the world.

Cooking Some Healthful Recipes

Throughout the book I have been emphasizing that it's possible to enjoy your food and still keep your diabetes under control. The following recipes verify this contention. They come from the best chefs and restaurants and prove that there are many chefs who not only want to feed you tasty and hardy food but healthful food as well.

Grilled Romaine Caesar Salad

Prep time: 10 min plus chilling time • **Cook time:** 5 min • **Yield:** 4 servings

Ingredients	*Directions*
½ **sheet toasted nori**	*1* Grind nori sheet in a blender or food processor to a fine powder. Add the tofu, 2 tablespoons olive oil, lemon juice, garlic, Worcestershire, salt, and pepper and puree until smooth. Refrigerate the dressing for 30 minutes.
1 **package silken tofu**	
3 **tablespoons olive oil, divided**	
1½ **ounces lemon juice**	
2 **cloves garlic**	*2* Meanwhile, wash the romaine hearts and slice off the ends. Cut each romaine heart in half. Drizzle each half with the remaining olive oil and season with salt and pepper.
1 **teaspoon vegan Worcestershire sauce**	
Salt and pepper to taste	
6 **romaine hearts**	*3* Place each romaine heart face down on hot grill (or grill pan) for 45 seconds or until lightly charred. Remove and serve on chilled plate with drizzled Caesar dressing. Garnish with grilled bread or croutons.
Grilled bread or croutons as garnish	

Per serving: Calories 104; Fat 7g (Saturated 1g); Cholesterol 0mg; Sodium 134mg; Carbohydrate 5g (Dietary Fiber 1g); Protein 6g.

Note: This delicious recipe is Vegetate's (Washington, D.C.) take on a classic Caesar salad; they replace the anchovies with toasted ground *nori* (seaweed sheets often used for making sushi rolls), and instead of eggs, they use silken tofu, a high-protein, cholesterol-free improvement.

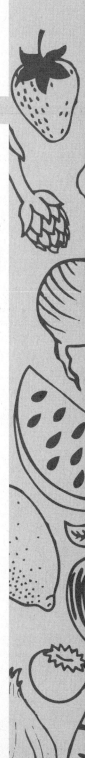

Summer Tomato Salad

Prep time: 10 min • **Cook time:** 0 min • **Yield:** 4 servings

Ingredients	*Directions*
4 medium tomatoes, diced small	*1* Combine all the ingredients in a large bowl and serve the salad at room temperature.
1 garlic clove, minced	
6 leaves basil, chiffonaded	
2 tablespoons olive oil	
1 tablespoon balsamic vinegar	
Salt and pepper to taste	

Per serving: Calories 99; Fat 7g (Saturated 1g); Cholesterol 0mg; Sodium 152mg; Carbohydrate 8g (Dietary Fiber 1g); Protein 1g.

Tip: Try a combination of tomatoes in this salad to add color and flavor. Look for Green Zebras, Yellow Teardrops, pear tomatoes, grape tomatoes, and everyone's first favorite tomato, the cherry. So many choices, so little time! Refer to Figure A-1 for how to seed and dice tomatoes.

Note: This dish, courtesy of Paley's Place in Portland, Oregon, is low in saturated fat and contains no cholesterol but still remains intense in flavor from the fresh basil and garlic.

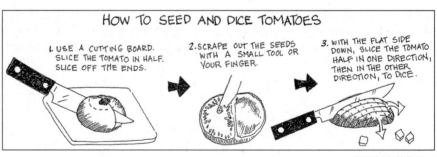

Figure A-1: How to seed and dice a tomato.

Illustration by Liz Kurtzman

Blood Orange, Beet, and Avocado Salad

Prep time: 25 min • **Cook time:** 1 hr or more • **Yield:** 6 servings

Ingredients	Directions

Ingredients

1 bunch yellow beets

3 tablespoons plus about 1 tablespoon extra-virgin olive oil

1 head red lettuce (or a small bag of mesclun)

4 blood oranges

2 avocados

¼ cup shelled pistachios or toasted pine nuts

½ teaspoon coarse salt

1½ tablespoons red wine vinegar

Freshly ground black pepper, to taste

Directions

1 Preheat the oven to 400 degrees. Cut the leaves and roots from the beets. Rub the beets with about 1 tablespoon of olive oil and wrap each one in foil. Bake until they're soft when pierced with a fork, at least 1 hour. When the beets are cool enough to handle, remove the skins and cut the beets into wedges.

2 Meanwhile, wash and dry the lettuce and place it in a large bowl.

3 Cut both ends off the oranges, lay them on a cut side, and with a knife, remove the rind in 1-inch strips around the orange, cutting down to the flesh. Squeeze any excess juice from the cuttings over the lettuce. Cut the skinned oranges into rounds.

4 Cut each avocado in half, and cut the flesh of each half into slices. Arrange the blood orange slices, the avocado slices, and the beets over the lettuce. Sprinkle with pistachios or pine nuts.

5 When ready to serve, mix salt in the bowl of a spoon with the vinegar. Toss vinegar mixture over the salad, and then add 3 tablespoons of olive oil and black pepper to taste. Toss salad gently so that all the ingredients are lightly coated with dressing. Arrange salad on individual salad plates.

Per serving: Calories 245; Fat 18g (Saturated 3g); Cholesterol 0mg; Sodium 159mg; Carbohydrate 21g (Dietary Fiber 9g); Protein 5g.

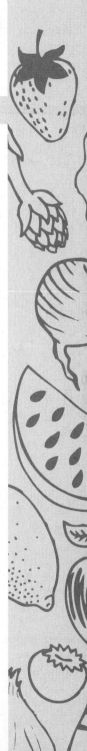

Shrimp Salad

Prep time: 15 min • **Cook time:** 0 min • **Yield:** 4 servings

Ingredients	Directions
1 pound medium shrimp, cooked	**1** In a bowl, combine the shrimp (refer to Figure A-2 to know how to peel and devein), the red and yellow peppers, half of the cilantro, and the chives.
¼ cup chopped red pepper	
¼ cup chopped yellow pepper	
1 tablespoon chopped fresh cilantro, divided	**2** In another bowl, whisk together the mayonnaise, mustard, lemon juice, and white pepper. Spoon over the shrimp mixture and toss together.
¼ cup chopped fresh chives	
¼ cup low-fat mayonnaise	
1 teaspoon Dijon mustard	**3** Arrange the salad greens on 4 large plates. Top the greens with equal portions of the shrimp mixture. Sprinkle with the remaining cilantro.
1 teaspoon lemon juice	
¼ teaspoon white pepper	
4 cups fresh mixed salad greens	

Per serving: Calories 154; Fat 3g (Saturated 0g); Cholesterol 221mg; Sodium 440mg; Carbohydrate 7g (Dietary Fiber 2g); Protein 25g.

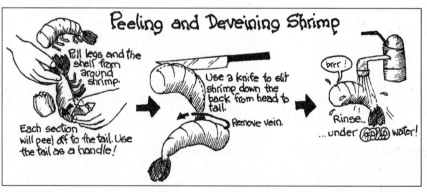

Figure A-2: How to peel and devein shrimp.

Illustration by Liz Kurtzman

Teriyaki Salmon Salad

Prep time: 15 min • **Cook time:** 10 to 12 min • **Yield:** 2 servings

Ingredients	*Directions*
1 tablespoon Dijon mustard	*1* Preheat the oven to 350 degrees. In a medium bowl, combine the mustard, wine, teriyaki sauce, soy sauce, honey, lemon juice, garlic powder, and white pepper. Place the salmon in the bowl and coat thoroughly.
1 tablespoon dry white cooking wine	
1 tablespoon low-sodium teriyaki sauce	*2* Place the salmon in a baking dish, pour the remaining liquid over the salmon, and place the dish in the oven. Bake for 10 to 12 minutes.
1 teaspoon low-sodium soy sauce	
1 teaspoon honey	*3* Arrange 1 cup of greens on each plate and place a salmon fillet on top. Sprinkle the red onion over the plate.
1 teaspoon lemon juice	
½ teaspoon garlic powder	
¼ teaspoon white pepper	
2 skinless salmon fillets, 6 ounces each	
2 cups field salad greens	
¼ small red onion, thinly sliced	

Per serving: Calories 256; Fat 7g (Saturated 1g); Cholesterol 97mg; Sodium 559mg; Carbohydrate 8g (Dietary Fiber 2g); Protein 39g.

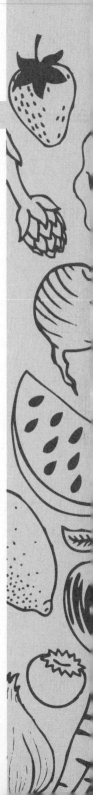

Avra Estiatorio's Traditional Greek Salad

Prep time: 6 min • **Yield:** 2 servings

Ingredients	Directions
1½ beefsteak tomatoes	**1** Cut tomatoes into pieces (about eight, depending on size).
1 Persian cucumber	
½ green bell pepper	**2** Slice cucumbers, onion, and bell pepper into bite-sized pieces.
¼ cup sweet Vidalia white onion and red onion mixed	
3 tablespoons extra virgin olive oil	**3** Toss all ingredients (except for the feta) in a bowl and mix.
1 teaspoon red wine vinegar	
½ teaspoon balsamic vinegar	**4** Serve in a bowl and top with crumbled feta cheese.
Pinch dried oregano	
Pinch sea salt	
Pinch black pepper	
3 black olives cut in half	
2 ounces feta cheese	

Per serving: Calories: 319; Fat 27g (Saturated 7g); Cholesterol 12.6mg; Sodium 176mg; Carbohydrate 14.5g (Dietary Fiber 3.5g); Protein 4.5g.

Border Grill's Cinnamon-Brandy Chicken

Prep time: 30 min plus marinating time • **Cook time:** 40 min • **Yield:** 6 servings

Ingredients	Directions
½ cup brandy 1 tablespoon cinnamon ¼ cup honey ½ cup lemon juice ½ cup orange juice 4 garlic cloves, minced 1 teaspoon salt ½ teaspoon freshly ground black pepper 1 frying chicken (2½ to 3 pounds), cut into pieces and seasoned 2 tablespoons vegetable oil	*1* In a medium bowl, mix the brandy, cinnamon, honey, lemon and orange juices, garlic (check out Figure A-3 for how to peel and mince the garlic), salt, and pepper. Add the seasoned chicken and toss to evenly coat. Cover and marinate in the refrigerator 8 hours or overnight. *2* Preheat the oven to 350 degrees. Remove the chicken from the bowl and shake off excess marinade. Pour the marinade into a small saucepan and bring to a boil. Boil until it begins to thicken and about 1 cup remains, 5 to 10 minutes. *3* Heat the oil in an ovenproof skillet over medium-high heat. Sear the chicken until golden on both sides. Pour the reduced marinade over the chicken and place in the oven. Bake about 20 minutes and serve.

Per serving: Calories 506; Fat 25g (Saturated 7g); Cholesterol 134mg; Sodium 502mg; Carbohydrate 16g (Dietary Fiber 0g); Protein 42g.

Note: Serve with the rice pilaf and roasted vegetable dishes, later in this section.

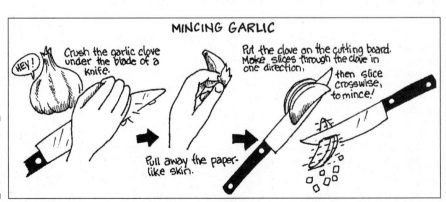

Figure A-3: How to peel and mince garlic.

Illustration by Liz Kurtzman

Border Grill's Green Rice Pilaf

Prep time: 40 min • **Cook time:** 25 min • **Yield:** 6 servings

Ingredients	Directions
1½ tablespoons vegetable oil 1 small onion, finely diced 1 cup long-grain white rice	**1** Heat the oil in a heavy saucepan over medium heat. Add the onion and rice and cook, stirring frequently, for about 7 minutes, until the onion is softened but not browned.
2 cups hot vegetable or chicken broth, preferably homemade ½ teaspoon salt	**2** Add the hot broth, salt, and chilies and bring to a boil. Reduce to a simmer and cook, covered, for about 10 minutes.
3 medium poblano chilies, roasted, peeled, seeded, and cut into strips	**3** Add the peas and simmer 5 minutes longer. Remove from heat and let stand, covered, for about 10 minutes.
1 cup fresh or frozen peas ½ cup crumbled Mexican queso fresco or feta cheese ½ bunch Italian parsley leaves, finely chopped ½ bunch cilantro, finely chopped	**4** Add the cheese, parsley, and cilantro. Evenly mix and fluff with a fork, and serve immediately.

Per serving: *Calories 202; Fat 7g (Saturated Fat 3g); Cholesterol 1mg; Sodium 948mg; Carbohydrate 28g (Dietary Fiber 2g); Protein 12g.*

Note: This dish can accompany the chicken in the preceding recipe, or it can be served with meat or fish.

Border Grill's Red Roasted Root Vegetables

Prep time: 35 min • **Cook time:** 40 min • **Yield:** 6 servings

Ingredients	Directions
½ pound turnips, peeled and cut into 1-inch chunks	**1** Preheat the oven to 450 degrees. In a large bowl, toss together all the ingredients until well mixed. Arrange the mixture in a single layer in an enamel cast-iron casserole or baking dish.
½ pound beets, peeled and cut into 1-inch chunks	
½ pound carrots, peeled and cut into 1-inch chunks	**2** Cover the casserole dish and roast for 30 to 40 minutes, stirring every 10 minutes. The vegetables are done when they're golden, lightly caramelized on the edges, and easily pierced with the tip of a knife.
½ pound butternut or other firm squash, peeled and cut into 1-inch chunks	
1 onion, coarsely chopped	
2 garlic cloves, minced	
½ bunch fresh oregano leaves, coarsely chopped	
⅓ cup olive oil	
1 teaspoon salt	
½ teaspoon freshly ground pepper	

Per serving: Calories 171; Fat 11g (Saturated Fat 2g); Cholesterol 0mg; Sodium 432mg; Carbohydrate 15g (Dietary Fiber 4g); Protein 2g.

Vary It! You can substitute any of your favorite root vegetables in this dish.

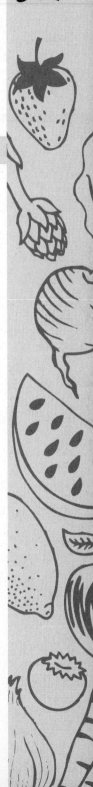

Border Grill's Baked Apples

Prep time: 35 min • **Cook time:** 1 hr • **Yield:** 6 servings

Ingredients	*Directions*
1 cup plus 2 tablespoons apple juice	*1* In a small saucepan, bring 2 tablespoons apple juice and the raisins to a simmer and remove from heat. Let them sit for 10 minutes.
¼ cup raisins	
¼ cup apple butter	*2* Preheat the oven to 350 degrees. In a bowl, stir together the apple butter, walnuts (refer to Figure A-4 for how to chop them), maple syrup, brandy, and raisins with their juice and mix well.
¼ cup toasted chopped walnuts	
2 tablespoons maple syrup	
2 tablespoons brandy	*3* Stuff the apples with the raisin mixture. Place the apples in a small roasting pan and top each with a dab of butter. Pour the remaining cup of apple juice into the pan and bake 50 to 60 minutes, or until the apples are tender but not split or mushy.
6 medium apples, cored and the top third peeled	
2 tablespoons unsalted butter	

Per serving: Calories 218; Fat 8g (Saturated Fat 3g); Cholesterol 11mg; Sodium 2mg; Carbohydrate 38g (Dietary Fiber 4g); Protein 2g.

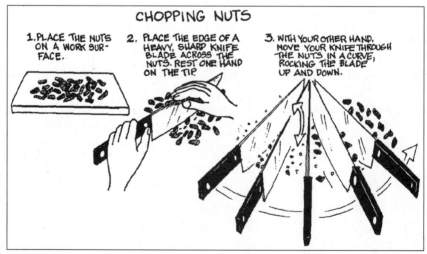

Figure A-4:
How to chop
walnuts.

Illustration by Liz Kurtzman

Greens' Romaine Hearts with Sourdough Croutons and Parmesan Cheese

Prep time: 10 min • **Cook time:** 10 min • **Yield:** 4 servings

Ingredients	Directions
4 small heads of romaine lettuce **2 garlic cloves, finely chopped** **6 tablespoons extra-virgin olive oil, divided** **4 thick slices of sourdough bread, cut into ½-inch cubes, about 1½ cups** **1¼ teaspoon minced lemon zest** **¼ teaspoon salt** **1½ tablespoons vinegar or lemon juice** **8 Geata or Nicoise olives, pitted and coarsely chopped** **1 ounce Parmesan cheese, grated, about ⅓ cup** **Freshly ground black pepper to taste**	*1* Discard the outer leaves of the romaine heads and use the whole leaves and the hearts, which should be pale green or yellow and firm. Wash the leaves, dry them in a spinner, and wrap them loosely in a damp towel and refrigerate. *2* Preheat the oven to 375 degrees. Add 1 garlic clove to 1 tablespoon olive oil and toss with the cubed bread. Spread the cubes on a baking sheet and bake for 7 to 8 minutes, until golden brown. Set aside to cool. *3* Make the vinaigrette by combining the lemon zest, salt, remaining garlic, and vinegar. Then whisk in 5 tablespoons olive oil. *4* When you're ready to serve the salad, place the lettuce in a large bowl. Add the olives and toss with the vinaigrette, coating all the leaves. Add the croutons and Parmesan; toss again. Sprinkle with freshly ground pepper and serve.

Per serving: Calories 355; Fat 23g (Saturated Fat 4g); Cholesterol 6mg; Sodium 696mg; Carbohydrate 31g (Dietary Fiber 3g); Protein 9g.

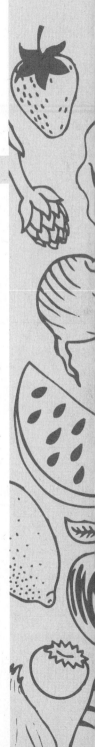

Greens' Summer Minestrone

Prep time: 30 min • **Cook time:** 45 min • **Yield:** 6 servings

Ingredients	*Directions*
½ cup dried red beans, sorted and soaked overnight	**1** Drain and rinse the beans, and then place them in a 2-quart saucepan with 6 cups of cold water, 1 bay leaf, sage leaves, and oregano. Bring to a boil; reduce heat and simmer, uncovered, until the beans are tender, about 30 minutes. Remove the herbs.
2 bay leaves	
2 fresh sage leaves	
1 fresh oregano sprig	
1 tablespoon extra-virgin olive oil	**2** While the beans are cooking, heat the oil in a soup pot. Add the onion, salt, dried basil, and a few pinches of pepper. Sauté the onion over medium heat until soft, 5 to 7 minutes.
1 medium red onion, diced (about 2 cups)	
½ teaspoon salt	**3** Add the garlic, carrots, bell pepper, and zucchini to the soup pot and sauté for 7 to 8 minutes, stirring often. Add the wine and cook for 1 to 2 minutes, until the pan is almost dry.
¼ teaspoon dried basil	
Black pepper to taste	
6 garlic cloves, finely chopped	
1 small carrot, diced (about ¼ cup)	**4** Add the tomatoes and then add the pasta, spinach or chard, and beans with their broth. Season with salt and pepper to taste. Add the fresh basil just before serving. Garnish each serving with a generous tablespoon of Parmesan cheese.
1 small red bell pepper, diced (about ¾ cup)	
1 small zucchini, diced (about ¾ cup)	
¼ cup red wine	
2 pounds fresh tomatoes, peeled, seeded, and coarsely chopped (about 3 cups)	
¼ cup small pasta, cooked al dente, drained, and rinsed	

½ bunch of fresh spinach or chard, cut into thin ribbons and washed, about 2 cups packed

2 tablespoons chopped fresh basil

Grated Parmesan cheese

Per serving: Calories 98; Fat 2g (Saturated Fat 0g); Cholesterol 1mg; Sodium 652mg; Carbohydrate 17g (Dietary Fiber 2g); Protein 4g.

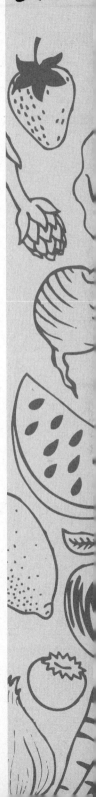

Greens' Sweet Pepper and Basil Frittata

Prep time: 30 min • **Cook time:** 30 min • **Yield:** 10 servings

Ingredients	Directions
2 tablespoons light olive oil	*1* Preheat the oven to 475 degrees. Heat 1 tablespoon olive oil in a large skillet; add the onion, ½ teaspoon salt, and a few pinches of pepper. Sauté the onion over medium heat until it begins to soften, about 4 to 5 minutes.
1 medium yellow onion, thinly sliced, about 2 cups	
¾ teaspoon salt	
Freshly ground black pepper	*2* Add the sweet peppers, garlic, and bay leaf; stew the onion and peppers together for about 15 minutes, until the peppers are tender. Set the vegetables aside to cool. Remove the bay leaf.
4 medium sweet peppers, preferably a combination of red and yellow, thinly sliced (about 4 cups)	
4 garlic cloves, finely chopped	*3* Beat the eggs in a bowl and add the onion-pepper mixture, cheeses, and basil. Season with ¼ teaspoon salt and ⅛ teaspoon pepper.
1 bay leaf	
6 eggs	*4* In a 9-inch nonstick, ovenproof sauté pan, heat the remaining tablespoon of olive oil until almost smoking. Swirl the oil around the side of the pan to coat. Turn the heat down to low and then immediately pour the egg mixture into the pan. The pan should be hot enough so that the eggs sizzle when they touch the oil. Cook the frittata over low heat for 2 to 3 minutes, until the sides begin to set.
3 ounces Fontina cheese, grated, about 1½ cups	
2 ounces Parmesan cheese, grated, about ¾ cup	
¼ cup fresh basil leaves, bundled and thinly sliced	
3 tablespoons balsamic vinegar	*5* Transfer the sauté pan to the oven and bake the frittata, uncovered, for 6 to 8 minutes, until firm and the eggs are completely cooked.

6 Loosen the frittata gently with a rubber spatula. Place a plate over the pan, flip it over, and put it on a plate. Brush the bottom and sides with the vinegar and cut into wedges. Serve warm or at room temperature.

Per serving: *Calories 149; Fat 10g (Saturated Fat 4g); Cholesterol 159mg; Sodium 349mg; Carbohydrate 45g (Dietary Fiber 1g); Protein 10g.*

Note: You can serve this dish right out of the oven as a main course or let it cool and serve as a light lunch. You can also refrigerate the dish and cut it into small squares to serve as an hors d'oeuvre.

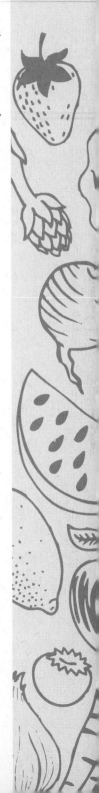

Gerald Hirigoyen's Lemon-Braised Sea Bass with Star Anise and Baby Spinach

Prep time: 30 min • **Cook time:** 15 min • **Yield:** 4 servings

Ingredients	Directions
4 sea bass fillets (about 4 ounces each)	**1** Preheat the oven to 475 degrees. Rub both sides of the sea bass fillets with salt and pepper and set aside.
Salt and freshly ground pepper to taste	
1 teaspoon olive oil	**2** Heat the olive oil in a large ovenproof sauté pan (preferably nonstick) over high heat. Add the celery root, fennel (check out Figure A-5 for how to cut and clean it), carrot, garlic, and star anise and sauté until slightly caramelized, 4 to 5 minutes. Soften the caramelization with the lemon juice and cook for 1 minute.
¼ cup finely diced celery root	
⅓ cup finely diced fennel	
¼ cup finely diced carrot	
3 garlic cloves, peeled and chopped	**3** Lay the sea bass fillets on top of the sautéed vegetables, add the water, and cover the pan. Place the pan into the preheated oven just until the fish is cooked though (5 to 6 minutes). Remove the pan from oven and remove the fillets of fish and set them aside, covered to keep warm.
4 star anise	
¼ cup freshly squeezed lemon juice	
1½ cups water	
⅓ cup finely diced cucumber	**4** Add the cucumber (refer to Figure A-6 for how to prepare the cucumber), tomato, and apple to the vegetables in the sauté pan and place over high heat. Bring to a boil and cook for 1 to 2 minutes.
⅓ cup finely diced tomato	
⅛ cup finely diced apple	
4 cups baby spinach	**5** Add the spinach, extra-virgin olive oil, mild cayenne, and salt and pepper to taste. Cook just until the spinach wilts (30 seconds to 1 minute).
2 teaspoons extra-virgin olive oil	
Pinch of mild cayenne powder	**6** In 4 shallow soup bowls, spread an even amount of the vegetables and juice from the pan. Lay a fillet on top of the vegetables in each bowl and place a star anise on top to garnish. Sprinkle the chives and parsley over the top of each dish and serve immediately.
2 tablespoons fresh chopped chives	
2 tablespoons fresh chopped parsley	

Per serving: Calories 236; Fat 6g (Saturated Fat 1g); Cholesterol 77mg; Sodium 240mg; Carbohydrate 17g (Dietary Fiber 3g); Protein 31g.

Note: This meal is low in total carbohydrate and total fat, so you can complete the meal with a couple servings of carbohydrate (such as a serving of French bread and rice) and a tossed green salad with vinaigrette dressing.

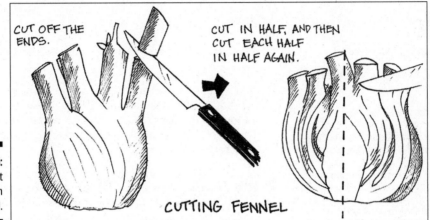

Figure A-5: How to cut and clean fennel.

Illustration by Liz Kurtzman

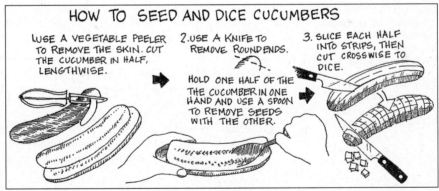

Figure A-6: How to peel, seed, and chop a cucumber.

Illustration by Liz Kurtzman

Gerald Hirigoyen's Onion Pie with Roquefort and Walnuts

Prep time: 1 hr • **Cook time:** 40 min • **Yield:** 8 servings

Ingredients	*Directions*
2 tablespoons olive oil	*1* Place a baking sheet with sides in the freezer.
2 white onions, very thinly sliced	*2* In a sauté pan over medium-high heat, warm the olive oil. Add the onions and sauté until golden brown (about 10 minutes). Add the water and continue to sauté until all the moisture evaporates, about 5 minutes.
¼ cup water	
3 ounces Roquefort cheese, crumbled into small pieces	
Salt and freshly ground pepper to taste	*3* Reduce heat to medium low. Add the Roquefort cheese and continue cooking, stirring occasionally, until melted, about 5 more minutes. Season lightly with salt, if needed, and add pepper to taste.
½ cup walnuts, coarsely chopped	
1 tablespoon melted butter	*4* Stir in the walnuts and then spread the mixture out onto the chilled sheet pan. Place in the freezer until the onions cool down completely (about 10 minutes).
2 puff pastry sheets (11-x -15-inch sheets), fresh or thawed frozen	
1 egg, lightly beaten	*5* Preheat the oven to 450 degrees and evenly brush a sheet pan with melted butter.
8 slices of prosciutto (about ½-ounce each)	
Mixed greens to garnish	*6* Place the puff pastry on a cutting board. Using the rim of a small plate about 5 inches in diameter as a guide, cut the pastry into 8 rounds. Discard scraps.
	7 Place the rounds onto the prepared baking sheet. Brush the outer rims and tops with the beaten egg. Evenly distribute the cooled onion mixture in the middle of each of the 8 rounds, leaving 1 inch uncovered all around the edges.

8 Place 1 prosciutto slice on top of each mound of the onion mixture. Fold over the pastry rounds to create half-moon shapes. Pinch down firmly around the edges to seal in the filling.

9 Brush the top of each pie with more of the beaten egg. Using a sharp knife, pierce the top of each pie with a small slit.

10 Bake until the pastry is pale golden and fully puffed, about 20 to 25 minutes.

Per serving: Calories 454; Fat 34g (Saturated Fat 7g); Cholesterol 47mg; Sodium 562mg; Carbohydrate 26g (Dietary Fiber 1g); Protein 13g.

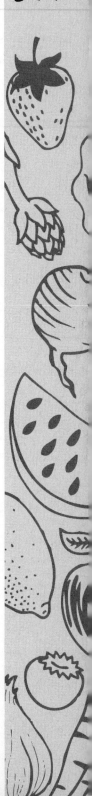

Luna Blu's Eggplant Roll

Prep time: 30 min • **Cook time:** 15 min • **Yield:** 4 servings

Ingredients	Directions
1 eggplant, peeled	**1** Thinly slice the eggplant from the top to the bottom, grill on high heat for each side until marked.
4 Roma tomatoes, cubed	
12 fresh basil leaves, chopped	**2** Place the basil leaves on top of the eggplant with one piece of bell pepper and a small ball of goat's cheese. Roll up tightly from top to bottom.
½ red pepper, julienne cut	
1½ ounces soft goat cheese	
½ cup of white wine	**3** Heat pan over a high heat, and add olive oil, salt, pepper and garlic. Infuse the oil with the garlic for a couple of minutes. Remove the garlic and add the chopped tomato.
1 clove of garlic, crushed	
5 tablespoons extra virgin olive oil to taste	
Salt and pepper to taste	**4** Cook for a couple more minutes and add the eggplant rolls.
	5 Add the wine and let the wine reduce until serving.

Per serving: Calories: 234; Fat 20.5g (Saturated 5g); Cholesterol 8mg; Sodium 36mg; Carbohydrate 4g (Dietary Fiber 2g); Protein 8.4g.

Luna Blu's Seafood Skewers

Prep time: 20 min • **Cook time:** 25–30 min • **Yield:** 4 servings

Ingredients	Directions

Ingredients

10 ounces swordfish

10 ounces wild salmon

7 ounces of calamari

8 medium sized prawns

2 bell peppers — 1 red
1 yellow, cut into 1 inch squares

2 medium sized zucchini, ⅕ inch slices

3 tablespoons of extra virgin olive oil

½ glass of white wine

Salt and pepper to taste

2 dry bay leaves, chopped

4 or 5 sprigs of thyme, chopped

1 sprig of dill, chopped

1 sprig of rosemary, chopped

2 sage leaves, chopped

8 cooking skewers

Directions

1 Cut the swordfish and salmon into 1-inch cubes.

2 Skewer a piece of zucchini, a cube of swordfish, red bell pepper, salmon, another slice of zucchini, a prawn, yellow bell pepper, calamari, another piece of red bell pepper, another swordfish, another slice of zucchini, and lastly another piece of yellow bell pepper. Repeat with all the skewers.

3 Use a pot large enough to lay all the skewers flat. Heat the pot at a high temperature and add the olive oil. After the oil is hot, add the herbs. Let the oil infuse with the herbs for a minute.

4 Add the skewers and let it cook for 2½ minutes each side.

5 Pour the white wine on top with the salt and pepper.

6 Cover with pan lid let it cook for 10–15 minutes at a low heat. Let it reduce until the sauce has almost disappeared and then serve.

Per serving: Calories: 356.6; Fat 17.7g (Saturated 2.9g); Cholesterol 101mg; Sodium 160mg; Carbohydrate 1.4g (Dietary Fiber 0g); Protein 45.1g.

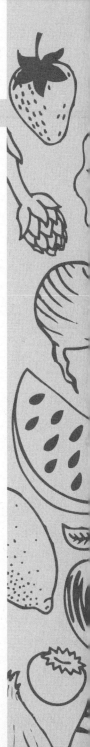

Luna Blu's Sicilian Salad

Prep time: 20 min • **Yield:** 6 servings

Ingredients	*Directions*
¾ **ounce of golden raisins**	**1** Put the golden raisins in a small bowl cover with warm water for 10 minutes.
2 fennel roots, sliced	
2 oranges	**2** Remove the outside leaves from the fennel root and slice thinly (with a mandolin slicer if possible). Place in a large bowl.
1¾ ounces of pine nuts	
1 teaspoon of pumpkin seeds	
1 handful of spinach	**3** Take one orange and squeeze the juice into a separate bowl.
5 tablespoons of extra virgin olive oil	**4** Peel the other orange and slice thinly cross sectionally. Put together with the fennel.
1 teaspoon of apple vinegar	
Salt and pepper to taste	**5** Squeeze the golden raisins and put together in the bowl with the other ingredients. Add the pumpkin seeds and the spinach; stir everything together.
	6 In a nonstick pan, toast the pine nuts until golden. Let them cool and then put them with the other ingredients.
	7 Take a bowl and put the orange juice, apple vinegar, olive oil, salt and pepper in it. Blend together with a hand blender until it becomes creamy dressing.
	8 Toss the ingredients together with the dressing and serve.

Per serving: Calories: 286; Fat 22.7g (Saturated 2.7g); Cholesterol 0mg; Sodium 42mg; Carbohydrate 20g (Dietary fiber 3.3g); Protein 3.3g.

Luna Blu's Tomato Soup

Prep time: 15 min • **Cook time:** 50 min • **Yield:** 4 servings

Ingredients	Directions
One can (28-ounce) of Roma tomatoes	**1** Slice the bread and put in oven 110°F. Bake for 5 minutes. Grate the garlic on top of the bread.
10 ounces of sliced Tuscan bread	**2** Place the tomatoes into boiling water for a minute.
One container (34-ounce) of vegetable stock	**3** Remove from water and peel skin from tomatoes. Pass through a vegetable mill and collect the juice.
1 bunch of fresh basil	
Ground black pepper and salt to taste	**4** Take the bread and put in a large nonstick frying pan, pour the tomato juice and the vegetable stock on top. Add sugar, salt, and pepper. Cook for 40–50 minutes on a low temperature to reduce the liquid, stirring occasionally until the bread dissolves into small pieces.
2 tablespoons extra virgin olive oil	
2 cloves of garlic	
1 teaspoon of sugar	
	5 Remove from heat and add the basil. Serve hot or serve chilled.

Per serving: Calories: 184: Fat 9g (Saturated 1.1g); Cholesterol 0mg; Sodium 566mg; Carbohydrate 25g (Dietary Fiber 2.1g); Protein 3.5g.

Tip: Mark the tomatoes lightly with a cross to aid peeling after.

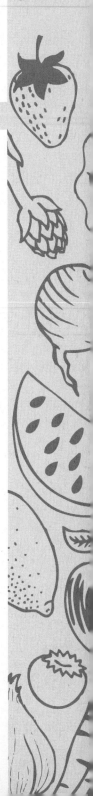

Paulette Mitchell's Beef and Broccoli Stir-Fry

Prep time: 15 min • **Cook time:** 10 min • **Yield:** 4 servings

Ingredients	Directions
Beef	
1 tablespoon soy sauce	**1** For the beef, stir together all the ingredients, except the beef, in a medium bowl. Add the beef and stir until the mixture is evenly combined.
1 tablespoon dark (Asian) sesame oil	
2 teaspoons finely chopped fresh ginger	**2** Stir together the sauce ingredients in a small bowl.
1 teaspoon cornstarch	**3** Heat 1 tablespoon of the oil in a large sauté pan over medium-high heat. Add the beef mixture. Cook, stirring constantly, for 3 minutes or until the beef is just cooked. Use a slotted spoon to transfer the beef to a bowl and cover to keep warm.
2 garlic cloves, minced	
8 ounces boneless beef sirloin, cut into 1/8-inch slices	

Sauce

¾ cup reduced-sodium beef broth

2 tablespoons Chinese oyster sauce

1 tablespoon soy sauce

¼ teaspoon red pepper flakes, or to taste

2 teaspoons cornstarch

2 tablespoons canola oil, divided

2 cups small broccoli florets

1 cup thinly sliced onion

½ red bell pepper, cut into ¼-inch strips

4 Heat the remaining 1 tablespoon oil in the pan. Add the broccoli, onion, and bell pepper; cook, stirring constantly, for 3 minutes or until the broccoli is crisp-tender.

5 Add the beef and sauce. Stir gently for 1 minute or until the sauce thickens.

Per serving: Calories 243; Fat 17g (Saturated 4g); Cholesterol 37mg; Sodium 634mg; Carbohydrate 8g; Dietary Fiber 2g; Protein 15g.

Tip: To speed up preparation, you can buy precut broccoli florets. Serve this colorful stir-fry over brown basmati rice that can cook on the stove as you prepare this dish.

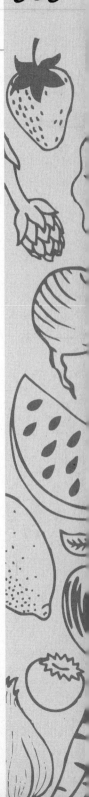

Paulette Mitchell's Cannellini Bean and Chicken Salad with Red-Wine Vinaigrette

Prep time: 20 min • **Cook time:** 0 min • **Yield:** 4 servings

Ingredients	*Directions*
Vinaigrette	
¼ cup red-wine vinegar	*1* Whisk together the vinaigrette ingredients, except the basil, in a medium bowl. Stir in the basil.
2 tablespoons extra-virgin olive oil	
1 tablespoon fresh lemon juice	*2* Add the salad ingredients and stir gently.
2 teaspoons Dijon mustard	
1 teaspoon minced garlic	
¼ teaspoon salt, or to taste	
¼ teaspoon pepper, or to taste	
¼ cup finely chopped fresh basil	
Salad	
2 cups coarsely chopped rotisserie chicken, skin removed, cooled	
One 15-ounce can cannellini beans, drained and rinsed	
1 tomato, coarsely chopped	
½ cup red onion, thinly sliced	

Per serving: Calories 253; Fat 13g (Saturated 3g); Cholesterol 50mg; Sodium 685mg; Carbohydrate 15g; Dietary Fiber 4g; Protein 20g.

Paulette Mitchell's Chunky Gazpacho

Prep time: 20 min plus chilling time • **Cook time:** 0 min • **Yield:** 4 servings

Ingredients	*Directions*
One can (15-ounce) tomato sauce	**1** Combine the tomato sauce, vinegar, oil, and honey in a medium bowl. Stir in the remaining ingredients.
2 tablespoons red-wine vinegar	
1 tablespoon extra-virgin olive oil	**2** To allow flavors to blend, refrigerate in a covered container for at least 2 hours, or until chilled.
1 tablespoon honey	
½ cucumber, seeded and coarsely chopped	
1 tomato, cut into ½-inch cubes	
½ green bell pepper, coarsely chopped	
1 rib celery, coarsely chopped	
2 tablespoons finely chopped red onion, or to taste	
1 teaspoon minced garlic, or to taste	
¼ teaspoon Tabasco sauce, or to taste	
¼ teaspoon pepper, or to taste	
Salt to taste	

Per serving: Calories 118; Fat 4g (Saturated 1g); Cholesterol 0mg; Sodium 495mg; Carbohydrate 23g; Dietary Fiber 4g; Protein 2g.

Tip: This gazpacho is best served in chilled bowls on a blistering-hot day, topped with whole-grain croutons.

Note: This soup will keep for up to five days in a covered container in the refrigerator. After storage, thin the soup with water or tomato juice to the desired consistency. You can spoon the thickened gazpacho over chilled grilled fish or chicken, or bring it to room temperature to serve over polenta or baked potatoes.

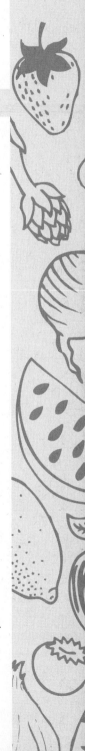

Paulette Mitchell's Fava Bean Salad with Manchego

Prep time: 10 min • **Yield:** 4 servings

Ingredients	Directions
Dressing	
3 tablespoons extra-virgin olive oil	**1** Whisk together the dressing ingredients In a medium bowl. Stir in the beans, bell pepper, and onion.
1 teaspoon lemon zest	
2 tablespoons fresh lemon juice	**2** To assemble each salad, arrange a layer of arugula leaves on a plate. Add a mound of the bean mixture. Top with two shaved slices of cheese.
2 tablespoons finely chopped fresh flat-leaf parsley	
½ teaspoon minced garlic	
Salt and pepper to taste	
Salad	
1 (19-ounce) can fava beans, drained and rinsed	
½ red bell pepper, finely chopped	
2 tablespoons finely chopped red onion	
2 cups arugula leaves	
8 very thin slices Manchego cheese	

Per serving: Calories: 235; Fat 13.7g (Saturated 3.2g); Cholesterol 6.8mg; Sodium 72mg; Carbohydrate 23.7g (Dietary Fiber 0g); Protein 12.2g.

Tip: Use a sharp vegetable peeler to shave very thin slices of firm cheeses.

Paulette Mitchell's Mediterranean Chicken with Penne

Prep time: 10 min • **Cook time:** 11 min • **Yield:** 4 servings

Ingredients	Directions
8 ounces penne	**1** Cook the penne, according to package instructions.
3 tablespoons olive oil, divided	**2** Meanwhile, heat 1 tablespoon olive oil in a large sauté pan over medium-high heat. Add the chicken, garlic, and a dash of salt and pepper; cook, stirring occasionally, for 5 minutes or until the chicken is lightly browned and thoroughly cooked. Transfer to a plate and cover to keep warm.
12 ounces chicken tenders, cut into 1-inch pieces	
1 teaspoon minced garlic	
Salt and pepper to taste	
2 small zucchini, cut into ¾-inch slices	**3** Heat 1 tablespoon olive oil in the skillet over medium-high heat. Add the zucchini; cook, stirring occasionally, for 2 minutes or until crisp-tender. Stir in the tomatoes spinach, chicken broth, and oregano. Reduce the heat to medium. Cover and cook for 3 minutes or until the zucchini is tender and the spinach is wilted. Add the chicken; stir gently for 1 minute or until warm. Season with additional salt and pepper.
2 plum tomatoes, cut into ¾-inch cubes	
1 cup packed coarsely shredded salad spinach	
¼ cup reduced-sodium chicken broth, dry red wine, or dry white wine	
1 tablespoon finely chopped fresh oregano	**4** When the penne is done, drain well and return to the pasta pan. Add the remaining 1 tablespoon olive oil and toss.
Freshly ground pepper and coarsely crumbled feta cheese for garnish	**5** To serve, spoon the penne into shallow pasta bowls. Top with the chicken-vegetable mixture and garnish with pepper and feta cheese.

Per serving: Calories: 206; Fat 4.6g (Saturated 0.5g); Cholesterol 48.8mg; Sodium 242mg; Carbohydrate 18.3g (Dietary Fiber 3.0g); Protein 22.9g.

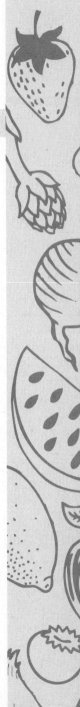

Paulette Mitchell's Mediterranean Seafood Stew

Prep time: 10 min • **Cook time:** 10 time • **Yield:** 4 servings

Ingredients	Directions
2 tablespoons olive oil	**1** Heat the oil in a Dutch oven over medium-high heat. Add the onion, carrot, and garlic; cook, stirring occasionally, for 4 minutes or until tender.
1 cup finely chopped onion	
1 carrot, peeled and finely chopped	
2 teaspoons minced garlic	**2** Meanwhile, mix the saffron with the hot water. Set aside.
¼ teaspoon saffron threads, crushed, or more to taste	
1 tablespoon hot water	**3** Pour the chicken broth and tomatoes into the Dutch oven. When the liquid comes to a boil, stir in the potatoes, red pepper flakes, and the saffron mixture. Reduce the heat to medium; cover and cook for 3 minutes or until the potatoes are nearly tender.
2 (14-ounce) cans reduced-sodium chicken broth	
1 (14-ounce) can diced tomatoes	
3 small red-skinned potatoes, peeled and cut into 1/2-inch cubes	**4** Stir in the fish; cook for 3 minutes. Stir in the scallops; continue to cook for 2 more minutes or until the potatoes are tender and the fish is thoroughly cooked.
1/8 teaspoon red pepper flakes, or to taste	
8 ounces firm white fish (such as sea bass, mackerel, or monk fish), remove and discard skin, cut flesh into 1-inch squares	**5** Garnish the servings with parsley.
8 ounces sea scallops	
Coarsely chopped fresh flat-leaf parsley for garnish	

Per serving: Calories: 266; Fat 59g (Saturated 0.9g); Cholesterol 81.7mg; Sodium 667.6mg; Carbohydrate 13.8g (Dietary Fiber 1.7g); Protein 34.6g.

Paulette Mitchell's Orange, Olive, and Arugula Salad

Prep time: 8 min • **Yield:** 4 servings

Ingredients	Directions
Vinaigrette	
¼ cup fresh orange juice	*1* Whisk together the vinaigrette ingredients in a medium bowl.
2 tablespoons hazelnut or walnut oil	
1 tablespoon honey	*2* Add the oranges and olives and toss.
Salt to taste	*3* To serve, arrange the arugula leaves on salad plates; top with the orange mixture. Garnish the servings with parsley.
Salad	
3 large oranges, peeled and thinly sliced	
12 black olives, pitted and coarsely chopped	
12 large arugula leaves	
Finely chopped flat-leaf parsley for garnish	

Per serving: Calories: 216; Fat 7g (Saturated 0.6g); Cholesterol 0mg; Sodium 48mg; Carbohydrate 35.3g (Dietary Fiber 3.8 g); Protein 1.3g.

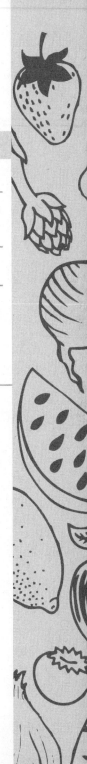

Paulette Mitchell's Spanish Garlic Shrimp with Sherry

Prep time: 10 min • **Cook time:** 3 min • **Yield:** 4 servings

Ingredients	Directions
2 tablespoons olive oil	*1* Heat the oil in a large sauté pan over medium heat. Add the onion and garlic; cook, stirring constantly for 15 seconds.
½ cup coarsely chopped onion	
6 cloves garlic, thinly sliced	
12 ounces medium (26 to 30 count) shrimp, peeled and deveined	*2* Add the shrimp, paprika, and cumin; cook, stirring constantly for 1 minute. Stir in the sherry, lemon juice, red pepper flakes, and salt. Continue to stir for 1 minute or until the shrimp turn pink.
½ teaspoon paprika or Spanish pimentón	
¼ teaspoon ground cumin	
⅓ cup dry sherry	*3* Transfer the shrimp and all juices to a serving dish or shallow bowls and garnish with parsley.
1 tablespoon fresh lemon juice	
¼ teaspoon red pepper flakes or to taste	
Salt to taste	
Finely chopped fresh flat-leaf parsley for garnish	

Per serving: Calories: 144; Fat 7.7g (Saturated 1.2g); Cholesterol 165.8mg; Sodium 190mg; Carbohydrate 0g (Dietary Fiber 0g); Protein 17.8g.

Index

● C ●

• F •

• S •

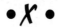

• X •

About the Author

Alan L. Rubin, MD, is one of the nation's foremost experts on diabetes. He is a professional member of the American Diabetes Association and the Endocrine Society and has been in private practice specializing in diabetes and thyroid disease for more than 35 years. Dr. Rubin was Assistant Clinical Professor of Medicine at the University of California Medical Center in San Francisco for 20 years. He has spoken about diabetes to professional medical audiences and nonmedical audiences around the world. He has been a consultant to many pharmaceutical companies and companies that make diabetes products.

Dr. Rubin was one of the first specialists in his field to recognize the significance of patient self-testing of blood glucose, the major advance in diabetes care since the advent of insulin. As a result, he has been on numerous radio and television programs, talking about the cause, the prevention, and the treatment of diabetes and its complications.

Since publishing *Diabetes For Dummies,* Dr. Rubin has had seven other bestselling *For Dummies* books — *Diabetes Cookbook For Dummies, Thyroid For Dummies, High Blood Pressure For Dummies, Type 1 Diabetes For Dummies, Prediabetes For Dummies, Vitamin D For Dummies,* and *Diabetes Meal Planning and Nutrition For Dummies* — all published by John Wiley & Sons, Inc. His eight books cover the medical problems of 150 million Americans.

Dedication

This book is dedicated to my wife, Enid. She has been the perfect helpmate, always there with a smile and encouragement. There is no question that she promotes all my books better than anyone else. She even listens to my recommendations. For this book she obtained all the new recipes and prepared them, resulting in many delicious evenings.

This edition is also dedicated to the thousands of people with diabetes who have written to thank me for helping them to understand what they are dealing with and for telling me where I need to provide more information and emphasis to make this an even better book.

Author's Acknowledgments

For this fourth edition, acquisitions editor Tracy Boggier deserves major thanks. I am also blessed with another great project manager, development editor, and copy editor Chad Sievers, who not only made sure that everything was readable and understandable, but also offered excellent suggestions to improve the information. My thanks also to Dr. Sandra Kammerman for reviewing the book for scientific accuracy.

Ronnie and Michael Goldfield should definitely be considered the godparents of this book.

My friends in the Dawn Patrol, a group of guys with whom I play squash and solve the problems of the world thereafter, kept me laughing throughout the production of this book. Their willingness to follow me convinced me that others would be willing to read what I wrote.

My teachers are too numerous to mention, but one group deserves special attention. They are my patients over the last 35 years, the people whose trials and tribulations caused me to seek the knowledge that you will find in this book.

This book is written on the shoulders of thousands of men and women who made the discoveries and held the committee meetings. Their accomplishments can't possibly be given adequate acclaim. We owe them big time.

Publisher's Acknowledgments

Acquisitions Editor: Tracy Boggier

Project Manager/Development Editor/Copy Editor: Chad R. Sievers

Technical Editor: Sandra Kammerman, MD

Art Coordinator: Alicia B. South

Production Editor: Kinson Raja

Illustrator: Kathryn Born

Recipe Tester: Emily Nolan

Nutritional Analyst: Patty Santelli

Cover Photos: ©iStock.com/ratmaner

Apple & Mac

iPad For Dummies,
5th Edition
978-1-118-72306-7

iPhone For Dummies,
7th Edition
978-1-118-69083-3

Macs All-in-One
For Dummies, 4th Edition
978-1-118-82210-4

OS X Mavericks
For Dummies
978-1-118-69188-5

Blogging & Social Media

Facebook For Dummies,
5th Edition
978-1-118-63312-0

Social Media Engagement
For Dummies
978-1-118-53019-1

WordPress For Dummies,
6th Edition
978-1-118-79161-5

Business

Stock Investing
For Dummies, 4th Edition
978-1-118-37678-2

Investing For Dummies,
6th Edition
978-0-470-90545-6

Personal Finance
For Dummies, 7th Edition
978-1-118-11785-9

QuickBooks 2014
For Dummies
978-1-118-72005-9

Small Business Marketing
Kit For Dummies,
3rd Edition
978-1-118-31183-7

Careers

Job Interviews
For Dummies, 4th Edition
978-1-118-11290-8

Job Searching with Social
Media For Dummies,
2nd Edition
978-1-118-67856-5

Personal Branding
For Dummies
978-1-118-11792-7

Resumes For Dummies,
6th Edition
978-0-470-87361-8

Starting an Etsy Business
For Dummies, 2nd Edition
978-1-118-59024-9

Diet & Nutrition

Belly Fat Diet For Dummies
978-1-118-34585-6

Mediterranean Diet
For Dummies
978-1-118-71525-3

Nutrition For Dummies,
5th Edition
978-0-470-93231-5

Digital Photography

Digital SLR Photography
All-in-One For Dummies,
2nd Edition
978-1-118-59082-9

Digital SLR Video &
Filmmaking For Dummies
978-1-118-36598-4

Photoshop Elements 12
For Dummies
978-1-118-72714-0

Gardening

Herb Gardening
For Dummies, 2nd Edition
978-0-470-61778-6

Gardening with Free-Range
Chickens For Dummies
978-1-118-54754-0

Health

Boosting Your Immunity
For Dummies
978-1-118-40200-9

Diabetes For Dummies,
4th Edition
978-1-118-29447-5

Living Paleo For Dummies
978-1-118-29405-5

Big Data

Big Data For Dummies
978-1-118-50422-2

Data Visualization
For Dummies
978-1-118-50289-1

Hadoop For Dummies
978-1-118-60755-8

Language & Foreign Language

500 Spanish Verbs
For Dummies
978-1-118-02382-2

English Grammar
For Dummies, 2nd Edition
978-0-470-54664-2

French All-in-One
For Dummies
978-1-118-22815-9

German Essentials
For Dummies
978-1-118-18422-6

Italian For Dummies,
2nd Edition
978-1-118-00465-4

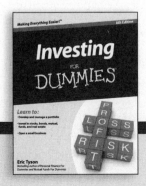 **Available in print and e-book formats.**

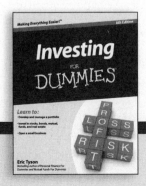
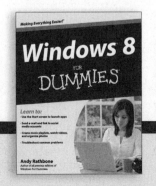
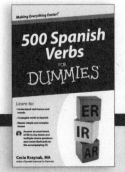
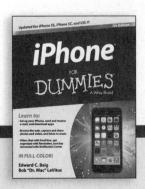

Available wherever books are sold. **For more information or to order direct visit www.dummies.com**

Math & Science

Algebra I For Dummies,
2nd Edition
978-0-470-55964-2

Anatomy and Physiology
For Dummies, 2nd Edition
978-0-470-92326-9

Astronomy For Dummies,
3rd Edition
978-1-118-37697-3

Biology For Dummies,
2nd Edition
978-0-470-59875-7

Chemistry For Dummies,
2nd Edition
978-1-118-00730-3

1001 Algebra II Practice
Problems For Dummies
978-1-118-44662-1

Microsoft Office

Excel 2013 For Dummies
978-1-118-51012-4

Office 2013 All-in-One
For Dummies
978-1-118-51636-2

PowerPoint 2013
For Dummies
978-1-118-50253-2

Word 2013 For Dummies
978-1-118-49123-2

Music

Blues Harmonica
For Dummies
978-1-118-25269-7

Guitar For Dummies,
3rd Edition
978-1-118-11554-1

iPod & iTunes
For Dummies, 10th Edition
978-1-118-50864-0

Programming

Beginning Programming
with C For Dummies
978-1-118-73763-7

Excel VBA Programming
For Dummies, 3rd Edition
978-1-118-49037-2

Java For Dummies,
6th Edition
978-1-118-40780-6

Religion & Inspiration

The Bible For Dummies
978-0-7645-5296-0

Buddhism For Dummies,
2nd Edition
978-1-118-02379-2

Catholicism For Dummies,
2nd Edition
978-1-118-07778-8

Self-Help & Relationships

Beating Sugar Addiction
For Dummies
978-1-118-54645-1

Meditation For Dummies,
3rd Edition
978-1-118-29144-3

Seniors

Laptops For Seniors
For Dummies, 3rd Edition
978-1-118-71105-7

Computers For Seniors
For Dummies, 3rd Edition
978-1-118-11553-4

iPad For Seniors
For Dummies, 6th Edition
978-1-118-72826-0

Social Security
For Dummies
978-1-118-20573-0

Smartphones & Tablets

Android Phones
For Dummies, 2nd Edition
978-1-118-72030-1

Nexus Tablets
For Dummies
978-1-118-77243-0

Samsung Galaxy S 4
For Dummies
978-1-118-64222-1

Samsung Galaxy Tabs
For Dummies
978-1-118-77294-2

Test Prep

ACT For Dummies,
5th Edition
978-1-118-01259-8

ASVAB For Dummies,
3rd Edition
978-0-470-63760-9

GRE For Dummies,
7th Edition
978-0-470-88921-3

Officer Candidate Tests
For Dummies
978-0-470-59876-4

Physician's Assistant Exam
For Dummies
978-1-118-11556-5

Series 7 Exam For Dummies
978-0-470-09932-2

Windows 8

Windows 8.1 All-in-One
For Dummies
978-1-118-82087-2

Windows 8.1 For Dummies
978-1-118-82121-3

Windows 8.1 For Dummies,
Book + DVD Bundle
978-1-118-82107-7

Available in print and e-book formats.

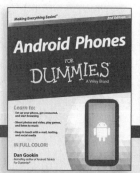
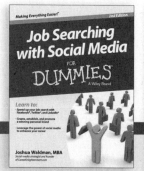
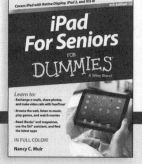
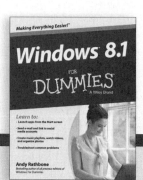

Available wherever books are sold. **For more information or to order direct visit www.dummies.com**

Take Dummies with you everywhere you go!

Whether you are excited about e-books, want more from the web, must have your mobile apps, or are swept up in social media, Dummies makes everything easier.

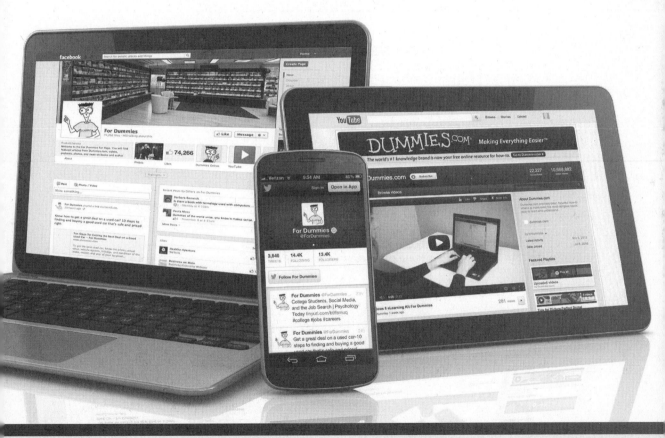

 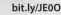

Leverage the Power

For Dummies is the global leader in the reference category and one of the most trusted and highly regarded brands in the world. No longer just focused on books, customers now have access to the For Dummies content they need in the format they want. Let us help you develop a solution that will fit your brand and help you connect with your customers.

Advertising & Sponsorships

Connect with an engaged audience on a powerful multimedia site, and position your message alongside expert how-to content.

Targeted ads • Video • Email marketing • Microsites • Sweepstakes sponsorship

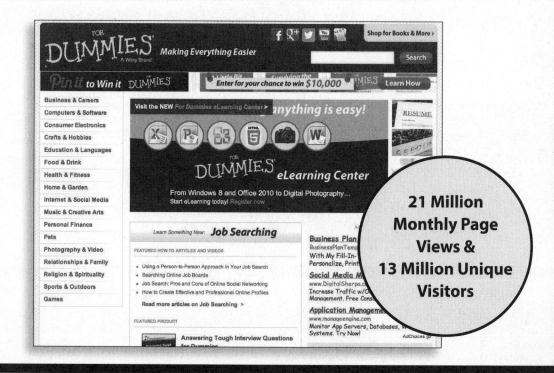

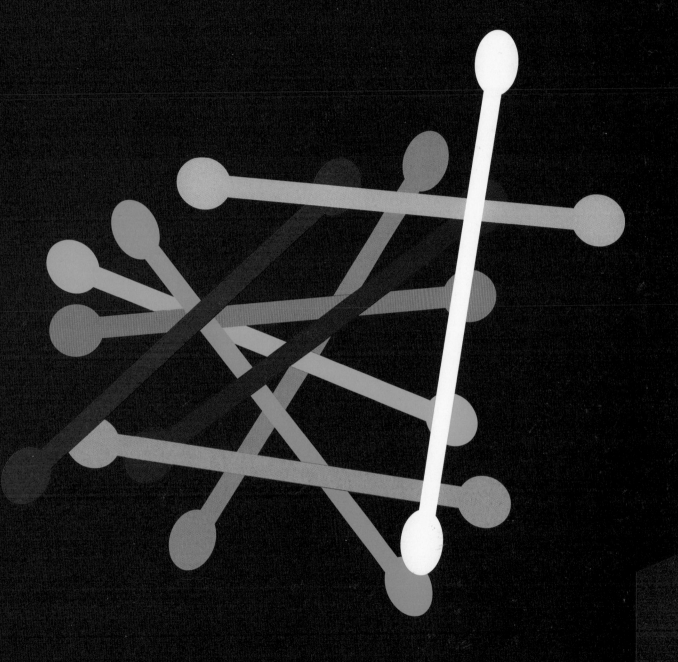

Thinking about PlayThinks

Japanese Temple

The inspiration for PlayThinks came from *sangaku,* the Japanese temple geometry that flourished in the seventeenth, eighteenth and nineteenth centuries. In those times *sangaku* (the Japanese word for mathematical tablet) was a national pastime enjoyed by everyone from peasants to samurai nobility. People would solve geometrical proofs and puzzles, then offer the solutions to the spirits in the form of elegantly designed and executed wooden tablets. Those tablets, engraved with geometrical problems, hung under the roofs of shrines and temples. Indeed, the best *sangaku* tablets were works of art that paid homage to the spirits that guided one to the answer.

Today only a few devotees remember *sangaku.* In 1989 Hidetoshi Fukagawa and Daniel Pedoe published the first collection of *sangaku* to be translated into English; that book was later publicized in a *Scientific American* article. But more than 880 *sangaku* tablets survive. The problems typically involved geometrical constructions, often circles within circles, triangles or ellipses. The level of difficulty ranged from quite simple to impossible, though all would be considered recreational mathematics by contemporary standards. The proofs of the problems or theorems were usually not provided, just the results.

During that period, many ordinary Japanese people loved and enjoyed mathematics, and were carried away by the beauty of geometry. The authors of *sangaku* were probably teachers and their students. The tablets were crafted with loving care and were intended to be visual teaching aids for mathematicians and nonmathematicians alike.

And that defines perfectly what a PlayThink is.

I've always been fascinated by all types of puzzles and games for the mind, but the ones I like best

> "**I**MAGINATION **I**S MORE IMPORTANT THAN KNOWLEDGE."
> —ALBERT EINSTEIN

are not always the hardest. Sometimes a puzzle that is quite easy to solve is elegant or meaningful enough to make it especially satisfying. Solving puzzles has as much to do with the way you think about them as with natural ability or some impersonal measure of intelligence. Most people should be able to understand all the problems in this book, although some problems will undoubtedly seem easier than others. Thinking is what they are all about: comprehension is at least as important as visual perception or mathematical knowledge. After all, our different ways of thinking set us apart as individuals and make each of us unique.

PLAYTHINK
1

DIFFICULTY: ●●●●●●○○○○
REQUIRED: ◉ ✎
COMPLETION: ☐   TIME: _____

HALVING SEVEN

Can you prove that seven is half of twelve?

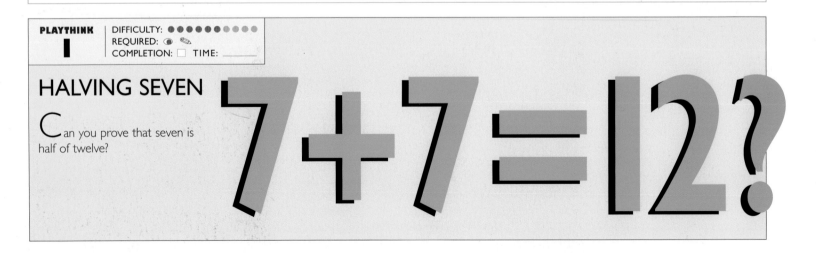

PLAYTHINK 2

DIFFICULTY: ●●●●●●●○○○
REQUIRED: ◉ ✎
COMPLETION: ☐ TIME: _____

A SANGAKU PROBLEM FROM 1803

Upon the diameter of the large green circle, place two shapes: an isosceles triangle and a smaller red circle. Position the triangle so that its base lies upon the diameter of the large circle. And position the smaller circle so that its diameter runs along the diameter of the large circle from the base of the triangle to the circumference of the large circle. Now add a third circle, inscribed so that it touches the other two circles and the triangle. If you draw a line from the center of the third circle to the point where the red circle and the triangle meet, can you prove that that line is in fact perpendicular to the diameter of the large green circle?

PLAYTHINK 3

DIFFICULTY: ●●○○○○○○○○
REQUIRED: ◉
COMPLETION: ☐ TIME: _____

AHMES'S PUZZLE

Seven houses each have seven cats. Each cat kills seven mice. Each of the mice, if alive, would have eaten seven ears of wheat. Each ear of wheat produces seven measures of flour.

How many measures of flour were saved by the cats?

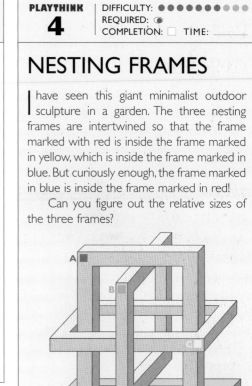

PLAYTHINK 4

DIFFICULTY: ●●●●●●○○○○
REQUIRED: ◉
COMPLETION: ☐ TIME: _____

NESTING FRAMES

I have seen this giant minimalist outdoor sculpture in a garden. The three nesting frames are intertwined so that the frame marked with red is inside the frame marked in yellow, which is inside the frame marked in blue. But curiously enough, the frame marked in blue is inside the frame marked in red!

Can you figure out the relative sizes of the three frames?

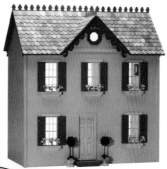

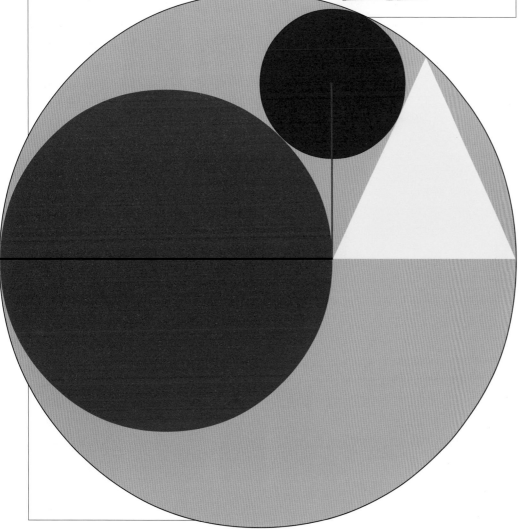

PLAYTHINK 5

DIFFICULTY: ●●●●○○○○○○
REQUIRED: ◉
COMPLETION: ☐ TIME: _____

FLAP DOOR

Study for a moment the drawing of the flap door. Now cover it and look at the drawings at the bottom. From memory can you choose the correct shape of the door?

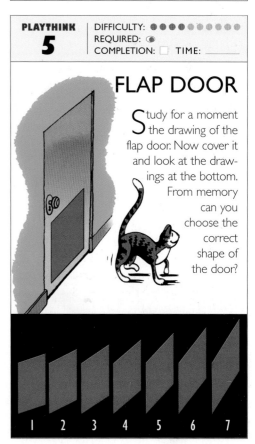

1 2 3 4 5 6 7

PLAYTHINK 6

DIFFICULTY: ●●●●○○○○○○
REQUIRED: ◉
COMPLETION: ☐ TIME: _____

CHICKEN OR EGG?

Can you answer the ancient question: Which came first, the chicken or the egg?

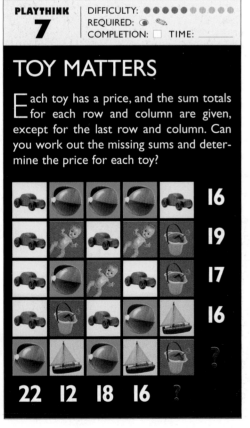

PLAYTHINK 7

DIFFICULTY: ●●●●●○○○○○
REQUIRED: ◉ ✎
COMPLETION: ☐ TIME: _____

TOY MATTERS

Each toy has a price, and the sum totals for each row and column are given, except for the last row and column. Can you work out the missing sums and determine the price for each toy?

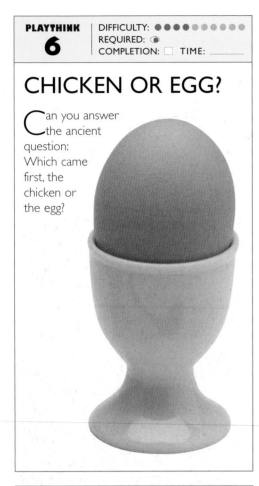

PLAYTHINK 8

DIFFICULTY: ●●●●●●●○○○
REQUIRED: ✎
COMPLETION: ☐ TIME: _____

CONSECUTIVE RECTANGLE SQUARES

This interesting question crops up in recreational mathematics literature: Using each of the first consecutive integers (1, 2, 3, 4, 5, 6, 7, 8, 9, 10) once each to create the dimensions of five rectangles, how many combinations of those five rectangles can be assembled into a square? In each of these four cases, place the colored rectangles at right on the grid at left.

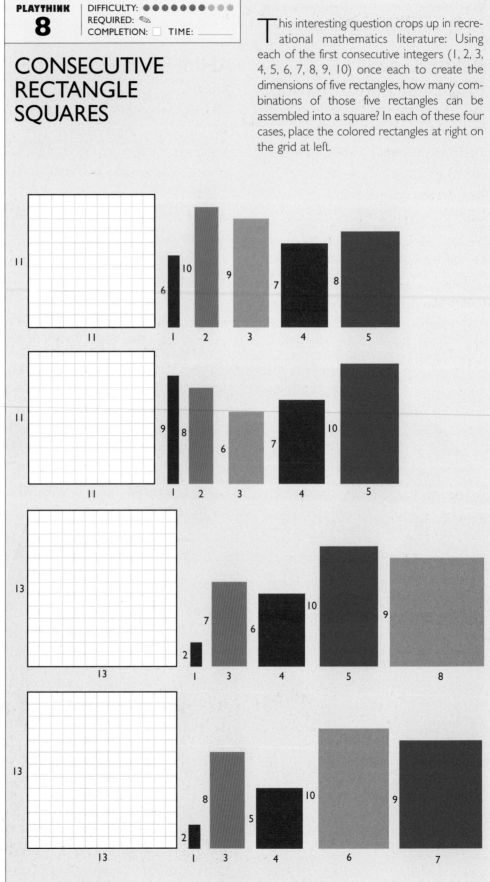

The Beauty of Patterns

For the ancient Greeks, mathematics was the science of numbers. But this definition of mathematics has been invalid for hundreds of years. In the middle of the seventeenth century, Isaac Newton in England and Gottfried von Leibniz in Germany independently invented calculus, the study of motion and change, and touched off an explosion in mathematical activity. Contemporary mathematics comprises eighty distinct disciplines, some of which are still being split into subcategories. So today, rather than focus on numbers, many mathematicians think their field is better defined as the science of patterns.

A love affair with patterns is something that starts very early in our lives. And those patterns may take many forms—numerical, geometric, kinetic, behavioral and so on. As the science of patterns, mathematics affects every aspect of our lives; abstract patterns are the basis of thinking, of communication, of computation, of society and even of life itself.

Patterns are everywhere and everyone sees them, but mathematicians see patterns within the patterns. Yet, despite the somewhat imposing language used to describe their work, the goal of most mathematicians is to find the simplest explanations for the most complex patterns.

Part of the magic of mathematics is how a simple, amusing problem can lead to far-ranging insights. Look at PlayThink 54 ("Handshakes 2"). Figure it out? Then imagine that the people are points on a graph, and that their handshakes represent interconnecting lines. Thought of this way, the problem can lead you to picture a graph in which every point is interconnected with all the others—a useful image for, say, airline flight coordinators.

Realizing the importance of this kind of thinking, many schools are mixing more geometry, topology and probability into the math curriculum. This is all to the good: Wherever there is relationship and pattern, there is mathematics.

> "THERE IS AN OLD DEBATE ABOUT WHETHER YOU CREATE MATHEMATICS OR JUST DISCOVER IT. IN OTHER WORDS, ARE THE TRUTHS ALREADY THERE, EVEN IF WE DON'T YET KNOW THEM? IF YOU BELIEVE IN GOD, THE ANSWER IS OBVIOUS."
>
> —PAUL ERDÖS

PLAYTHINK **9**	DIFFICULTY: ●●●●●●●●●●
	REQUIRED: ◉
	COMPLETION: ☐ TIME: _____

SAD CLOWN

Can you find the clown with a frown?

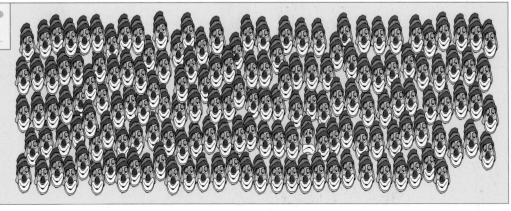

PLAYTHINK
10
DIFFICULTY: ●●●●●○○○○○○
REQUIRED: ◉
COMPLETION: ☐ TIME: _____

PICK-UP STICKS I

This puzzle works just like the familiar children's game. Remove one stick at a time from the pile, making sure that no other stick lies on top of it. To clear the entire pile, what color sequence must be chosen?

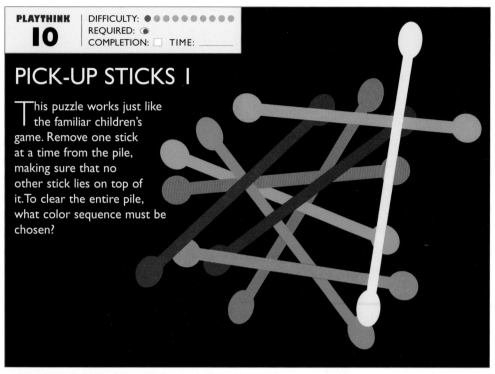

PLAYTHINK
11
DIFFICULTY: ●●●●●○○○○○○
REQUIRED: ◉ ✎
COMPLETION: ☐ TIME: _____

MATCH SQUARES

Twenty-four matchsticks can be arranged to create the pattern illustrated below. Can you remove eight matchsticks from the configuration so that you are left with two squares that do not touch each other?

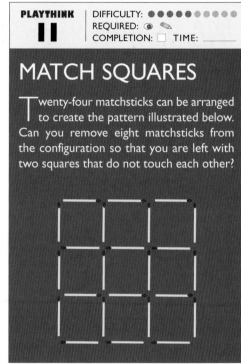

PLAYTHINK
12
DIFFICULTY: ●●●●●●○○○○○
REQUIRED: ✎
COMPLETION: ☐ TIME: _____

ARROW NUMBER BOXES

The object of this sort of puzzle is to place arrows in the boxes according to the following rules: The arrows must point in one of the eight main compass directions (north, south, east, west, northeast, southeast, northwest, and southwest); the number of arrows pointing to each number in the outer boxes must equal the value of that number; and each box must have an arrow in it. The sample shown (upper right) is a flawed attempt at a solution, since no arrow can be placed on the blank square within the rules of the game, and one of the outer squares has no arrow pointing at it.

Can you find complete solutions for the arrow number boxes of order 4 (upper left), order 5 (lower left), and order 6 (lower right)?

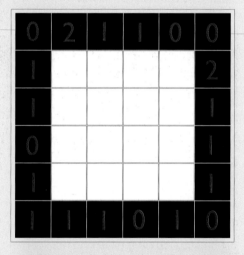

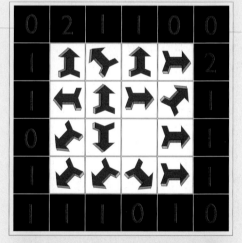

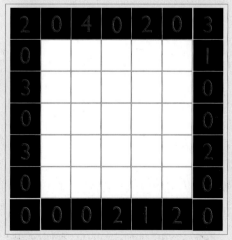

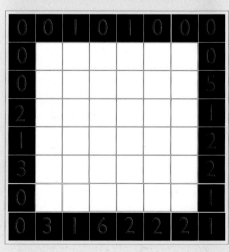

Thinking as a Skill

We constantly use intuition in our everyday life. Yet until recently the scientific study of intuition was largely ignored. New research has found that intuition springs from a set of important human skills that all act together to give a so-called gut reaction. The more you use these skills, the better your intuition becomes.

PlayThinks includes problems that will sharpen your ability to recognize and perceive patterns, to stretch your imagination, to make the most of trial and error. And as you do these problems, you will improve your creativity, insight and intuition.

Thinking is a learnable skill, like cooking or golf. If you make even a small effort to develop it, you will see improvement. As Nob Yoshigahara, the editor of the famous *Puzzletopia Newsletter,* once said: "What jogging is to the body, thinking is to the brain. The more we do it, the better we become."

PLAYTHINK 13 | DIFFICULTY: ●●●●●●●○○○
REQUIRED: ◉
COMPLETION: ☐ TIME: _____

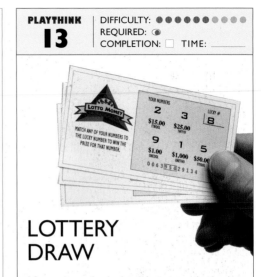

LOTTERY DRAW

If you draw the lucky ticket, you win the lottery jackpot. You are given the option to draw one ticket out of a box of 10, or draw ten times out of a box of 100. Which choice gives you the best odds?

PLAYTHINK 14 | DIFFICULTY: ●●●●●●○○○○
REQUIRED: ◉ ✎
COMPLETION: ☐ TIME: _____

PATTERN 15

Five different whole numbers add up to 15.

Multiply those same five numbers together, and the result is 120.

Can you determine what those five numbers are?

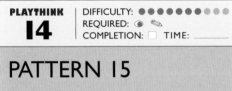

$$\blacksquare + \blacksquare + \blacksquare + \blacksquare + \blacksquare = 15$$
$$\blacksquare \times \blacksquare \times \blacksquare \times \blacksquare \times \blacksquare = 120$$

PLAYTHINK 15 | DIFFICULTY: ●●●●●●●●○○
REQUIRED: ◉ ✎
COMPLETION: ☐ TIME: _____

PATTERN 30

Five different single-digit whole numbers add up to 30. Two of them are given as 1 and 8.

Multiply those same five numbers together, and the result is 2,520.

Can you determine what the other three numbers are?

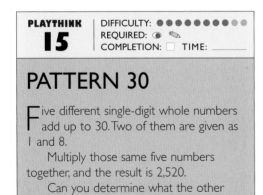

$$\blacksquare + \blacksquare + \blacksquare + 1 + 8 = 30$$
$$\blacksquare \times \blacksquare \times \blacksquare \times 1 \times 8 = 2,520$$

PLAYTHINK 16 | DIFFICULTY: ●●●●●●●○○○
REQUIRED: ◉ ▤ ✂
COMPLETION: ☐ TIME: _____

HORSE AND RIDER

With only your powers of mental manipulation, can you figure out how to position the strip with the cowboys onto the square with the horses so that it looks as if the cowboys were riding the horses? This problem (based on the classic Trick Donkeys puzzle created by Sam Loyd) looks deceptively simple, but one soon realizes that the obvious answer is wrong. If you can't solve this in your mind, try copying and cutting out the strip to experiment with paper. Hint: The solution makes the horses look much faster.

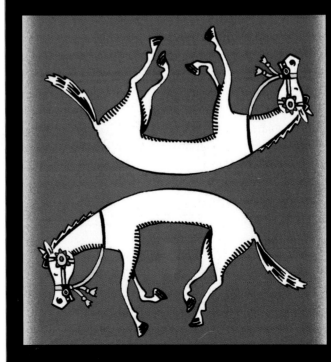

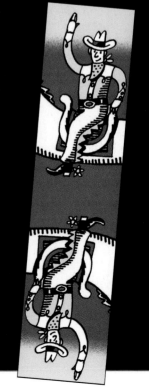

PLAYTHINK
17

DIFFICULTY: ●●●●●○○○○○
REQUIRED: ◉
COMPLETION: ☐ TIME: _____

IMPOSSIBLE DOMINO BRIDGE

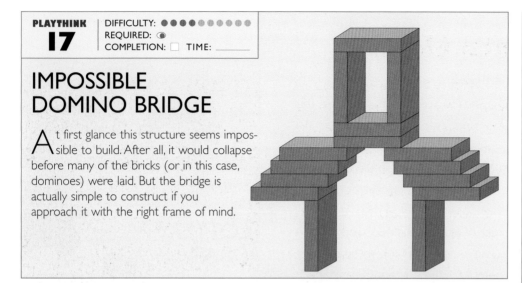

At first glance this structure seems impossible to build. After all, it would collapse before many of the bricks (or in this case, dominoes) were laid. But the bridge is actually simple to construct if you approach it with the right frame of mind.

PLAYTHINK
18

DIFFICULTY: ●●●●●●○○○○
REQUIRED: ◉ ✎
COMPLETION: ☐ TIME: _____

GLOVES IN THE DARK

There are twenty-two gloves in a drawer: five pairs of red gloves, four pairs of yellow and two pairs of green. If the lights are out and you must select the gloves in the dark, how many must you choose to ensure that you have at least one matching pair?

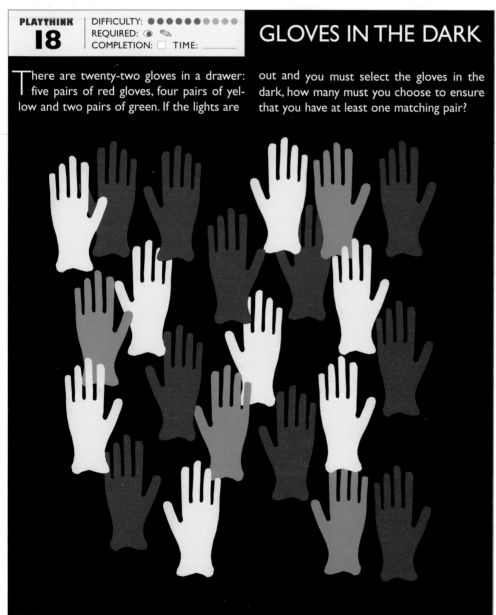

PLAYTHINK
19

DIFFICULTY: ●●●●●●●●○○
REQUIRED: ✎
COMPLETION: ☐ TIME: _____

OVERLAPPING SQUARES 2

Can you fit the six squares into the big gray square to create a pattern of eighteen squares of four different sizes formed by their outlines? The white grid lines are provided only to help in the alignment of the overlapping squares.

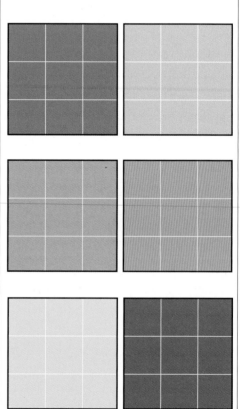

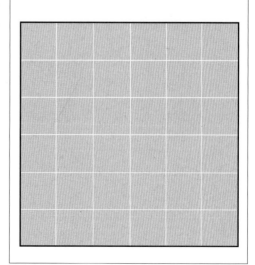

Getting Around Mental Blocks

Your brain works much better than you might think. It is capable of making a virtually unlimited number of synaptic connections, each of which is a pattern of thought. (The number of possible connections has been calculated, but the result is so large—1 followed by 60 million miles of typewritten zeros—it might as well be infinity.)

In spite of the vast number of possible thoughts to think, thinking can be hard work, and there is a natural human tendency to do as little of it as possible. This tendency is seen in the hit-and-run approach many people take to problem solving: they pick the first solution that comes to mind and run with it. Such an approach generally fails to take into account the full range of possible solutions. People can become trapped in their own preconceptions, not so much neglecting information that might solve the problem as simply not perceiving it.

Problem solving works best with the fewest self-imposed blinders. The greater the choice of creative concepts, the better chance there is to find an answer. If your first idea fails to solve the problem, try another. It is important to avoid the mental walls known as conceptual blocks, which can shield us from even the simplest and most obvious answer. Sometimes the conceptual block is of one's own creation, while others stem from incomplete information, emphasis on the wrong detail or deliberately misleading directions. Inventors of puzzles and magic tricks exploit such conceptual blocks to lead suggestible minds up blind alleys. But in spite of the universal tendency to suffer from blocks, most people at one time or another can tackle a problem of bewildering complexity, penetrate to its core and extract an insight of startling simplicity and elegance that solves the problem at a stroke.

> "IT ISN'T THAT THEY CAN'T SEE THE SOLUTION. IT IS THAT THEY CAN'T SEE THE PROBLEM."
> —G. K. CHESTERTON

The best puzzles are seldom what they seem. The solutions may demand that a common item be used in an unfamiliar way or that a conventional assumption be abandoned or that components be assembled in an unusual arrangement. The direct, head-on approach often leads nowhere, while a lengthy detour can sometimes be the fastest route to a solution. When you are faced with a mental wall, the best approach is not to tunnel through it but to walk around.

PLAYTHINK 20

DIFFICULTY: ●●●●●○○○○○
REQUIRED: ◉ 📄 ✂
COMPLETION: ☐ TIME: _____

T-PUZZLE

In this classic puzzle the four red pieces can be placed together to form a perfect capital T. Can you visualize how they fit together?

Copy and cut out the pieces to experiment with different possible solutions before you look at the answer in the back.

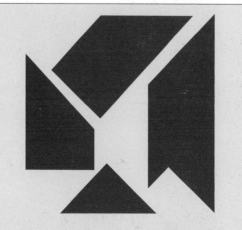
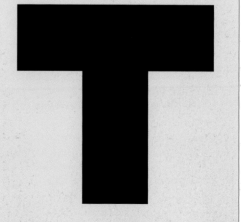

PLAYTHINK
21
DIFFICULTY: ●●●●●●●●○○
REQUIRED: ✏ 📄 ✂
COMPLETION: ☐   TIME: _____

RALLY

Conventional sliding-block or sliding-disk puzzles have an empty space into which the pieces can move. Knowing how to move pieces into the space is usually the key to solving such puzzles. Rally is a sliding-disk puzzle with no empty spaces. The thirty-two disks move like a chain through two elliptical channels, one vertical and one horizontal. Each chain is composed of eighteen disks, and there are four disks common to both chains. Moving one disk in the chain moves all the other disks in its channel; by switching the movement from one channel to another, disks can be transferred from one chain to another.

There are twelve red disks, twelve blue disks and eight yellow disks. Initially, the red disks form a square in the middle of the puzzle. How many moves will it take you to transform the red square in the middle to a blue square?

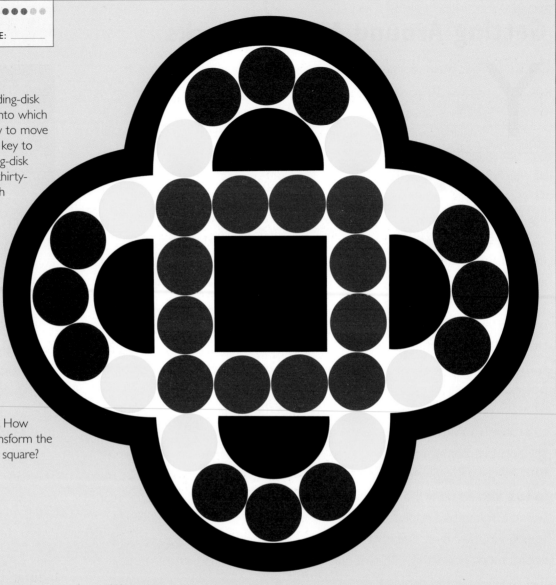

PLAYTHINK
22
DIFFICULTY: ●●●●●●●○○○
REQUIRED: ◉ ✏
COMPLETION: ☐   TIME: _____

ALIEN ABDUCTION

Four UFOs hover above a man they plan to abduct. To catch the man, the four aliens must create a rectangular energy field around him. Each alien fires a laser randomly, either to the left of the man or to his right. Out of all the possible random combinations of the four laser shots, what is the probability that each will form a side of a rectangle around the man? (In the example shown, all rays are directed to the right of the man.)

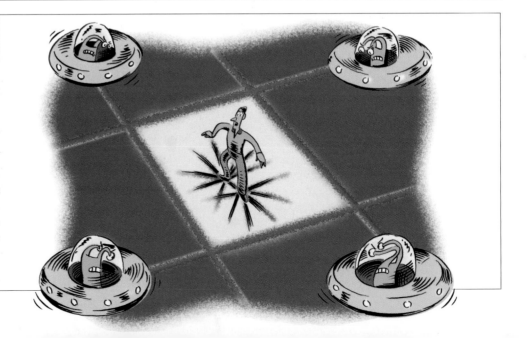

PLAYTHINK 23

DIFFICULTY: ●●●●●●●○○○
REQUIRED: ◉ ✎
COMPLETION: ☐ TIME: _____

INVENTOR PARADOX

Three friends talked about Ivan, but only one of them knew the truth.

"Ivan has invented hundreds of toys," Gerry said.

"No, he hasn't," George said. "He has invented fewer than that."

"Well, he has invented at least one toy," Anitta said.

If only one of those statements is true, can you figure out how many toys Ivan has invented?

Also, Ivan is pictured on this page. Can you find him?

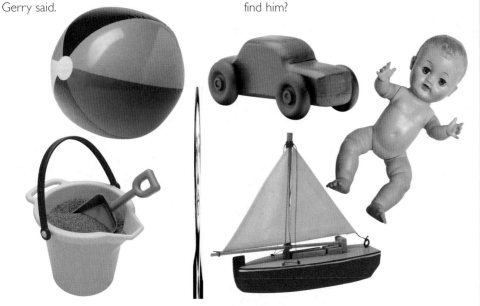

PLAYTHINK 24

DIFFICULTY: ●●●●●●●●○○
REQUIRED: ◉
COMPLETION: ☐ TIME: _____

TREASURE ISLAND

To confuse his enemies, the pirate who made this map made only one of the statements false. Can you still figure out where the treasure is buried?

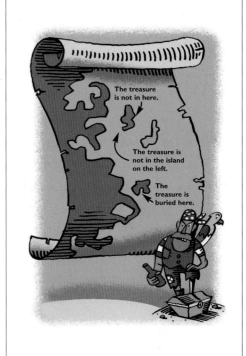

The treasure is not in here.

The treasure is not in the island on the left.

The treasure is buried here.

PLAYTHINK 25

DIFFICULTY: ●●●●●●○○○○
REQUIRED: ◉ ✎
COMPLETION: ☐ TIME: _____

CIRCUS RIDERS

Each of the horses is a different color. How many different ways can the seven horses be arranged to circle the circus area?

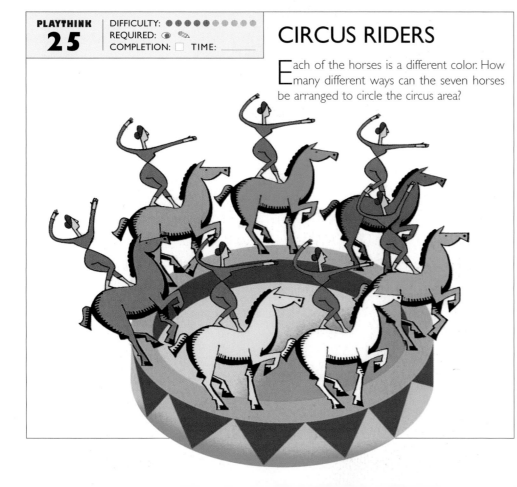

> "THE SIMPLEST SCHOOLBOY IS NOW FAMILIAR WITH FACTS FOR WHICH ARCHIMEDES WOULD HAVE SACRIFICED HIS LIFE."
>
> —ERNEST RENAN

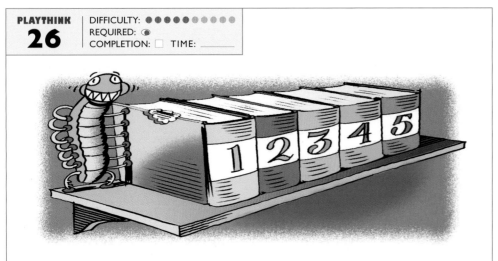

BOOKWORM

A bookworm finds itself on page 1 of volume 1 and begins eating straight through to the last page of volume 5. If each book is 6 centimeters thick, including the front and back covers, which are half a centimeter each, what is the distance the bookworm travels?

HALLOWEEN MASK

You have five different colors of paint. How many different ways can you paint the Halloween mask if you make the eyes, nose and mouth each a different color?

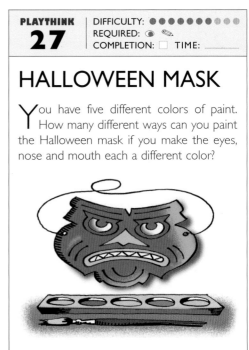

BINARY TRANSFORMATIONS

This puzzle involves swapping pairs of rows or pairs of columns or flipping one row or column end to end to transform one pattern to another. A move constitutes one exchange of rows or columns or a reorientation (flipping) of a single row or column.

From the initial patterns on the left, create the patterns on the right. How many moves will it take?

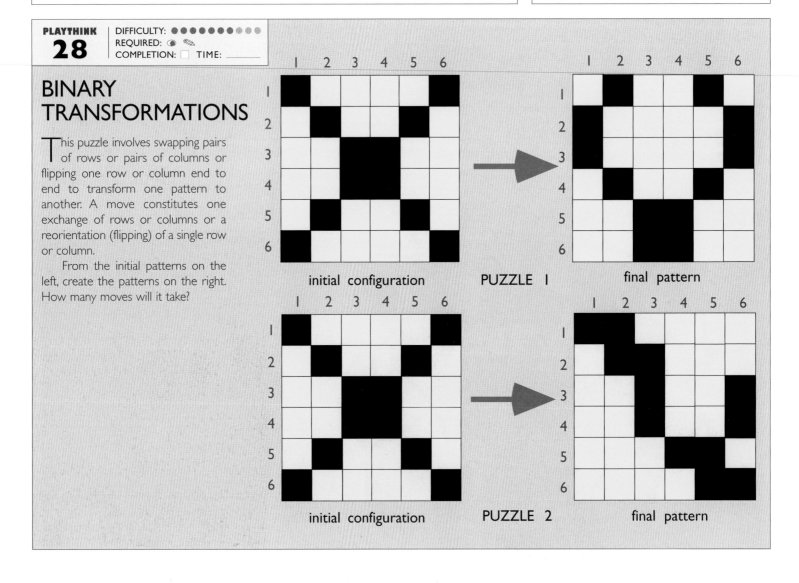

initial configuration   PUZZLE 1   final pattern

initial configuration   PUZZLE 2   final pattern

PLAYTHINK
29
DIFFICULTY: ●●●●●●●○○○
REQUIRED: ✎
COMPLETION: ☐ TIME: _____

JUMPING PEGS PUZZLE

Can you jump from point to point across the board to connect the matching numbers along the edge? Only jumps that are equal to the segments shown below are valid. To illustrate the concept, the series of jumps connecting the two points marked 5 are shown above.

The three allowable lengths:

_____

_____

_____

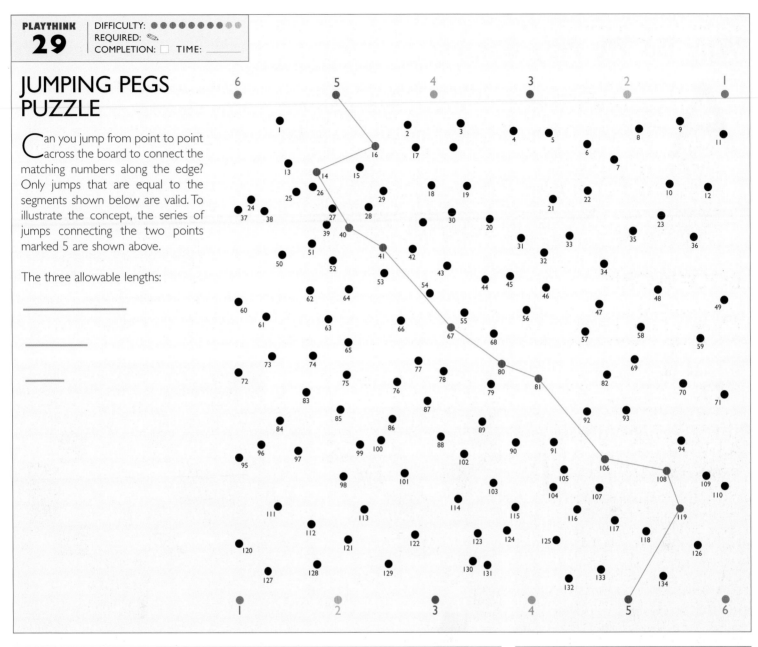

PLAYTHINK
30
DIFFICULTY: ●●●●●●●○○○
REQUIRED: ◉ ✎
COMPLETION: ☐ TIME: _____

THREE-COIN FLIP

You ask a friend about probability, and he tells you the following: "The odds of three tossed coins turning up all heads or all tails is one in two, that is, fifty-fifty. That's because anytime you toss three coins, at least two must match, either two heads or two tails. So that means the third coin— which is equally likely to be heads or tails— determines the odds."

Is your friend right? If not, what are the odds of three tossed coins turning up all heads or all tails?

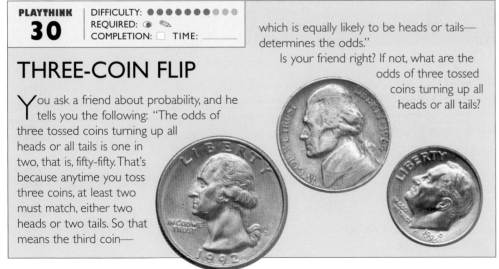

PLAYTHINK
31
DIFFICULTY: ●●○○○○○○○○
REQUIRED: ◉
COMPLETION: ☐ TIME: _____

SCRAMBLED MATCHSTICKS

It takes just a couple of little twists to turn these matchsticks into a message. Can you find the word?

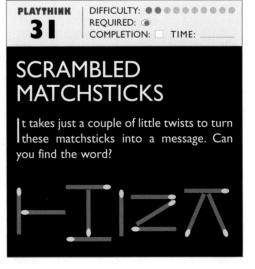

Why Do We Play Games?

As living, intelligent organisms, we humans possess curiosity about our environment, about one another, about ourselves—and putting that curiosity to use through an exploration of the unknown energizes us. No one knows why really, but we can feel that it's true. Likewise, playing games that engage our curiosity makes us feel more alive. Again, we don't really know why, but I think it has a lot to do with the risk of losing.

I believe that each person seeks out stimuli just slightly more complex than his or her preferred level of stimulation. What could be a better way to find stimulating uncertainties than in a game in which the outcome is never known? But games do much more than provide stimulation, ego satisfaction and fun. They help the mind develop by teaching cooperation and competition, exploration and invention. They encourage us to devise strategies for victory and, ultimately, for loss. Indeed, games duplicate, in model form, almost every human condition, aspiration and social structure. How else to explain that gaming has become one of our most potent metaphors: the money game, the marketing game, the survival game, the dating game? The meaning is always clear: games require players who want to win and know they may not.

PLAYTHINK 32
DIFFICULTY: ●●●●●○○○○○
REQUIRED: ◉
COMPLETION: ☐   TIME: _____

INTERSTELLAR GREETING

Can you decipher this simple message?

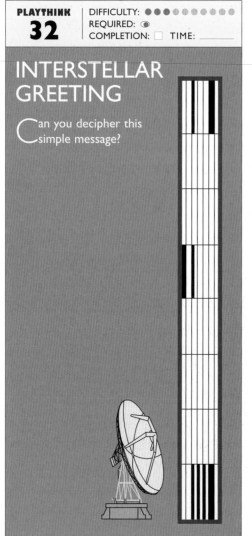

PLAYTHINK 33
DIFFICULTY: ●●●●●●○○○○
REQUIRED: ◉
COMPLETION: ☐   TIME: _____

INTERSTELLAR MESSAGE 1

Astronomers have sent messages like this one into outer space in order to establish communication with intelligent life on other planets. Researchers hope that even if such alien life forms cannot understand our written or spoken languages or make sense of images of our culture, they might use radio for communication and be adept at mathematics. For that reason messages have been sent that incorporate binary codes and simple mathematical principles.

Can you decipher the message shown below?

PLAYTHINK 34
DIFFICULTY: ●●●●●●○○○○
REQUIRED: ◉
COMPLETION: ☐   TIME: _____

INTERSTELLAR MESSAGE 2

Let's say the alien beings received the previous message and answered back with this series of dots and geometric figures. Can you work out the meaning of the message?

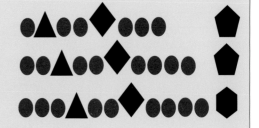

Communicating with Numbers

The most important thing a person inherits is the ability to learn a language. Language—especially written language—makes connection possible between people living in vastly different circumstances, places and times. What humans know of the past and can foretell of the future comes from language.

To get a true sense of how significant language is, consider this: is it possible to get meaning from something without the use of words or signs? Indeed, some philosophers believe that a world without language would be a world devoid of meaning.

Language is carried visually by either signs, which are written marks that stand for units of language, or symbols, which represent an object itself. In the 20,000 years since humans first scratched simple tallies on a bone, the visual aspect of language has flourished. First objects, then words were abstractly represented. By 300 B.C. the library of Alexandria contained some 750,000 papyrus scroll books, the greatest storehouse of knowledge the world had ever seen—possible only through the use of signs and symbols.

Later, technological developments such as block printing (by the Chinese) and movable type (by Johannes Gutenberg) enabled written language to reach virtually every person on the planet. Although attempts to replace the some 3,000 languages and dialects with one "invented" language, such as Esperanto, have consistently failed, the use of symbols to supplement spoken language has proliferated. Indeed, the modern world is awash in signs and symbols.

Symbolic language promotes a type of visual thinking that today's designers and communication engineers must take into account. Older ways of presenting complex ideas and more verbal forms of recalling information are quickly being rendered obsolete. Change is happening so quickly that even written language may not be the most trustworthy means of communicating with future generations. It is no exaggeration to say that anyone trying to send a message to the future—be it a memorial to a great leader or a warning about a toxic waste site—ought to look at the efforts that have been made by astronomers to communicate with intelligent life forms on other planets.

If such aliens existed, they would be unfamiliar with any human language, written or spoken. Astronomers involved with the Search for Extra-Terrestrial Intelligence, or SETI, are scanning the heavens with radio telescopes in search of a scrap of message—intentional or accidental—amid the natural noise of the stars, although no one knows what such a message might look like. Other astronomers have tried to send messages to distant stars in the form of pictographs symbolizing everything from the human form to the lightest chemical elements. But even such simple pictures would require some ingenuity to decode.

Perhaps mathematics will provide the key.

Only mathematics can be a language universal enough for both humans and extraterrestrials to understand. The interstellar greeting may not be "hello" but "one, two, three. . . ."

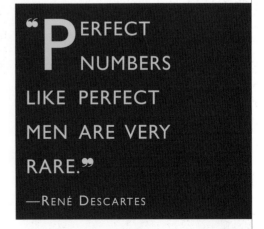

"**P**ERFECT NUMBERS LIKE PERFECT MEN ARE VERY RARE."

—RENÉ DESCARTES

PLAYTHINK	DIFFICULTY: ●●●●●●○○○○
35	REQUIRED: 👁 ✎
	COMPLETION: ☐ TIME: _____

HIGH CROSSING

The gap between the two skyscrapers is 5 meters at the narrowest point. On the roof of the L-shaped building, there are two steel girders, each 1 meter wide and 4.8 meters long. Is there a way to cross from the roof of the L-shaped building to the roof of the square building without jumping across or welding the two girders together?

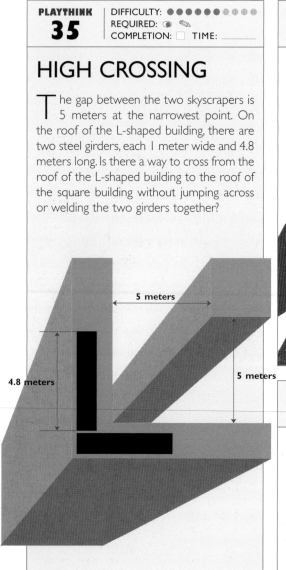

5 meters

4.8 meters

5 meters

PLAYTHINK	DIFFICULTY: ●●●●●●○○○○
36	REQUIRED: 👁
	COMPLETION: ☐ TIME: _____

HOG-TIED

Two hostages are tied together by their wrists, as shown. Can they separate themselves without cutting the rope or untying the knots?

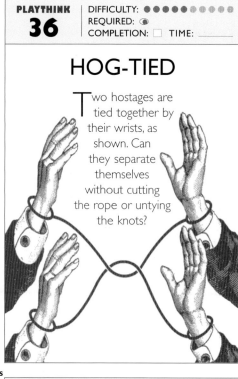

PLAYTHINK	DIFFICULTY: ●●●●●●●○○○
37	REQUIRED: 👁 ✎
	COMPLETION: ☐ TIME: _____

SIX–SEVEN

Is there a way to use three 6s to make a 7?

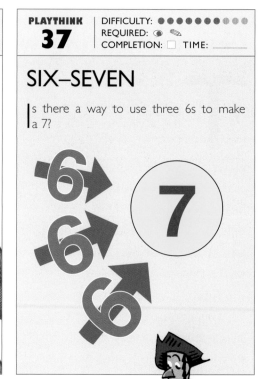

PLAYTHINK	DIFFICULTY: ●●●●●●○○○○
38	REQUIRED: ✎
	COMPLETION: ☐ TIME: _____

PACKING SWORD

A soldier needs to store his 70-centimeter-long sword, but the only chest available measures 40 centimeters long, 30 centimeters wide and 50 centimeters high. Will the sword fit in the chest?

PLAYTHINK	DIFFICULTY: ●●●●●●○○○○
39	REQUIRED: 👁 ✎
	COMPLETION: ☐ TIME: _____

DIVISION INTO FIVE

The colored shape is divided into four identical pieces. Can you divide the white square into five identical pieces?

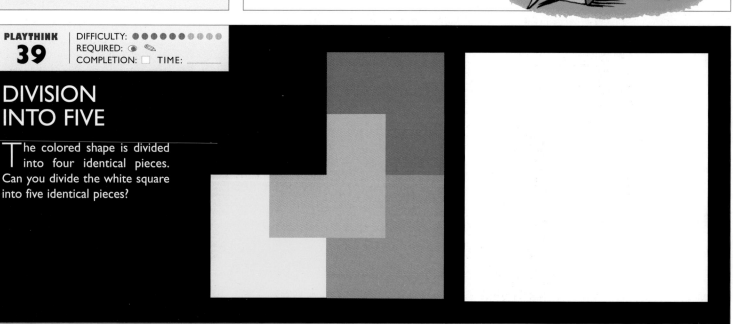

PLAYTHINK 40

DIFFICULTY: ●●●●●●●○○○
REQUIRED: 👁 ✏
COMPLETION: ☐ TIME: _____

STRANGE VIEWS

The two drawings below are two views of a three-dimensional object. The drawing at left is the view from the front; the drawing on the right shows the object directly from above.

Can you work out the shape of this strange object and make a sketch of it?

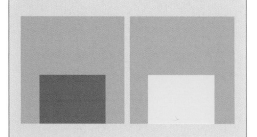

PLAYTHINK 41

DIFFICULTY: ●●●●●●○○○○
REQUIRED: 👁
COMPLETION: ☐ TIME: _____

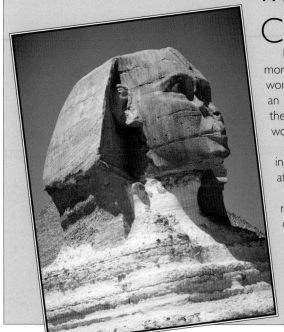

RIDDLE OF THE SPHINX

Can you solve one of the greatest puzzles of antiquity?

In Greek mythology the Sphinx was a monster who possessed the head of a woman, the body of a lion and the wings of an eagle. The Sphinx guarded the gates of the city of Thebes, challenging all who would enter with this simple riddle:

"What goes on four legs in the morning, on two legs at noon, and on three legs at dusk?"

The Sphinx killed anyone who could not answer the riddle and vowed to destroy herself should anyone solve it. She had to make good on her word when Oedipus told her the answer. Can you?

PLAYTHINK 42

DIFFICULTY: ●●●●●●●●●○
REQUIRED: 📄 ✂
COMPLETION: ☐ TIME: _____

HEPTAGON MAGIC

Copy the large heptagon shown on this page and carefully cut out the twenty subdivisions.

Puzzle 1:
Reassemble the twenty pieces to form two identical seven-pointed stars.

Puzzle 2:
Reassemble the twenty pieces to form four smaller heptagons.

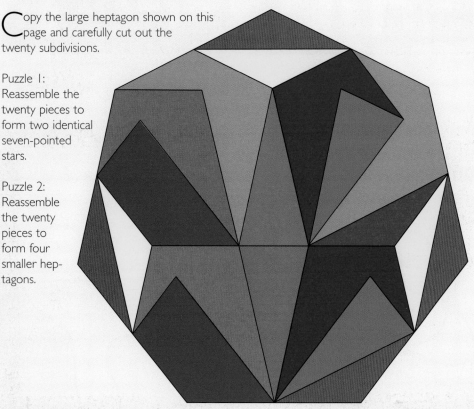

PLAYTHINK 43

DIFFICULTY: ●●●●○○○○○○
REQUIRED: 👁
COMPLETION: ☐ TIME: _____

LADYBUG RENDEZVOUS

Mister Ladybug meets Miss Ladybug on the petal of a flower.

"I'm a boy," says the one with red dots.

"I'm a girl," says the one with yellow dots.

Then they both laugh because at least one of them is lying. From that information can you tell which one has the red dots and which has the yellow?

Four Stages of Problem Solving

There is no recipe for creativity. But research on the subject has identified four essential steps to creative problem solving:

Stage 1: Preparation—This requires both a short-term reading up on the problem at hand and a broader understanding that only a commitment to a well-rounded education can bring. After all, you never know where the unexpected solution to a difficult problem might lie.

Stage 2: Incubation—No one knows why getting away from a problem is useful. Some psychologists see it as a period of rest; others, as a time when you subconsciously select and discard various pieces of information. Whatever the reason, creative thinking requires some quiet, unstructured time.

Stage 3: Illumination—This is the sudden flash of insight, the proverbial light bulb glowing overhead. Some call it the "Aha!" moment.

Stage 4: Elaboration—Sometimes a flash of insight is really just the flicker of a bad idea. One must always check the validity of an answer. And then comes the most important part: explaining the solution in a way that can be understood by others.

PLAYTHINK 44

DIFFICULTY: ●●●●●○○○○○○
REQUIRED: ◉
COMPLETION: ☐ TIME: _____

SKYLINE

Can you match the skylines, shown above, with their corresponding skies?

1   2   3   4   5   6

7   8 9   10   11   12

PLAYTHINK 45

DIFFICULTY: ●●●●●●●●●○○
REQUIRED: ◉ ✏
COMPLETION: ☐ TIME: _____

ODD INTERSECTION

The red closed line is drawn so that it crosses a black closed line from inside to outside or vice versa exactly ten times.

Can you draw a new red closed line over the same black line so that it makes only nine crossings?

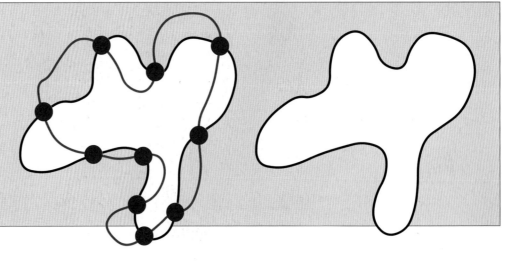

PLAYTHINK
46
DIFFICULTY: ●●●●●○○○○○○
REQUIRED: ◉ ✐
COMPLETION: ☐ TIME: _____

OVERLAPPING RUGS

A square rug that is 2 meters on a side overlaps a smaller square rug that is only 1 meter on a side. The corner of the larger rug falls exactly on the center of the smaller one. Not counting the fringe, what percentage of the smaller rug is hidden?

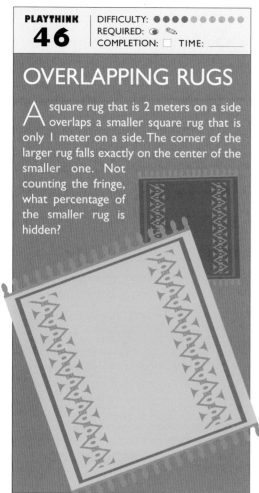

PLAYTHINK
47
DIFFICULTY: ●●●●●●○○○○○
REQUIRED: ◉ 📄 ✂
COMPLETION: ☐ TIME: _____

DOCKING POLYGONS

Leaving the two black triangles in place, can you arrange the polygons side by side so that they form a bridge from one triangle to the other? The polygons should not be rotated when moved.

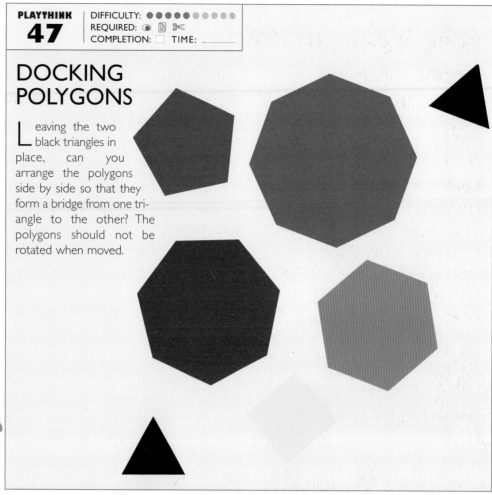

PLAYTHINK
48
DIFFICULTY: ●●●●●●○○○○○
REQUIRED: ◉ ✐
COMPLETION: ☐ TIME: _____

MURPHY'S LAW OF SOCKS

Imagine that after washing five pairs of socks you discover that two socks are missing. Which scenario is more likely:

A. The two missing socks make a complete pair and you are left with four complete pairs.

B. You are now left with three pairs of socks and two orphan socks.

Captain Edward A. Murphy stated, "Anything that can go wrong will, and at the worst possible time." Does Murphy's law rule the sock drawer?

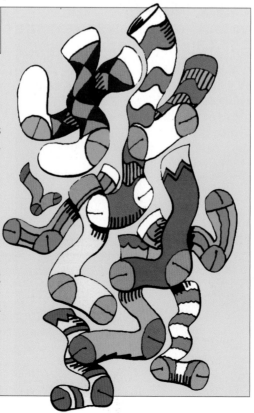

PLAYTHINK
49
DIFFICULTY: ●●●○○○○○○○○
REQUIRED: ◉ 📄 ✂
COMPLETION: ☐ TIME: _____

HOLE IN A POSTCARD

Can you make a hole in a postcard large enough for a man to step through?

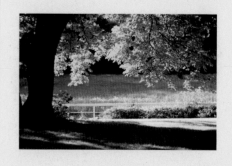

PLAYTHINK 50

DIFFICULTY: ●●●●●●●○○○
REQUIRED: 👁 ✏
COMPLETION: ☐ TIME: _____

PHONE NUMBER

A man and a woman meet at a bar. After a long conversation they agree to have dinner the next day if the man remembers to call the woman to confirm the date. The next morning the man discovers that he can remember the digits in her number—2, 3, 4, 5, 6, 7 and 8—but he has completely forgotten their order.

If he decides to arrange the seven digits in random order and dial every combination, what are the chances that any given phone number will be hers?

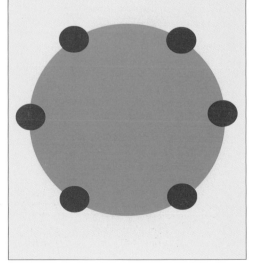

IMPERFECT HEXAGON

A regular hexagon can be subdivided into exactly six identical equilateral triangles. But what about this irregular hexagon? The shape can be divided into as few as fifteen equilateral triangles of different sizes. Using the hexagonal grid as a guide, can you find the right pattern? Some of the triangles in the solution can be identical.

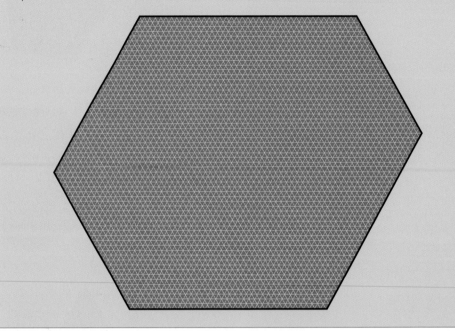

PLAYTHINK 51

DIFFICULTY: ●●●●●●●○○○
REQUIRED: ✏
COMPLETION: ☐ TIME: _____

PLAYTHINK 52

DIFFICULTY: ●●●●●●●●○○
REQUIRED: 📄 ✂
COMPLETION: ☐ TIME: _____

THE COLORED DODECAGONS

Can you rotate the nine multicolored umbrellas so that the color panels of neighboring umbrellas match up?

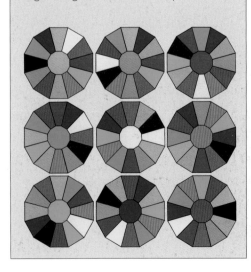

PLAYTHINK 53

DIFFICULTY: ●●●○○○○○○○
REQUIRED: ✏
COMPLETION: ☐ TIME: _____

HANDSHAKES 1

At a business meeting each person shook hands with every other person exactly once. If there were fifteen handshakes, can you tell how many people attended the meeting?

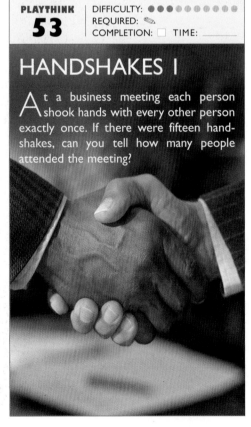

PLAYTHINK 54

DIFFICULTY: ●●●●●○○○○○
REQUIRED: ✏
COMPLETION: ☐ TIME: _____

HANDSHAKES 2

Six people are sitting at a round table. How many combinations of simultaneous, noncrossing handshakes are possible?

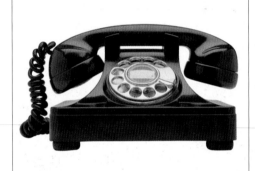

PLAYTHINK 55

DIFFICULTY: ●●●●●●●●●○
REQUIRED: 📄 ✂
COMPLETION: ☐ TIME: _____

TANGRAM POLYGONS

A tangram is a set of seven three- and four-sided puzzle pieces that can be combined to form a number of complex shapes. In 1942 the Chinese mathematicians Fu Traing and Chuan Chih proved that the seven tangram pieces can form exactly thirteen different convex polygons: one triangle, six quadrilaterals, two pentagons and four hexagons. The thirteen polygons are shown and the tangram pieces have been placed on one of the quadrilaterals (a square) to demonstrate the principle. Can you arrange the tangram pieces to form the other twelve polygons?

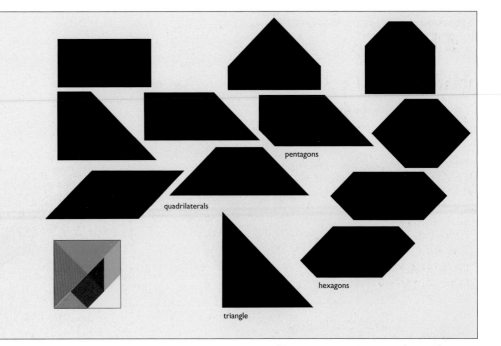

pentagons

quadrilaterals

hexagons

triangle

PLAYTHINK 56

DIFFICULTY: ●●●●●●●○○○
REQUIRED: 👁 ✎ 📄 ✂
COMPLETION: ☐ TIME: _____

DOMINO PATTERNS

The patterns at the right were each formed from the complete set of twenty-eight dominoes shown at left. Through careful observation, can you determine exactly how the dominoes were assembled? Tracing the domino pieces and cutting them out may help.

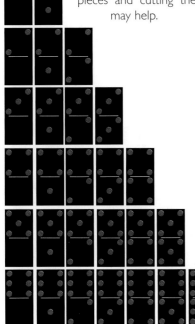

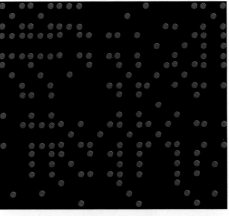

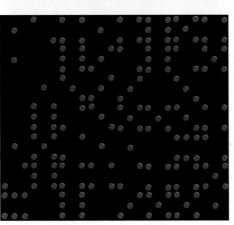

PLAYTHINK 57

DIFFICULTY: ●●●●●●●●●●
REQUIRED: 👁
COMPLETION: ☐ TIME: _____

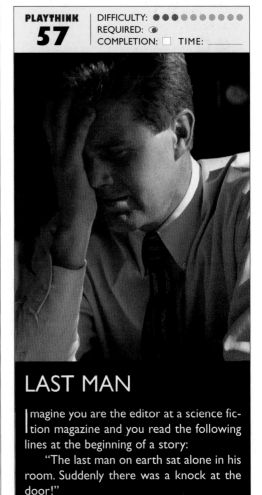

LAST MAN

Imagine you are the editor at a science fiction magazine and you read the following lines at the beginning of a story:

"The last man on earth sat alone in his room. Suddenly there was a knock at the door!"

Can you change one word in the first sentence to make the man's isolation before the knock at the door more complete?

PLAYTHINK
58
DIFFICULTY: ●●●●●●●○○○
REQUIRED: ◉ ✎
COMPLETION: ☐ TIME: _____

HOTEL KEYS

A porter leads eight guests to their hotel rooms, rooms 1 through 8. Unfortunately, the keys are unlabeled and the porter has mixed up their order. Using trial and error, what is the maximum number of attempts the porter must make before he opens all the doors?

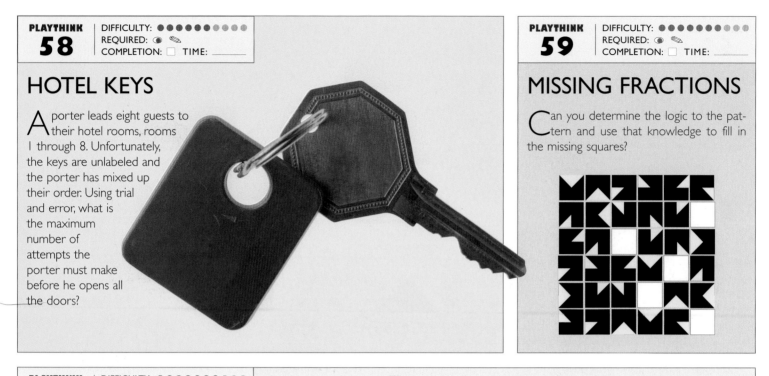

PLAYTHINK
59
DIFFICULTY: ●●●●●●●●○○
REQUIRED: ◉ ✎
COMPLETION: ☐ TIME: _____

MISSING FRACTIONS

Can you determine the logic to the pattern and use that knowledge to fill in the missing squares?

PLAYTHINK
60
DIFFICULTY: ●●●●●●●○○○
REQUIRED: ✎ 📄 ✂
COMPLETION: ☐ TIME: _____

SQUARE SPLIT

Can you rearrange the twenty-two square pieces that comprise the square on the left to make the two squares at the right?

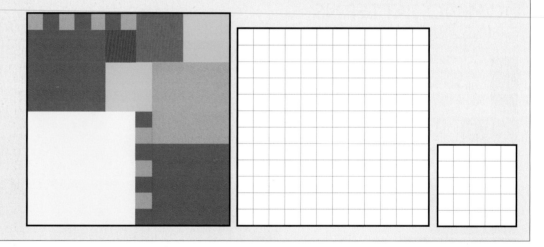

PLAYTHINK
61
DIFFICULTY: ●●●●●●●○○○
REQUIRED: ◉ ✎
COMPLETION: ☐ TIME: _____

FAULT-FREE SQUARE

The manner in which the one-by-two bricks were packed into a square has created a so-called fault line—a straight line of edges that runs from one side to the other. To create a stronger structure, can you repack the bricks into the square so that it is free of faults?

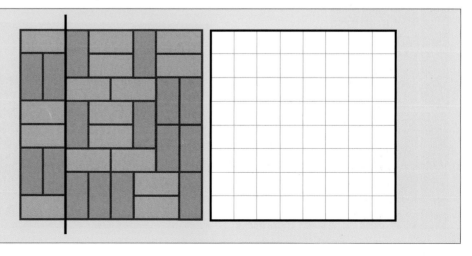

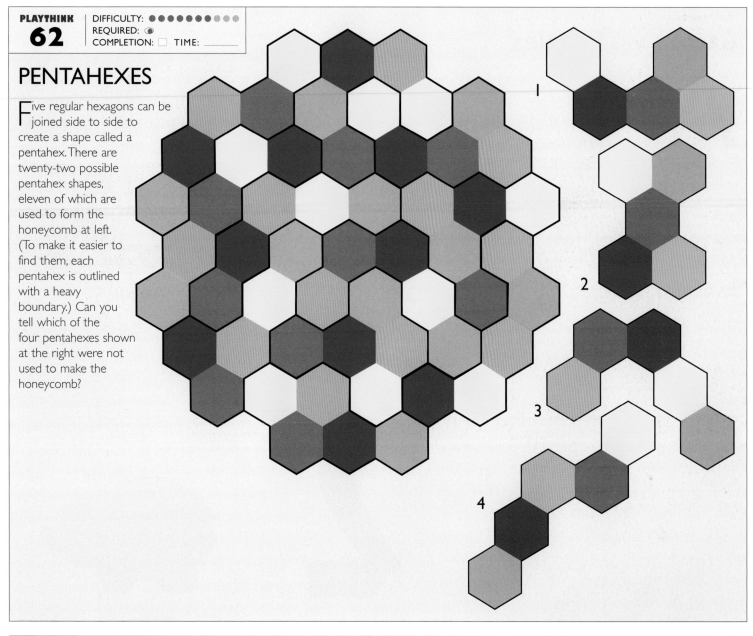

PLAYTHINK 62

DIFFICULTY: ●●●●●●●○○○
REQUIRED: ◉
COMPLETION: ☐ TIME: _____

PENTAHEXES

Five regular hexagons can be joined side to side to create a shape called a pentahex. There are twenty-two possible pentahex shapes, eleven of which are used to form the honeycomb at left. (To make it easier to find them, each pentahex is outlined with a heavy boundary.) Can you tell which of the four pentahexes shown at the right were not used to make the honeycomb?

PLAYTHINK 63

DIFFICULTY: ●●●●●●●○○○
REQUIRED: ◉ ✎
COMPLETION: ☐ TIME: _____

FRUIT BASKETS

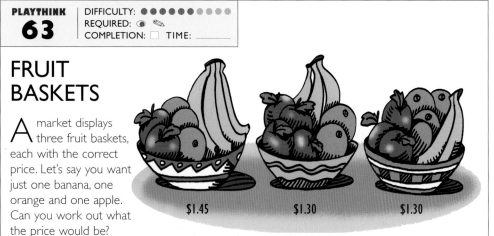

A market displays three fruit baskets, each with the correct price. Let's say you want just one banana, one orange and one apple. Can you work out what the price would be?

$1.45 $1.30 $1.30

PLAYTHINK 64

DIFFICULTY: ●●●●●●○○○○
REQUIRED: ◉ ✎
COMPLETION: ☐ TIME: _____

FAMILY REUNION

One grandfather, one grandmother, two fathers, two mothers, four children, three grandchildren, one brother, two sisters, two sons, two daughters, one father-in-law, one mother-in-law and one daughter-in-law attended a family reunion. If both halves of each relationship attended (i.e., the father *and* the son), how many people showed up?

Games vs. Puzzles

Adults can continue to delight in the science of patterns by solving puzzles (which, if well constructed, have one solution) and playing games (which can end in many ways). The boundary between the two, however, is not entirely clear-cut. Mathematicians have studied many simple games and found strategies that never fail to bring victory to one player. For example, if he or she plays properly, the first player will never lose a game of tic-tac-toe. Indeed, when fully understood, simple, well-designed games can seem very much like puzzles.

PLAYTHINK 65

DIFFICULTY: ●●●●●●○○○○
REQUIRED: ◉ ✎
COMPLETION: ☐ TIME: _____

FASHION SHOW

Three models—Miss Pink, Miss Green and Miss Blue—are on the catwalk. Their dresses are solid pink, solid green and solid blue.

"It's strange," Miss Blue remarks to the others. "We are named Pink, Green and Blue, and our dresses are pink, green and blue, but none of us is wearing the dress that matches her name."

"That *is* a coincidence," says the woman in green.

From that information, can you determine the color of each model's dress?

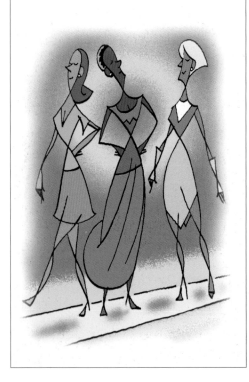

PLAYTHINK 66

DIFFICULTY: ●●●●●●●○○○
REQUIRED: ◉ ✎
COMPLETION: ☐ TIME: _____

NETWORK OF TWOS

How many numbers can you write using three 2s and no other symbols?

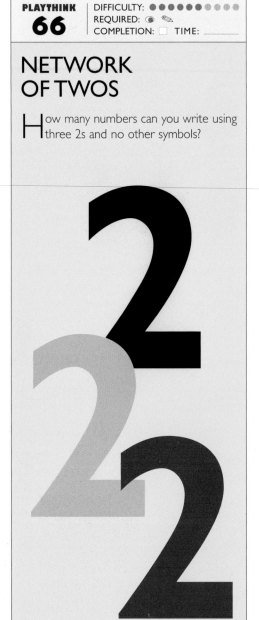

PLAYTHINK 67

DIFFICULTY: ●●●●●●●○○○
REQUIRED: ◉
COMPLETION: ☐ TIME: _____

PIGGY BANKS

Three nickels and three dimes are distributed among three piggy banks so that each bank holds two coins. Although each bank has a number of cents printed on its side, all three banks are mislabeled. Is it possible to determine how to correctly relabel the banks simply by shaking one of the banks until one of the coins drops out? If so, explain how.

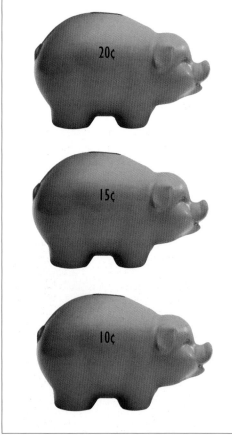

PLAYTHINK
68
DIFFICULTY: ●●●●●●●●○○
REQUIRED: ◉
COMPLETION: ☐ TIME: _____

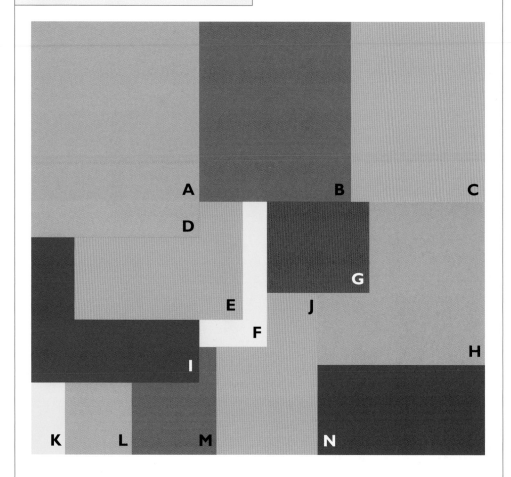

OVERLAPPING SQUARES

Fourteen identical squares have been placed one on top of the other to form this rectangular pattern. Can you determine the order in which the squares must have been laid down? Start with the bottommost and work your way up.

"WHENEVER YOU LOOK AT A PIECE OF WORK AND YOU THINK THE FELLOW WAS CRAZY, THEN YOU WANT TO PAY SOME ATTENTION. . . . ONE OF YOU IS LIKELY TO BE, AND YOU HAD BETTER FIND OUT WHICH ONE. . . . IT MAKES AN AWFUL LOT OF DIFFERENCE."

—CHARLES FRANKLIN KETTERING

PLAYTHINK
69
DIFFICULTY: ●●●●●○○○○○
REQUIRED: ◉
COMPLETION: ☐ TIME: _____

TETRAHEDRON

A tetrahedron is a regular pyramid made of four equilateral triangles. It is possible to paint each face a different color—in this case red, green, yellow and blue. Five views of the tetrahedron are shown below. Can you tell which one is inconsistent with the other four?

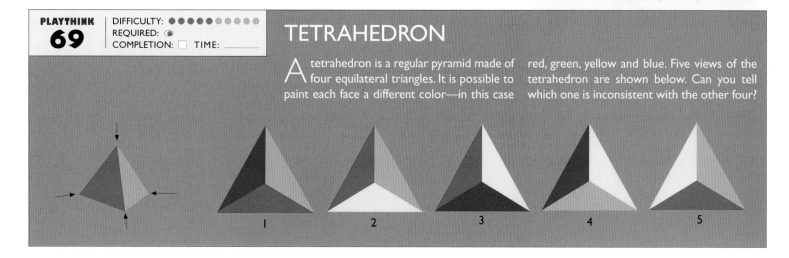

PLAYTHINK 70

DIFFICULTY: ●●●●●●●○○○
REQUIRED: ◉ 📄 ✂
COMPLETION: ☐ TIME: _____

FOLDING STAMPS

Six stamps, each of which is the same color both front and back, are joined along their edges to form a two-by-three sheet. That sheet, however, can be folded along the perforations to create a stack of stamps. Of the four stacks shown, which is impossible to form by folding the sheet?

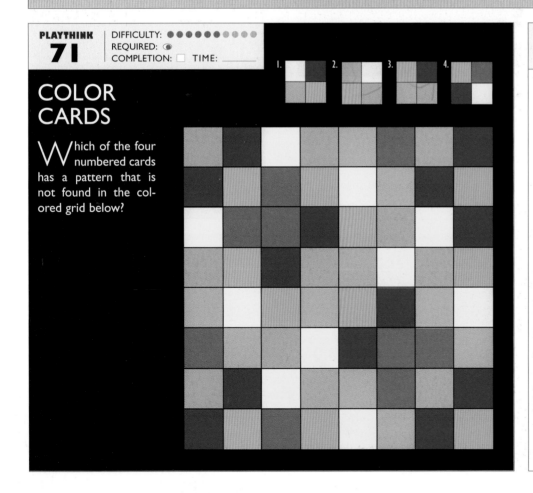

1   2   3   4

PLAYTHINK 71

DIFFICULTY: ●●●●●●○○○○
REQUIRED: ◉
COMPLETION: ☐ TIME: _____

COLOR CARDS

Which of the four numbered cards has a pattern that is not found in the colored grid below?

PLAYTHINK 72

DIFFICULTY: ●●●●●●●○○○
REQUIRED: ◉
COMPLETION: ☐ TIME: _____

CRYPTOGRAM

This message has been encrypted with a simple cipher. Can you break the code to discover the three secret words?

POF UIPVTBOE QMBZUIJOLT

PLAYTHINK 73

DIFFICULTY: ●●●●●●○○○○
REQUIRED: ◉
COMPLETION: ☐ TIME: _____

PYRAMID ART SCULPTURE

Four cloth sails are fixed to the wire structure of a three-dimensional sculpture, as shown. What pattern do you see when you look down on the sculpture from above?

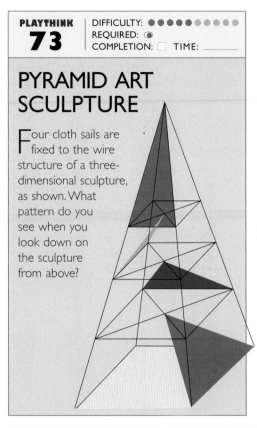

PLAYTHINK 74

DIFFICULTY: ●●●●●○○○○○
REQUIRED: ◉
COMPLETION: ☐ TIME: _____

STAR STRIPS

Can you make a perfect star from three identical strips of translucent paper?

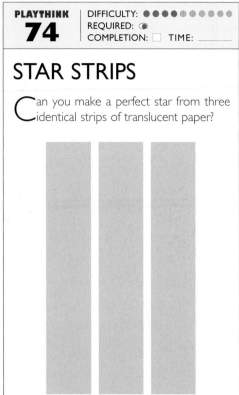

PLAYTHINK 75

DIFFICULTY: ●●●●●●●○○○
REQUIRED: ◉ ✎
COMPLETION: ☐ TIME: _____

OUTLINE PATTERNS

The three blank outlines are all composed of the five rectangles that make up the square on the top. Can you draw in their outlines along the grids?

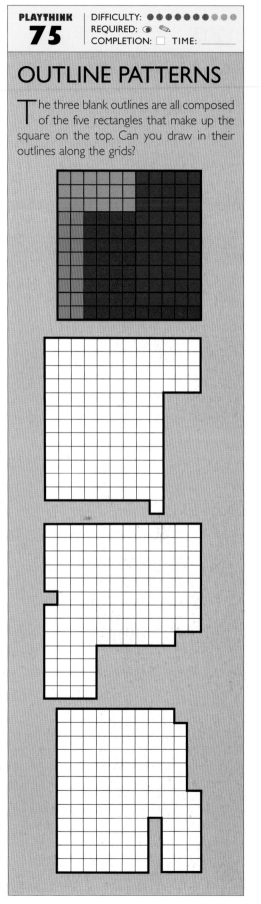

PLAYTHINK 76

DIFFICULTY: ●●●●●●○○○○
REQUIRED: ◉ ✎
COMPLETION: ☐ TIME: _____

MATCHSTICK TRIANGLES

Starting with the equilateral triangle shown, can you create two smaller equilateral triangles by moving just four matchsticks?

Then can you create four even smaller equilateral triangles by moving just four matchsticks?

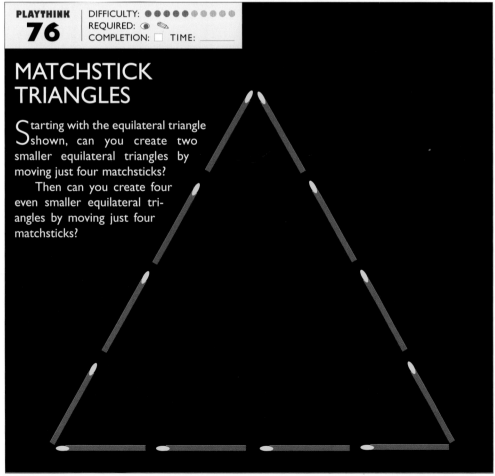

PLAYTHINK 77

DIFFICULTY: ●●●●●●●○○○
REQUIRED: ◉ ✎
COMPLETION: ☐ TIME: _____

PAIRS IN ROWS AND COLUMNS

The object of this game is to place twenty-one small coins on the game board so that they satisfy the following conditions:

Each row must contain three coins.

Each column must contain three coins.

When you compare any two rows or columns, there can be only one pair of adjacent coins vertically (for rows) or horizontally (for columns).

How quickly can you win this game?

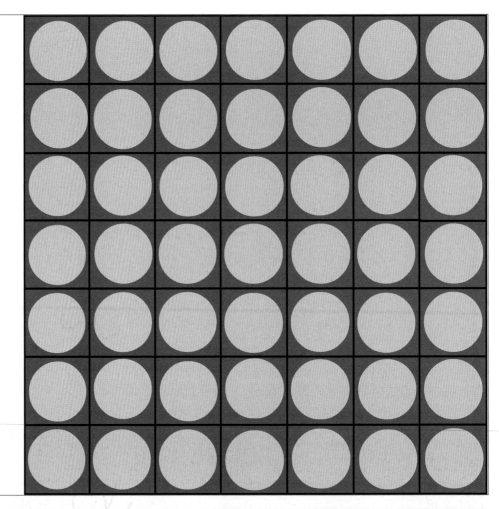

PLAYTHINK 78

DIFFICULTY: ●●●●●●○○○○
REQUIRED: ◉
COMPLETION: ☐ TIME: _____

ORDER LOGIC

Can you uncover the logic of the pattern and add the missing animal?

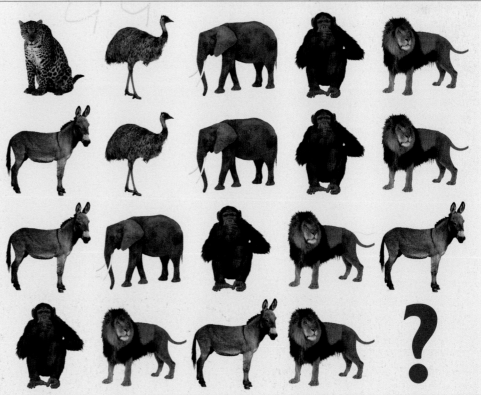

PLAYTHINK
79

DIFFICULTY: ●●●●●○○○○○
REQUIRED: ◉
COMPLETION: ☐ TIME: _____

CIRCLE ART MEMORY GAME

Pairing games have been long popular the world over. In this one, match all the like pairs of cards to discover the odd one out. How long will it take you to solve this?

One interesting note: These game cards employ simple color variations of a single pattern that can be constructed by a compass and ruler. It is similar to decorative patterns made by the ancient Greeks.

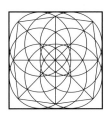

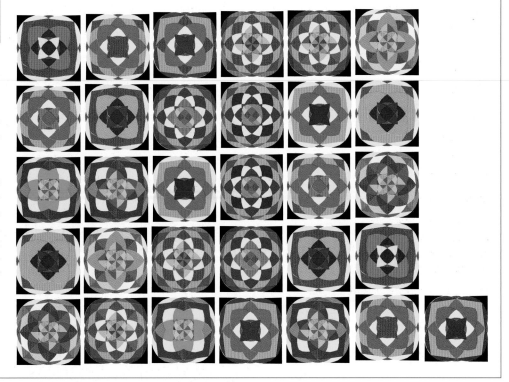

PLAYTHINK
80

DIFFICULTY: ●●●●●●●○○○
REQUIRED: ◉ ✎
COMPLETION: ☐ TIME: _____

KNIGHTS ATTACK

Twenty knights are placed on a chessboard so that each one can attack one and only one other knight. (As you know, the knights move in an L-shaped manner, two squares up and one square over, or two squares over and one square up.) Is it possible to pack even more knights on the board and still follow the one-attack rule?

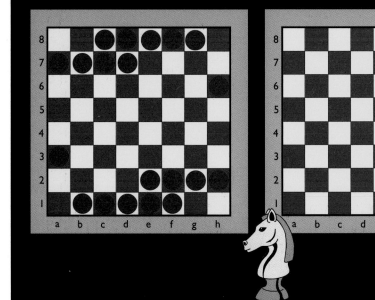

PLAYTHINK
81

DIFFICULTY: ●●●●●●●●○○
REQUIRED: ◉ ✎
COMPLETION: ☐ TIME: _____

HAT MIX

Three men check their hats at the theater, but the attendant mixes up the checks as she hands them out. When the three men return after the performance to claim their hats, what are the chances that they all will have their own hats returned to them?

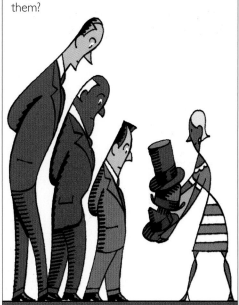

PLAYTHINK 82

DIFFICULTY: ●●●●●●●○○○
REQUIRED: 👁 ✎
COMPLETION: ☐   TIME: _____

WORD PATTERN

Can you find the secret message from Socrates?

AFGTRYT	SUGYUJO	SDNYTVB	MKRRDVB	UPMPLKM	SVFETVH
ATGTRHT	SEGYURO	SDEY–IB	MKSRDVB	U–OPLNM	SVLETYH
HGNDCTY	RTUIOMK	LMCZSTU	WETYUNV	OKPLMNH	SEFTCVG
–ONDNTY	REUI–GK	LOCZOTU	WDTY–KV	ONPLMOH	SWFTCLG
FJWBNMK	DEVNKOL	LPNMSGE	KERTYUN	SEFTRYV	XDCVFRE
FEWBDMK	DGVNEOL	L–AMSNE	KDRT–ON	SNFTREV	X–EVFVE
SEDCFVG	YUOPLKM	VBRHTRF	CDFRTYU	DEVBPKO	POUKJHY
SIDCFVG	YLOP–IM	VBGHTNF	COFRTRU	DAVBNKO	POCKJEY
WERTYFD	DFGYHUO	BNMKOPX	CVBNJUY	FRGVBHU	VBNJKOP
W–STYFD	DOGYCUO	BRMKAPX	CTBNJEY	FRGSBHU	VBNJKOP

PLAYTHINK 83

DIFFICULTY: ●●●●●●●●○○
REQUIRED: 👁 ✎
COMPLETION: ☐   TIME: _____

COIN ON A CORNER

If you randomly toss a coin (smaller than a square on this game board), what is the probability of the coin landing on a corner of one of the squares?

Puzzles and Intelligence

Most of us grew up with a concept of intelligence that is driven by tests: the person who can answer the most questions is thought to be the most intelligent. But imagining that intelligence can be boiled down to a single number—the IQ—is an obsolete notion. If you find yourself having difficulty with some of these PlayThinks, don't worry that you are not "smart" enough to do the puzzles. It is all a matter of freeing up your latent creativity. With the proper mind-set, anyone can do these puzzles.

And if you find the puzzles easy, congratulations. But remember, that fact by itself does not mean you are smart. It just means you are especially attuned to this style of thinking.

> " IN THESE DAYS, A MAN WHO SAYS A THING CANNOT BE DONE IS QUITE APT TO BE INTERRUPTED BY SOME IDIOT DOING IT. "
>
> —ELBERT GREEN HUBBARD

PLAYTHINK 84

DIFFICULTY: ●●●●●●●○○○
REQUIRED: 👁 ✏
COMPLETION: ☐ TIME: _____

FACTORS

At the chalkboard the teacher demonstrates the four factors of the number 6—that is, the whole numbers that can divide into 6 and leave no remainder. (Remember, a number is always its own factor, as is 1.) Between 1 and 100, there are five numbers that have exactly twelve factors. How quickly can you find all five?

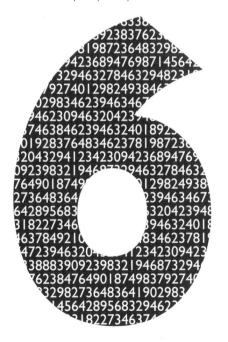

PLAYTHINK 85

DIFFICULTY: ●●●●●●●○○○
REQUIRED: 👁 ✏
COMPLETION: ☐ TIME: _____

NECKLACE PAIRS

Can you place beads on the necklace so that each two-color pair shown at left appears exactly once in either direction?

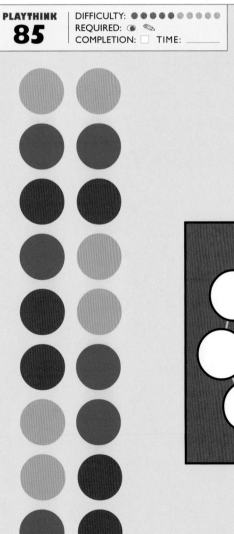

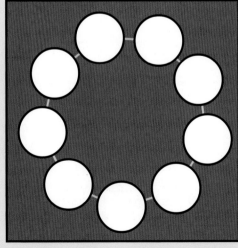

PLAYTHINK 86

DIFFICULTY: ●●●●●○○○○○
REQUIRED: 👁 ✎
COMPLETION: ☐   TIME: _____

GOLD BAR

This gold bar is exactly 31 centimeters long. If you want to divide the bar into smaller segments so that one or a combination of segments can add up to every whole number of centimeters from 1 to 31, how many cuts must you make?

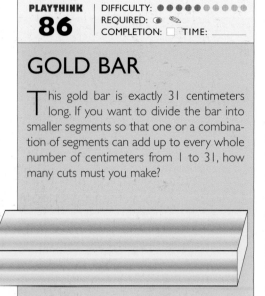

PLAYTHINK 87

DIFFICULTY: ●●●●○○○○○○
REQUIRED: ✎
COMPLETION: ☐   TIME: _____

TRAVERSING SQUARES

Can you trace a path along all five yellow squares without picking up your pencil, going over the same segment twice or crossing a line you've already laid down?

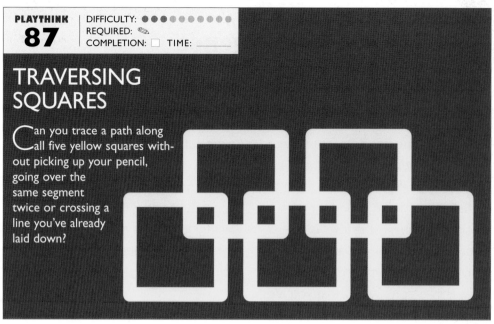

PLAYTHINK 88

DIFFICULTY: ●●●●●●●●○○
REQUIRED: 👁 ✎
COMPLETION: ☐   TIME: _____

LOST IN CAVES

Five hapless tourists are lost in a labyrinth of caves. The path from one cave to another is marked with either a red arrow or a blue arrow. Their guide is outside and doesn't know where any of the five tourists is. Nonetheless, he shouts a sequence of red and blue arrows for the tourists to follow. Amazingly, all the tourists follow that sequence and arrive at the same cave, and the guide is there to pick them up.

Can you work out the sequence of reds and blues the guide shouted and which cave the tourists ended up in?

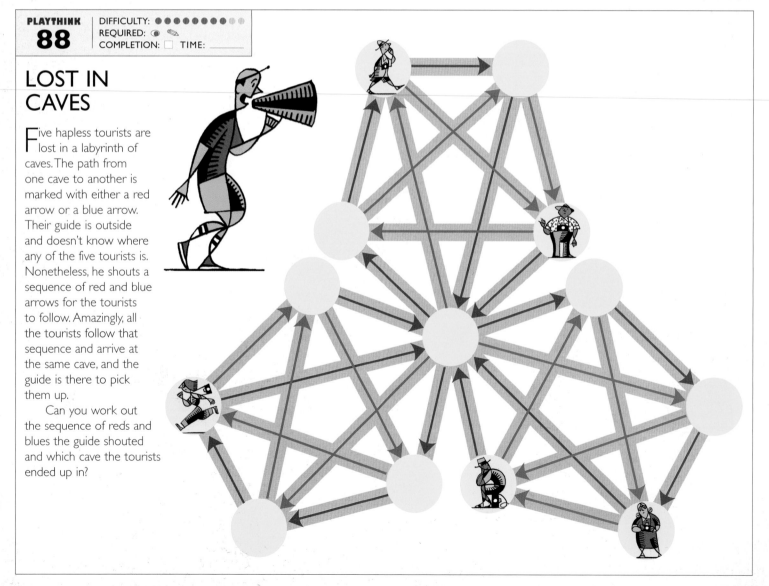

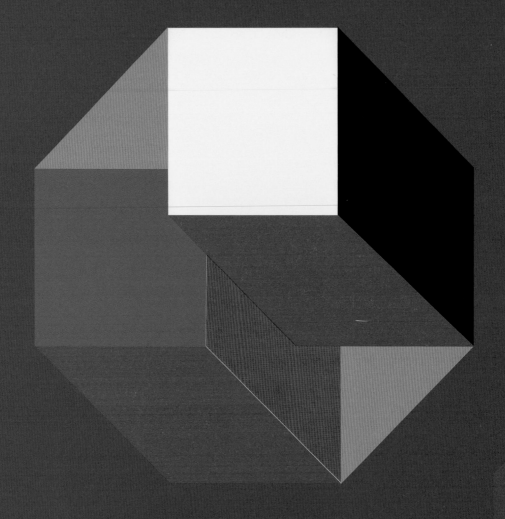

Geometry

In the Beginning . . .

There is an old debate among mathematicians: Is mathematics something they create or a truth they discover? The answer depends upon one's idea of truth. Some people believe that mathematical concepts are tools that were created in response to otherwise unsolvable questions, much the way screws were invented to hold pieces of wood together, or telephones to carry voices over long distances. Others view mathematics as a truth that exists regardless of whether anyone finds it: Mathematicians do not invent solutions to problems; they discover them.

Although the debate often divides the mathematical community, some mathematicians are so sure in their view that they give the matter little thought. As the famous Hungarian mathematician Paul Erdös declared, "If you believe in God, the answer is obvious."

To me the answer is also obvious. Mathematics was not invented. Mathematical forms existed before the advent of life on our planet or, indeed, before the earth was formed. When the sun with its solar system was just a cloud of dust and gas, galaxies, stars and other planets had developed configurations and motions based on simple geometric forms and principles. Some galaxies, for instance, possess a striking

beauty derived from their form: an exact logarithmic spiral. The motions of stars, planets, comets and other bodies through space follow trajectories that can be described by geometric curves: ellipses, parabolas and hyperbolas.

And let us not forget that the first time three dinosaurs joined two other dinosaurs at a watering hole, there were five dinosaurs, whether or not anyone was there to count them.

When trying to trace the history of mathematics, it is important to keep those facts in mind. Mathematics started with the beginning of the universe itself. In many cases historians limit themselves to the dictionary definition of mathematics— an abstract science that investigates deductively the conclusions implicit in the elementary conceptions of spatial and numerical relations—and so begin their discussion with Thales, the great Greek mathematician who lived some 2,600 years ago. But although Thales helped invent the language by which we describe mathematics, humans had been using math long before that. The oldest mathematical textbook is an Egyptian papyrus scroll written by the scribe Ahmes in 1850 B.C. And even that may not be the beginning—4,000-year-old clay bricks found in the Tigris River valley bear numbers inscribed by Babylonian priests.

Even our prehistoric, cave-dwelling ancestors had a good grasp of many mathematical concepts. Prehistoric art, which reduced the complex shapes found in nature to simple, abstract forms, paved the way for geometry. And a hunt that produced fewer killed animals than there were hunters—so that the leaders needed to figure out how to divide the spoils—helped develop the concepts of division and inequality. The constant northern stars provided a reliable clue to direction, and finger counting progressed into arithmetic.

Some mathematics, notably anything that depends upon the use of the base ten number system, is undeniably a human invention. But most mathematics does not rely upon that sort of human ingenuity. It was a truth that existed before it was discovered. Take, for example, the Pythagorean theorem: although it is forever linked to the great Greek mathematician Pythagoras, it has been independently discovered several times, by various civilizations, throughout history. If our present society were to disappear, the Pythagorean theorem would eventually be discovered again. And if there is some other form of intelligent life on some distant planet, it, too, has probably discovered that the sum of the squares of the lengths of the sides of a right triangle is equal to the square of the hypotenuse.

> **"I** HAVE AN INFAMOUSLY LOW CAPACITY FOR VISUALIZING RELATIONSHIPS, WHICH MADE THE STUDY OF GEOMETRY AND ALL SUBJECTS DERIVED FROM IT IMPOSSIBLE FOR ME."
>
> —SIGMUND FREUD

PLAYTHINK 89

DIFFICULTY: ●●●●●●●○○○
REQUIRED: 👁 ✎
COMPLETION: ☐ TIME: _____

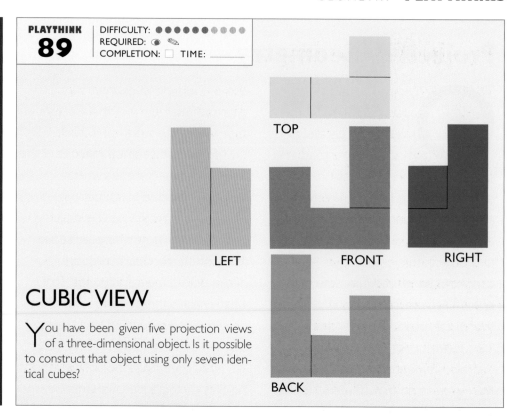

TOP

LEFT   FRONT   RIGHT

BACK

CUBIC VIEW

You have been given five projection views of a three-dimensional object. Is it possible to construct that object using only seven identical cubes?

PLAYTHINK 90

DIFFICULTY: ●●●●●●○○○○
REQUIRED: 👁 ✎
COMPLETION: ☐ TIME: _____

MULTIVIEWS

Imagine flying over a city in an airplane. As seen from above, the buildings seem quite different from the way they look when you are standing in front of them. And yet nothing about the buildings has changed. This is the concept that architects tap into when they represent their building plans in two different ways: the plan, which represents the way the building will be laid out on the ground, and the front elevation, which is derived directly from the plans to represent the way the building will look from the front. A third type of architectural drawing, the perspective, combines those two views to create a more realistic view of the building.

This puzzle is based on the same concept. There are sixteen objects, yet seen from the front, they present only four different types of views. And seen from the top, they present four different types of views. But every object with a similar front view has a different overhead view—sixteen unique objects.

Can you match each object with its proper overhead and front views? Write your answers in the boxes provided.

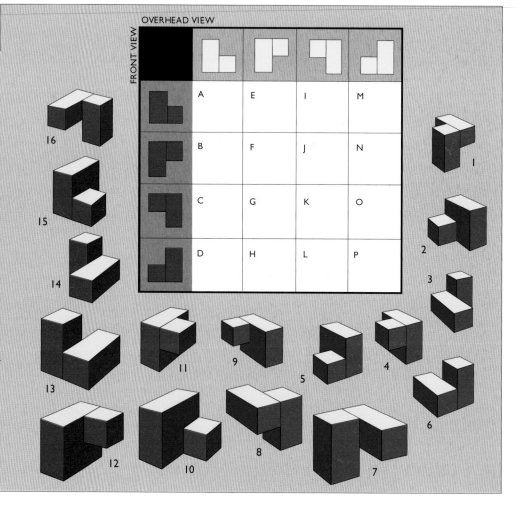

Projective Geometry

Our eyes present a distorted view of the world. The parallel tracks of a railroad should never meet, but rails in the distance do look as if they come to a point. Large things look small when they are far off, and distance can make two objects that are of equal size appear to be on radically different scales. The reverse is true as well: a thumb can obscure the largest galaxy.

Even though human perception of scale is a given, it was only during the Renaissance that painters solved the problem of representing the perspective of a three-dimensional space on a two-dimensional plane. That solution, called projection, created not only a breakthrough in art but also a new type of geometry— a form of mathematics that closely approaches the world of illusion.

Projective geometry studies what happens to shapes when they are distorted in special ways. Although the results can be startling, projective transformations preserve many of the geometric properties of the objects being projected. That's what enables three-dimensional objects to be recognizable in their two-dimensional form.

Maps are projections. The Flemish cartographer Gerardus Mercator employed projective geometry to produce the first modern map of the world in 1569. The so-called Mercator projection was made from the center of the earth; the surface was projected onto an imaginary cylinder tangent to the equator. Although the resulting map was quite useful for navigation, Mercator's projection distorted the areas near the poles. That's why Greenland, which has an area comparable to Mexico, appears on a Mercator map to be the same size as South America.

These days we see the uses of projective geometry all around us. Photographs are images of projections, as are many mechanical and architectural drawings. And video games in realistic 3-D are possible because sophisticated computer programs can calculate the projection of imaginary three-dimensional objects.

PLAYTHINK 91

DIFFICULTY: ●●●●●●●○○○
REQUIRED: 👁 ✏️
COMPLETION: ☐   TIME: _____

SHADOW GARDEN

All twelve walls of a dodeca-gonal garden are illuminated by a single lamp, which is positioned in the garden's center. Can you redesign the garden so that even though a lamp is placed at its center, each of the twelve walls is partly or entirely in shadow? The walls must be straight, but they don't have to be the same length.

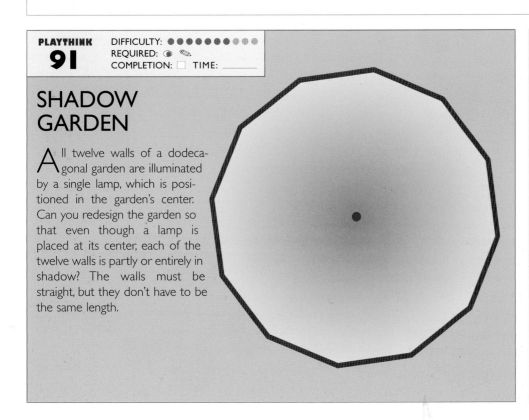

PLAYTHINK 92

DIFFICULTY: ●●●●●●○○○○
REQUIRED: 👁 ✏️
COMPLETION: ☐   TIME: _____

THE CIRCULAR-TRIANGULAR SQUARE

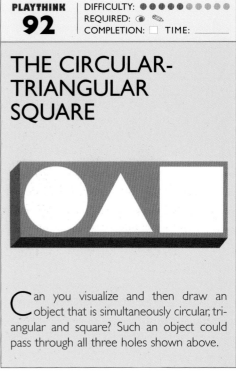

Can you visualize and then draw an object that is simultaneously circular, triangular and square? Such an object could pass through all three holes shown above.

PLAYTHINK
93

DIFFICULTY: ●●●●○○○○○○
REQUIRED: 👁 ✏
COMPLETION: ☐ TIME: _____

CUBES IN PERSPECTIVE

These eight colored figures represent cubes that have been drawn by tracing along the lines in the center grid. Through careful observation, can you retrace the lines to re-create each figure?

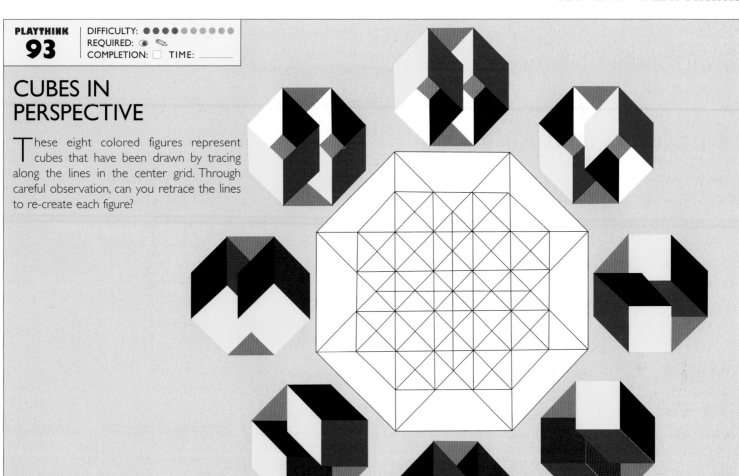

PLAYTHINK
94

DIFFICULTY: ●●●●●●○○○○
REQUIRED: 👁 ✏
COMPLETION: ☐ TIME: _____

COLORING SOLIDS

Each of the sixteen objects seen in outline is formed from two blocks and one wedge. Fill in the colors of the objects, using the colors and orientation of the cubes and wedge shown in the inset as a guide. Both parallel sides of the wedge are green, and the two hidden sides are white.

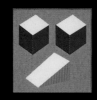

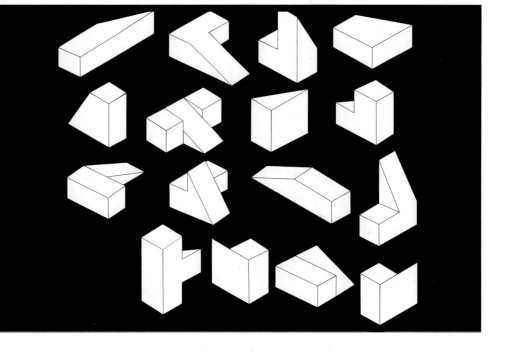

"**G**EOMETRY **G**ENLIGHTENS THE INTELLECT AND SETS ONE'S MIND RIGHT. ALL ITS PROOFS ARE VERY CLEAR AND ORDERLY. . . . IN THIS CONVENIENT WAY, THE PERSON WHO KNOWS GEOMETRY ACQUIRES INTELLIGENCE. IT HAS BEEN ASSUMED THAT THE FOLLOWING STATEMENT WAS WRITTEN UPON PLATO'S DOOR: '**N**O ONE WHO IS NOT A GEOMETRICIAN MAY ENTER OUR HOUSE.'"

—IBN KHALDUN

PLAYTHINK 95

DIFFICULTY: ●●●○○○○○○○
REQUIRED: ◉
COMPLETION: ☐ TIME: _____

BLUEPRINT AND SOLIDS

For each group of objects, can you find the one that was constructed by folding the pattern provided?

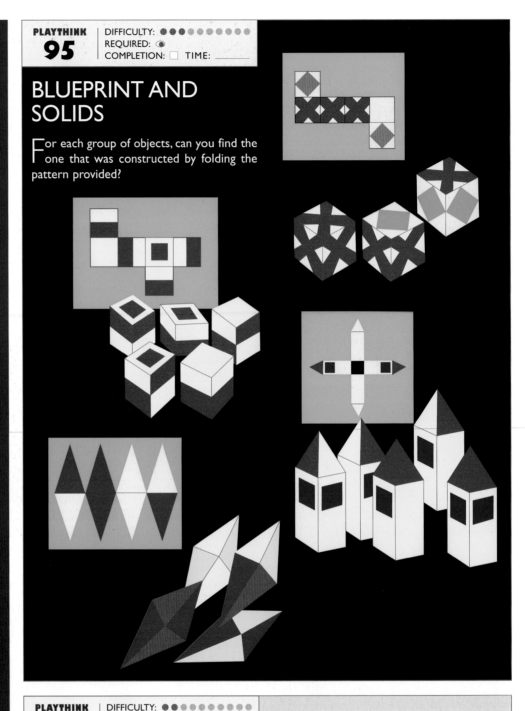

PLAYTHINK 96

DIFFICULTY: ●●○○○○○○○○
REQUIRED: ◉
COMPLETION: ☐ TIME: _____

ANOTHER POINT OF VIEW

This is a form of anamorphic projection, in which the image is distorted in such a way that it makes sense only when seen from the proper angle. Can you tell what this image is?

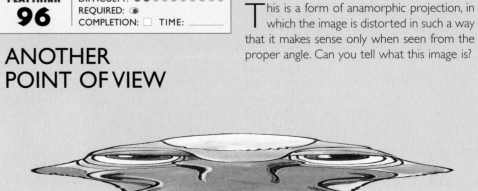

PLAYTHINK
97
DIFFICULTY: ●●●●●●○○○○
REQUIRED: 👁 ✎
COMPLETION: ☐ TIME: _____

WHAT'S IN THE SQUARE?

An artist has constructed a sculpture from colored plastic sheets attached to a three-dimensional wire frame. From most perspectives the sculpture looks chaotic. But can you envision what it looks like if seen from the red point on the left of the image? You can use the empty frame at right as a guide to solving the puzzle.

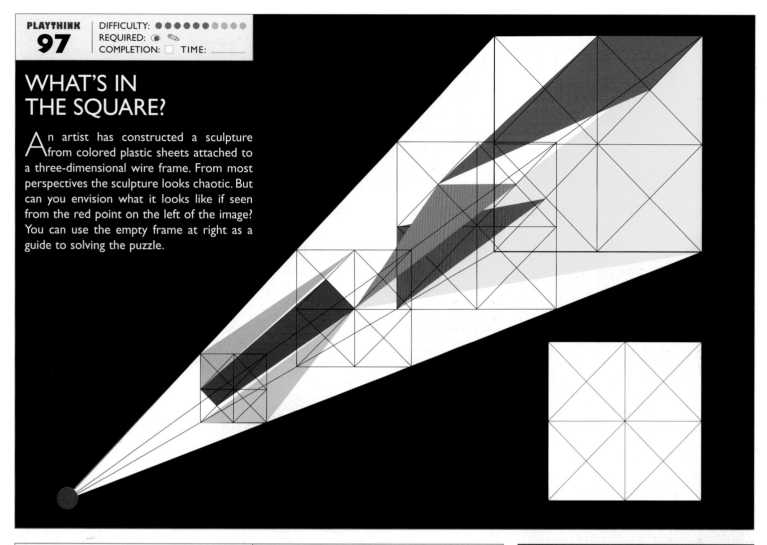

PLAYTHINK
98
DIFFICULTY: ●●○○○○○○○○
REQUIRED: 👁 ✎
COMPLETION: ☐ TIME: _____

PASCAL'S TRIANGLE

Can you uncover the logical basis for the triangular number pattern shown here and complete the last two rows? Can you add even more rows?

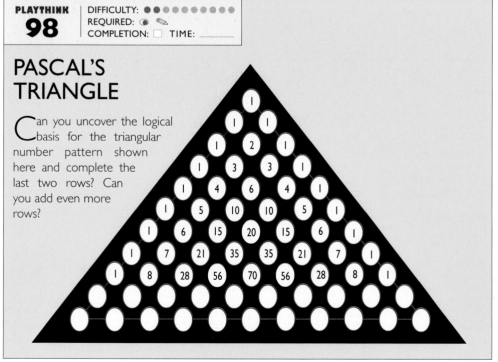

> **"U**BI MATERIA, UBI GEOMETRIA. (WHERE THERE IS MATTER, THERE IS GEOMETRY.)"
> —JOHANNES KEPLER

PLAYTHINK
99
DIFFICULTY: ●●●●●●○○○○
REQUIRED: ◉ ✎
COMPLETION: ☐ TIME: _____

TAXICAB GEOMETRY SQUARES

In Euclidean geometry squares can have only one shape. Does that rule hold up in taxicab geometry?

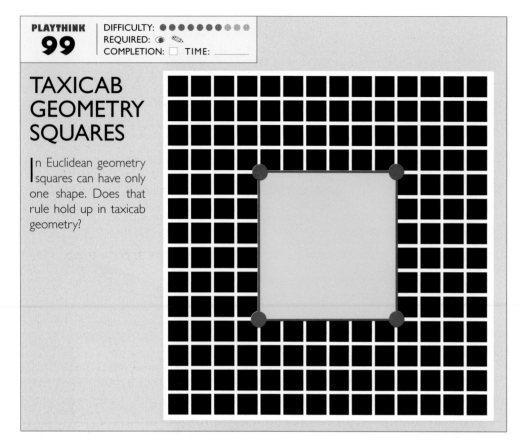

PLAYTHINK
100
DIFFICULTY: ●●●●●●●○○○
REQUIRED: ◉ ✎
COMPLETION: ☐ TIME: _____

TAXICAB ROUTES

Imagine you drive a taxicab in Gridlock City. Your cab is called to visit three places in succession and return back to the garage. The points on the map are marked 1 for the garage and 2, 3 and 4 for the pick-up points. Can you find the shortest route that will accomplish this task? Are there alternative routes you could take?

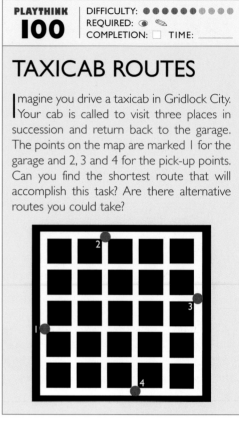

Early Geometry

Early humans learned how to build structures more efficiently by simple trial and error. And when the ancient Egyptians added a great deal of ingenuity to the mix, they accomplished wondrous feats of architecture and engineering—and in the process developed the first form of geometry.

Later in antiquity, Greek geometers were absorbed in the study of simple forms—the circle, the square, the triangle. Armed with only compass and ruler, they set out to find geometric truths; by 350 B.C. Euclid had compiled a set of rules concerning space and shapes that dominated geometry for 2,000 years.

Although early Greek geometers made huge theoretical advances, the mathematician Eratosthenes, who lived in Alexandria, Egypt, in the third century B.C., accomplished perhaps the greatest practical achievement. He learned that on a day in midsummer in the town of Syene (near present-day Aswan), the reflection of the noonday sun was visible on the water of a deep well. For that to occur, the sun had to be directly overhead, with its rays pointed directly toward the center of the earth. On the same day the noonday sun cast shadows in Alexandria that measured 7.5 degrees, or about one part in fifty of a full circle. Eratosthenes knew that sunbeams travel in parallel straight lines and so deduced that the difference in the angles was caused by the curvature of the earth. Once Eratosthenes found the distance north to south between Alexandria and Syene, which is about 480 miles, he multiplied that distance by fifty to determine the circumference of the circle that passes through those two towns and the North and South Poles—in other words, the circumference of the earth. His estimate, about 24,000 miles, was remarkably accurate.

Taxicab Geometry

Understanding non-Euclidean geometries can be a formidable task. One approachable non-Euclidean geometry is the so-called taxicab geometry, which you can explore with a city map or even ordinary graph paper. Imagine Gridlock City, in which the streets run either north-south or east-west. (Many cities established in the nineteenth century possess just that sort of grid.) To get around Gridlock City by taxicab, one must measure distances not "as the crow flies" but "as the cab drives"—along the lines of the square grid. Taxicab distances are in general longer than ordinary distances except when you drive from one end of a street to the other.

If Gridlock City is made up of straight lines on a plane, how can it be non-Euclidean? One of Euclid's axioms states that the shortest distance between two points is a straight line. Is that the case in Gridlock City? In fact, the shortest path in most cases is a series of short lines, since travel is restricted to the street grid. You must drive around blocks, not through them.

PLAYTHINK	DIFFICULTY: ●●●●●○○○○○
101	REQUIRED: ◉ ✎
	COMPLETION: ☐ TIME: _____

GRIDLOCK CITY

Aman who lives at the top right corner of this city district works in the bottom left corner. What is the shortest path to his office? How many different routes can he take?

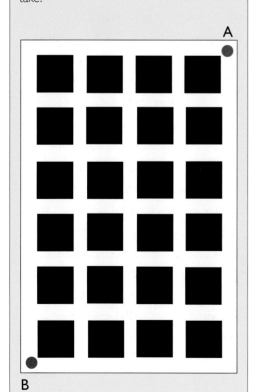

PLAYTHINK	DIFFICULTY: ●●●●●●○○○○
102	REQUIRED: ◉ ✎
	COMPLETION: ☐ TIME: _____

TAXICAB GEOMETRY CIRCLES

In Gridlock City you can move around only in blocks. Does that mean it is impossible to have a circle?

By definition a circle is a shape in which all points are equidistant from a fixed point. Suppose that there are six blocks to a kilometer in Gridlock City and you travel a kilometer by taxi from the center of the city. Where do you end up?

You could travel six blocks due east and stop. Or you could go five blocks east and one block north, or four blocks east and two blocks north. All those points lie on the "taxicab circle" of radius I kilometer.

Can you plot the shape of such a circle?

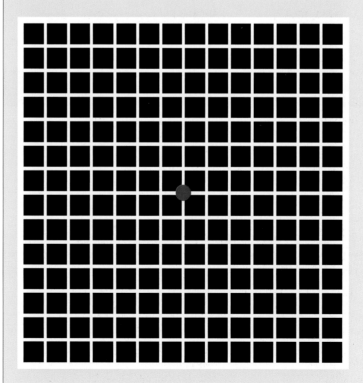

PLAYTHINK 103

DIFFICULTY: ●●●●●●●●●●
REQUIRED: ◉ 📄 ✂
COMPLETION: ☐ TIME: _____

FACE IT: THE PUZZLE OF VANISHING FACES

Copy and cut out the thirty-six tiles and place them on a six-by-six game board. In the configuration shown here, there are twelve complete faces—five smiling, seven frowning. Can you rearrange the tiles so that you add a thirteenth face and make nine frowning faces and four smiling ones? Can you change the mood so that there are nine smiling faces and only four frowning ones? Or nine smiling faces and only three frowning ones?

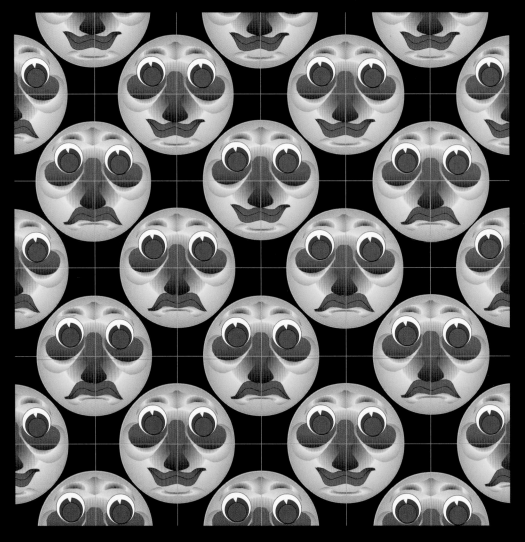

PLAYTHINK 104

DIFFICULTY: ●●●●●●●●●●
REQUIRED: ◉
COMPLETION: ☐ TIME: _____

FACE IT: THE GAME OF VANISHING FACES

The "Face It" puzzle tiles lend themselves to making a simple but subtly rewarding game. The object of the game is for each player to form smiling faces looking in his or her direction. Up to four persons may play, each sitting on a different side of the board. The tiles are mixed and placed face down. Players take turns selecting a tile and placing it on the board

alongside one or more tiles already played. Each tile played must create a proper face match with one of the tiles next to it. The scores are tallied at the end of play. Each smile facing a player counts as one point; each frown facing the player costs a point.

In the sample game shown here, play has ended because no more pieces can be placed on the board. There is no single winner. Player 1 is faced by two smiles and three frowns, for a score of minus one. All the other players are faced by one smiling face, for a score of one a piece. Note that some of the faces are mixed or incomplete and thus don't count toward the final scores.

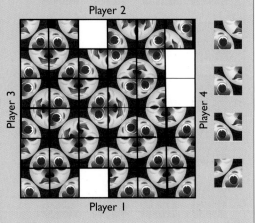

Worlds of Two Dimensions

Astrophysicists say that the universe possesses four dimensions—three of space and one of time—and some recent theories have suggested that there may be even more dimensions exerting an influence at the subatomic scale.

How can we begin to understand hypothetical higher dimensions? By getting outside our normal system. In this case, try to imagine a world that has only *two* dimensions.

In 1884 Edwin A. Abbott, an English clergyman and popularizer of science, made a beautiful attempt to describe a world made up of only two dimensions. In his satirical novel, called *Flatland,* the characters are basic geometric figures gliding over the surface of an infinite two-dimensional plane—a vast tabletop. Apart from a negligible thickness, Flatlanders have no perception of the third or any higher dimension.

Although Abbott did not describe any of the physical laws or technological innovations of Flatland, his book spawned sequels that tackle those issues. One such book, *An Episode of Flatland,* written by Charles Howard Hinton in 1885, cleverly extends Abbott's original.

The action in Hinton's book takes place on the apparently two-dimensional planet Astria. Astria is simply a giant circle, and its inhabitants live on the circumference, forever facing in one direction. All males face east, and all females face west. To see what is behind him, an Astrian must bend over backward, stand on his or her head or use a mirror.

Astria is divided between two nations, the civilized Unaeans in the east and the barbaric Scythians in the west. When the two nations go to war, the Scythians have an enormous advantage: they can strike the Unaeans from the back. The unfortunate and helpless Unaeans are driven to a narrow region bordering the great ocean. Facing complete extinction, the Unaeans are saved by a scientific advance: their astronomers have discovered that the planet is round. A group of Unaeans cross the ocean and carry out a surprise attack on the Scythians, who have never before been attacked from the rear. The Unaeans are thus able to defeat their foes.

Over the course of the book, Hinton fleshed out the details of his world. Houses in Astria can have only one opening. A tube or pipe is impossible. Ropes cannot be knotted, although levers, hooks and pendulums can be used.

In Alexander Dewdney's 1984 book, *The Planiverse,* the ideas of *Flatland* are taken to their contemporary conclusion. Dewdney, a computer scientist at the University of Western Ontario, lays down the complete theoretical base for a possible two-dimensional world in a beautiful synthesis of science, art and mathematics.

PLAYTHINK 105

DIFFICULTY: ●●●●●●○○○○
REQUIRED: ◉
COMPLETION: ☐   TIME: _____

FLATLAND HIERARCHY

In *Flatland,* Edwin Abbott describes a society of geometric shapes subject to a strict hierarchy. Ladies are sharp straight lines; soldiers and workmen are isosceles triangles; middle-class people are equilateral triangles; professionals are either squares or pentagons; the wealthy are hexagons; and the top of the class system—the high priests—are circles.

Of course, since ladies are one-dimensional lines, they are invisible from some directions and may be hazardous to run into. How do you think the Flatlanders avoid this problem?

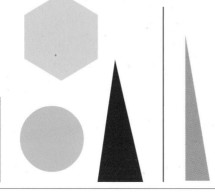

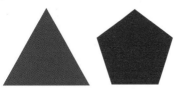

PLAYTHINK 106

DIFFICULTY: ●●●●●○○○○○
REQUIRED: ◉
COMPLETION: ☐ TIME: _____

FLATLAND CATASTROPHE

The senses of Flatlanders are limited to two dimensions. So if someone were to observe them from a point just "above" their world, the Flatlanders would have no way of seeing that observer.

But what if you tossed a ball through the two-dimensional plane of Flatland? Would the Flatlanders perceive the event as some sort of astronomical catastrophe? Can you describe exactly what they would see?

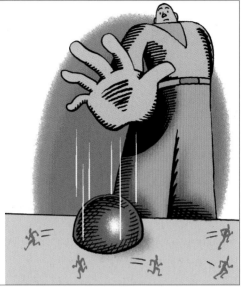

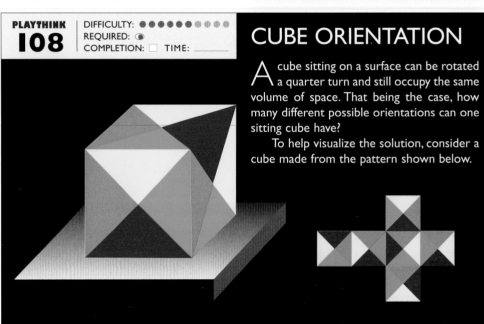

"*GEOMETRIA EST GARCHETYPUS PULCHRITUDINIS MUNDI.* (GEOMETRY IS THE ARCHETYPE OF THE BEAUTY OF THE WORLD.)"

—JOHANNES KEPLER

PLAYTHINK 107

DIFFICULTY: ●●○○○○○○○○
REQUIRED: ◉
COMPLETION: ☐ TIME: _____

FLATLAND PLAYPEN

The two toddlers on the facing pages of this book will cry until they can play together. How can you make them happy without removing one from the crib or the other from the high chair?

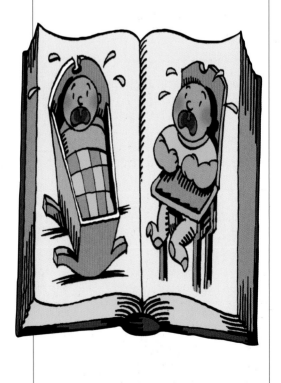

PLAYTHINK 108

DIFFICULTY: ●●●●●●○○○○
REQUIRED: ◉
COMPLETION: ☐ TIME: _____

CUBE ORIENTATION

A cube sitting on a surface can be rotated a quarter turn and still occupy the same volume of space. That being the case, how many different possible orientations can one sitting cube have?

To help visualize the solution, consider a cube made from the pattern shown below.

PLAYTHINK 109

DIFFICULTY: ●●●●●●●●○○
REQUIRED: ◉
COMPLETION: ☐ TIME: _____

DODECAHEDRON ORIENTATION

A dodecahedron is a regular polyhedron made up of twelve pentagonal sides. When the ancient Pythagoreans discovered the dodecahedron, they guarded it as a great secret—and anyone who disclosed its existence was punished by death.

If a dodecahedron that sits on a surface makes a 72-degree turn, it will occupy the same volume of space. That being the case, how many different possible orientations can one sitting dodecahedron have?

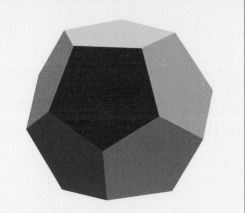

Symmetry

Objects that possess symmetry—the ability to undergo certain geometric transformations without changing form—are found throughout nature. The most perfect natural examples of symmetry are in the arrangements of atoms and molecules in crystals; a common example is the snowflake, which possesses many axes of symmetry. Biological creatures also display a remarkable amount of symmetry. Fivefold or pentagonal symmetry is found in many marine flowers and animals, such as the sea star, or starfish, which has five, ten or even twenty-three symmetric arms.

We human beings, who are roughly symmetric about one axis, the spine, display bilateral symmetry—the most common form of symmetry in nature. (Biologists believe we are programmed to recognize symmetry, which is why we judge highly symmetrical faces and bodies to be more beautiful than asymmetrical ones.)

Objects that look the same as they are rotated about an axis have rotational symmetry; an equilateral triangle, for instance, will appear identical in three different positions as it rotates around a point at its center. Objects with lateral symmetry can be reflected on either side of a line or axis without appearing different.

We can easily make symmetrical patterns by folding and cutting paper or by using plane mirrors—what child hasn't made snowflakes or paper dolls that way?—but symmetry is also an enormously important mathematical tool. Scientists could never have determined the structure of viruses and molecules without a full understanding of symmetry; neither could they have built the standard model of particle physics.

> "SYMMETRY IS ONE IDEA BY WHICH MAN THROUGH THE AGES HAS TRIED TO COMPREHEND AND CREATE ORDER, BEAUTY AND PERFECTION."
> —HERMANN WEYL

PLAYTHINK 110

DIFFICULTY: ●●●●●●●●●●
REQUIRED: 👁 ✎
COMPLETION: ☐ TIME: _____

SYMMETRY SQUARES

Both of these images are symmetrical—but some of the squares have been erased.

In the near image, by carefully observing the position of the black squares in relation to the red line, which is the axis of vertical symmetry, you should be able to fill in the rest of the picture.

In the far image, by carefully observing the position of the blue squares in relation to the two red lines, which are the axes of vertical and horizontal symmetry, you should be able to fill in the rest of the picture.

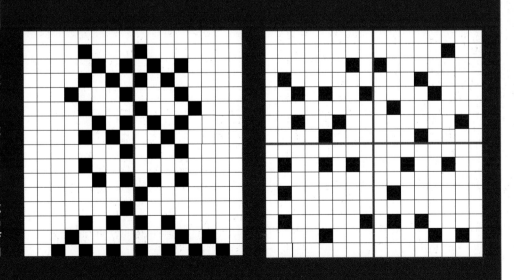

PLAYTHINK
111

DIFFICULTY: ●●●●●○○○○○
REQUIRED: ◉ ✎ 📄 ✂
COMPLETION: ☐ TIME:

SYMMETRY OF THE SQUARE AND STAR

Cut out a square and a star and color them as shown on both sides, making sure that the red areas are red both front and back and that the yellow areas are yellow both front and back.

How many different ways can you place the square and the star in their respective outlines at right? Mathematicians call this sort of movement a transformation.

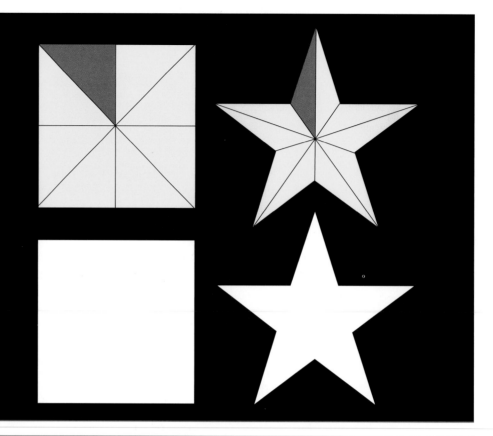

PLAYTHINK
112

DIFFICULTY: ●●●●●●●○○○
REQUIRED: ◉
COMPLETION: ☐ TIME: _____

PLACING COINS

Two players take turns placing identical coins on a perfectly round table. The first player who cannot put a coin on the table without overlapping an existing coin loses. Can you devise a strategy so that one of the players will always win, no matter how large the table is?

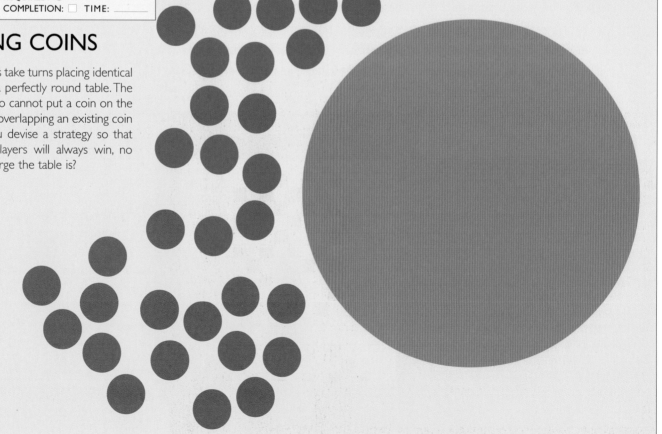

Isometries of the Plane

A transformation of the plane is a movement of its points. There are many types of transformations, but the most important are the rigid motions, or isometries, which move figures but do not change their size or shape. (Note that an isometry that leaves the object looking the same is called a symmetry.) There are four basic types of isometries of the plane:

Translation

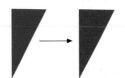

The red and blue triangles are congruent, which means they are exactly identical and that one transformation may superimpose one upon the other. In this case the blue triangle may slide onto the red one without turning. That is called translation.

Rotation

In this instance the congruent triangles can be superimposed by turning one of them around a point at one vertex. That is called rotation.

Reflection

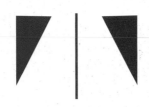

The red and blue triangles are mirror images of each other. No motion within the plane of the triangles will allow one to be superimposed on the other. But what if you could lift one off the plane and turn it over, much like turning a page in a book? That is what occurs during reflection.

Glide Reflection

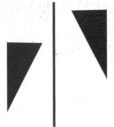

Glide reflection is simply the combination of reflection and translation.

SYMMETRICAL FLOOR

This floor is made of identical square tiles, each of which is diagonally divided into red and yellow. If the floor is symmetrical about the red axes, can you fill in the rest of the tiles to find the overall pattern?

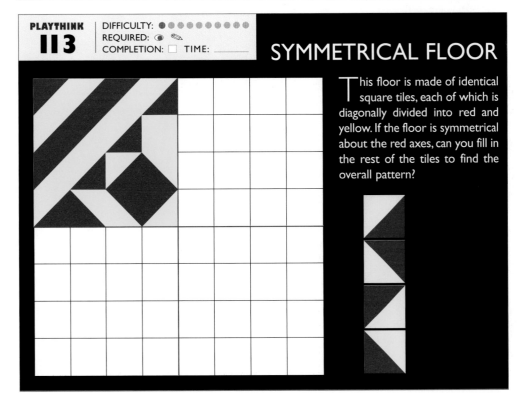

REFLECTION-REVERSAL

In each row the tiles in this pattern are supposed to be the reflected and inverted image of the tiles to their left. That is, the colors are to be reversed and the tile flipped along the vertical axis. Which tile does not follow that rule?

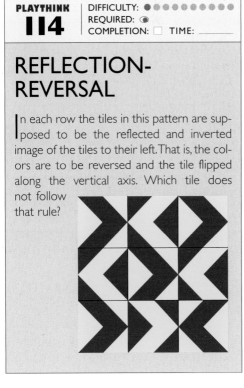

PLAYTHINK 115

DIFFICULTY: ●●●●●●●○○○○
REQUIRED: ◉
COMPLETION: ☐ TIME: _____

FITTING HOLES

How many different ways can the seven flat shapes fit into the holes at right? Treat each piece like a three-dimensional object of considerable thickness that can undergo every sort of normal manipulation.

isosceles triangle			
scalene triangle			
equilateral triangle			
square			
greek cross			
rhombus			
parallelogram			

PLAYTHINK 116

DIFFICULTY: ●●●●●○○○○○○
REQUIRED: ◉
COMPLETION: ☐ TIME: _____

ALPHABET I

What do the red letters have in common? What do the blue letters have in common?

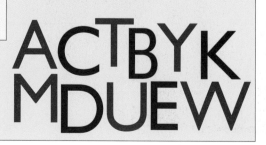

ACTBYK
MDUEW

PLAYTHINK 117

DIFFICULTY: ●●●●●●●●○○○
REQUIRED: ◉ ✎
COMPLETION: ☐ TIME: _____

SYMMETRY AXES

Symmetrical patterns can be found by folding and cutting paper or by using a plane mirror. For each of the thirteen shapes shown below, find and draw the symmetry axes. Are some figures not symmetrical? Which shape has the most symmetry axes?

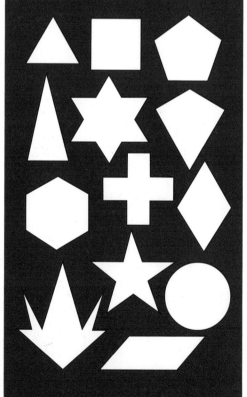

PLAYTHINK
118

DIFFICULTY: ●●●●●●○○○○○
REQUIRED: 👁 ✎
COMPLETION: ☐ TIME: _____

SYMMETRY CRAFT

This image with three red lines as an indication of rotational and reflectional symmetry (the axis of which points straight up) has had most of its colored tiles removed. Even so, enough remain for you to reconstruct the original image by following the rules of symmetry. Can you color the tiles correctly?

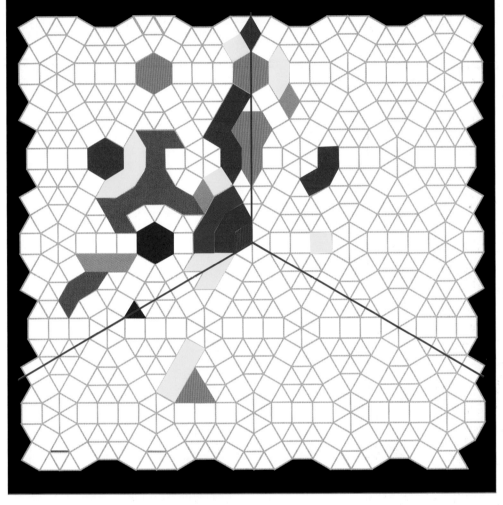

PLAYTHINK
119

DIFFICULTY: ●●●○○○○○○○○
REQUIRED: 👁 ✎
COMPLETION: ☐ TIME: _____

SYMMETRY ALPHABET

Can you draw the symmetry axes for the capital letters of the alphabet? If the letter is rotationally symmetrical, draw the point of rotation. Leave asymmetrical letters unmarked.

ABCD EFGH IJKL MNO PQRS TUVW XYZ

PLAYTHINK
120

DIFFICULTY: ●●○○○○○○○○○
REQUIRED: 👁
COMPLETION: ☐ TIME: _____

MYSTERY SIGNS

Can you decipher the mystery signs and read the secret word? A small mirror may help.

PLAYTHINK
121

DIFFICULTY: ●●●○○○○○○○○
REQUIRED: 👁
COMPLETION: ☐ TIME: _____

ALPHABET 2

What's the difference between the red letters and the blue letters?

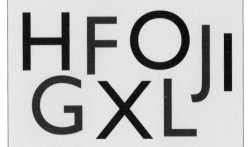

PLAYTHINK 122

DIFFICULTY: ●●●○○○○○○○
REQUIRED: ◉
COMPLETION: ☐ TIME: _____

ALPHABET 3

What is the difference between the red letters and the blue letters?

NpSRZQ

PLAYTHINK 123

DIFFICULTY: ●○○○○○○○○○
REQUIRED: ◉ 📄 ✂
COMPLETION: ☐ TIME: _____

TRANSCLOWN: GAME OF A THOUSAND FACES

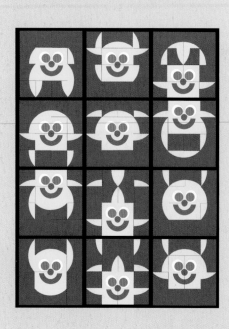

Create a set of tiles like the fourteen shown below and place them in the basic starting configuration.

The object of the game is to transform the starting image into one of the twelve faces on the cards shown below left. Players take turns sliding two or more tiles horizontally or vertically into the empty spaces—taking care to preserve the symmetry of the picture at all times. No piece can leave the four-by-four grid, but several pieces may move at once, with some of the pieces filling the void left by other pieces as they move into the empty spaces.

During each turn a player may make five moves. Every time a player re-creates one of the faces on the card, that player takes the card. The winner is the player who has taken the most cards.

According to the rules of the game, which of the twelve faces is it impossible to re-create?

The Golden Rectangle

The ancient Greeks discovered a rectangle with unique properties. If you subtract from the rectangle a square with sides equal to the short side of the rectangle, you are left with a new, smaller rectangle whose sides are in the same ratio as the original. The Greeks believed that the two sides of that rectangle bore a divine relationship and called the proportion from one to another the golden ratio. That ratio, approximately 1.6180037, is often symbolized by the Greek letter φ, much the same way the number 3.14159 . . . is symbolized by π.

The golden ratio shows up in the growth patterns of many plants and animals. For example, the growth of the nautilus shell follows the same pattern as the logarithmic spiral formed by the golden rectangle.

PLAYTHINK
124
DIFFICULTY: ●●●●●●●●○○
REQUIRED: ◉ ✎
COMPLETION: ☐ TIME: _____

GOLDEN TRIANGLE

Draw all the diagonals in a regular penta-gon. You have created a five-pointed pentagonal star known as the pentagram. Since pentagonal symmetry is found through-out nature—in plants and in animals such as the starfish—it is sometimes called the sym-metry of life.

Because the secret from which the golden rectangle and golden triangle could be created lies within the pentagram, it was the secret symbol of Pythagoras and his followers. To begin to understand its mystery, figure out the proportion of the sides of the pentagon to the sides of the pentagram.

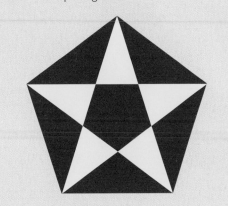

PLAYTHINK
125
DIFFICULTY: ●●●●●●●●○○
REQUIRED: ◉ ✎
COMPLETION: ☐ TIME: _____

SYMMETRY OF THE CUBE

The cube has many more rotational symmetries than a two-dimensional figure. Can you find them all?

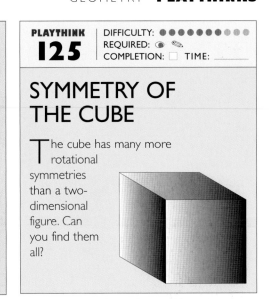

PLAYTHINK
126
DIFFICULTY: ●●●●●●●●○○
REQUIRED: ◉ ✎
COMPLETION: ☐ TIME: _____

ISOMETRIX: THE SHAPE GAME

There are two boards used in this game: a stationary base with holes cut into it (bottom right) and a similar board (bottom left) that is placed atop the base and revolves around its center point. Initially there are sixty-four shapes that fit in the holes of the revolving board: sixteen squares, sixteen right isosceles triangles, sixteen circles and sixteen semicircles.

See if you can use your mind's eye to track the revolving board as it makes one complete turn. Some of the shapes will fall through the board right away; others will fall through after the first quarter turn in the clockwise direction. Still more will fall through after a full half turn. Can you fill in the table at right for the number of each type of shape that falls after each quarter turn? Can you discover which shape or shapes will stay on after a whole turn?

Number of shapes initially on top	16	16	16	16
SHAPES	■	◪	●	◗
Number of shapes initially falling through	☐	☐	☐	☐
Number of shapes falling through after ¹/₄ turn clockwise	☐	☐	☐	☐
Number of shapes falling through after ¹/₂ turn clockwise	☐	☐	☐	☐
Number of shapes falling through after ³/₄ turn clockwise	☐	☐	☐	☐
Number of shapes falling through after one full turn clockwise	☐	☐	☐	☐
Number of shapes staying on top	☐	☐	☐	☐

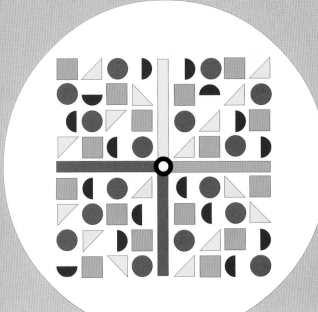

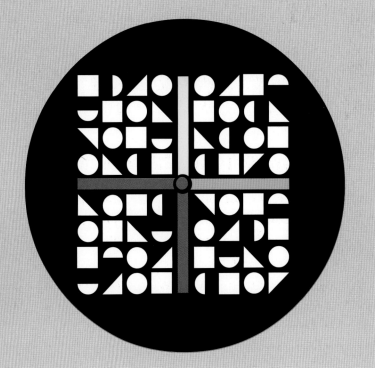

PLAYTHINK
127

DIFFICULTY: ●●○○○○○○○○○
REQUIRED: ✎ 📄 ✂
COMPLETION: ☐   TIME: _____

BILATERAL SYMMETRY GAME

■ *For one or more players*

Copy and cut out ten each of the shapes shown at right: an equilateral triangle, a square, a regular pentagon and a regular hexagon. (Note that the sides of every shape must be identical.) Mix the shapes and stack them in one pile.

The object is to build a symmetrical pattern. The players take turns picking the top two shapes from the pile and placing them next to the pieces already laid down, sides touching, so that they preserve the pattern's overall symmetry along the vertical symmetry axis. If the pieces cannot be placed symmetrically, they must go into the player's discard pile. The game continues until all the pieces have been used or no other pieces may be added to the pattern. The player with the fewest pieces in his or her discard pile wins.

In this sample game, one of the players loses by not being able to place the last blue square in his discard pile.

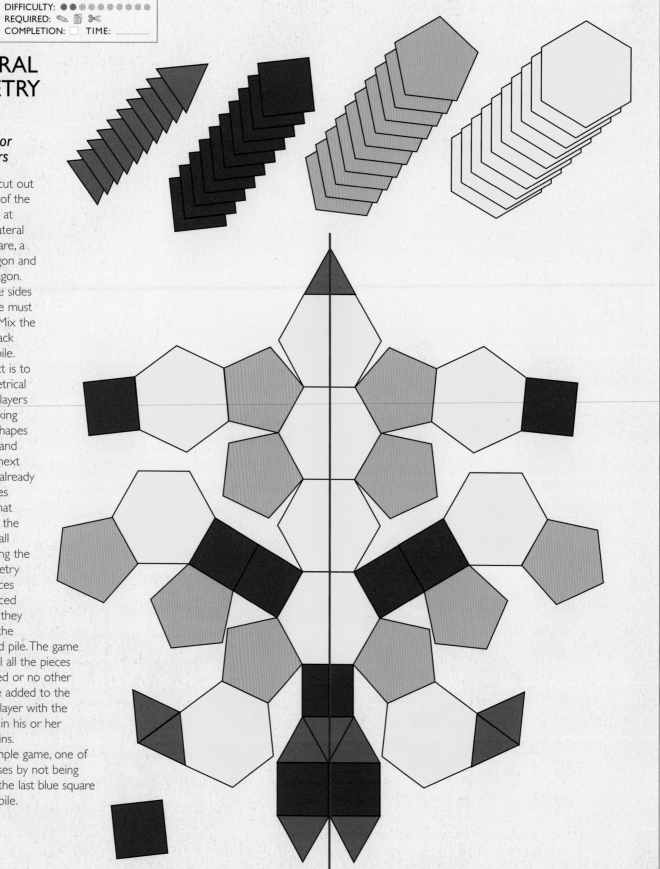

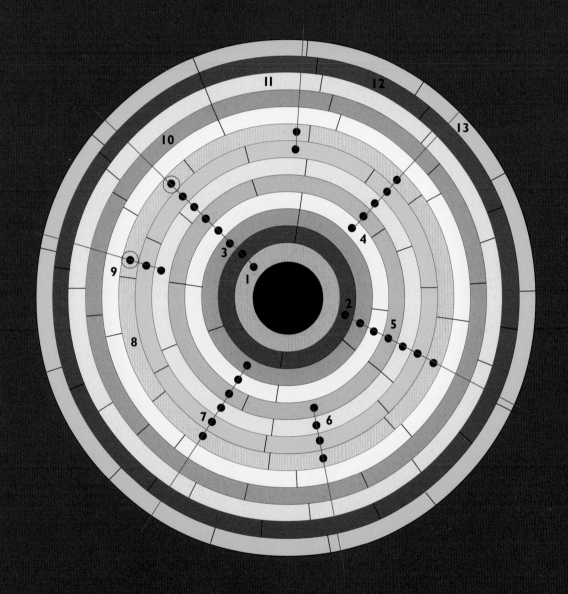

The Basic Tools of Geometry

Points are not just marks—they are mathematical symbols that define position. And lines are not only the fundamental elements of drawn images but also mathematical symbols that link points, indicate distance and direction and define space. Points and lines—and the relationships between them—are the basic tools of geometry.

The ancient Greeks had to turn geometry from the practical study of measuring land to the science of abstract form before they could produce mathematical proofs. They "idealized" points and lines, thereby creating an abstract world to which the laws of geometry could apply with perfect accuracy. And they understood that they could obtain real conclusions from that idealized world only by making geometry deductive—that is, based on axioms. Euclid's *Elements*, the greatest work of Greek geometry, was for centuries the ultimate textbook of human reasoning. Indeed, it was not until well into the nineteenth century that Georg Cantor took the final step of including every possible form and shape into geometry.

PLAYTHINK 128

DIFFICULTY: ●●●●●●●●●○○
REQUIRED: ◉ ✎
COMPLETION: ☐ TIME: _____

THE THIRTEEN-POINT GAME

Imagine that there is a circular strip of land on which someone has planted one tree. Divide the strip in half and plant a tree somewhere on the half that doesn't have a tree. Then divide the strip into thirds and plant a tree on the third of the strip that is treeless.

How long can you keep this up? Can you divide the strip thirteen times so that each plot has its own tree?

The image shown at bottom left depicts thirteen concentric circles, but this is only for convenience. It is really the same strip of land seen after successive divisions.

A challenging two-player game can be played following this sequence: players can alternate placing marks (which symbolizes planting trees). Play continues until one player cannot plant a tree in an empty section.

The sample game at right ended after the eighth move because two marks wound up in the same section.

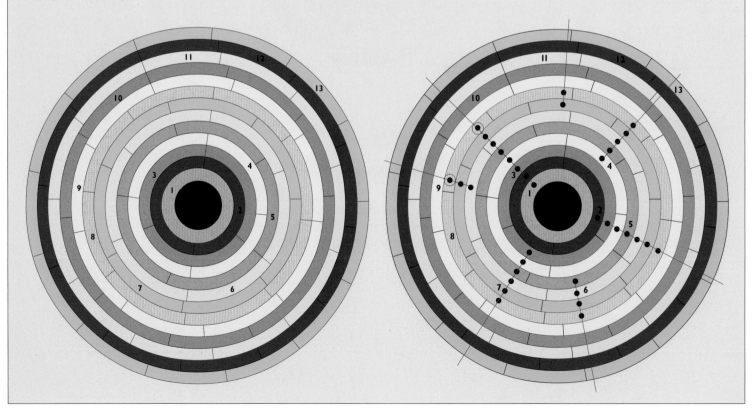

PLAYTHINK
129

DIFFICULTY: ●●●●●●●●●●
REQUIRED: ◉
COMPLETION: ☐ TIME: _____

MATCH THE LINES MATRIX

The patterns of lines at the top of the matrix were combined with the patterns of lines to the left of the matrix to create a new alphabet. Unfortunately, several errors crept into the combining process. Can you find them all?

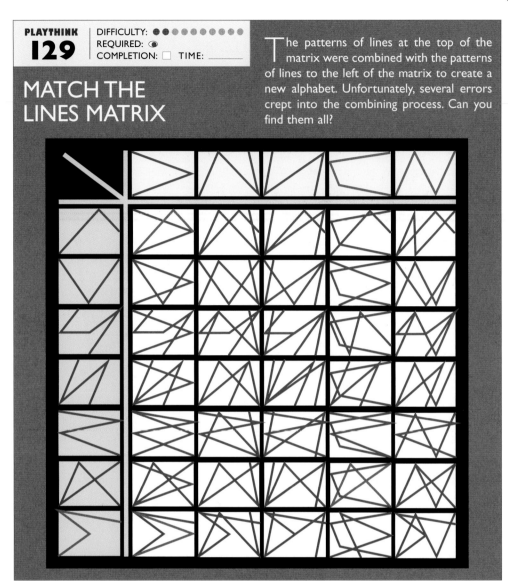

PLAYTHINK
130

DIFFICULTY: ●●●●●●●●●●
REQUIRED: ◉ ✎
COMPLETION: ☐ TIME: _____

THE SIX-LINE PROBLEM

The six lines in the figure to the right enclose eight triangles of three different sizes. Can you devise a way to draw six straight lines so that they enclose eight triangles of only two different sizes?

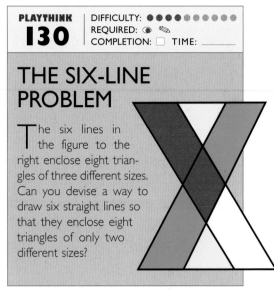

PLAYTHINK
131

DIFFICULTY: ●●●●●●●●●●
REQUIRED: ◉ ✎
COMPLETION: ☐ TIME: _____

LINES AND TRIANGLES

With three lines you can enclose one triangle; with four lines, four triangles. Can you enclose ten triangles by adding two more straight lines to the three shown here?

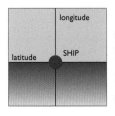

Dimensions

All of geometry begins with the point, which indicates a position on a two-dimensional plane or in three-dimensional space. The point, which is the intersection of two or more lines, is a pure abstraction. You must imagine that it is there.

The most fundamental concept in geometry is the idea of dimension.

The position of a car on a road can be indicated by a single number, its distance from some location—a milestone.

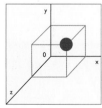

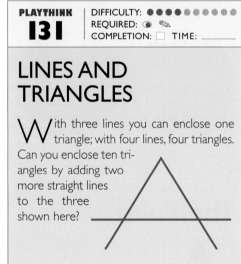

The location of a ship at sea can be determined by noting its latitude and longitude. Two dimensions, two numbers.

The position of a point in a room can be pinned down with three numbers, or coordinates—say, the distance from two of the walls and its height off the floor. Three-dimensional coordinates are usually given as x, y, and z.

PLAYTHINK
132
DIFFICULTY: ●●●●●●○○○○
REQUIRED: ◉
COMPLETION: ☐ TIME: _____

MYSTERY WHEELS

■ *Revolving Lines*

These straight colored lines have been taped to a turntable. When the turntable revolves, the lines will blur into new patterns. Can you envision what each of the four patterns will look like?

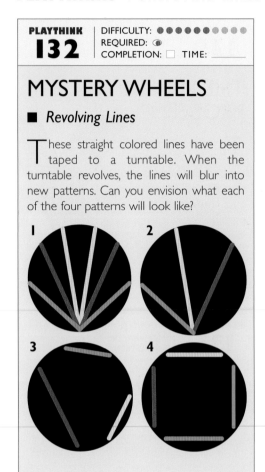

PLAYTHINK
133
DIFFICULTY: ●●●●●●●○○○
REQUIRED: ◉ ✎
COMPLETION: ☐ TIME: _____

KOBON TRIANGLES I

How many nonoverlapping triangles can you form by drawing six continuous straight lines? Can you do better than this example?

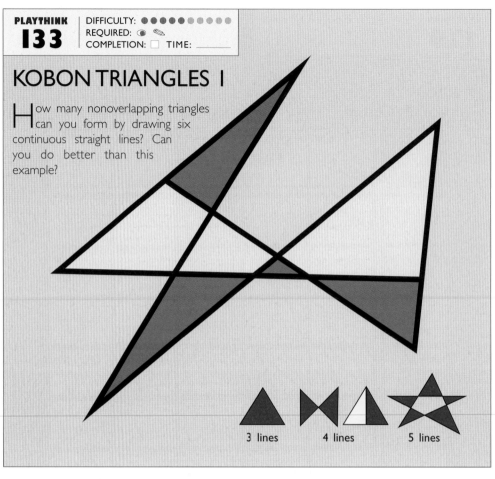

3 lines   4 lines   5 lines

The Point

At some point something must have come from nothing.

Inside the white box at right there is a point. Can you see it?

No, there's no printing error. Just because you cannot see the point doesn't mean it isn't there. The point

is an imaginary object, a purely abstract idea.

A point has no dimension and occupies no space. If a plane exists in two dimensions and a line in one dimension, then a point is a zero-dimensional object. Since it is difficult to refer to something you can't see, the point is usually represented by a dot, which is a small circle on a plane or a small sphere in three-dimensional space.

So a point is "nothing," but it is the fundamental particle from which all of geometry is built. Can it be said that geometry is built on an imaginary foundation?

Now that you have been introduced to the point, we can start constructing the beautiful and playful structure of geometry. For instance, it is now clear that within the white box there is not simply one point but an infinite number of points. That observation will soon be very important.

> " **A**T SOME POINT **A**SOMETHING MUST HAVE COME FROM NOTHING. "

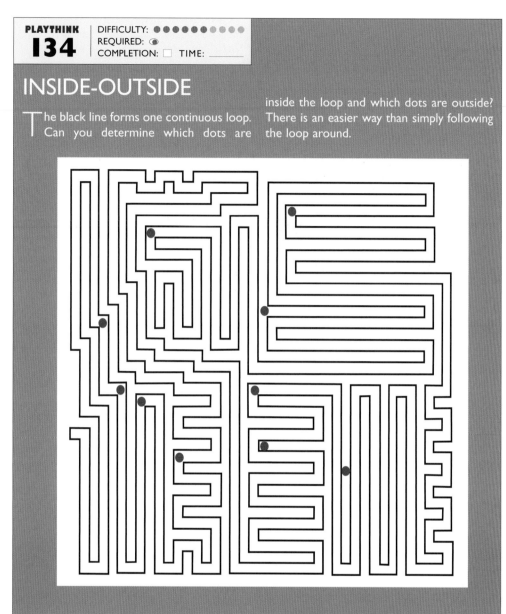

INSIDE-OUTSIDE

The black line forms one continuous loop. Can you determine which dots are inside the loop and which dots are outside? There is an easier way than simply following the loop around.

PAPPUS'S THEOREM

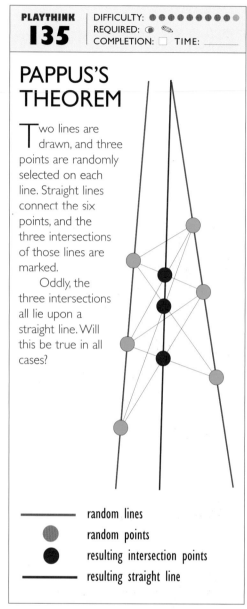

Two lines are drawn, and three points are randomly selected on each line. Straight lines connect the six points, and the three intersections of those lines are marked.

Oddly, the three intersections all lie upon a straight line. Will this be true in all cases?

—— random lines
● random points
● resulting intersection points
—— resulting straight line

CONVEX OR SIMPLE?

A convex polygon is one in which every point in the interior can be connected to any point on the perimeter with a straight line that does not cross the perimeter. A simple polygon is one in which no lines or sides cross each other. Working with that basic information, can you figure out how many convex polygons are shown in the drawing at right?

One of the lines or polygons depicted is different from all the others. Can you tell which one it is?

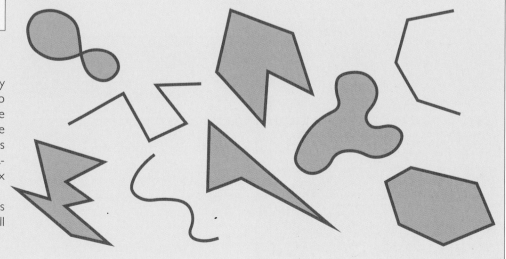

The Eighteen-Point Problem

Mathematicians sometimes invent seemingly simple, trivial-looking problems that prove much more difficult to solve than anyone dare think. One such conundrum is the eighteen-point paradox, first mentioned by Martin Gardner in his "Mathematical Games" section in *Scientific American* magazine.

The object is to distribute eighteen points along a line according to some simple rules. Lines, of course, comprise a multitude of points—indeed, an infinite number of points are on a line. So you might imagine that with sufficient foresight, one could place an infinite number of points on a line. That intuition, however, turns out to be wrong.

The rules of the game are quite simple: Place a point anywhere on the line. Now place a second point so that each of the two points lies on a different half of the line.

Then place a third point so that each of the three points is in a different third of the line. At this stage it becomes clear that the first two points cannot be just anywhere; the points must be placed carefully so that when the third point is added, each will be in a different third of the line.

The game follows a predictable pattern—place the fourth point so that all are on different quarters, the fifth so that all are on separate fifths, and so on. You can proceed with this process as carefully as you wish, but it turns out, astonishingly, that you cannot go beyond seventeen points. The eighteenth point will always violate the rules of the game.

Even when you choose the locations of your points very carefully, placing ten points is a good result. You are doing even better if you can solve the version of this paradox in "The Thirteen-Point Game" (page 54).

PLAYTHINK
137
DIFFICULTY: ●●●●●○○○○○
REQUIRED: ◉
COMPLETION: ☐ TIME: _____

CHEESE CUT

Can you cut this wheel of cheese into eight identical pieces with only three straight cuts?

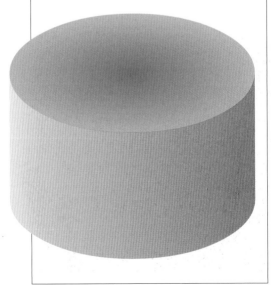

PLAYTHINK
138
DIFFICULTY: ●●●●●●○○○○
REQUIRED: ◉ ✎
COMPLETION: ☐ TIME: _____

KOBON TRIANGLES 2

How many nonoverlapping triangles can be enclosed by seven straight lines? The illustration shows a six-triangle solution. Can you do better?

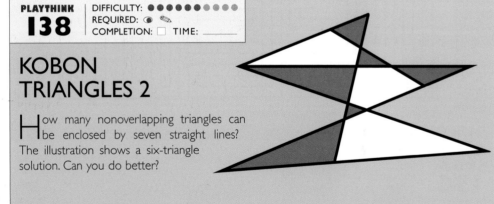

PLAYTHINK
139
DIFFICULTY: ●●●●●●●○○○
REQUIRED: ◉ ✎
COMPLETION: ☐ TIME: _____

KOBON TRIANGLES 3

How many nonoverlapping triangles can be enclosed by eight straight lines? The illustration shows a six-triangle solution. Can you do better?

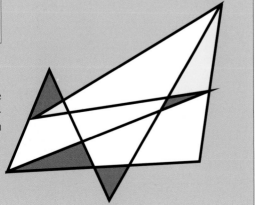

PLAYTHINK 140

DIFFICULTY: ●●●●●○○○○○
REQUIRED: 👁 ✎
COMPLETION: ☐ TIME: _____

GREAT DIVIDE 1

Four straight cuts can divide a cake into ten pieces, as shown below. Is it possible to go one better and divide the cake into eleven pieces?

Can you determine the general rule for finding the greatest number of regions that can be formed by a given number of straight cuts in a single plane?

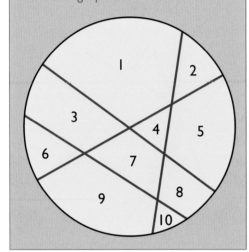

PLAYTHINK 141

DIFFICULTY: ●●●●●●○○○○
REQUIRED: 👁 ✎
COMPLETION: ☐ TIME: _____

GREAT DIVIDE 2

Five straight cuts are used to cut a cake into fifteen pieces. Can you cut the cake into sixteen pieces with only five cuts?

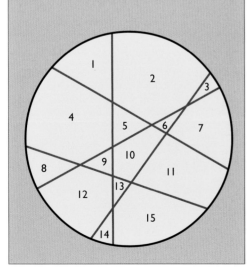

PLAYTHINK 142

DIFFICULTY: ●●●●●●●○○○
REQUIRED: 👁 ✎
COMPLETION: ☐ TIME: _____

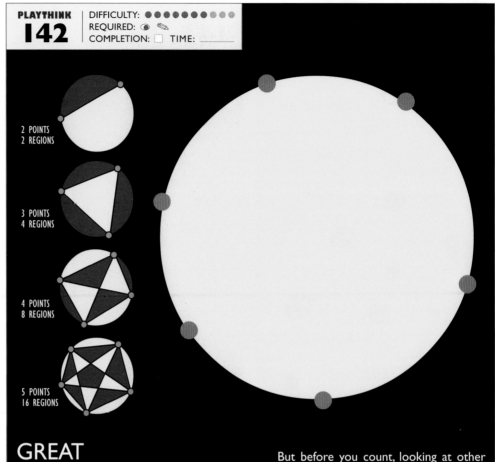

2 POINTS
2 REGIONS

3 POINTS
4 REGIONS

4 POINTS
8 REGIONS

5 POINTS
16 REGIONS

GREAT DIVIDE 3

The circle above has six points on its circumference. Join all the points with straight lines and count the number of regions those cords have partitioned.

But before you count, looking at other cases may help you estimate the answer. Illustrated are the solutions for two, three, four and five randomly selected points on the circle. Based on that simple doubling series, what would your estimate be for the problem of six points?

PLAYTHINK 143

DIFFICULTY: ●●●●●●○○○○
REQUIRED: 👁 ✎
COMPLETION: ☐ TIME: _____

CROSSED BOX

A ten-by-fourteen box is divided into 140 one-by-one compartments. A laser beam shines from the top left-hand corner of the box to the lower right-hand corner.

Without counting, can you work out how many compartments the laser will pass through?

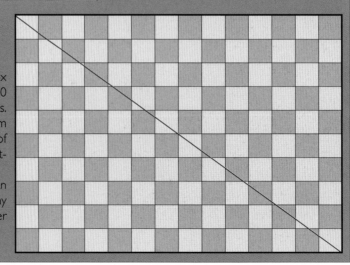

PLAYTHINK 144

DIFFICULTY: ●●●●●●○○○○
REQUIRED: ◉ ✎
COMPLETION: ☐ TIME: _____

LADYBUGS IN THE FIELD

Drawing just four straight lines across the circle, can you separate the eleven ladybugs into eleven individual compartments?

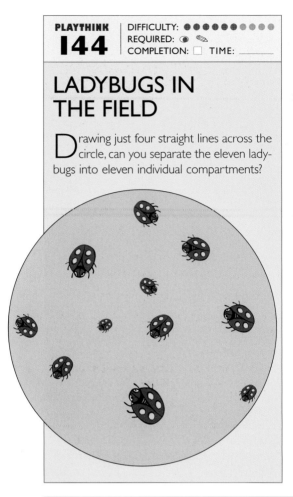

PLAYTHINK 145

DIFFICULTY: ●●●○○○○○○○
REQUIRED: ◉ ✎
COMPLETION: ☐ TIME: _____

LINE MEETS LINE

■ *Intersections*

The five lines shown below intersect at nine different points. Can you draw five lines that intersect at a total of ten points? What is the greatest number of intersections possible with just five lines?

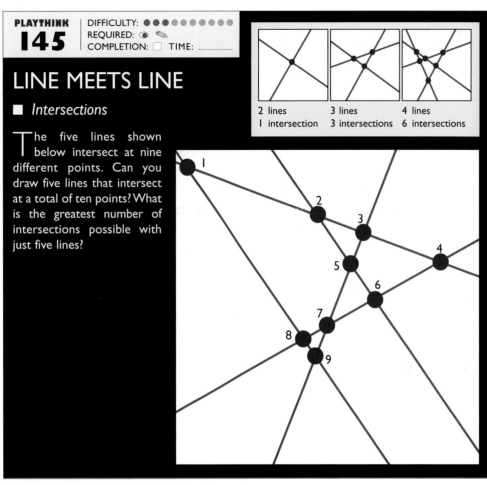

| 2 lines | 3 lines | 4 lines |
| 1 intersection | 3 intersections | 6 intersections |

Pappus's Theorem: The Power of the Moving Point

The great fourth-century mathematician Pappus of Alexandria first recognized that space could be filled with a moving point. A point moving in one dimension produces a straight line. That line moving in a direction perpendicular to the point defines a rectangle. And that rectangle moving in a direction at right angles to the point and the line creates a rectangular prism. This same concept can be extended to include points that move along curves to define complex areas and volumes. What's more, Pappus's theorem is the basis for the scanning mechanism that produces television images.

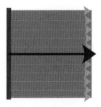

The dot creates a line when moving in one unit in some direction.

The line creates a square when moving one unit in a direction perpendicular to itself.

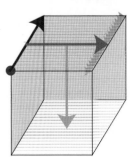

The square creates a cube when moving one unit in a direction perpendicular to itself.

Lines Through Dots

Let's see just how imaginative you are. Draw nine dots in a three-by-three square configuration. Then take your pencil and, without lifting it from the paper, draw a single line broken into no more than four straight segments that passes through all nine dots.

This problem appears to be impossible at first glance. Connecting eight of the nine points is easy, but connecting nine defies logic.

If you haven't discovered how to solve the problem, it may be because you have run into a conceptual block. Too often people confine themselves to a small number of possible solutions to a problem. For example, many people assume that the answer to this problem must consist of vertical and horizontal lines and that the lines must be confined to the "box" formed by the nine dots. But none of those

restrictions were mentioned as part of the problem.

Diagonals and lines that extend beyond the visual boundary of the problem provide a way toward a solution.

In the 1990s business consultants and politicians often referred to the search for innovative solutions as "thinking outside the box." That was an allusion to the solution to this seemingly impossible puzzle.

PLAYTHINK 146 | DIFFICULTY: ●●●●●○○○○○ REQUIRED: ◉ ✎ COMPLETION: ☐ TIME: _____

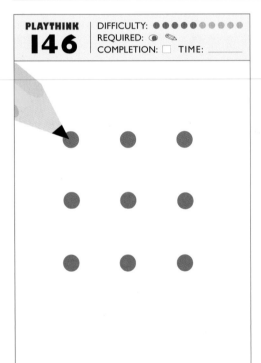

NINE-POINT PROBLEM

Can you connect the nine points with four straight lines without lifting your pencil?

Can you solve this problem using only three straight lines?

PLAYTHINK 147 | DIFFICULTY: ●●●●●●●○○○ REQUIRED: ◉ ✎ COMPLETION: ☐ TIME: _____

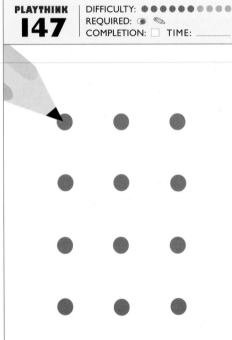

TWELVE-POINT PROBLEM

Can you connect these twelve dots with a series of straight lines without lifting your pencil? What is the least number of lines necessary?

PLAYTHINK 148 | DIFFICULTY: ●●●●●●●●○○ REQUIRED: ◉ ✎ COMPLETION: ☐ TIME: _____

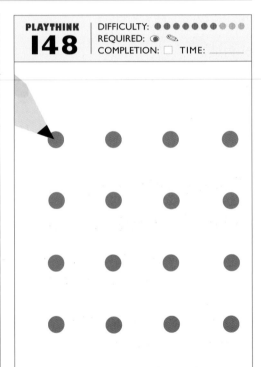

THE SIXTEEN-POINT PROBLEM

Can these sixteen dots in a square be connected with a series of straight lines without lifting your pencil? What is the least number of lines necessary?

Coordinates

Shapes are not simply physical objects—they are also mathematical creations that can be described by numbers. And like all numbers they can be manipulated in different ways to get new results, a form of math known as geometric algebra.

The concept of geometric algebra dates back to about 300 B.C., when Euclid used a form of it for proofs in his *Elements*. The field came into its own in the mid-seventeenth century, when René Descartes and Pierre de Fermat began describing the position of points with a pair of numbers. Cartesian coordinates, named after Descartes, use axes at right angles to the point where the axes cross. In coordinates such as (2,3), the first number represents the distance along the horizontal (*x*) axis, and the second shows the distance along the vertical (*y*) axis.

With Cartesian coordinates, equations can be used to plot shapes. If an equation has two variables, the shape is two-dimensional; if it has three, the shape is three-dimensional. Cartesian coordinates can be used to analyze curves. They can also help to solve simultaneous equations; the point or points where the equations' lines cross provide the numerical solutions. These powerful tools have made geometric algebra a valuable asset to science, engineering and data analysis.

PLAYTHINK 149

DIFFICULTY: ●●○○○○○○○○
REQUIRED: ◉ ✎
COMPLETION: ☐ TIME: _____

COORDINATE CRAFT

A point on a plane can be defined by the intersection of two lines, known as coordinates. Use the coordinates numbered one through twenty-four to define points on this grid. If you connect the dots in order, you will find a hidden picture.

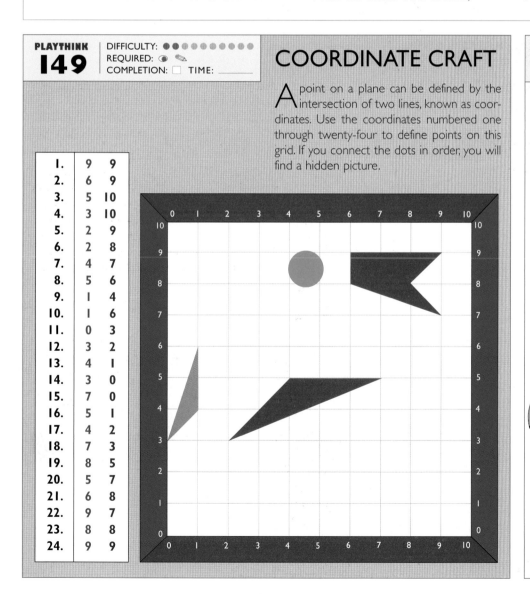

1.	9	9
2.	6	9
3.	5	10
4.	3	10
5.	2	9
6.	2	8
7.	4	7
8.	5	6
9.	1	4
10.	1	6
11.	0	3
12.	3	2
13.	4	1
14.	3	0
15.	7	0
16.	5	1
17.	4	2
18.	7	3
19.	8	5
20.	5	7
21.	6	8
22.	9	7
23.	8	8
24.	9	9

PLAYTHINK 150

DIFFICULTY: ●●●●○○○○○○
REQUIRED: ◉
COMPLETION: ☐ TIME: _____

EQUIDISTANT TREES

These three trees are equidistant—that is, each is at an equal distance from every other tree. Is this the maximum number of trees that can be equidistant?

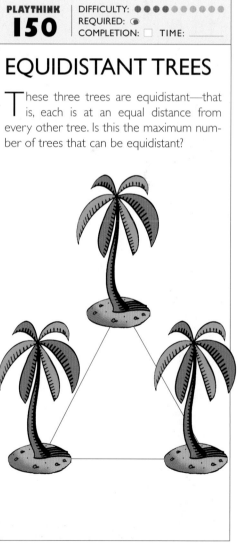

PLAYTHINK 151

DIFFICULTY: ●●●●●○○○○○○○
REQUIRED: ◉
COMPLETION: ☐ TIME: _____

DOG TIED

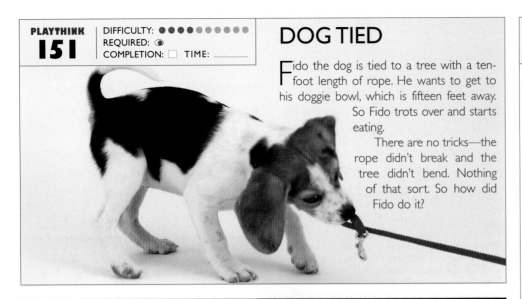

Fido the dog is tied to a tree with a ten-foot length of rope. He wants to get to his doggie bowl, which is fifteen feet away. So Fido trots over and starts eating.

There are no tricks—the rope didn't break and the tree didn't bend. Nothing of that sort. So how did Fido do it?

PLAYTHINK 152

DIFFICULTY: ●●●●●●●○○○○○
REQUIRED: ◉ ✎
COMPLETION: ☐ TIME: _____

LONGEST LINE

Can you find the longest line connecting two points on the two intersecting circles that passes through the point marked A? (Points A and D are the points at which the two circles intersect.)

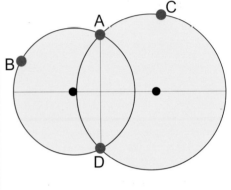

PLAYTHINK 153

DIFFICULTY: ●●●●○○○○○○○○
REQUIRED: ✎
COMPLETION: ☐ TIME: _____

INTERSECT

■ A Two-Person Game

The object of the game is to form as many intersections as possible. Players take turns drawing lines connecting the dots along the sides of the game board; each player uses a different color pencil or pen. Each time a player's line crosses a previously drawn line, that intersection gets a dot with the color corresponding to that player.

At the end of the game, the intersections are added up. Every intersection where a player crossed a line he or she drew counts as two points; every intersection where a player crossed a line drawn by the opponent counts as one point.

PLAYTHINK 154

DIFFICULTY: ●●●●●●●●○○○○
REQUIRED: ◉
COMPLETION: ☐ TIME: _____

SERPENTS

There are nine snakes—three red, three green and three blue—coiled in closed loops under a rock. The snakes do not touch one another, nor do their loops intersect.

Eight of the snakes are partly uncovered. Just by studying the image, can you tell what color snake is fully hidden by the rock?

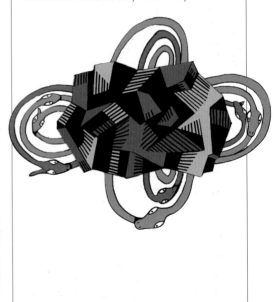

Electronic Imaging

Early in the twentieth century engineers discovered that they could deliver moving pictures to a screen by breaking up the image into very small pieces called pixels. Each pixel was encoded with information about its brightness and color, which was sent electronically to television receivers, where the pixels were combined to create a TV image. Modern computer screens employ much the same technology. If you look closely, you will see that even the most complex computer images are made of minuscule dots. That concept was simplified to produce the "Pixel Craft" puzzles below.

PLAYTHINK 155 | DIFFICULTY: ●●●●●●●●●● REQUIRED: ◉ ✎ COMPLETION: ☐ TIME: _____

PIXEL CRAFT 1

Study the two grid patterns below. Can you determine what the image would be if the two patterns were fused together?

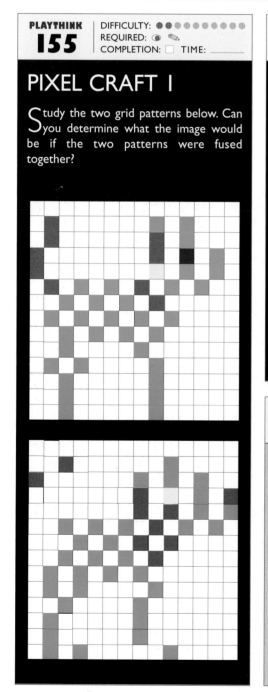

PLAYTHINK 156 | DIFFICULTY: ●●●●●●●●●● REQUIRED: ◉ ✎ COMPLETION: ☐ TIME: _____

PIXEL CRAFT 2

Can you use your imagination to combine the two patterns below into one image? If not, try transferring the pixels from each pattern onto the blank grid at the right. Be careful to match up the exact colors and positions.

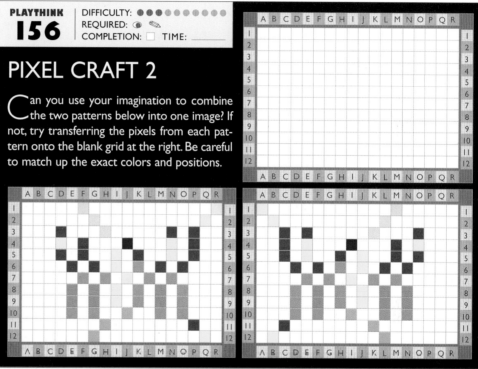

PLAYTHINK 157 | DIFFICULTY: ●●●●●●●●●● REQUIRED: ◉ ✎ COMPLETION: ☐ TIME: _____

PLANTING SIX TREES

A garden is planted with five trees along six straight paths—two paths have three trees, and four paths have two trees. Can you design a new garden with six trees and four paths so that each path has exactly three trees?

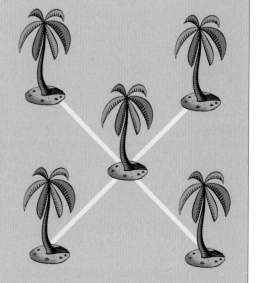

PLAYTHINK 158

DIFFICULTY: ●●●●●●●○○○
REQUIRED: 👁 ✏️
COMPLETION: ☐ TIME: _____

TWO-DISTANCE SETS

Points on a plane can be any distance apart. But there is a limited set of points that are exactly one or two discrete distances from every other point in the set. For example, two given points are exactly one distance from each other, and each of the three points that form the vertices of an equilateral triangle are also the same distance from the other two points. Those two sets of points are the only one-distance sets.

An isosceles triangle is an example of a two-distance set. Within a plane, how many other two-distance sets can you find?

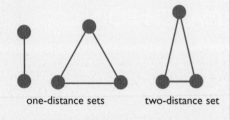

one-distance sets   two-distance set

PLAYTHINK 159

DIFFICULTY: ●●●●●●●●○○
REQUIRED: 👁 ✏️
COMPLETION: ☐ TIME: _____

THREE-DISTANCE SETS

The four points shown below are connected by six lines, each of a different length. This is an example of a six-distance set.

Can you arrange four points so that the interconnections form only three different, discrete distances—one distance three times, one distance twice, and one distance only once? How many examples of this sort of three-distance set can you find?

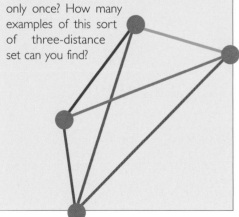

PLAYTHINK 160

DIFFICULTY: ●●●●●●●○○○
REQUIRED: 👁 ✏️
COMPLETION: ☐ TIME: _____

ROWS OF ROSES

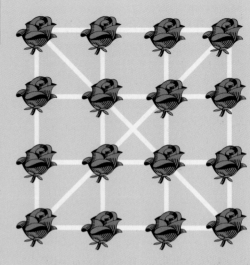

Mr. Rose wanted to plant sixteen rosebushes in his garden, and he began to plan how he wanted them laid out. At first he designed his rose garden so that there would be four rows of four roses each, which would result in ten straight lines—four vertical lines, four horizontal lines and two diagonal lines—each of which would have four bushes.

Then Mr. Rose hit on an even better plan: he would plant the sixteen bushes along fifteen straight lines with four bushes in each line. Can you figure out how he planted them?

PLAYTHINK 161

DIFFICULTY: ●●●●●●●●●○
REQUIRED: 👁 ✏️
COMPLETION: ☐ TIME: _____

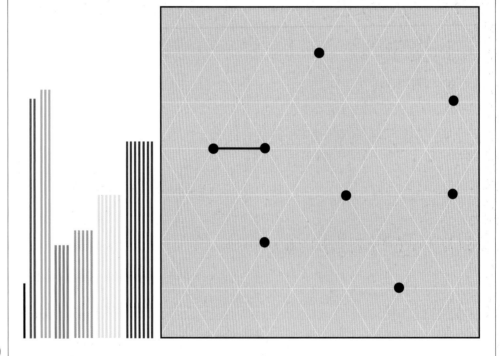

MULTI-DISTANCE SET

Connect points on this triangular grid so that the interconnecting lines have lengths that have a special property: one length should occur only once, another should occur twice, another three times and so on.

Begin with the black segment shown. How far can you carry on?

PLAYTHINK
162
DIFFICULTY: ●●●●●●●○○○
REQUIRED: ◉
COMPLETION: ☐ TIME: _____

SQUARE THE MATCH

These puzzles involve moving matches (or any other short, straight objects of the same length, such as soda straws) to create new patterns made up of squares.

Each column directs you to the number of matches to be moved; each row tells you the number of squares that you must create. (Squares may overlap or have common corners.) Can you solve all twelve puzzles?

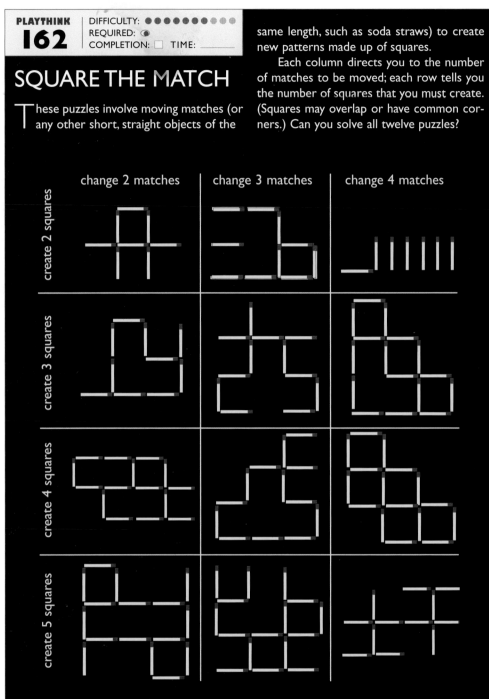

PLAYTHINK
164
DIFFICULTY: ●●●●●●●○○○
REQUIRED: ◉
COMPLETION: ☐ TIME: _____

MATCH FISH

Can you change the direction of the fish by moving just three matchsticks?

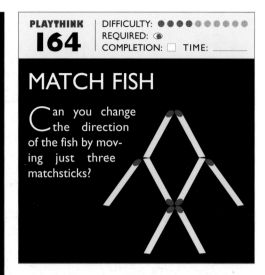

PLAYTHINK
165
DIFFICULTY: ●●●●●●●●●●
REQUIRED: ◉
COMPLETION: ☐ TIME: _____

MATCH POINT

In the figure below, the three matchsticks come together at a point. Can you create a figure out of matchsticks so that both ends of every matchstick are connected with exactly two other matchsticks in this way? Note that the matchsticks may meet only at their ends, and there can be no overlapping. What shape conforms to this rule and yet possesses the fewest number of matchsticks?

This problem was first posed by the German mathematician Heiko Harborth and was described by Nob Yoshigahara in his famous *Puzzletopia* newsletter. A variant of this problem demands that four matchsticks meet at every point; the best solution known requires 104 matchsticks meeting at 52 points. It has been determined that no solution exists for the variant requiring five matchsticks to meet at every point.

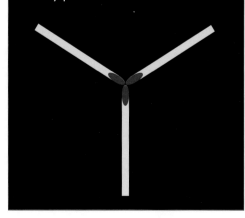

PLAYTHINK
163
DIFFICULTY: ●●●●●●○○○○
REQUIRED: ◉
COMPLETION: ☐ TIME: _____

CHERRY IN THE GLASS

Can you empty the glass and remove the cherry by moving just two matchsticks? (In your solution the glass must retain its original shape.)

PLAYTHINK
166
DIFFICULTY: ●●●●●●●○○○
REQUIRED: ◉
COMPLETION: ☐ TIME: _____

MATCH CONFIGURATIONS

This puzzle is based on an old solitaire game. How many topologically different configurations can you make with a given number of matchsticks on a flat surface? Certain restrictions apply:

1. An edge consists of a single matchstick, and the only point where two matchsticks may touch is at their ends.

2. The matchsticks must lie flat on the surface, but two figures are considered identical if one can be deformed in three-dimensional space without separating the joints (as if the figure were picked up and moved) to resemble the other.

All the possible configurations for one, two and three matchsticks are shown below. How many different configurations can you make with four matchsticks? Five matchsticks?

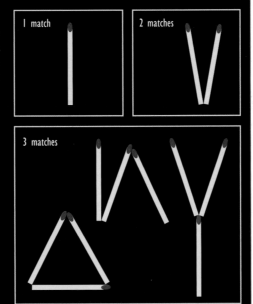

PLAYTHINK
167
DIFFICULTY: ●●●●●●●○○○
REQUIRED: ◉
COMPLETION: ☐ TIME: _____

TOUCHING DAGGERS

Can you arrange these eight daggers so that each one touches at least five others?

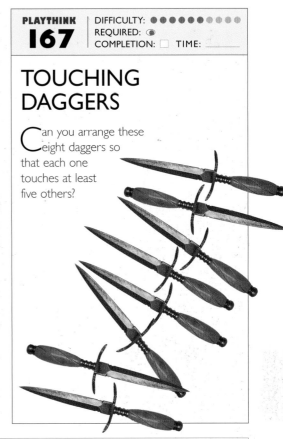

Lines and Linkages

A line is the idealization of a rigid rod. Conversely, problems about linked rods are really just studies in the geometry of lines.

A linkage is a system of rods, or lines, either connected to one another by movable joints or fixed to the plane by pivots around which the rods can turn freely. If you pivot a single rod at one end, the free end moves in a circle around that point.

Circular motion is easy and natural for linkages. The trick is to construct straight-line motion in the absence of a fixed straight line. That isn't just a theoretical problem in geometry. The natural motion

produced by a steam engine is rotary, and though it can be converted to straight-line motion by a piston, pistons require bearings that are subject to wear. A linkage would be a better way to harness the power of a steam engine.

James Watt, the inventor of the steam engine, devised the first practical solution—an approximate straight-line linkage. Rather than a straight line, Watt's linkage (as it came to be known) produced a complex mathematical curve known as Bernoulli's lemniscate—an elongated figure eight—a segment of which was close enough to a straight line for Watt's purposes. Ironically, such

a complex curve is more easily generated by a linkage than is a straight line.

The first mechanical device to produce exact straight-line motion was Peaucellier's linkage, invented in 1864. It is based on a general geometrical principle called inversion. Six links, four of equal length, form an inverter: if a particular point in the linkage follows one curve, then another point follows the inverse curve. Since the inverse curve to a straight line is a circle, a final, seventh, link constrains one of the points in Peaucellier's linkage to a circle. Another point is then forced to follow the inverse, the straight line.

PLAYTHINK **168** | DIFFICULTY: ●●●○○○○○○○
REQUIRED: ◉ ✎
COMPLETION: ☐ TIME: _____

PARALLELOGRAM LINKAGE

Four strips are linked by four flexible joints to form the four-sided polygon known as the parallelogram. Such a four-bar linkage can transform a square or rectangle into other parallelograms, such as rhombuses and rhomboids. During the transformations shown at right, can you tell which elements and relationships change and which remain constant? Fill in the chart with your answers.

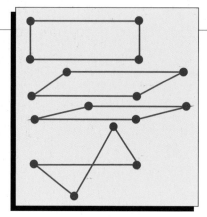

	CONSTANT	CHANGE
AREA		
PERIMETER		
SIDES		
ANGLES		

PLAYTHINK **169** | DIFFICULTY: ●●●●●●○○○○
REQUIRED: ◉ ✎
COMPLETION: ☐ TIME: _____

WATT'S LINKAGE

Examine the mechanical linkage shown below. The arms are anchored to the mounts on one end but may move freely on the other. And the red link connects the blue arms and constrains their motion. Given that information, can you determine the path of the white point in the middle of the red linkage through a full cycle of motion?

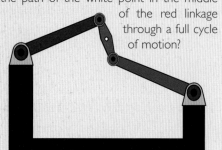

PLAYTHINK **170** | DIFFICULTY: ●●●●●●●○○○
REQUIRED: ◉ ✎
COMPLETION: ☐ TIME: _____

SWING TRIANGLE

In this mechanical linkage, the green arms are anchored to the blue base but both the arms and the red triangle, though linked, are otherwise free to swing back and forth. Can you trace the path of the white dot through one full swing of the linkage?

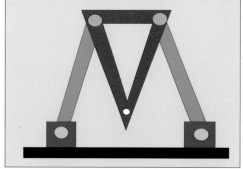

PLAYTHINK **171** | DIFFICULTY: ●●●●●●○○○○
REQUIRED: ◉ ✎ ✂
COMPLETION: ☐ TIME: _____

MOVING ALONG CIRCLES

Imagine a straight linkage as shown here, with each end constrained to one of two intersecting circles. Can you puzzle out the path traced by the middle dot of one linkage as it moves through one full cycle? Note: It may be necessary to make this linkage yourself and trace the path with a pencil.

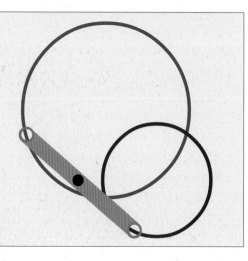

PLAYTHINK **172** | DIFFICULTY: ●●●●●●●●○○
REQUIRED: ◉ ✎ ✂
COMPLETION: ☐ TIME: _____

CRANKSHAFT

Cut six strips—three long and three short—from heavy paper or card stock. Pin the ends of the long strips to a sheet of paper so that the pinned points form the vertices of an equilateral triangle. The arms should swing freely about those points. Then attach the short strips to the free ends of the long strips so that the short strips are able to swing around the end of the long arms. Finally, attach the ends of the short strips together and punch a hole through that joint large enough for a pencil to fit through. Place a pencil through the hole.

The motion of the central joint will be constrained to a certain area. Using the pencil to trace the joint's path, can you find those limits?

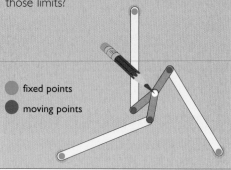

● fixed points
● moving points

PLAYTHINK **173** | DIFFICULTY: ●●●●○○○○○○
REQUIRED: ◉ ✎ ✂
COMPLETION: ☐ TIME: _____

MOVING TRIANGLE

Two points of the triangle illustrated below may move along the circumferences of the intersecting circles. The third point has a hole for a pencil tip to pass through. As the triangle points follow their circular paths, the pencil traces out a complex shape. Can you determine what the shape looks like? It may be useful to construct a replica of this triangular linkage and trace out the path yourself.

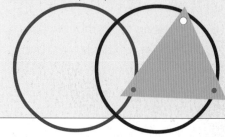

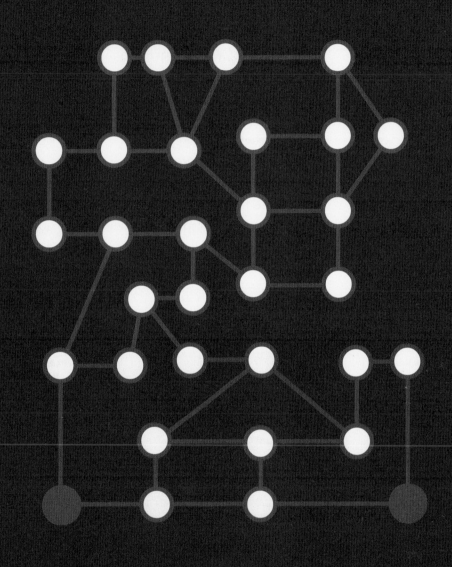

Graphs and Networks

Graph Theory

Imagine you are a traveling salesperson. You have a certain number of cities to visit in a short amount of time. Can you find the route that will allow you to visit all the cities while traveling the least distance?

Or imagine you are given a dodecahedron and are presented with the following challenge: move your finger along the edges so that it traces a path on the surface of the three-dimensional form that visits each of the vertices just once.

Those two challenges are related and are part of a field of study called graph theory. Both the real-life itinerary and the three-dimensional dodecahedron can be represented by a graph: a two-dimensional system of dots, vertices or nodes that are connected by lines or edges. Graphs embody an abstract form of a seemingly more complicated construct. For example, specific points on a graph may represent the various tasks necessary to manufacture a certain product, while the lines connecting those points show all the different orders in which those tasks may be performed. By analyzing such a graph, an engineer can find the most efficient way to order the tasks.

Two graphs are considered the same—or topologically equivalent—if the corresponding nodes are joined in a corresponding way. The exact position of the nodes or shape of the edges is unimportant; the only thing that matters is the pattern of connections.

Neither the problem of the traveling salesperson nor the puzzle involving the dodecahedron, called the Icosian Game (PlayThink 184), has a general solution; solutions for these sorts of problems must be found through trial and error. Perhaps that's part of the reason graph theory not only leads to satisfying puzzles and challenging games but is one of the most active frontiers of mathematics today.

PLAYTHINK 174

DIFFICULTY: ●●●●●●○○○○
REQUIRED: ◉
COMPLETION: ☐ TIME: _____

INTELLIGENT LADYBUG

The ladybug at the bottom of the diagram wants to meet up with her friend at the top. To get there, she'll have to cross the field of colored flowers. Each color represents a different direction—either up, down, left or right. The black squares are deep pits that must be avoided.

Can you figure out the directions represented by each color and find the path the ladybug must take to cross the field?

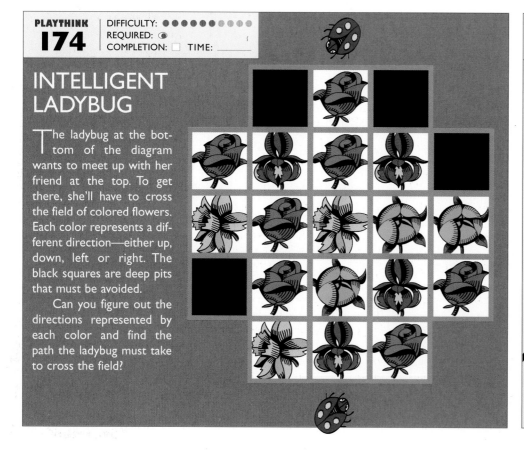

PLAYTHINK 175

DIFFICULTY: ●○○○○○○○○○
REQUIRED: ◉
COMPLETION: ☐ TIME: _____

MYSTERY TRACKS

Can you figure out what could have made these tracks in the sand?

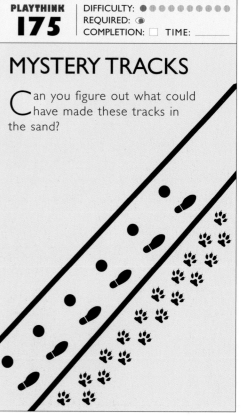

Euler's Problem

The eighteenth-century Swiss mathematician Leonhard Euler was enormously prolific, but he is best remembered for devising the solution to a recreational math problem: the Seven Bridges of Königsberg. At one time, it was fashionable to stroll through the Prussian town of Königsberg and ponder this problem: Could one cross each of the seven bridges that traversed the Pregel River and connected the various districts *once and only once?*

Although the problem itself was simple—was it possible to walk a circuit that crossed each bridge only once?—Euler found the solution by making the situation even simpler. He replaced the bridges and islands of Königsberg with lines and points.

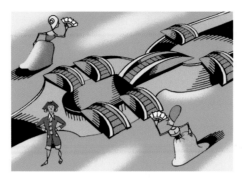

The four landmasses (two islands and both riverbanks) became special points, or nodes, that were connected by seven lines representing the bridges. Using that abstract graph, Euler demonstrated that to complete a circuit, there would have to be a maximum of two places where an odd number of lines met, and if a return to the start was required, there would have to be no places where an odd number of lines met. The reasoning is simple, once seen: a continuous journey will enter each such junction exactly as often as it leaves except at the start and finish. Since the graph of Königsberg had four nodes, each of which possessed an odd number of lines, no solution could exist.

Euler's problem is really one of topology, the branch of mathematics that deals with the properties of figures that are preserved during continuous distortions. Two networks are topologically equivalent if one can be distorted to give the other, as can the city of Königsberg and Euler's graph of the city. If a network can be traversed by a single continuous path, so can any topologically equivalent network.

Euler's work on the bridges of Königsberg founded the field of graph theory. Not bad for one recreational math puzzle!

FOUR-POINTS GRAPH

Disregarding rotations and reflections, can you find all the different ways some or all of the four points shown below may be connected?

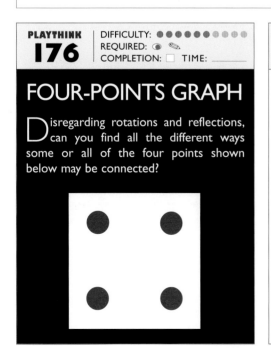

PILLAR GAME

When I was young, I often played in a small, enclosed courtyard adorned with eight pillars near the perimeter. In the center, a low fence surrounded an octagonal flowerbed. One of my favorite games involved running in a straight line from pillar to pillar for as long as possible. I could cross my previous tracks and, if needed, hop over the fence and cut across the flowerbed. I could keep running until I had only two options: repeating a track or running in a line that ran along any side of the octagonal fence around the flowerbed. When those were my choices, I had to stop.

At right is a diagram of one of my games.

In this game, I ran thirteen legs without any problem, but after that my only free move would take me alongside the fence, so the game ended.

Can you run even more legs following my childhood rules?

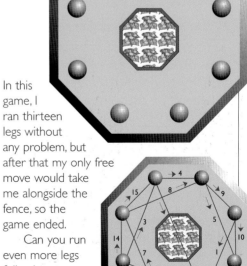

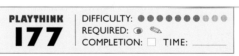

Defining Graphs and Networks

• A *route* is a path that can be drawn with one continuous line.

• A route is *circular* if following its entire length brings you back to the starting point.

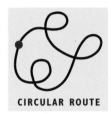

CIRCULAR ROUTE

• A route is *noncircular* if it terminates (that is, it has two end points) or if it is partially circular (it has only one end point).

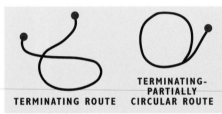

TERMINATING ROUTE   **TERMINATING-PARTIALLY CIRCULAR ROUTE**

• A *junction* is a point at which two or more routes meet.

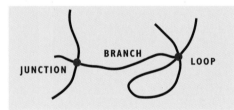

JUNCTION   **BRANCH**   **LOOP**

• The *power* of a junction is the number of routes leading from it.

• A *branch* is a section of a route between two consecutive junctions.

• A *loop* is a section of route that begins and ends at the same junction without passing through another junction. It is a circular section. To determine the power of a junction that possesses a loop, count both arms of the loop as a separate branch.

• The *order* of a pair of junctions is the number of branches connecting them.

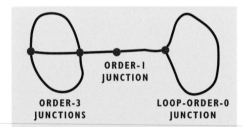

ORDER-1 JUNCTION

ORDER-3 JUNCTIONS   **LOOP-ORDER-0 JUNCTION**

• A network is *connected* if there are at least two completely distinct routes between any two junctions.

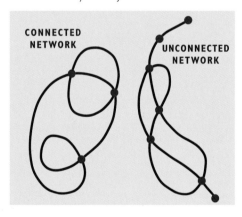

CONNECTED NETWORK   **UNCONNECTED NETWORK**

• A *region* is the space bounded by one or more branches of a network.

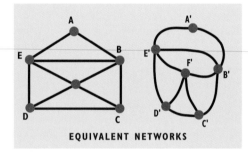

3-REGIONS NETWORK

• The *rank* of a network is the minimum number of arcs needed to draw it completely if each branch is drawn just once.

• Two networks are considered *equivalent* if they have the same number of similarly powered junctions occurring in the same order.

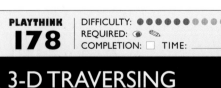

EQUIVALENT NETWORKS

• *Tree networks* are points connected by lines that don't contain closed loops.

• The *valency* is the number of edges that meet at a given node.

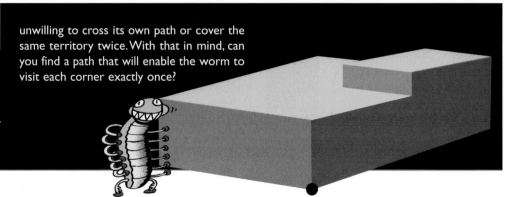

3-D TRAVERSING PROBLEM

The worm can climb along the edges of the solid figure shown at right, but it is unwilling to cross its own path or cover the same territory twice. With that in mind, can you find a path that will enable the worm to visit each corner exactly once?

Crossing Numbers

If the lines that connect the nodes of a graph were not allowed to cross, there would be serious restrictions on the kinds of graphs mathematicians could draw; in fact, a complete graph containing just five points would be impossible. But if the lines were permitted to cross, then any graph could be drawn in the plane. (You can think of the crossed lines as edges of a solid that have been projected onto the plane.) Such an "extra" meeting of two edges is called a crossing point. Topological

deformation of a graph may change the number of crossings: for example, the complete graph on four nodes can be drawn as a square with its diagonals, with nodes at its corners. The intersection of the two diagonals is a crossing point. That same graph can be drawn in the plane in a way that avoids any crossings (see "Planar Graph").

There may be dozens of ways to draw a given graph, but there is at least one that has the fewest number of crossings. That minimal

number of crossings is called, naturally enough, the crossing number, and it does not change even as the graph is topologically deformed. Graphs with crossing number zero are called planar graphs. The crossing number is remarkably difficult to calculate, and it is not known in general even for complete graphs. The crossing number for the complete graph with five nodes is one (see "Complete Graphs of Five Points").

Complete Graphs

A graph is complete if there are at least two completely distinct routes between any pair of nodes (points). These are complete graphs of three to six points.

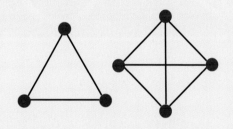

Planar Graph

A planar graph of four points has no crossing point.

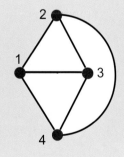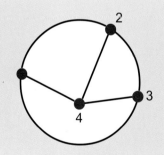

Complete Graphs of Five Points

This visual proof demonstrates that a complete graph of five points must have at least one pair of crossing branches.

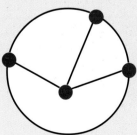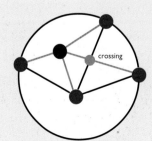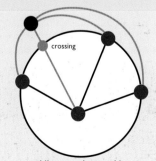

a four-point graph   adding a point in the middle   adding a point outside

PLAYTHINK 179

DIFFICULTY: ●●●●●●○○○○
REQUIRED: ◉ ✎
COMPLETION: ☐ TIME: _____

EULER'S PROBLEM

The object of these puzzles is to trace the complete pattern marked out by the white lines without picking up your pencil or backtracking over any sections. Your lines may cross only at the red points.

Can you do all eleven? If not, which ones do you find impossible to solve?

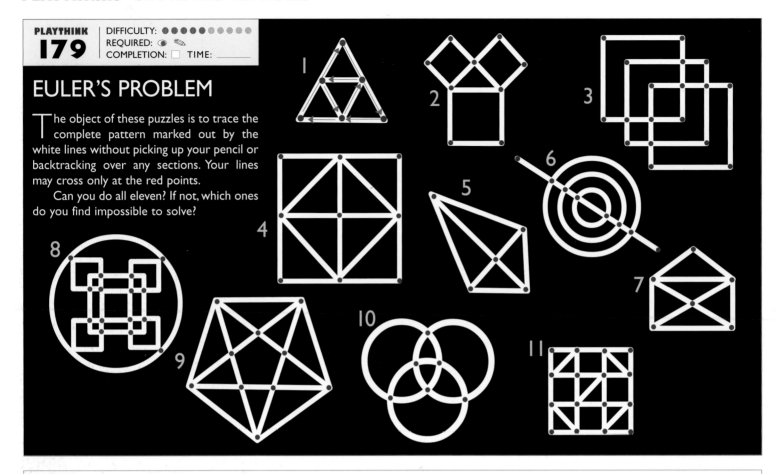

Euler Circuits

Think of a drawing of one continuous line that returns to the point where it started—a circle, for instance. Then think of a route along a graph that covers every edge just once and ends at the same vertex. That's an Euler circuit, named after Leonhard Euler. There are two obvious questions to ask about Euler circuits: Is it possible to tell by calculation (rather than by trial and error) whether a particular graph has an Euler circuit? And how can one find the possible Euler circuit without resorting to trial and error?

Euler examined such issues by using the concepts of valence and connectedness. The valence of a vertex in a graph is the number of edges that meet at that point. And a connected graph has at least one path between each potential pair of vertices.

According to those terms, then, a graph possesses an Euler circuit if it is connected and each of its valences is even.

You have only to check how many lines are going into or out of every intersection point to see if an Euler circuit is possible. If there are more than two intersection points from which an odd number of lines emanate, the pattern is impossible to trace.

A slightly different take on the Euler circuit is the Hamiltonian circuit: a route along the edges of a graph that visits each vertex once and only once. Hamiltonian circuits typically run over some, but not all, of the edges of a graph. Though different, the concepts of the Euler and Hamiltonian circuits are similar, in that both forbid reuse: for Euler circuits, of edges; for Hamiltonian circuits, of vertices. Hamiltonian circuits, it turns out, are far more difficult to determine than are Euler circuits.

PLAYTHINK
180
DIFFICULTY: ●●●●●○○○○○
REQUIRED: ◉ ✎
COMPLETION: ☐ TIME: _____

DIFFERENT ROUTES

This puzzle has one rule: Always follow the arrows. Can you find all the allowable routes from "in" to "out" that adhere to the rule?

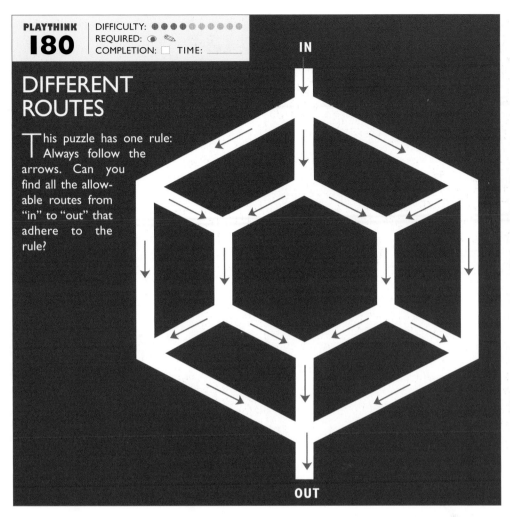

PLAYTHINK
181
DIFFICULTY: ●●●●●●●●○○
REQUIRED: ◉ ✎
COMPLETION: ☐ TIME: _____

HAMILTONIAN CIRCUIT

A Hamiltonian circuit is a continuous path that passes once through each point of a graph. Can you find the Hamiltonian circuit for the eleven-point graph illustrated below?

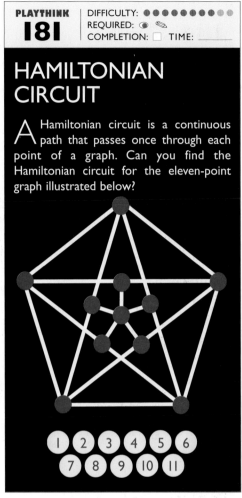

PLAYTHINK
182
DIFFICULTY: ●●●●●●○○○○
REQUIRED: ◉ ✎
COMPLETION: ☐ TIME: _____

TRAVERSING STARS

Can you walk along all the yellow paths outlining the four interconnected stars in one continuous line? You may cross your path and visit each red dot a number of times, but you may not retrace any path.

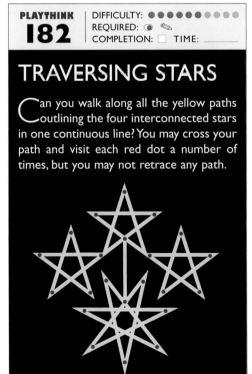

PLAYTHINK
183
DIFFICULTY: ●●●●●●○○○○
REQUIRED: ◉ ✎
COMPLETION: ☐ TIME: _____

NEIGHBORS

Three neighbors live in a gated compound. Each of their houses is painted a different color, and each has a private gate that is painted to match the house. Ideally, all three houses would be connected to their own gates by paths that didn't cross any of the other paths, but as you can see, there is a problem: the red and green paths intersect.

Can you draw new paths that would make the neighbors happy?

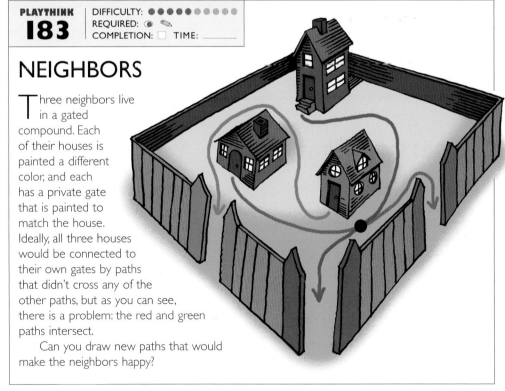

PLAYTHINK
184
DIFFICULTY: ●●●●●●●●○○○
REQUIRED: ◉ ✎
COMPLETION: ☐ TIME: _____

THE ICOSIAN GAME

■ *A Journey Around a Dodecahedron*

A classic of recreational geometry, the Icosian game was invented by the mathematician W. R. Hamilton in 1859. Hamilton's original took the form of a dodecahedron, a three-dimensional solid with twelve pentagonal faces. But the game can be played on the two-dimensional diagram shown above, which is topologically equivalent to the dodecahedron.

To play, move from circle to circle following the paths marked in white. You can start at any circle you wish, but you may visit each circle only once. And you must return to where you started. To keep track of which circles you have visited, you can mark each one with consecutively numbered disks, such as those at the left.

Graphs such as this one, which project three-dimensional problems and puzzles onto the two-dimensional plane and thereby make them easier to solve, are called Schlegel diagrams.

Hamilton himself devised a branch of mathematics to solve similar path-tracing problems on two-dimensional solids. He called it Icosian calculus.

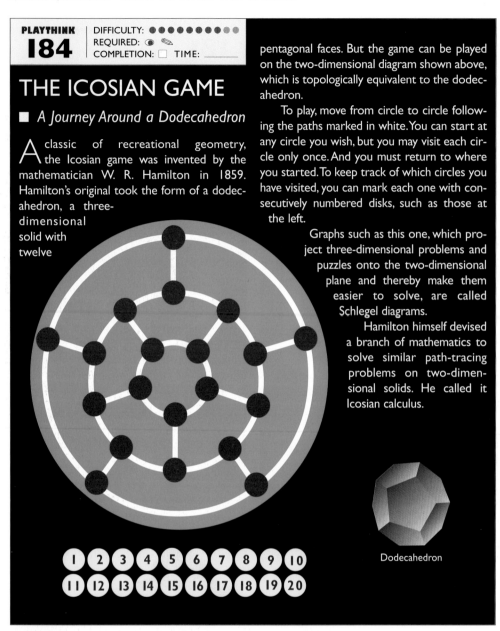

Dodecahedron

PLAYTHINK
185
DIFFICULTY: ●●●●○○○○○○○
REQUIRED: ◉ ✎
COMPLETION: ☐ TIME: _____

FOUR SCHOOLS

Four children from four different families attend four different schools. Each school is a different color and gives its students notebooks that are the color of the school. Can you lead each student to his or her school without letting any one path cross another?

Bipartite Graphs

Some graphs don't require connecting every point to every other point. One example of such a graph is a complete bipartite graph. Its nodes are divided into two sets, with *m* and *n* nodes each, and all the nodes in one set are joined to all the nodes in the other set, but no two nodes in the same set are joined. (Such a graph is a generalized version of the "Utilities" puzzles on the following page.)

Although the crossing number for certain complete bipartite graphs is known, it has not been worked out for a general *m* and *n*. For example, if m=n=7, then it is known that the crossing number is either 77, 79 or 81. But nobody knows which of these three is the correct answer.

Many other simple properties of graphs prove equally elusive. Combinatorial mathematics is still in its infancy, and it is a fertile ground for challenging puzzles and problems.

PLAYTHINK 186

DIFFICULTY: ●●●●●○○○○○
REQUIRED: ◉ ✎
COMPLETION: ☐ TIME: _____

UTILITIES 1

Before they can be occupied, these three houses must each be connected to the telephone, electricity and water lines. Nine lines are needed in total. Can you draw lines to connect each house to each utility without allowing any of the lines to intersect?

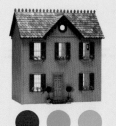
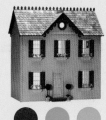
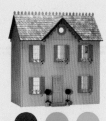

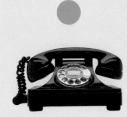

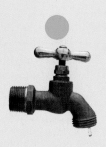

PLAYTHINK 187

DIFFICULTY: ●●●●●●●○○○
REQUIRED: ◉ ✎
COMPLETION: ☐ TIME: _____

UTILITIES 2

The object of this puzzle is to draw lines connecting each animal to all the animals that are different in color without connecting any animals that are the same color. For example, a red fish could be connected to a green fish and a yellow nautilus but not a red clam. Can you draw all the lines connecting the appropriate animals without allowing any of the lines to cross?

This problem and the two that follow turn out to be more complicated than Utilities 1, which has two sets of points based on a bipartite graph. These problems possess what are called multipartite graphs; here there are three sets of points, making for a tripartite graph.

PLAYTHINK 188

DIFFICULTY: ●●●●●●●○○○
REQUIRED: ◉ ✎
COMPLETION: ☐ TIME: _____

UTILITIES 3

Draw lines connecting each animal to all the animals different in color without connecting any animals that are the same color. How many interconnecting lines can you draw without allowing any of the lines to cross?

PLAYTHINK 189

DIFFICULTY: ●●●●●●●●●○
REQUIRED: ◉ ✎
COMPLETION: ☐ TIME: _____

UTILITIES 4

Draw lines connecting each animal to all the animals that are different in color without connecting any animals that are the same color. How many interconnecting lines can you draw without allowing any of the lines to cross?

PLAYTHINK 190
DIFFICULTY: ●●●●●●●○○○
REQUIRED: ◉
COMPLETION: ☐ TIME: _____

WORM TRIP

A worm crawls only along the edges of a box measuring 2 by 2 by 3 centimeters. What is the longest distance the worm can travel without retracing any of its steps?

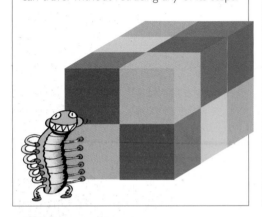

PLAYTHINK 191
DIFFICULTY: ●●●●●●●○○○
REQUIRED: ◉ ✎
COMPLETION: ☐ TIME: _____

EVEN NUMBER ROUTE

This is another simple route problem with a small twist: the only allowable path from the circle marked "start" to the one marked "finish" involves traveling over an even number of segments. Can you find the shortest allowable path?

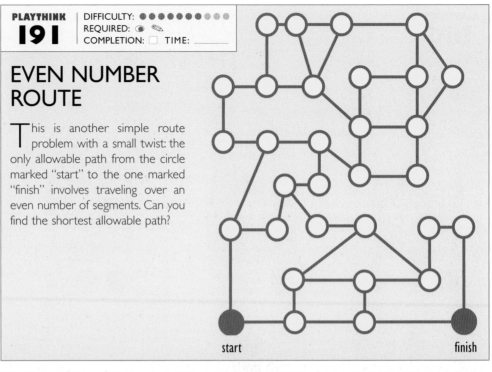

start   finish

PLAYTHINK 192
DIFFICULTY: ●●●●●●●●○○
REQUIRED: ◉ ✎
COMPLETION: ☐ TIME: _____

SUBWAY

The subway is designed to be the quickest way across town—and for many trips it is. But in cities with several subway lines that have only a handful of interconnecting stations, travelers spend a lot of time waiting around. And they also have to take time simply to walk from one subway platform to another. In fact, for many subway systems the time needed to change trains is more or less equivalent to the time it takes to travel by subway from one station to another. That statistic is at the heart of this puzzle.

The object is to find the fastest route between specific stations. You have to stay on the same line, which is designated by a distinct color, unless you make a transfer at a station where two lines meet. You count each station you pass (as well as the one where you start) as one minute and any station where you change lines as two minutes. Given those rules, can you find the fastest routes from A to B, C to D, E to F and G to H?

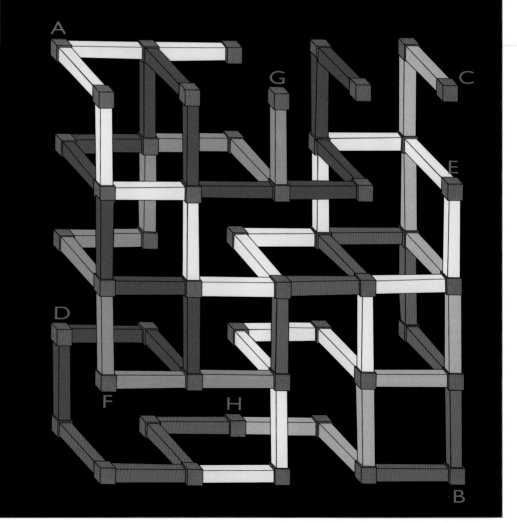

PLAYTHINK
193
DIFFICULTY: ●●●●●●●●○○
REQUIRED: ◉ ✎
COMPLETION: ☐ TIME: _____

STAR TOURS

There are fourteen stars in the constellation shown here, each of which is connected to at least three of its neighbors by an interstellar guideway. Can you follow the guideways to visit each star once and only once?

Sixteen of the guideways have been assigned a number and will be closed for repairs, one at a time, in numerical order. Can you complete the task of visiting each star without the use of guideway 1? How about guideway 2?

Try to find routes connecting all the stars consecutively without the use of one of the sixteen numbered guideways in succession. You will find that in two of the sixteen instances, there will be no solution. Can you figure out which two?

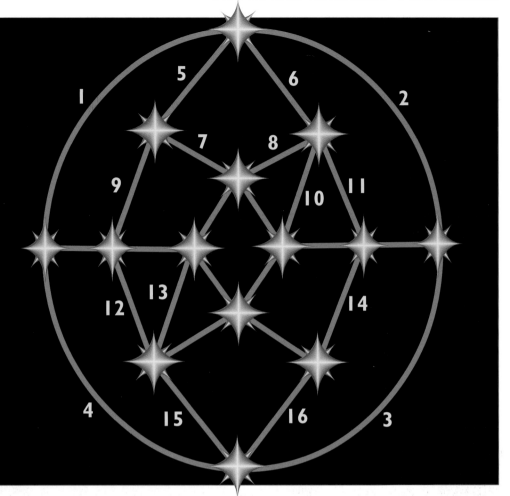

PLAYTHINK
194
DIFFICULTY: ●●●●●●●●○○
REQUIRED: ◉ ✎
COMPLETION: ☐ TIME: _____

MARS PUZZLE

There are twenty scientific outposts scattered on the surface of Mars, each marked with a letter and each linked by a canal to at least two other stations. Starting at the outpost marked T and visiting each station just once, follow the various canals to spell out a complete English sentence.

Can you find a solution?

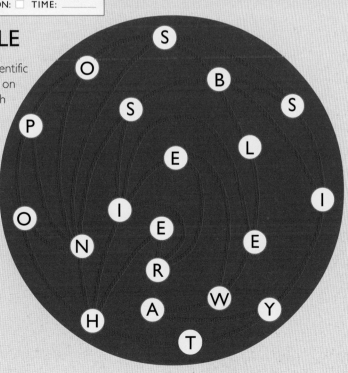

PLAYTHINK
195
DIFFICULTY: ●●●●●●○○○○
REQUIRED: ◉
COMPLETION: ☐ TIME: _____

MISSING ARROWS 1

Two arrows are missing from the pattern shown below. Can you add the missing arrows so that they help create a consistent pattern throughout the grid?

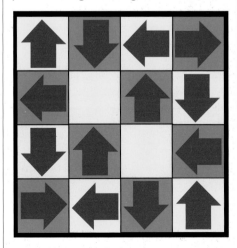

PLAYTHINK
196
DIFFICULTY: ●●●●●●○○○○○
REQUIRED: ◉ ✎
COMPLETION: ☐ TIME: _____

PRINTED CIRCUITS 1

Printed circuits are two-dimensional graphs—the junctions carry out electronic operations, while the lines carry electrical signals from place to place. If the lines cross, there will be a short-circuit and the device will fail.

Can you connect the five pairs of colored circuits on this circuit board without crossing any lines? The connecting lines must remain in the gray area.

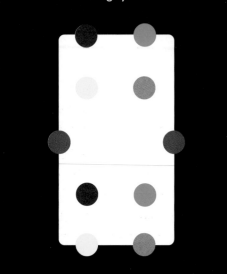

PLAYTHINK
197
DIFFICULTY: ●●●●●●●○○○○
REQUIRED: ◉ ✎
COMPLETION: ☐ TIME: _____

PRINTED CIRCUITS 2

Can you draw five lines to connect the five pairs of colored circles? All connecting lines must run along the white lines of the grid, and no connecting lines may intersect.

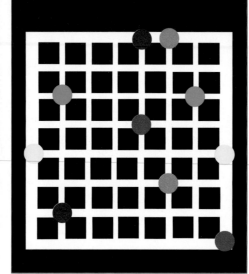

PLAYTHINK
198
DIFFICULTY: ●●●●●●●●○○○
REQUIRED: ◉ ✎
COMPLETION: ☐ TIME: _____

PRINTED CIRCUITS 3

Can you draw eight lines to connect the eight pairs of colored circles? All connecting lines must run along the white lines of the grid, and no connecting lines may intersect.

This puzzle can become a two-player game. The players take turns connecting the circles; play continues until one player is unable to make a connection.

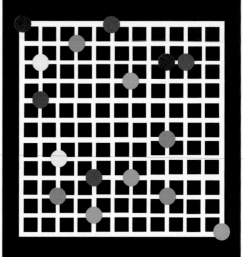

PLAYTHINK
199
DIFFICULTY: ●●●●●○○○○○○
REQUIRED: ◉
COMPLETION: ☐ TIME: _____

LIGHTING THE LAMPS

The three lamps and three batteries shown below are arranged around an empty space for a triangular circuit board.

Using just your eyes and imagination, can you work out which of the three numbered circuit boards can be placed into the empty space so that each lamp will be powered by its own battery?

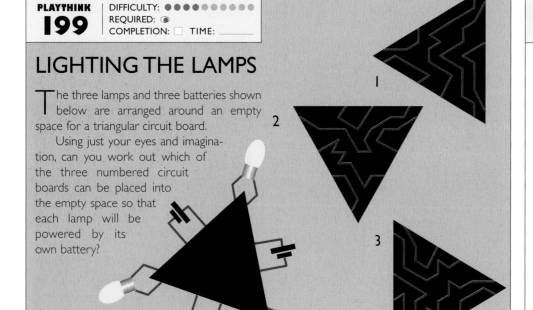

PLAYTHINK
200
DIFFICULTY: ●●●●●●●●●○○
REQUIRED: ◉ ✎
COMPLETION: ☐ TIME: _____

DICE ARROWS

How many different ways can you put six arrows on the faces of a cube?

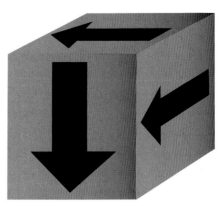

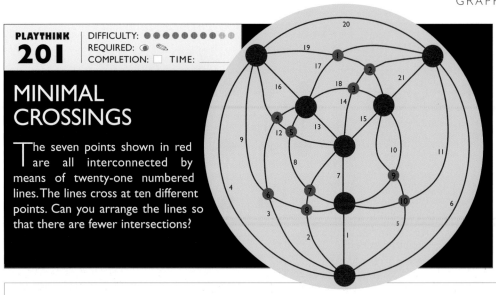

PLAYTHINK 201 | DIFFICULTY: ●●●●●●●○○○ REQUIRED: ◉ ✎ COMPLETION: ☐ TIME: ___

MINIMAL CROSSINGS

The seven points shown in red are all interconnected by means of twenty-one numbered lines. The lines cross at ten different points. Can you arrange the lines so that there are fewer intersections?

PLAYTHINK 202 | DIFFICULTY: ●●●●●○○○○○ REQUIRED: ◉ COMPLETION: ☐ TIME: ___

FIVE ARROWS

Rearrange the four arrows to form five arrows.

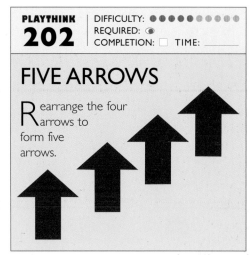

Topology and the Tree Graph

Take a shape such as a triangle and start to deform it: change the angles, lengthen the sides, add extra corners. What, from the geometric point of view, remains unchanged from the original figure? That is the kind of question answered in the field of study called topology.

Little of what is important in traditional geometry is of any use in topology. Instead, topology looks at such facts as (a) a triangle has an inside and an outside and (b) it is impossible to pass from one to the other without crossing an edge. No matter how you deform a triangle in the plane, it will still possess an inside and outside—that's a defining point in topology. In fact, to a topologist a triangle is the same as a square, a parallelogram or even a circle. The torus—the shape of an inner tube or a doughnut—has a hole in the middle and retains the hole no matter how much it is distorted; that's a property

that sets it apart from triangles but gives it something in common with a coffee mug. In topology, the number 8 and the letter B are equivalent: each has two holes.

Many topological properties concern the way objects are connected; whether a loop of string is knotted is a topological property. The basic concepts of topology include many ideas infants learn: insideness and outsideness, right- and left-handedness, linking, knotting and disconnectedness.

Topological ideas are crucial to the understanding of graphs. When nodes are joined by edges, what matters is not the precise position of the edges and nodes but, rather, the way they connect up. For example, a graph is connected if it is "all in one piece," that is, there's a continuous path from any node to any other node. The precise shape of the edges is irrelevant; all that matters in topology is the connectedness of the

graph. Similarly, if a graph contains a circuit—a closed loop with distinct edges—it is topologically equivalent to any other graph possessing a loop.

Graphs that possess no loops are called trees (because, like real trees, these graphs have branches that never link except through a trunk). Many processes that branch may be represented as trees. For example, the positions in a game of chess form a tree whose edges are the moves of the game. The strategy in many games is generally based on viewing the game as a tree, and computer programs that play such games as chess, checkers and backgammon make essential use of this idea. Indeed, the advanced chess-playing computers that are capable of beating human grand masters work out trees of possible moves; the computer then selects the move at the present point that will ensure the best possible outcome many moves in the future.

PLAYTHINK 203

DIFFICULTY: ●●●●●●●○○○
REQUIRED: 👁 ✏
COMPLETION: ☐ TIME: _____

FOUR-POINT TREE GRAPH

Tree graphs are points connected by lines that don't possess closed loops. How many different tree graphs can you find that connect the four points shown below?

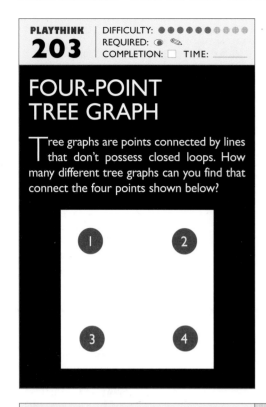

PLAYTHINK 204

DIFFICULTY: ●●●●●●●●○○
REQUIRED: 👁 ✏
COMPLETION: ☐ TIME: _____

TREE GRAPHS

If you combine all the graphs that are topologically equivalent, only one tree graph connects a set of two points, and only one connects three points. Two tree graphs can connect four points, and three can connect five points. All those graphs are illustrated at right.

How many different, topologically distinct tree graphs can connect six points? Seven points?

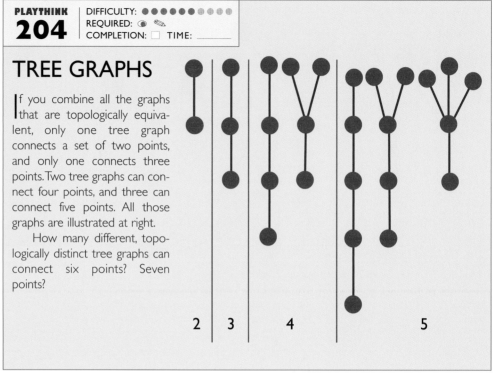

PLAYTHINK 205

DIFFICULTY: ●●●●●●●●○○
REQUIRED: 👁 ✏ 📄 ✂
COMPLETION: ☐ TIME: _____

TREE GAME

This simple stick figure game requires each player to match specific arrangements of matchsticks to patterns on playing cards.

To play the game, you need the following simple materials:

a set of cards that depicts stylized versions of tree graphs possessing three, four, five and six nodes (see PlayThink 206)

and a set of six identical sticks—matches, drinking straws or whatever is on hand— to re-create the graphs shown on the cards

The object is to reproduce the patterns on the cards in the fewest number of moves. To play, shuffle the cards and place them all face down in a pile. Place five sticks in a straight line on the table. (The sixth stick is held in a reserve pile.)

The first player takes the top three cards from the pile and places them face up. That player then has two moves to change the positions of the sticks to match the graphs shown on the exposed cards. A move consists of picking up a stick from the table and laying it in a

new position, or adding a stick from the reserve pile to the graph, or removing a stick from the graph and placing it in the reserve pile. A player may also rotate as many sticks on the graph as possible, as long as the end that is attached to the graph remains fixed. (Obviously, if both ends are attached to the graph, a stick cannot be rotated.)

If a player succeeds in forming one of the graphs, he or she takes the card that depicts it and keeps it until the end of the game. Cards that the player could not duplicate remain on the table.

The second player, if necessary, draws cards to replace the cards captured by the first player and tries to duplicate one or more of the cards with just two moves of the sticks. The game continues until all the cards have been taken. The winner is the player with the most cards.

You can play two forms of the game: classical and topological. In the classical game a card may be taken only if the tree formed by the sticks is exactly the same as that depicted on the card; the topological game allows trees that are topologically equivalent. Playing both versions of the game will help drive home the difference between exact similarity and topological equivalence.

SAMPLE GAME

Three cards drawn by a player are shown at top. The cards are laid face up.

The player then makes moves according to the cards drawn. In this case the player earns a score of three points.

gray = removed stick
yellow = rotated stick

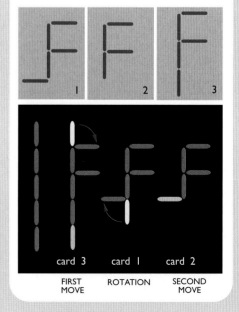

PLAYTHINK
206
DIFFICULTY: ●●●●●●○○○○
REQUIRED: ◉
COMPLETION: ☐ TIME: _____

TREE GAME CARDS AND VARIANT

These are the sixty-four cards used to play the "Tree Game": sixteen sets of topolog-ically equivalent cards, with four variations in each set. For example, one set is made up of cards 1, 20, 35 and 61.

You can also use them to play a variant game: namely, how long will it take you to identify all sixteen sets?

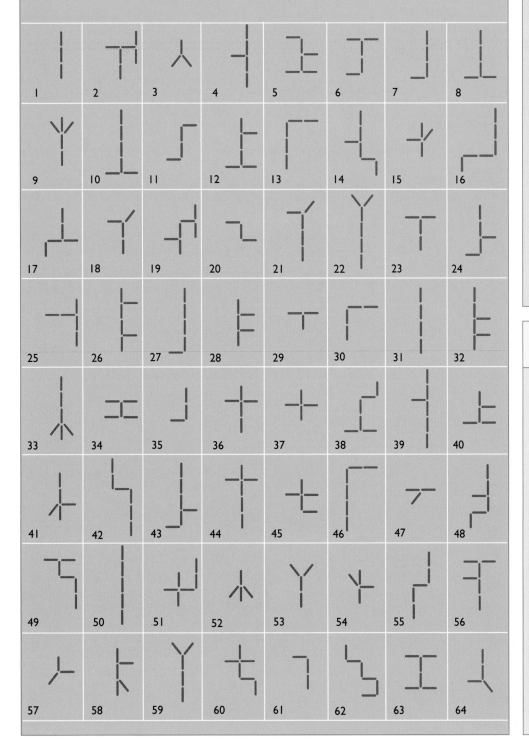

PLAYTHINK
207
DIFFICULTY: ●●●●●●○○○○
REQUIRED: ◉ ✎
COMPLETION: ☐ TIME: _____

TREE CHAIN

Nineteen beads lie on a table. Can you join them with string to create a tree graph?

What is the smallest number of branches you can draw between nineteen beads, or nineteen points? Remember that since it is one graph, each point must be linked to every other point by some number of branches. And since it is a tree graph, there can be no closed loops. Is there a general rule for the minimum number of branches needed?

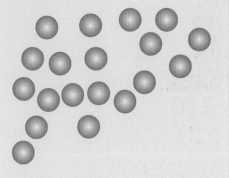

PLAYTHINK
208
DIFFICULTY: ●●●●●●○○○○
REQUIRED: ◉
COMPLETION: ☐ TIME: _____

MISSING ARROWS 2

Can you work out where the four miss-ing arrows should point?

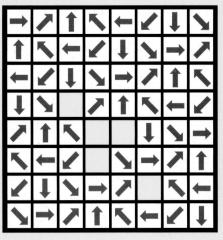

PLAYTHINK 209

DIFFICULTY: ●●●●●●○○○○
REQUIRED: ◉ ✎
COMPLETION: ☐ TIME: _____

ARROWS PUZZLE AND GAME 1

The puzzle: Place sixteen arrows on the four-by-four game board so that each row, each column and each main diagonal contains four arrows pointing in four different directions—north, south, east and west.

The game: The object of the game is to place sixteen arrows so that no row, column or main diagonal has two or more arrows pointing in the same direction. Two players take turns placing an arrow of their color on the board. The arrows must point in one of the four main directions (north, south, east or west, or perhaps up, down, right or left). After

each move the board is checked to see if any squares are blocked from receiving arrows; that is, any arrows placed on such a square would violate the rules. A player whose moves create such blocked squares can mark them in her or his color before the next player's turn.

The game ends when no legal moves remain. Players receive a point for each row, column or diagonal consisting of at least three boxes of his or her color, of which at least two are arrows. A row in which a player has one arrow and two blocked squares in his or her color yields no points.

In the sample game illustrated at right, the game ended in a tie, with each player getting three points.

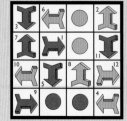

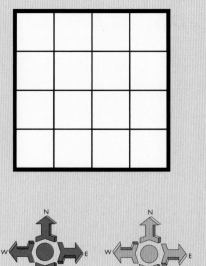

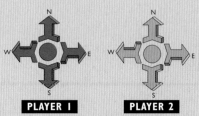

PLAYER 1   **PLAYER 2**

PLAYTHINK 210

DIFFICULTY: ●●●●●●●○○○
REQUIRED: ◉ ✎
COMPLETION: ☐ TIME: _____

ARROWS PUZZLE AND GAME 2

The puzzle: On the eight-by-eight game board, fit sixty-four arrows so that each row and column contains eight arrows, each pointing in a different direction—north, northeast, east, southeast, south, southwest, west and northwest.

The game: The object of the game is to place arrows on the board so that no row or column has two or more arrows pointed in the same direction. Two players take turns placing arrows of their color on the game board. The arrows must be in one of the eight orientations used in the puzzle version. Play continues until no legal moves are possible. Each player receives one point for every row or column in which he or she has placed five or more arrows. In the game illustrated at right, red wins with two points versus green's one point.

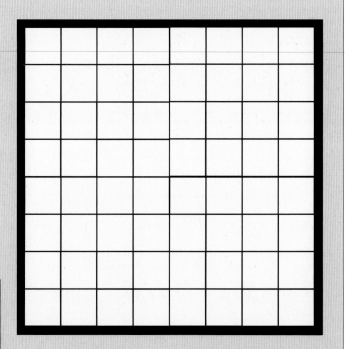

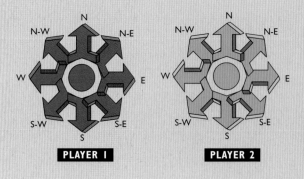

PLAYER 1   **PLAYER 2**

Digraphs

Add an arrowhead to each line of a graph and it becomes a directed graph, or digraph. A complete digraph, in which every edge has a direction and every pair of points is joined by a line, is called a tournament. No matter how you place the arrows, every tournament will have a Hamiltonian path—that is, a route that visits every node once. A path that returns to its starting point after visiting all the other points is called a Hamiltonian circuit; such a route is not possible for every tournament.

PLAYTHINK 211
DIFFICULTY: ●●●●●●●●●●
REQUIRED: ◉ ✎
COMPLETION: ☐ TIME:

DIGRAPH PENTAGON

Each path between two of the numbered points allows travel in just one direction, which is marked with an arrow. With that in mind, can you find the route that will allow travel to all five points?

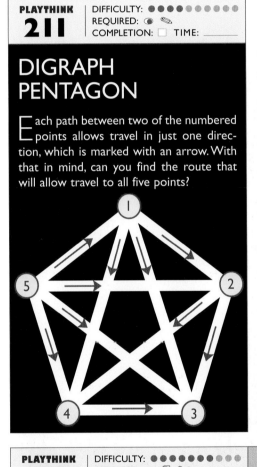

PLAYTHINK 212
DIFFICULTY: ●●●●●●●●●●
REQUIRED: ◉ ✎
COMPLETION: ☐ TIME:

DIGRAPH HEXAGON

Each path between two of the numbered points allows travel in just one direction, which is marked with an arrow. With that in mind, can you find a route that will allow travel to all six points?

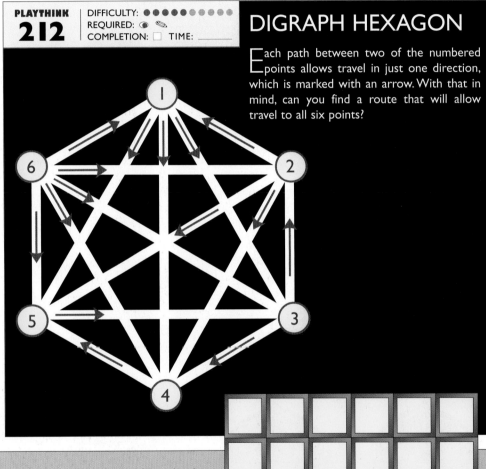

PLAYTHINK 213
DIFFICULTY: ●●●●●●●●●●
REQUIRED: ◉ 📄 ✂
COMPLETION: ☐ TIME:

ARROWS TOUR

In this puzzle the arrows below are numbered; each number tells you how many spaces to move. For example, an arrow marked 3 means you may move three places in that direction.

Can you place the nine arrows on the board so that each arrow points at another arrow to create a continuous loop? That is, after nine jumps, you should end up where you started.

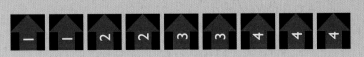

PLAYTHINK
214
DIFFICULTY: ●●●○○○○○○○
REQUIRED: ◉ ✎ 📄 ✂
COMPLETION: ☐ TIME: _____

HAMILTON GAME 1

Cut out fifteen airplanes that match the ones at right and place them in a random fashion along the fifteen route lines in the diagram below. Can you find a path that visits each of the six cities exactly once by following the directions of the arrows?

In each random placement of the planes, can you name the order of the cities to be visited just by looking at the layout?

PLAYTHINK
215
DIFFICULTY: ●●●●●●●○○○
REQUIRED: ◉ ✎ 📄 ✂
COMPLETION: ☐ TIME: _____

HAMILTON GAME 2

In this advanced version of the previous game, you visit a total of nineteen intersection points exactly once. To do this, you must find a continuous path that interconnects all nineteen intersection points. At each point, you may continue only in the directions the arrows allow.

You can play this as a two-player game. One of the players distributes the arrows along the fifteen lines, establishing the directions in which travel may occur. Then the second player tries to create a continuous path connecting the intersection points, marking the first point visited as 1 and numbering the points in the order of visit.

You might want to remember this: taking into consideration the nine intersection points rather than simply the nodes on the outside, even a Hamiltonian path is not found every time. Depending on how the arrows are placed, there are 32,786 different configurations, of which 27,846 have a Hamiltonian path (190 of those also make Hamiltonian circuits) and 4,940 have no complete solutions.

Nine specially selected puzzles of the "Hamilton Game 2," with the complete sets of arrows laid out on their lines, are illustrated here.

There are hundreds of possible combinations.

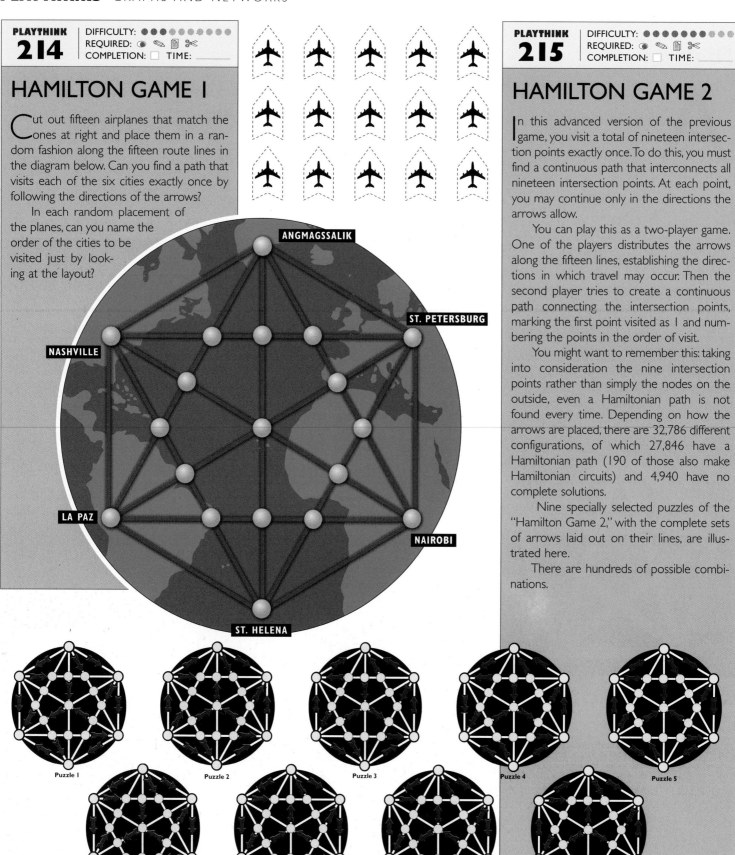

ANGMAGSSALIK

ST. PETERSBURG

NASHVILLE

LA PAZ

NAIROBI

ST. HELENA

Puzzle 1   Puzzle 2   Puzzle 3   Puzzle 4   Puzzle 5

Puzzle 6   Puzzle 7   Puzzle 8

Puzzle 9

Ramsey Theory

Although Frank Ramsey made considerable contributions to economics and philosophy, he is remembered more for his brilliance as a mathematician. The Englishman's best-known work was in set theory; indeed, a branch of that field now carries his name—quite an accomplishment for a man who died in 1930 at twenty-seven!

The appearance of disorder is really a matter of scale: a mathematical structure can be found if you look widely enough. Ramsey wanted to find the smallest set of objects that would guarantee that some of those objects would share certain properties. For example, the smallest number of people that will always include two people of the same sex is three. If there are only two, you might have a man and a woman; since the third person would be either a man *or* a woman, adding him or her guarantees at least two of one sex.

Or take this question: Can a complete graph have its edges colored using only two colors, so that no three edges of the some color form a triangle? Ramsey proved some general theorems on this question, but instances with four, five or six nodes are simple enough to analyze using pencil and paper. The famous Party Puzzle (which we present as "Love-Hate Relationships," PlayThink 216) is based on Ramsey's work.

To appreciate how elegant graphs are for solving this sort of problem, imagine listing all possible combinations of acquaintanceship among six people—a total of 32,768—and having to check if each combination included the desired relationship.

A more advanced Ramsey problem would be to imagine a party in which there must be a foursome in which everyone is a mutual friend or everyone is a mutual stranger. How large must the party be? Ramsey's work demonstrated that eighteen guests are necessary. If you draw a complete graph with eighteen nodes, no matter how you color the lines using two colors, you will inevitably create a quadrilateral formed by connecting four points (persons) in one of the colors.

The party size required to ensure at least one fivesome of mutual friends or strangers is still unknown. The answer lies between 43 and 49.

PLAYTHINK 216

DIFFICULTY: ●●●●●●●○○○
REQUIRED: ◉ ✎
COMPLETION: ☐ TIME: _____

LOVE-HATE RELATIONSHIPS

You and your friends feel your emotions very strongly—at any given time you either love someone or you hate that person. To avoid bloodshed, when you all get together, you like to arrange it so there is no group of three who all mutually hate one another and no group of three who all mutually love one another.

Four, five and six of you need to get together on successive evenings. Is trouble inevitable? Or is it possible to avoid both love triangles and hate triangles?

For each group, color in the lines between points in one of two colors: red for love or blue for hate. How many lines can you color before you are forced to create a love or hate triangle? Is it possible to color the lines so that, when all the relationships have been accounted for, there are no triangles?

● **you**
   your friends
red lines - love
blue lines - hate

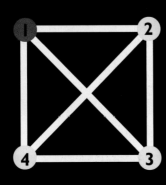
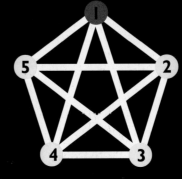
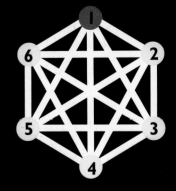

PLAYTHINK
217

DIFFICULTY: ●●●●○○○○○○
REQUIRED: 👁 ✏
COMPLETION: ☐ TIME: _____

SPIDER TRACK PUZZLE GAMES

This game can be played as a two-player competition or as a solitaire game.

In a two-player game the players take turns filling in the white lines between the numbered points with one of two colors—say, red and blue. Each player can use either color; the goal is to avoid creating a solid-color triangle. The game continues until one player must create a solid-color triangle. As a variant, each player can try to maneuver the other to draw a quadrilateral.

To play the game alone, fill in as many white lines as you can until you are forced to form a triangle whose vertices are the numbered points on the perimeter.

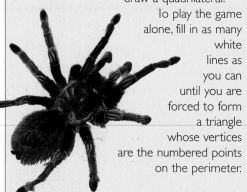

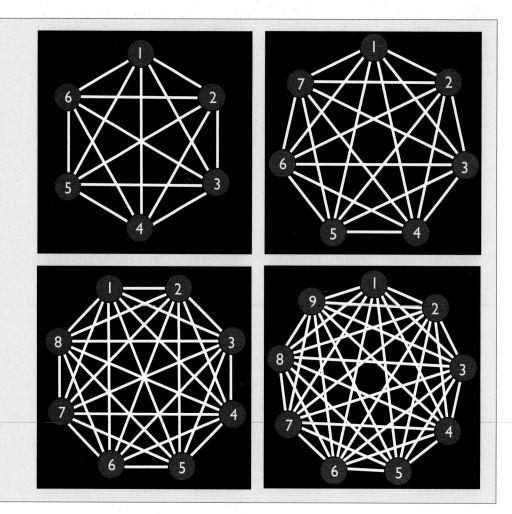

PLAYTHINK
218

DIFFICULTY: ●●●●●●●○○○
REQUIRED: 👁 ✏
COMPLETION: ☐ TIME: _____

TRAFFIX PUZZLE

Getting across town in Gridlock City can be a nightmare for motorists. It's not the traffic that is the problem—it's the crazy road signs that always seem to keep you from making the turn you want to make. Recently the town authorities made the problem worse by increasing the number of signposts and even inventing some new ones. The result is that at nearly every intersection there is at least one possible turn that is now forbidden. Getting from one side of town to the other now involves some surprising twists and turns.

Can you find the route across town for these three cars? For each color, enter at the left and exit at the right where indicated. And be sure to follow the road signs at each intersection.

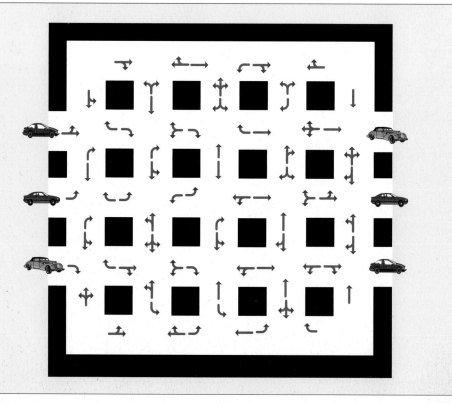

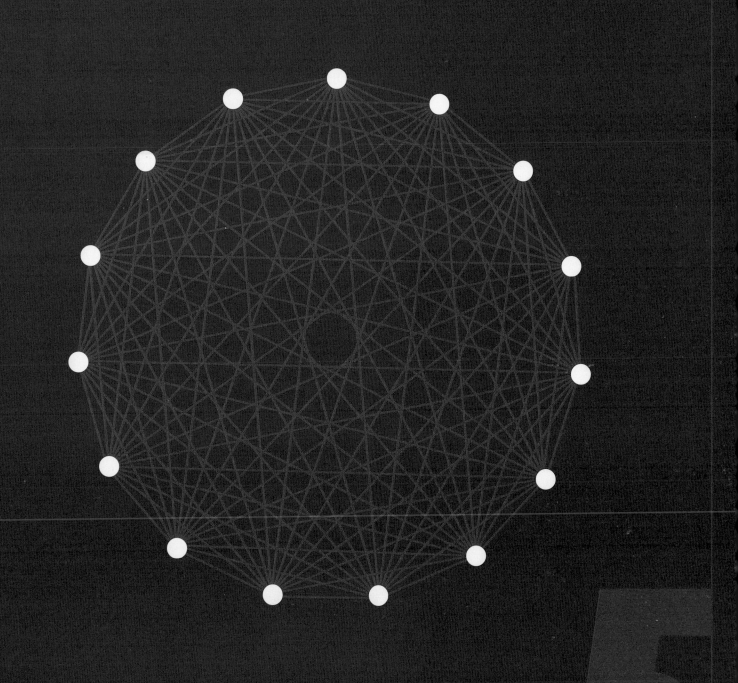

Curves and Circles

The Curves Around Us

The endless geometric pattern of a river's turns, called meanders, has a fascinating beauty. Over centuries of research, mathematicians and scientists have learned that a meander is the form a river takes in order to use the least amount of work when turning. That gives a new meaning to the phrase "lazy river"!

A thin steel strip can be bent into various configurations—all analogous to river meanders. When held firmly at two points, a strip takes on the shape in which the bend is as uniform as possible. And what is that bend? A curve—a line that continuously bends but has no angles.

Some curves, such as parabolas, are open: the line never returns to its starting point. Others join up with themselves to form closed curves, such as the circle and the ellipse. Some curves are like the helix and twist through three dimensions.

Although there are curves that are quite simple in form, others are so complex that they must be discovered experimentally. Such curves have been found through the study of soap films stretched over wire hoops. The complicated but beautiful curving glass roof over the Olympic stadium in Munich was designed in just that manner.

PLAYTHINK 219

DIFFICULTY: ●●●●●●●●●○○
REQUIRED: ◉ 📄 ✂
COMPLETION: ☐ TIME: _____

SERPENT

The eight segments shown at right form the body of a snake that has eaten its tail. Can you reassemble them into a continuous loop? (If you don't want to make a color copy, here's a challenge: try to do the puzzle totally in your head.)

This puzzle is not as easy as it looks. There are many possible ways the segments can be combined, but only one gives you the closed loop; the rest produce convoluted but "open" serpents. Trial and error will take a long time, but some careful observation will shorten the process considerably. Here's a hint: each part of the puzzle contains the key to its solution.

Once you've discovered the secret of the serpent, the solution will come easily. You can keep the serpent puzzle around as a conversation piece and astound your friends with how quickly you can put the pieces together.

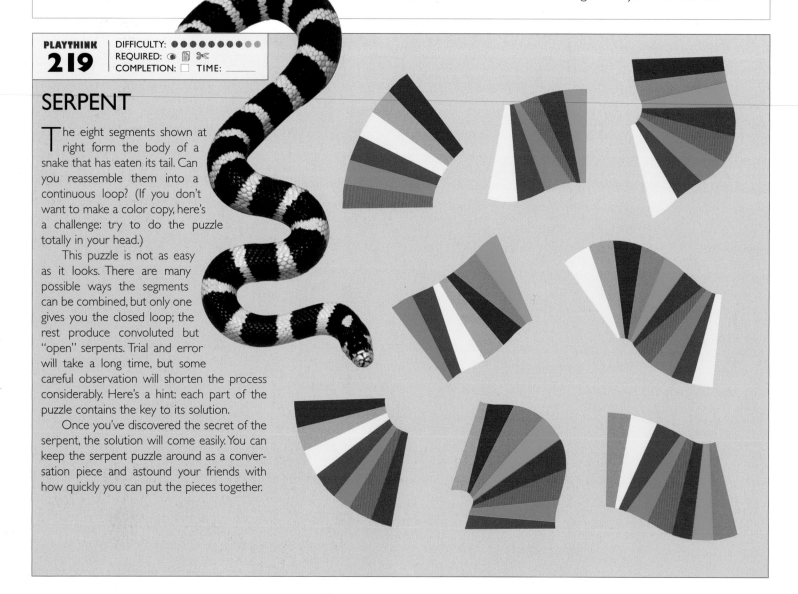

Ouroboros

In ancient Egyptian and Greek mythology, the Ouroboros is a serpent with its tail in its mouth, constantly devouring itself and yet constantly reborn. A gnostic and alchemical symbol, the Ouroboros represents the unity of all things—material and spiritual—and the eternal cycle of destruction and creation.

The nineteenth-century German chemist Friedrich August Kekule von Stradonitz took inspiration from the Ouroboros when he uncovered the true nature of benzene—a molecule made of a ring of carbon atoms.

PLAYTHINK 220

DIFFICULTY: ●●●●●●○○○○○
REQUIRED: ◉ ✎
COMPLETION: ☐ TIME: _____

SPIDERWEB GEOMETRY 1

Three diagonals have been drawn across a circle that is divided into equal segments along its circumference. If you continue drawing lines according to the pattern set by the first three lines, what type of pattern will emerge? Will it look much like a spider's web?

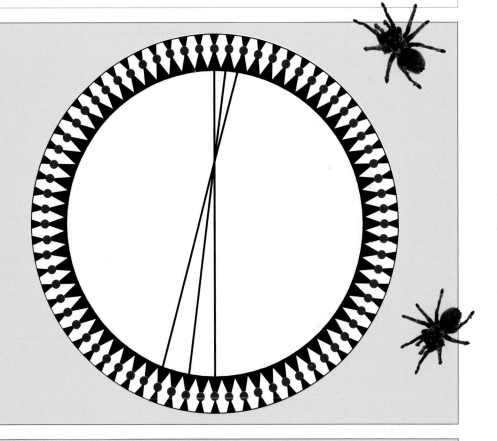
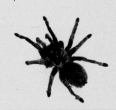

PLAYTHINK 221

DIFFICULTY: ●●●●●●○○○○○
REQUIRED: ◉ ✎
COMPLETION: ☐ TIME: _____

SPIDERWEB GEOMETRY 2

As before, three diagonals have been drawn across a circle that is divided into equal segments along its circumference. If you continue drawing lines according to the pattern set by the first three lines, what type of pattern will emerge?

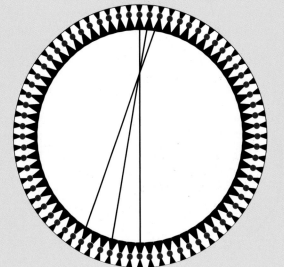

Nature's Basic Plan

Every living thing—every shell, plant or insect—embodies geometry. And little wonder: nature seems to delight in creating a multitude of geometrical shapes. Completely unrelated structures often show a surprising similarity, indicating the presence of both a basic order and basic principles in nature: the circle, the square, the triangle and the spiral.

The basic shapes of nature may be compared to the letters of an alphabet; they can be combined to establish more elaborate forms with new and unique properties. Systems that consist of a minimum number of components that can be combined to yield a great diversity of structural forms are called minimum inventory/maximum diversity systems.

The best example of such a system is nature itself, where we can find a great number of examples. Consider the endless variety of substances formed by the combinations and permutations of a relatively small number of chemical elements. Or think of music: all the songs and symphonies ever written use a relative

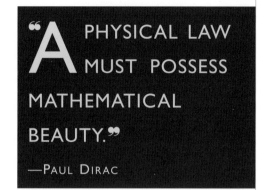

"A PHYSICAL LAW MUST POSSESS MATHEMATICAL BEAUTY."

—PAUL DIRAC

handful of notes. It is the way the elements are combined that is the hallmark of creativity.

PLAYTHINK **222**	DIFFICULTY: ●●●●●●○○○○ REQUIRED: 👁 ✎ COMPLETION: ☐ TIME: ___

DRUNKEN SPIDER I

Imagine drawing many circles, all of which have their centers on the circumference of the base circle, and all of which pass through the base point. What sort of pattern will emerge?

PLAYTHINK **223**	DIFFICULTY: ●●●●●●●○○○ REQUIRED: 👁 ✎ COMPLETION: ☐ TIME: ___

DRUNKEN SPIDER 2

Imagine drawing many circles, all of which have their centers on the circumference of the base circle and all of which touch the diameter of the base circle. What kind of pattern will emerge? You can use the illustration below to help figure this one out.

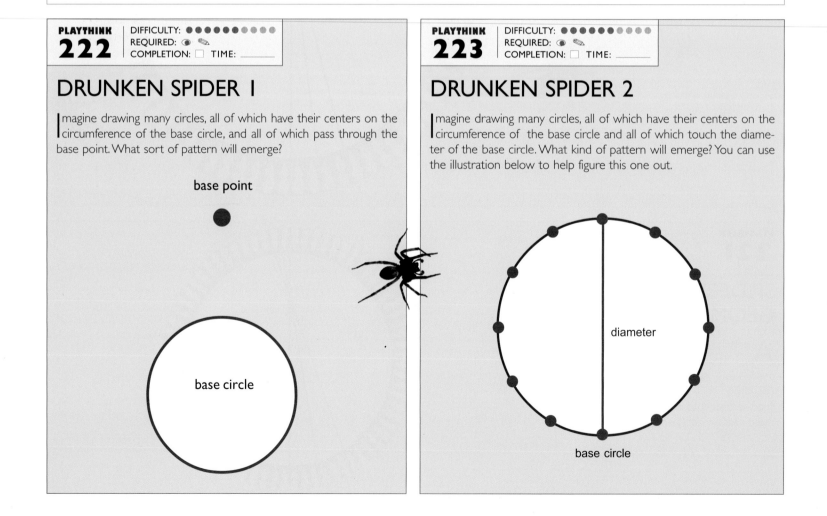

base point

base circle

diameter

base circle

CIRCLE ANATOMY

Can you name the parts of the circle marked in red?

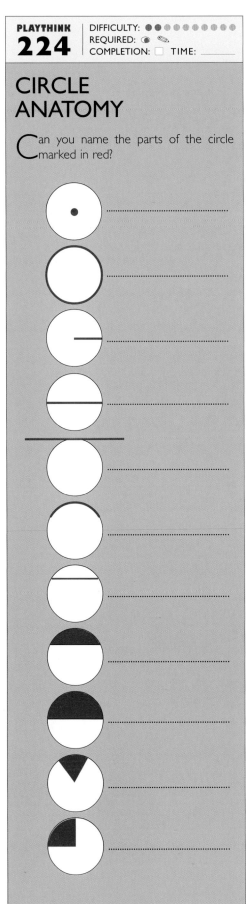

Beauty of the Spheres

Because their curvature is uniform, circles and spheres are considered the most perfect geometric shapes. With no beginning and no end, they symbolize the divine form. With that fact as his only evidence, Aristotle decreed that the paths of the planets must therefore be circular. Nearly 2,000 years later Copernicus, who understood that the sun, and not the earth, is the center of the solar system, uncritically accepted Aristotle's declaration. Even the brilliant German astronomer Johannes Kepler (1571–1630) was burdened by the "truth" of that idea until he discovered that planetary paths are actually elliptical.

Astronomers are not the only ones who have fixated on circles. Early humans certainly saw the roundness of the moon and the ripples made by a stone cast in water. Prehistoric cave paintings display a love of the form; a circle is almost always one of the first figures that a child draws.

Geometrically speaking, a circle is a plane figure bounded by a curved line (called the circumference) that at every point is equally distant from a point called the center. Like many other complex curves, all circles are similar: no matter how big or how small, they are essentially the same.

PURSUIT

A horse runs in a straight line; a person runs toward the horse at all times. Can you determine the shape of the path the runner takes in pursuit of the horse?

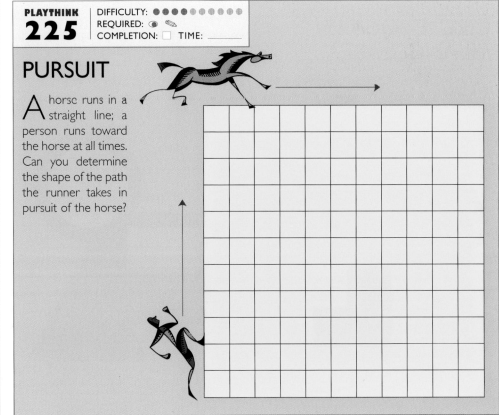

The Wheel

Our civilization runs on wheels, but there is little agreement on how the technology was developed. The best available evidence indicates that, unlike the alphabet or agriculture, the wheel was invented only once in human history: in Mesopotamia about 5,000 years ago. The first vehicles probably had four wheels and were derived from platforms that originally were moved on rollers to transport heavy objects. The rollers had to be constantly picked up from the rear of the platform and moved to the front end.

Notching the underside of such a platform to keep the rollers in place eliminated the need to cycle the rollers from back to front. Eventually rollers held in place evolved into the wheel and axle. The invention of proper wheels had to wait for the discovery of metals, with which more useful tools could be made. (Copper came into use about 4000 B.C. and bronze some time before 2500 B.C.)

The introduction of the wheel represented an event of enormous importance in technical history. It took thousands of years for humans to conceive the idea of a form of motion not evident in their immediate surroundings. After all, no animal uses wheels for moving about. The discovery of the wheel required a capacity for abstract thinking and the ability to pass from the object itself to the idea of it—from phenomenon to theory.

Once this problem was solved, the wheel remained fairly static. The only essential difference between the first wheel of Mesopotamia and the contemporary wheel is the widespread use of pneumatic tires.

PLAYTHINK 226	DIFFICULTY: ●●●●●●●○○○
	REQUIRED: ◉ ✎
	COMPLETION: ☐ TIME: _____

CIRCLE-SQUARE-TRIANGLE AREA

A three-chambered vessel for holding liquids is illustrated here. As the vessel rotates, the red fluid moves from chamber to chamber, filling one of them completely at each turn.

Based on this illustration, can you work out the relationship between a circle, a square and a triangle all possessing the same diameter, height and sides? (Don't forget: the area of a circle is r2π.) Also, can this demonstration give you a way to evaluate the number π? (See page 96.)

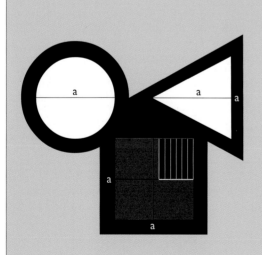
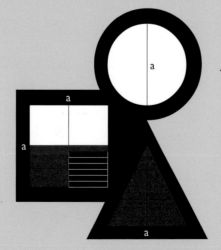
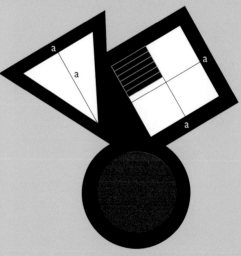

PLAYTHINK
227

DIFFICULTY: ●●●●●●●○○○
REQUIRED: ◉ 📄 ✂
COMPLETION: ☐ TIME: _____

AROUND

There are many classic circle dissection puzzles, such as the old circular tangram, parts of which are combined to make many different patterns and figures.

Our circle dissection puzzle is much more subtle. It consists of ten parts that when combined will form a perfect circle. The subtlety lies in the fact that the circle was dissected using a compass set at the radius of the circle itself—so that every curve is identical.

How long will it take you to reassemble the circle?

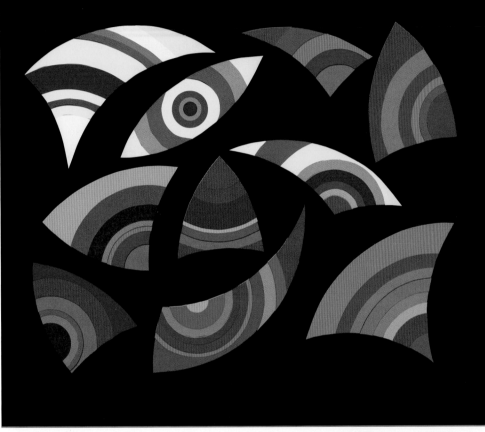

PLAYTHINK
228

DIFFICULTY: ●●●○○○○○○○
REQUIRED: ◉
COMPLETION: ☐ TIME: _____

WHY ROUND?

Why are manhole covers round? Can you find three reasons why round is the best possible shape? And the answer "Because manholes are round" doesn't count!

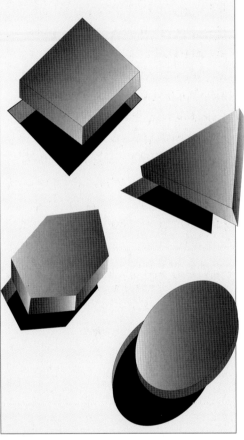

PLAYTHINK
229

DIFFICULTY: ●●●●●●○○○○
REQUIRED: ◉ ✎
COMPLETION: ☐ TIME: _____

ROLLING STONE

People once moved heavy weights by means of rollers made of logs. The circumference of the two identical logs shown here is exactly 1 meter. If the logs roll one whole turn, how far will the weight be carried forward?

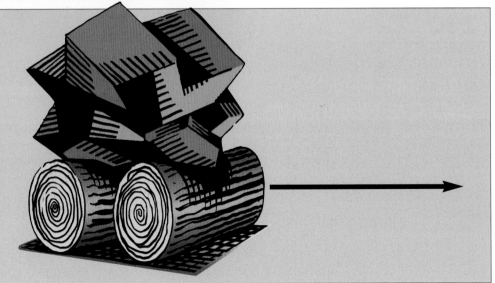

The Number π: 3.14159265358979323846264338327950288...

The ratio between the circumference of a circle and its diameter is one of the most fascinating numbers in mathematics. The Babylonians gave the ratio as simply 3, as does the Bible, though other ancient mathematicians strove for greater precision. The Egyptians, for instance, arrived at a ratio of 3.16 (which has an accuracy of 1 percent) as early as 1500 B.C. In 225 B.C., the Greek mathematician Archimedes inscribed and circumscribed a circle with a ninety-six-sided polygon and found that the ratio lies between 3¹⁄₇ and 3¹⁰⁄₇₁. Ptolemy in A.D. 150 found a value of 3.1416, which is sufficiently accurate for most practical purposes.

These days π (the Greek letter pi), as that ratio is known, has been calculated to millions of decimal places. Why should anyone bother to carry π to such fantastic lengths

through the ages, let alone today? There are three good reasons:

• π is there. Its mere existence, not to mention its great fame, is cause enough for mathematicians to tackle the problem.

• Such calculations often have useful spin-offs. Today the calculation of π provides a way to test new computers and train programmers.

• The more digits of π are known, the more mathematicians hope to answer a major unsolved problem of number theory: Is the sequence of digits behind the decimal place completely random? Thus far there seems to be no hidden pattern, but π does contain an endless variety of remarkable patterns that are the result of pure chance. For example, starting with the 710,000th decimal

place, π begins to stutter 3333333. Similar runs occur of every digit except 2 and 4.

The ratio was named π in 1737 by none other than Leonhard Euler (see page 71). In 1882 the German mathematician Ferdinand von Lindenmann proved that π is a transcendental number; that is, neither π itself nor any of its whole powers can be expressed as a simple fraction. No fraction, with integers above and below the line, can exactly equal π, and no straight line of length π can be constructed with compass and ruler alone.

The importance of π lies not simply in its role as a geometric ratio; π appears in the formulas engineers use to calculate the force of magnetic fields and physicists use to describe the structure of space and time.

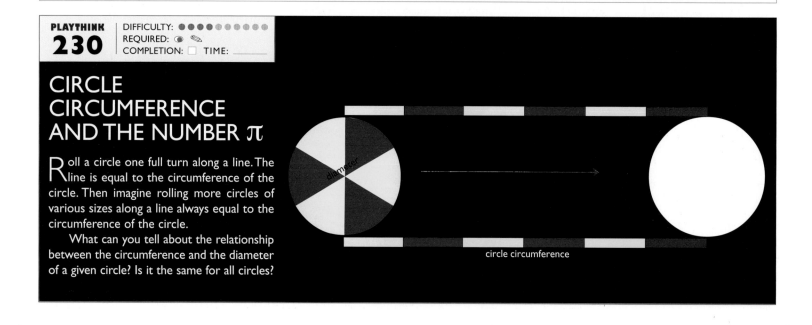

PLAYTHINK 230 | DIFFICULTY: ●●●●○○○○○○ | REQUIRED: ◉ ✎ | COMPLETION: ☐ TIME: _____

CIRCLE CIRCUMFERENCE AND THE NUMBER π

Roll a circle one full turn along a line. The line is equal to the circumference of the circle. Then imagine rolling more circles of various sizes along a line always equal to the circumference of the circle.

What can you tell about the relationship between the circumference and the diameter of a given circle? Is it the same for all circles?

circle circumference

Squaring the Circle

One of the most famous geometric problems of antiquity was that of squaring the circle. The problem was to construct a square with an area equal to that of a given circle, using only a straightedge and a compass. The ancient Greek mathematicians, with their great geometrical skill, tried hard but were unable to solve such an apparently simple problem. Ironically, in their trials in squaring the circle, the ancient Greeks succeeded in squaring many more complex curves, which made for exciting discoveries and theorems.

For more than 2,000 years mathematicians and amateurs devoted untold hours to solving this problem. Ferdinand von Lindenmann's proof that π is a transcendental number—and thus cannot be constructed with a compass and ruler—finally made official what all mathematicians who have tackled the problem have declared in frustration: Squaring the circle is impossible!

PLAYTHINK 231
DIFFICULTY: ●●●●●●●○○○
REQUIRED: ◉
COMPLETION: ☐ TIME: _____

CRESCENTS OF HIPPOCRATES

The ancient Greek geometer Hippocrates of Chios discovered this problem while trying to square the circle. He constructed overlapping semicircles on the sides of a right triangle, as shown below. Can you determine the total area of the two red crescents?

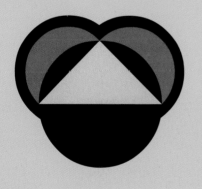

PLAYTHINK 232
DIFFICULTY: ●●●●●●●○○○
REQUIRED: ◉
COMPLETION: ☐ TIME: _____

CIRCLE IN THE SQUARE

Which is greater, the sum of the black areas or the sum of the red areas?

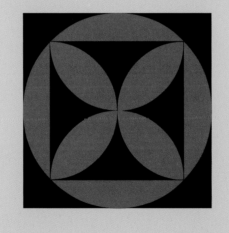

PLAYTHINK 233
DIFFICULTY: ●●●●●●●●○○
REQUIRED: ◉ ✎
COMPLETION: ☐ TIME: _____

SQUARE VASE

Can you divide the red vase and reassemble the parts to form a perfect square? This is possible in two different ways, one that divides the vase into three parts and another that divides it into four parts.

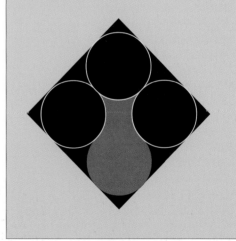

PLAYTHINK 234
DIFFICULTY: ●●●●●●●○○○
REQUIRED: ◉
COMPLETION: ☐ TIME: _____

SICKLE OF ARCHIMEDES

A circle is divided in half along its diameter, and two additional semicircles are constructed along that diameter, as shown here. A line (L) is drawn from the point on the diameter where the two circles meet and extended perpendicularly from the diameter to the circumference of the large semicircle.

The area of the large semicircle that is not covered by the smaller semicircles has the form of a sickle, an ancient tool used for harvesting grain. Can you guess what the area of the sickle might be?

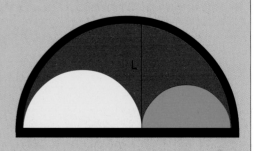

Mystic Roses

To create a mystic rose, a set of points is evenly spaced along the circumference of a circle, and each point is connected to every other point by a straight line. A small number of points leads to a relatively simple rose. As the number of points increases, the complexity rises substantially.

In 1809 the French mathematician Louis Poinsot asked what was the minimum number of continuous lines needed to draw mystic roses of various sizes. (A continuous line is drawn without lifting the pen from the paper or retracing any of the lines.) A three-point mystic rose can be drawn with one continuous line, but it is impossible to draw a four-point rose in one continuous line. Two continuous lines will always be needed.

PLAYTHINK
235

DIFFICULTY: ●●●●●●○○○○○
REQUIRED: ◉
COMPLETION: ☐ TIME: _____

MYSTIC ROSE ON FIFTEEN POINTS

Fifteen points are equally spaced around a circle. Each point is joined to every other point by a straight line. Can you work out how many lines there are? Can this pattern be drawn in a continuous manner without lifting pencil from paper or retracing any lines?

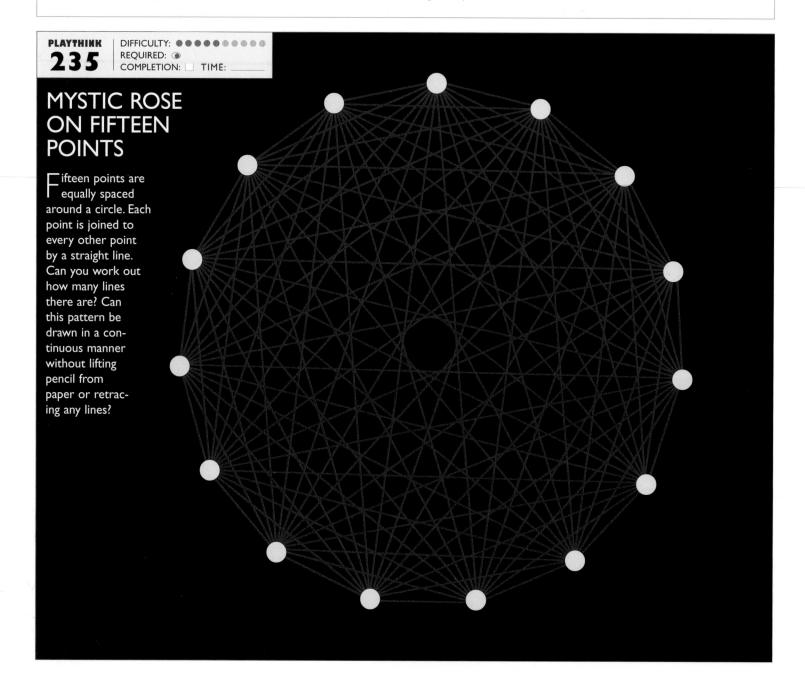

CIRCLE AREA

How can you demonstrate the formula for finding the area of a circle?

Imagine you have a circle of radius r and circumference 2πr. Cut that circle into sectors and arrange them into a parallelogram, as shown in the illustration. The more sectors you cut the circle into, the more each sector will resemble a triangle and the closer the figure will approach the shape of a rectangle with one side r and the other side πr. Can you now calculate the area?

"In the limit," as mathematicians say, the polygons inscribed in the circle become the circle itself. That limit can never be reached, but approaching it as nearly as we like is the foundation of the mathematical discipline known as calculus.

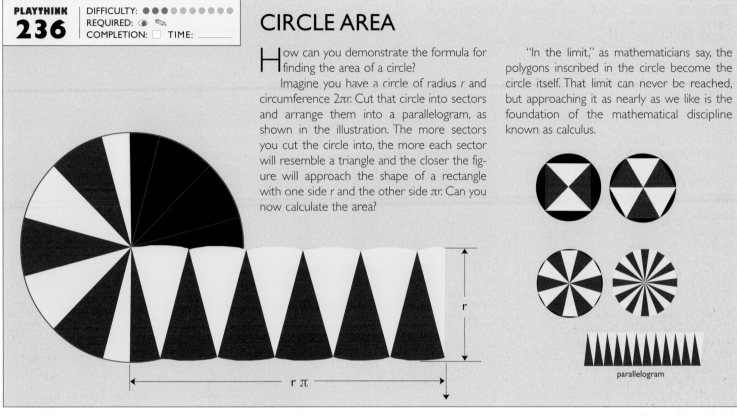

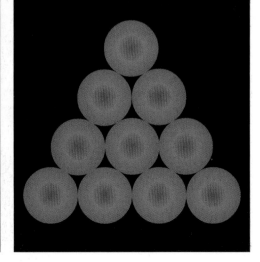

parallelogram

THREE CIRCLES

Three identical equilateral triangles are inscribed with circles, as shown. Which case provides the circles with the largest total area?

1. An incircle (the largest circle that can be inscribed on a triangle) and two smaller circles **2.** Three identical circles of the largest size possible **3.** One big circle and two smaller ones

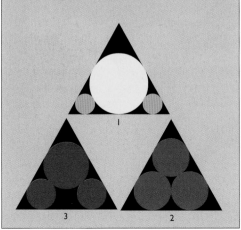

COIN MATTERS

You must rearrange the pyramid of six coins into a hexagon that possesses a hole large enough for a seventh coin. Can you do this in just five moves?

A move consists of sliding a single coin along a flat surface to a new position so that it is in contact with at least two other coins. When moving a coin, you cannot move or jostle any other coin.

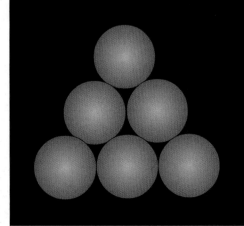

UPSIDE-DOWN COINS

The object is to turn the pyramid of ten coins upside-down, moving one coin at a time to a new position in which it touches two or more coins.

It is easy to do this in six moves. Can you do it in three?

PLAYTHINK 240

DIFFICULTY: ●●●●●○○○○○
REQUIRED: 👁 ✏
COMPLETION: ☐ TIME: _____

CIRCLES AND TANGENTS

How many essentially different ways can you find to arrange two circles of unequal size on a plane?

If a tangent is a straight line touching a curve at a single point, and a common tangent is a straight line tangent to two circles, can you find the total number of common tangents to the two circles for all the arrangements of two circles?

Would it make any difference if the circles were the same size?

PLAYTHINK 241

DIFFICULTY: ●●●●●○○○○○
REQUIRED: 👁 ✏
COMPLETION: ☐ TIME: _____

SEVEN CIRCLES PROBLEM

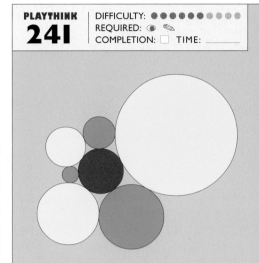

Start with any circle. (Use the red one in the diagram as a reference.) Add six circles around the circumference of the circle so that each of the new circles touches two other new circles and the red circle. Imagine that three of the circles (yellow in the diagram) become larger and larger and the green circles become smaller and smaller, though the green and yellow still remain in contact. Imagine that the yellow circles become so large that they even intersect. What will be the ultimate outcome?

PLAYTHINK 242

DIFFICULTY: ●●●●●●●●●○
REQUIRED: 👁 ✏
COMPLETION: ☐ TIME: _____

APOLLONIUS'S PROBLEM

How many different ways can you add a fourth circle to three existing circles so that the three circles all touch the circumference of the fourth one?

This is one of the classic problems from Greek antiquity. It relates to the general question about the maximum number of mutually tangent circles in a flat plane.

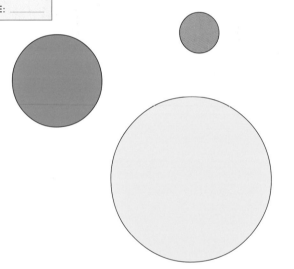

PLAYTHINK 243

DIFFICULTY: ●●○○○○○○○○
REQUIRED: 👁 ✏
COMPLETION: ☐ TIME: _____

CIRCLES COLORING

The pattern of colored circles on the left contains all the logical clues for filling in the blank circles on the right. Size has nothing to do with color, since circles of equal size have different colors.

Can you figure out the pattern, and color in the circles properly?

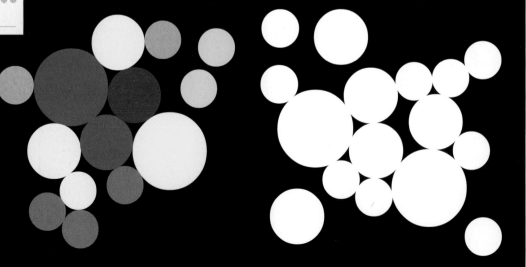

CIRCLE REGIONS

One circle can divide a plane into two regions: inside the circle and outside the circle. Two intersecting circles can divide a plane into four regions, as illustrated below.

Now consider five intersecting circles in which no three circles pass through the same point. Into how many regions can those five intersecting circles divide a plane? Is there a general rule for *n* circles?

1 circle
2 regions

2 circles
4 regions

3 circles
8 regions

4 circles
14 regions

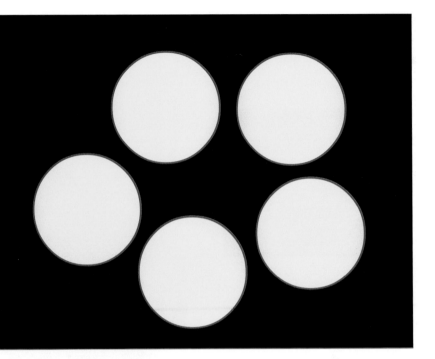

POLYGONS IN A CIRCLE

Five points are randomly distributed on the circumference of a circle. From any of those points, a continuous line may be drawn that connects the other points in the polygon before returning to the original point.

How many different polygons can be drawn with these five points?

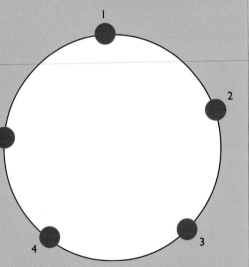

TOUCHING CIRCLES 2

Three differently colored circles of identical size can be arranged in a way so that all three are in contact but no two circles of the same color touch. (See the inset for an example of this.) Can you arrange identical circles in a way so that four colors are needed to avoid contact between two circles of the same color? What is the smallest number of circles needed for this to occur?

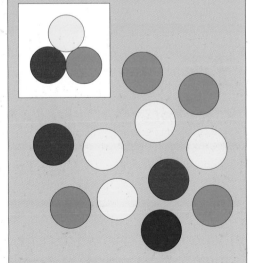

TOUCHING COINS 16

Can you arrange these sixteen coins flat on a table so that each coin touches exactly three other coins? Each coin must lie flat—no overlapping!

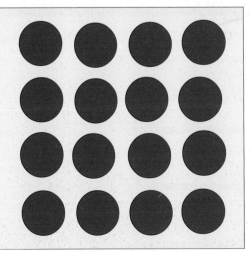

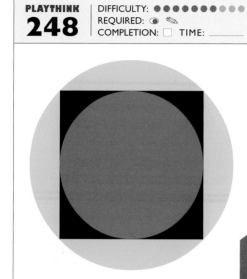

CIRCLE RELATIONSHIP

One circle is circumscribed around a square; another circle is inscribed within the same square. How are the areas of the two circles related?

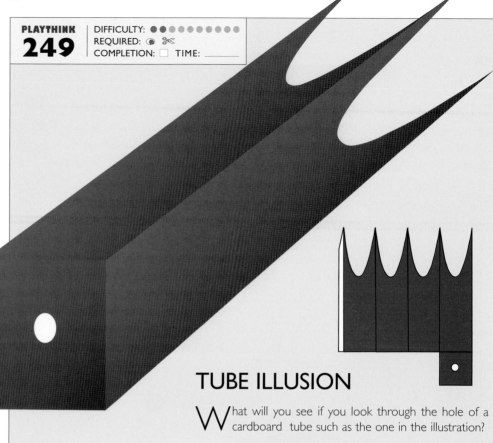

TUBE ILLUSION

What will you see if you look through the hole of a cardboard tube such as the one in the illustration?

ORANGE AND YELLOW BALLS

Can you stack six yellow balls and four orange balls in a triangle so that no three yellow balls form the corners of an equilateral triangle? The example at left is obviously wrong because the three yellow balls do, in fact, form such a triangle.

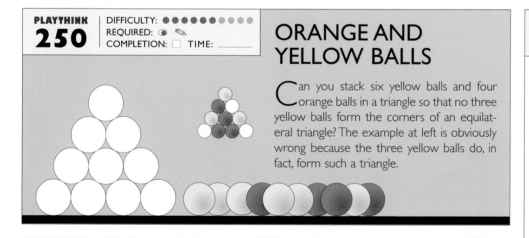

ROLLING CIRCLES PARADOX

Two identical rollers between two parallel rails can roll and retain their relative positions, one over the other. Would that be possible if one roller were twice as big as the other?

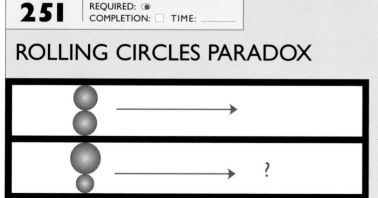

JUMPING COINS

You must stack the six numbered coins into two piles of three coins each. But in order to do so, you must move each coin by jumping over exactly three other coins. As an example of an allowable first move, coin 2 can jump over 3, 4 and 5 to stack on coin 6.

Can you stack the coins in five moves or less?

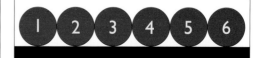

PLAYTHINK
253
DIFFICULTY: ●●●●●○○○○○
REQUIRED: ◉ ✎
COMPLETION: ☐ TIME: _____

TOUCHING CIRCLES

Three circles touch at three points, shown here with black circles. Can you find the minimum number of identical circles in a plane that are required to create nine touching points?

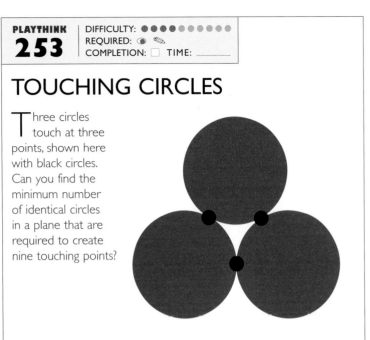

PLAYTHINK
254
DIFFICULTY: ●●●●●●●○○○
REQUIRED: ◉ ✎
COMPLETION: ☐ TIME: _____

INSCRIBED CIRCLES

The large black circle has a diameter of 1 unit. It is inscribed by an equilateral triangle and a square, as shown.

Can you determine the diameters of the three inscribed circles?

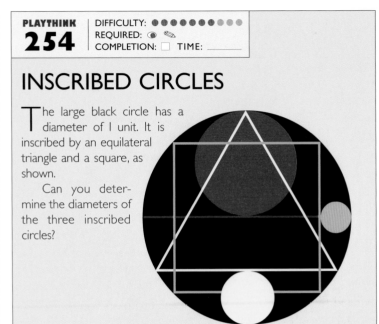
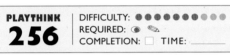

PLAYTHINK
255
DIFFICULTY: ●●●●●●●●○○
REQUIRED: ◉ 📄 ✂
COMPLETION: ☐ TIME: _____

SEMICIRCLE CHAIN

Can you attach the eight semicircles to the pegs on the line below so that no two semicircles cross? Although semicircles may be placed on either side of the line, no two are allowed to share a peg.

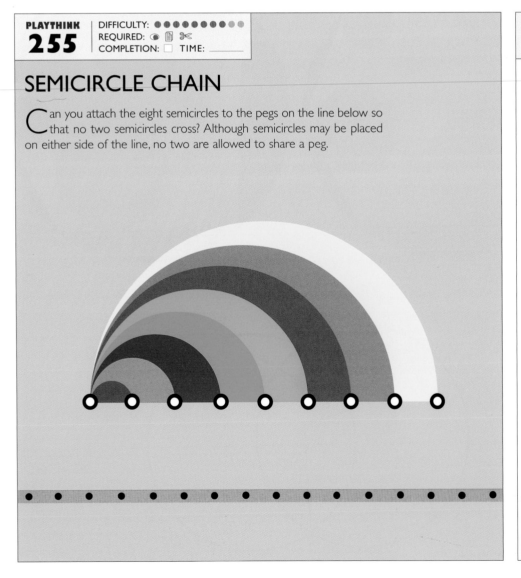

PLAYTHINK
256
DIFFICULTY: ●●●●●●●○○○
REQUIRED: ◉ ✎
COMPLETION: ☐ TIME: _____

ROSETTE CIRCUMFERENCE

When a number of circles of the same radius are drawn through a point, the result is a shape called a rosette. Can you tell which is greater, the perimeter of a rosette formed by circles of radius equal to 1 unit, or the circumference of a larger circle with a radius equal to 2? The illustration below may be helpful.

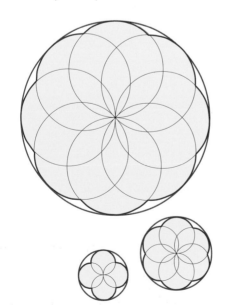

PLAYTHINK
257

DIFFICULTY: ●●●●●●●●●○
REQUIRED: ◉ ✎
COMPLETION: ☐ TIME: _____

● midpoints of sides
● bases of the altitudes
● midpoints to orthocenter

NINE-POINT CIRCLE

The white triangle has some interesting properties: the midpoints of the sides, the bases of the altitudes and the midpoints of the line joining the vertices to the orthocenter (the common intersection of all three altitudes of the triangle) all line up on the circumference of a circle.

Does every triangle form that sort of nine-point circle?

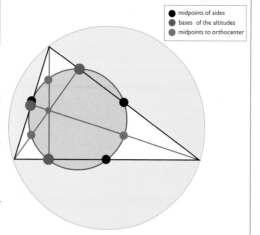

PLAYTHINK
258

DIFFICULTY: ●●●●●●●○○○
REQUIRED: ◉
COMPLETION: ☐ TIME: _____

INDIANA ESCAPE

Jones is running down a square tunnel, desperately trying to avoid being crushed by a giant round stone that is rolling toward him. The width of the tunnel is just about the same as the diameter of the sphere; both are 20 meters.

The end of the tunnel is too far for Jones to reach in time. Is he doomed?

PLAYTHINK
259

DIFFICULTY: ●●●●●●●●○○
REQUIRED: ◉ ✎
COMPLETION: ☐ TIME: _____

JAPANESE TEMPLE TABLET

The same polygon is inscribed in two identical circles, but it is triangulated in different ways. The biggest circle that can be inscribed is placed in each resultant triangle.

Can you compare the sum of the diameters of the two sets of circles? Is one set larger than the other?

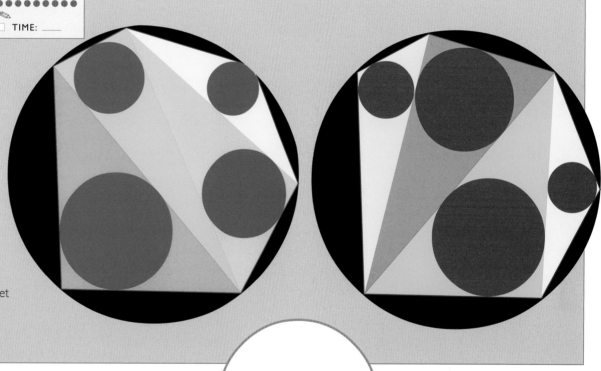

PLAYTHINK
260

DIFFICULTY: ●●●●●●●●●○
REQUIRED: ◉ ✎
COMPLETION: ☐ TIME: _____

THREE INTERSECTING CIRCLES

We interconnected three intersecting circles of random size by their common chords, as shown. The result should surprise: the common chords passed through a single point.

Will this happen regardless of the size and position of the three circles?

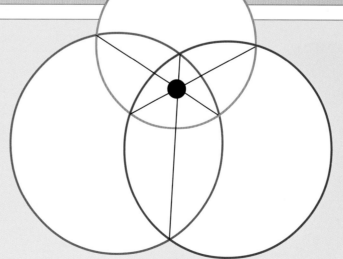

PLAYTHINK
261
DIFFICULTY: ●●●●●●●○○○
REQUIRED: ◉ ✎
COMPLETION: ☐ TIME: _____

TANGENTS TO THE CIRCLE

Three circles of different sizes are distributed randomly, as shown. Pairs of tangents are drawn around the circles, with a surprising result: the three intersection points for the tangents lie along a straight line.

Is this just a coincidence, or will it always happen?

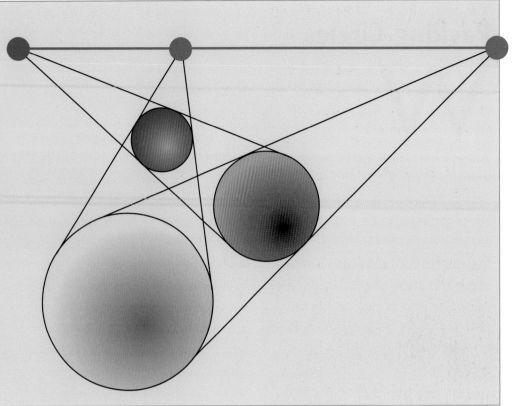

PLAYTHINK
262
DIFFICULTY: ●●●●●●○○○○
REQUIRED: ◉ ✎
COMPLETION: ☐ TIME: _____

COINS REVERSE

Seven coins are placed heads up in a circle. You would like them all to be tails up, but you are allowed to move them only if you turn five over at a time. Can you follow that rule repeatedly to eventually wind up with all seven coins tails up? How many moves will it take?

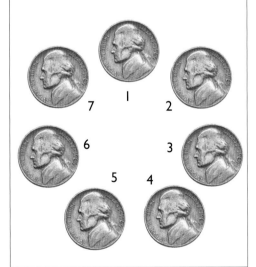

PLAYTHINK
263
DIFFICULTY: ●●●●●●●●○○
REQUIRED: ◉ ✎
COMPLETION: ☐ TIME: _____

ROLLING INSIDE OUT

Two identical circles touch the same point of a rectangle—one from the inside, one from the outside. Both circles begin rolling in the plane along the perimeter of the rectangle until they return to the starting point.

If the height of the rectangle is twice the circumference of the circles, and if the width is twice the height, how many revolutions will each circle make?

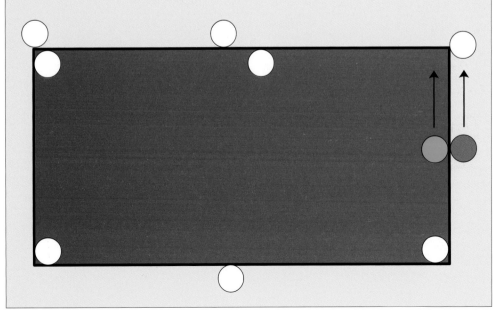

Packing Circles

Walk down the halls of some prestigious universities, and you will find grown men and women trying to figure out how to pack steel balls into boxes. This isn't a case of adults getting in touch with their inner children: What they are trying to do has a direct impact on such cutting-edge fields as information theory and solid state physics. Packing regular objects—circles on a plane or spheres in a space—is one of the most important problems in mathematics.

Balls of equal size do not fill a space completely, nor do circles in a plane. It is fairly easy to show that the densest possible configuration—a packing similar to a honeycomb, called a hexagonal lattice—is the most efficient regular packing of circles. It is enormously more difficult—though it

has been done nonetheless—to show that no irregular packing can be denser.

The analogous problem of spheres packed into a volume has proven to be even more difficult. The densest regular packing is known, but whether any irregular packing can do better is still a mystery. The best guess is no, but there is no proof.

A more recent problem involves packing a given number of circles into a specific boundary of the smallest area—a square, say, or a circle. No general solution is yet known, even when the boundary of the region is very simple; the best solutions that have been found apply to only a very few circles packed in a very regular space. For example, the solution for packing circles within a larger circle has been proved up to only ten circles. The densest packings

for instances up to ten circles are illustrated here. The numbers next to each example are the diameters of the outer circles, in terms of the unit circles they contain.

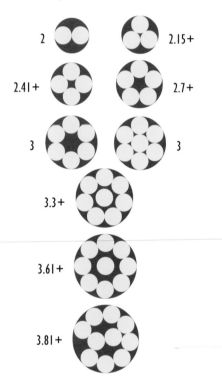

2
2.15+
2.41+
2.7+
3
3
3.3+
3.61+
3.81+

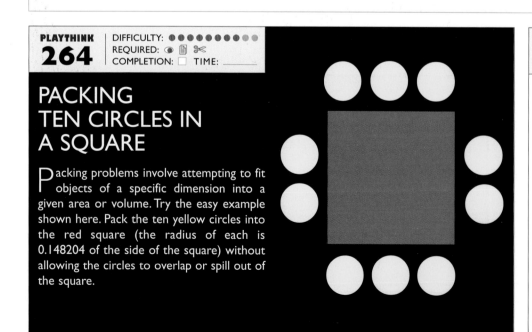

PACKING TEN CIRCLES IN A SQUARE

Packing problems involve attempting to fit objects of a specific dimension into a given area or volume. Try the easy example shown here. Pack the ten yellow circles into the red square (the radius of each is 0.148204 of the side of the square) without allowing the circles to overlap or spill out of the square.

PACKING TWELVE CIRCLES IN A CIRCLE

Twelve identical circles can be packed into a circle with a diameter just 4.02 times larger than that of the packing circles. This is the densest possible packing for twelve circles. Can you find the optimal packing configuration?

Spheres

To get their marbles exceedingly smooth and round, glassmakers have devised a simple and yet ingenious process. They melt the glass at the top of a tower and allow small amounts to dribble off into a shaft. As the globs of glass fall, they contract to form nearly perfect spheres. By the time the globs reach the bottom of the shaft, they have cooled to become hard and round.

Although the traditional icon for a drop is the "teardrop" shape, photography using a strobe flash has shown that most drops in midfall are spherical. Drops of liquid are spherical in shape because electrical forces pull the loose materials toward the middle. Molecules moving in from the outer parts of the drop fill in any open space close to the center of mass. Once the drop has reached its most compact form, it has taken on the shape of a sphere.

A sphere, or ball, is perhaps the simplest solid shape that one can imagine. It has no corners or edges. Every spot on the outside of a ball is exactly the same distance from the center as every other spot. A sphere is also one of the most common shapes in the universe. Stars and planets are subject to the constant pull of their own gravity and take on nearly spherical shapes; indeed, astronauts in orbit find that any spilled liquids quickly form little quivering balls.

PLAYTHINK 266 | DIFFICULTY: ●●●●●●○○○○ | REQUIRED: ◉ | COMPLETION: ☐ TIME: _____

ROLLING COIN 1

The yellow coin rolls over seven immovable coins in the configuration shown below. By the time the yellow coin returns to its starting position, how many complete revolutions will it have made? And which direction will the coin be facing?

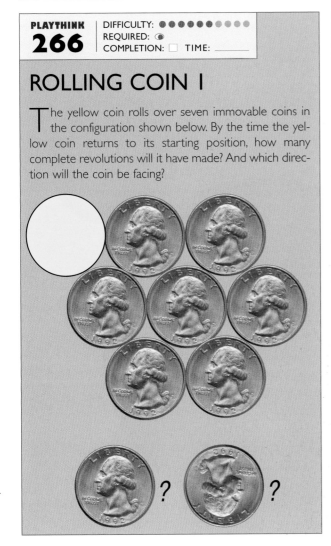

PLAYTHINK 267 | DIFFICULTY: ●●●●●●●●●○ | REQUIRED: ◉ ✎ | COMPLETION: ☐ TIME: _____

ROLLING CIRCLE

A small circle rolls over the perimeter of a circle that has a diameter three times that of the smaller one. How many revolutions of the small circle will it take for that circle to return to its starting point?

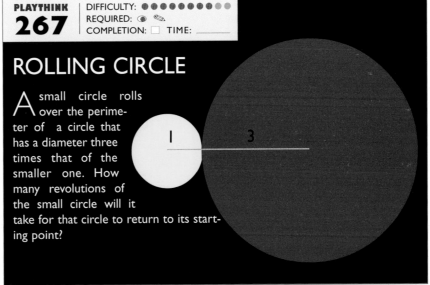

PLAYTHINK 268 | DIFFICULTY: ●●●●●●○○○○ | REQUIRED: ◉ | COMPLETION: ☐ TIME: _____

ROLLING COIN 2

Two identical coins are placed side by side, as shown at the right. Keeping the coin on the right motionless, roll the coin on the left over the top of the fixed coin until it reaches the opposite side of the coin. Will the figure on the rolling coin be facing left, right or upside-down?

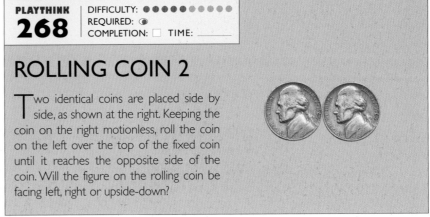

Packing Spheres

The astronomer Johannes Kepler revolutionized the study of the orbits of planets. He also researched the problem of packing spheres. Kepler found that there are two ways to arrange spheres in a plane: the square lattice and the hexagonal (or honeycomb) lattice. Those two arrangements can then be stacked to fill a volume in several ways.

Square layers, for example, can be stacked so that the spheres are vertically above each other, or the spheres in one layer can nestle into the gaps between the four spheres in the layer below—the so-called face-centered cubic lattice. Hexagonal layers also have two possibilities, either aligned or staggered, although this last instance is essentially no different than the face-centered cubic lattice.

One way to tell which arrangement is the most compact is by imagining that the spheres were allowed to expand to fill in the available space. What shape would the spheres then have? Spheres in a cubic lattice would simply form cubes, while spheres in a hexagonal lattice would form hexagonal prisms. But spheres packed in a face-centered cubic lattice, as Kepler found, would form a rhombic dodecahedron, which leads to the tightest possible packing.

The efficiency of a packing lattice is measured in the proportion of space that is filled with spheres. For spheres in a plane, the efficiency for a square lattice is 78.54 percent; for a hexagonal lattice, 90.69 percent. For spheres in a three-dimensional volume, the efficiency for a cubic lattice is 52.36 percent; for a hexagonal lattice, 60.46 percent; for a face-centered cubic lattice, 74.04 percent.

PLAYTHINK | DIFFICULTY: ●●●●●●●●○○
269 | REQUIRED: ◉ ✎
| COMPLETION: ☐ TIME: _____

PACKING DISKS

There are two ways to fill a plane with disks; both are shown below. Can you find the percentage of the total area of the plane covered by disks in both the hexagonal and rectangular packings?

hexagonal (triangular) packing

rectangular (square) packing

PLAYTHINK | DIFFICULTY: ●●●●●●○○○○
270 | REQUIRED: ◉ ✎
| COMPLETION: ☐ TIME: _____

KISSING SPHERES

How many identical spheres can you pack into a sphere that has a diameter three times as large?

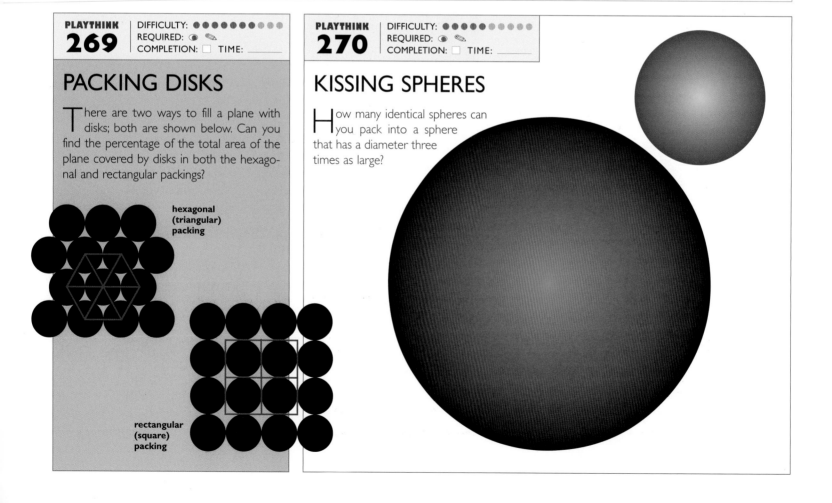

Cycloids

No point in the universe is truly fixed. A point that remains stationary within a car may be tracing a linear path as the car speeds down the highway. A point on a mountain follows the earth around the sun. And even the sun and the Milky Way galaxy have their own paths through an ever-expanding universe.

The motion of a fixed point on a moving body traces a curve that can have very unusual properties. For example, the curve traced by a point on a rotating circle is called a cycloid. The cycloidal curve appears in many places in modern society: mechanical gears have teeth whose sides possess a cycloidal curve; a machine engraves an elaborate cycloid on the plates used for printing bank notes; a popular science toy known as the Spirograph produces an endless variety of cycloidal shapes with just a few round parts.

Other similar curves include the spiral and the involute—the line traced by the end of a taut thread as it is unwound off a spool.

| PLAYTHINK **271** | DIFFICULTY: ●●●●●●○○○○ REQUIRED: ◉ ✎ COMPLETION: ☐ TIME: _____ |

ROLLING CIRCLE: HYPOCYCLOID

A smaller circle rolls inside a fixed circle twice its diameter. What path will the red point trace as the small circle completes one circuit?

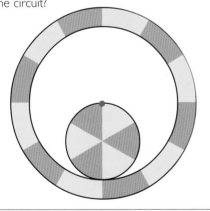

| PLAYTHINK **272** | DIFFICULTY: ●●●●●○○○○○ REQUIRED: ◉ COMPLETION: ☐ TIME: _____ |

NORTH POLE TRIP

An airplane leaves the North Pole and flies due south for 50 kilometers. Then it turns and flies east for another 100 kilometers.

At the end of that journey, how far is the plane from the North Pole?

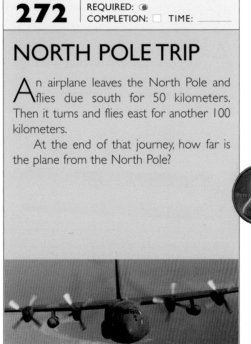

| PLAYTHINK **273** | DIFFICULTY: ●●●●○○○○○○ REQUIRED: ◉ COMPLETION: ☐ TIME: _____ |

ROWS OF FIVE COINS

Can you move just one coin to make two rows of five coins each?

| PLAYTHINK **274** | DIFFICULTY: ●●●●●●●○○○ REQUIRED: ◉ ✎ COMPLETION: ☐ TIME: _____ |

ROLLING WHEEL

The wheel of a train rolls along a rail. To keep the train on the tracks, each wheel has a flange that extends below the circumference of the point of contact with the train. Can you envision the path traced by these three points?

- A point on the inside of the rolling wheel
- A point on the circumference of the rolling wheel
- A point on the outer flange of the rolling wheel

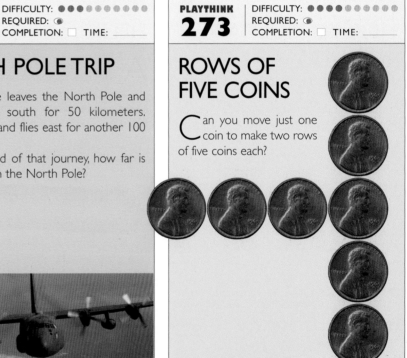

PLAYTHINK
275
DIFFICULTY: ●●●●●●●○○○
REQUIRED: 👁 ✏
COMPLETION: ☐ TIME: _____

CUTTING A SPHERE

Imagine that this sphere has been divided with four straight cuts, all of which go right through the sphere. Can you determine the maximum number of pieces into which the sphere has been divided?

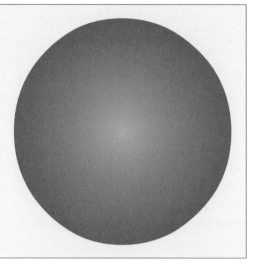

PLAYTHINK
276
DIFFICULTY: ●●●●●●●●○○
REQUIRED: 👁 ✏ ✂
COMPLETION: ☐ TIME: _____

REULEUX'S TRIANGLE

A curiously shaped triangle revolves inside a fixed square frame. To construct such a shape, begin with an equilateral triangle; with each of the three corners as centers, draw a circular arc passing through the other two corners. What you will have is called Reuleux's triangle, named after the man who discovered it in 1875. The width of the curve in every direction is equal to the side of an equilateral triangle.

Imagine the triangle rolling along the inside of the square, as shown here. Can you imagine the path traced by the blue dot through several complete rotations?

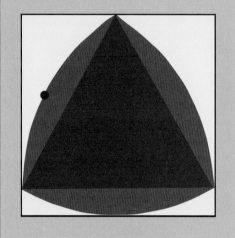

PLAYTHINK
277
DIFFICULTY: ●●●●●●●○○○
REQUIRED: 👁 📄 ✂
COMPLETION: ☐ TIME: _____

HEXSTEP SOLITAIRE: A SLIDING DISK PUZZLE

In this game the object is to transfer the red disk at the bottom to the space marked with the red dot at the top. To do so, you must slide disks one at a time into one of the two empty spaces (shown in the illustration as white circles). For example, the two possible first moves would be to slide either the green disk down or the blue disk up into one of the empty spaces. The yellow disks cannot reach the white spaces on the first move because the gap for them to move through is too narrow. As a rule, only two moves are possible at any given time.

Can you accomplish the goal in fewer than fifty moves?

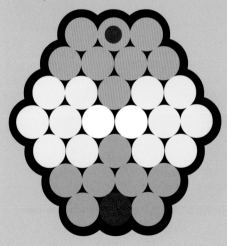

PLAYTHINK
278
DIFFICULTY: ●●●●●●●●○○
REQUIRED: 👁 ✏
COMPLETION: ☐ TIME: _____

HELIX

A rope winds around a large cylindrical pipe, making four complete turns, as shown. The circumference of the pipe is 4 meters and its length is 12 meters. Can you figure out how long the rope is?

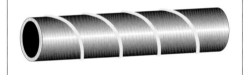

PLAYTHINK
279
DIFFICULTY: ●●●●●●●○○○
REQUIRED: 👁 ✏
COMPLETION: ☐ TIME: _____

LOOPED EARTH

Imagine the earth as a perfect sphere. (It is not, but picture it this way for the sake of this puzzle.) Then imagine the equator is a long belt that has been looped around the earth and fastened snugly.

If you loosened that belt by 2 meters and pulled the belt away from the surface, how much slack would there be? In other words, how high could you pull the belt? The answer is either .03 meters, .33 meters or 3.3 meters—but which?

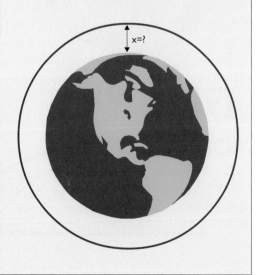

PLAYTHINK
280

DIFFICULTY: ● ● ● ● ● ● ● ○ ○ ○
REQUIRED: ◉
COMPLETION: ☐ TIME: _____

SPHERE SURFACE AREA

A sphere fits exactly inside a thin-walled cylinder that has a height and diameter equal to the diameter of the sphere. Which object has more surface area, the sphere or the cylinder?

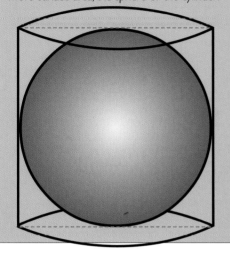

PLAYTHINK
281

DIFFICULTY: ● ● ● ● ● ● ● ○ ○ ○
REQUIRED: ◉ ✏
COMPLETION: ☐ TIME: _____

SPHERE VOLUME

A cylinder, a sphere and a cone are identical in height and width. Do their volumes have any sort of special relationship?

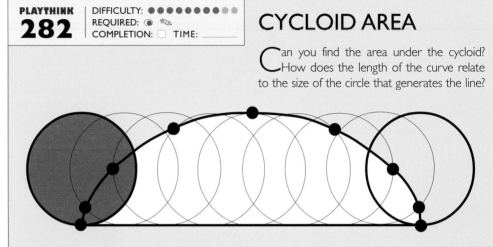

PLAYTHINK
282

DIFFICULTY: ● ● ● ● ● ● ● ● ○ ○
REQUIRED: ◉ ✏
COMPLETION: ☐ TIME: _____

CYCLOID AREA

Can you find the area under the cycloid? How does the length of the curve relate to the size of the circle that generates the line?

PLAYTHINK
283

DIFFICULTY: ● ● ● ● ● ● ● ○ ○ ○
REQUIRED: ◉
COMPLETION: ☐ TIME: _____

PACKING BOX

Is this story possible?

The king has a rectangular chest filled tightly with twenty golden spheres. Each sphere is held securely by the spheres touching it, so that when picked up, the spheres do not move about in the box.

How many spheres can be removed without disrupting the tightness of the fit?

...Once upon a time the king had all his money made into identical gold spheres. He packed the money into a big chest tightly. He knew that the chest was full, because it didn't rattle.

Soon the queen took out some money, repacked the chest, and still the chest didn't rattle. Then the treasurer took out some more money, repacked the chest, and still the chest didn't rattle. Then the prime minister took out some more money and still it didn't rattle. ...

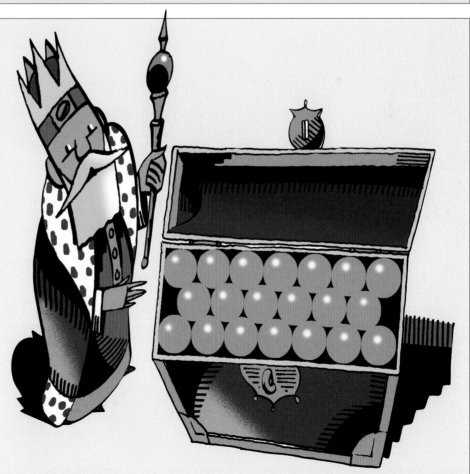

Curves of Constant Width

Curves that have the same width in every direction are called curves of constant width. Any curve of constant width can turn between two fixed parallel lines or within a square. Although some curves of constant width, such as the circle, are smooth, others have corners; and while some are highly symmetrical, others are quite irregular. As a matter of fact, any regular polygon with an odd number of sides can be rounded up to create a curve of constant width.

But every curve of constant width has one thing in common: the length of the curve is equal to π times that constant width. This is known as Minkowski's theorem and is seen most obviously in the formula for the circumference of a circle, which is π times the diameter.

PLAYTHINK 284

DIFFICULTY: ●●●●●●●○○○
REQUIRED: ◉
COMPLETION: ☐ TIME: _____

QUICKEST DESCENT

Four identical balls on four different tracks are released simultaneously. Which of the tracks—bent, straight, circular or cycloidal—will deliver its ball to the end of the slope the fastest?

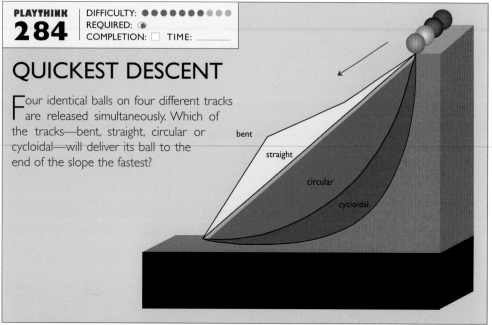

PLAYTHINK 285

DIFFICULTY: ●●●●●●●○○○
REQUIRED: ◉
COMPLETION: ☐ TIME: _____

CURVES OF CONSTANT WIDTH

As a circle revolves between two parallel rails, the rails remain the same distance apart. On the other hand, as an ellipse revolves, the rails move up and down twice over the course of a full rotation.

Examine the five curves below. Can you tell which ones will turn like a circle and which ones will turn like an ellipse?

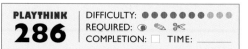

circle   ellipse

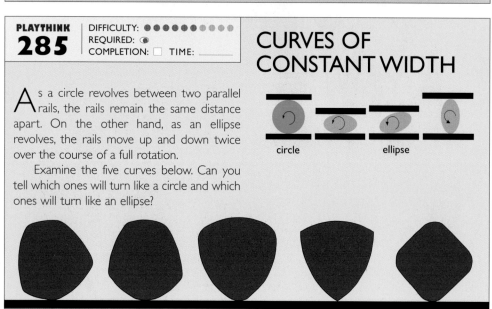

PLAYTHINK 286

DIFFICULTY: ●●●●●●●○○○
REQUIRED: ◉ ✎ ✂
COMPLETION: ☐ TIME: _____

POLYGON WHEELS

Can you describe the paths traced by the points on the rolling polygons illustrated below?

You may be unfamiliar with how some of the shapes might roll. Cutting the shapes out of cardboard and rolling them on a line may help you visualize the problem.

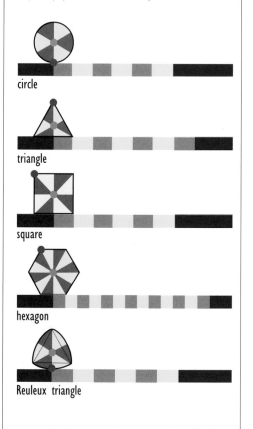

circle

triangle

square

hexagon

Reuleux triangle

Conic Sections and Spirals

The curves formed by passing a plane through a cone—known as conic sections—were a subject of intense study in ancient Greece. The aesthetic properties of ellipses, hyperbolas and parabolas fascinated Euclid and other geometers of that era. But they could find no uses for them and regarded conic sections as merely interesting geometrical recreations.

Mathematicians have a habit of studying utterly useless objects just for fun. But often those studies become enormously important to scientists in later centuries. That is what happened with conic sections. The work of Johannes Kepler and Isaac Newton relied on the study of conic sections to describe the paths traced by celestial bodies moving through space. Planets, comets and even galaxies move exclusively in ellipses, hyperbolas and parabolas.

The same is true of objects in flight on earth. The path of a ball through the air is a parabola. In fact, every projectile—every bullet, arrow, rocket or stream of water emerging from a nozzle—follows a parabolic path. The reason for this, Newton discovered, is that gravity's pull affects the path of an object at every point in its flight. Rather than being straight, the line traced by an object in flight is constantly curved, approaching but never reaching a perfectly vertical path over time. If the object is thrown fast enough, however—as in the case of a satellite launched by a rocket—the path will curve in such a way that the object (satellite) doesn't fall; instead, it orbits the earth.

PLAYTHINK 287

DIFFICULTY: ●●●●○○○○○○
REQUIRED: ◉
COMPLETION: ☐ TIME: _____

SWORDS AND SCABBARDS

As they prepare for battle, four warriors draw their swords from their scabbards. One sword is completely straight. Another is a semicircle. A third sword has the form of a wavy curve. And the fourth has the three-dimensional form of a helicoid spiral, as shown.

Something isn't right about this story. What is it?

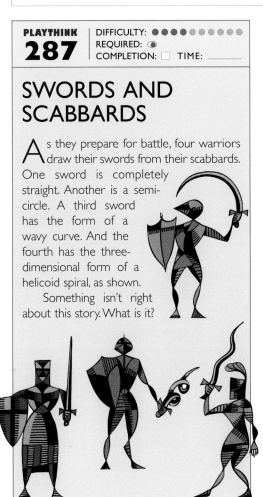

PLAYTHINK 288

DIFFICULTY: ●●●●●●○○○○
REQUIRED: ◉
COMPLETION: ☐ TIME: _____

CONICS

In his book *Conics,* dated 225 B.C., the Greek scholar Apollonius revealed that a cone with a circular base can be cut to form a family of curved shapes. For the cuts marked 1 through 4 in the illustration, which curved shapes will result?

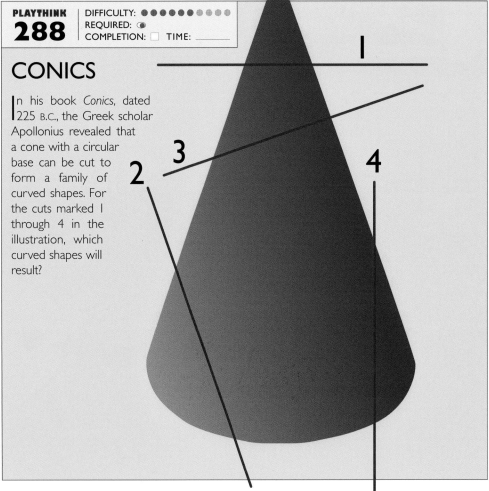

PLAYTHINK 289

DIFFICULTY: ●●●●○○○○○○
REQUIRED: ◉
COMPLETION: ☐ TIME: _____

ELLIPSE WHERE?

The man in the illustration desperately needs to see an ellipse. How can he make one while sitting at the table without touching his pen, compass, ruler or computer?

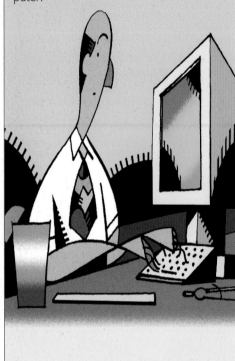

PLAYTHINK 290

DIFFICULTY: ●●●●●●○○○○
REQUIRED: ◉ ✎
COMPLETION: ☐ TIME: _____

ROLLING CIRCLE: EPICYCLOID

The radius of the smaller circle is exactly half that of the larger circle.

As the small circle rolls along the outside of the big circle, the green point will trace a curve. Can you envision the shape of that curve? There is no need to draw it exactly— a rough approximation of the shape will do.

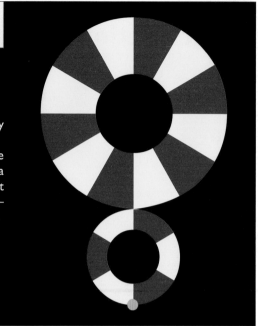

PLAYTHINK 291

DIFFICULTY: ●●●●●●●○○○
REQUIRED: ✄
COMPLETION: ☐ TIME: _____

ELLIPSE BY PAPER FOLDING

How can you create an ellipse from a circular piece of paper without using a pen or any other object?

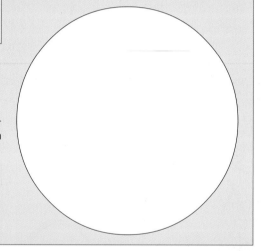

PLAYTHINK 292

DIFFICULTY: ●●●●●○○○○○
REQUIRED: ◉
COMPLETION: ☐ TIME: _____

ELLIPTICAL POOL TABLE

This elliptical pool table has a pocket at one focal point and a ball at the other focal point. Is it possible to strike the ball so that it lands in the pocket despite the obstacle in between?

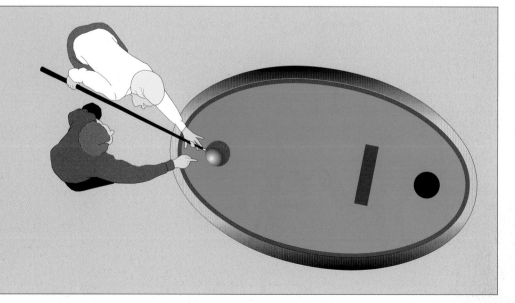

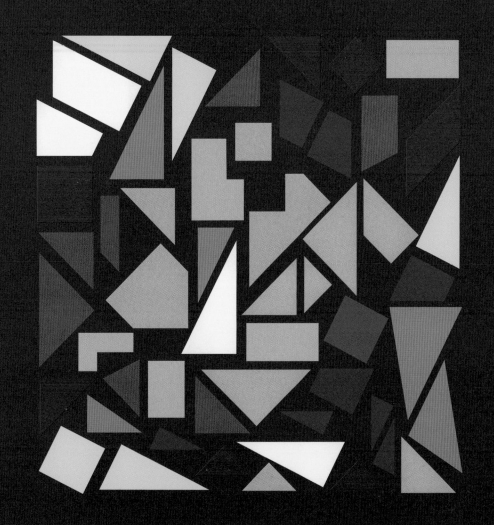

Shapes and Polygons

PLAYTHINK 293

DIFFICULTY: ●●●○○○○○○○
REQUIRED: ◉
COMPLETION: ☐ TIME: _____

ODD SHAPE

One of these seven shapes shown is not like the others. Which shape? And why?

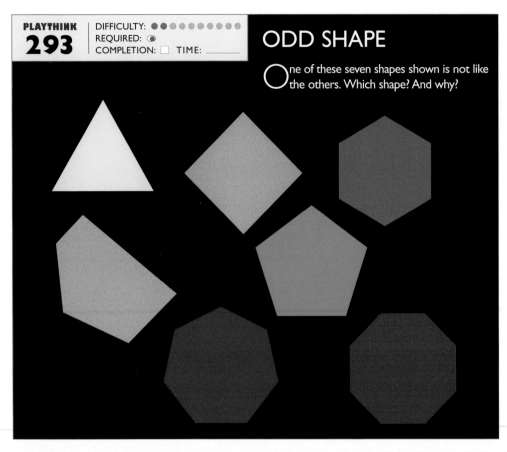

PLAYTHINK 294

DIFFICULTY: ●●●●●●○○○○
REQUIRED: ◉ ✎ ✂
COMPLETION: ☐ TIME: _____

POLYGONS FROM TRIANGLES AND SQUARES

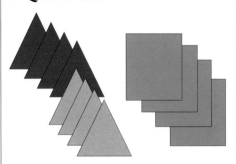

Starting with a supply of squares and equilateral triangles that all have sides of identical length, put the pieces together to form convex polygons. Can you form polygons that have a number of sides ranging from five to ten? How many triangles and squares do you need to form each polygon?

PLAYTHINK 295

DIFFICULTY: ●●●○○○○○○○
REQUIRED: ◉
COMPLETION: ☐ TIME: _____

ODD ONE OUT

Which of these shapes is different from the other four?

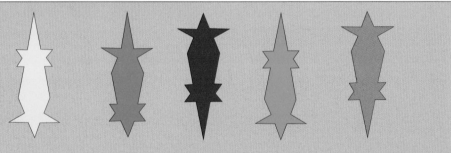

PLAYTHINK 296

DIFFICULTY: ●●●●○○○○○○
REQUIRED: ◉ ✎
COMPLETION: ☐ TIME: _____

CONVEX-CONCAVE

There's a number missing from the middle of the red polygon. What should it be?

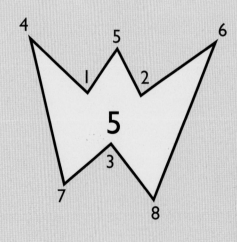

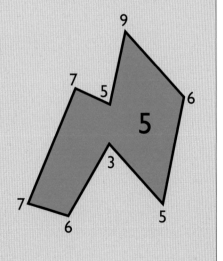

PLAYTHINK 297

DIFFICULTY: ●●●●●●○○○○○
REQUIRED: ◉
COMPLETION: ☐ TIME: _____

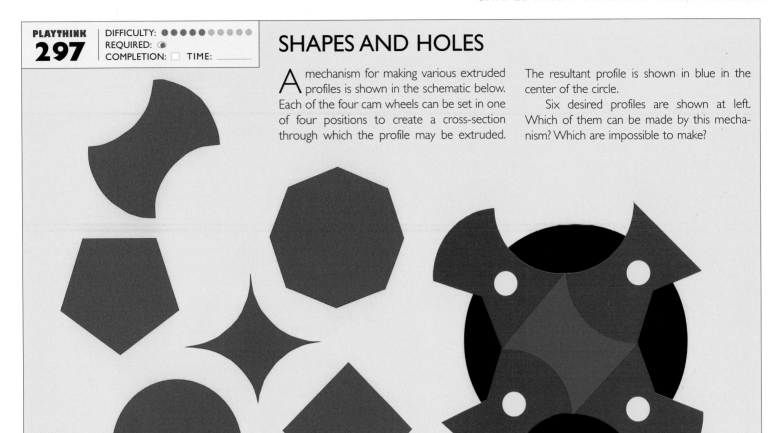

SHAPES AND HOLES

A mechanism for making various extruded profiles is shown in the schematic below. Each of the four cam wheels can be set in one of four positions to create a cross-section through which the profile may be extruded.

The resultant profile is shown in blue in the center of the circle.

Six desired profiles are shown at left. Which of them can be made by this mechanism? Which are impossible to make?

PLAYTHINK 298

DIFFICULTY: ●●●●●●●●○○○
REQUIRED: ◉ ✎
COMPLETION: ☐ TIME: _____

EULER'S FORMULA

Examine the complex polygonal map illustrated below. Then count the number of points represented by the black dots. From that number, subtract the number of sides, and add to that result the number of regions.

What is the number? Will it be the same for every polygon, regardless of its size, shape and complexity?

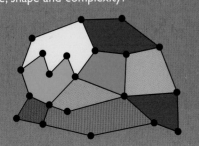

PLAYTHINK 299

DIFFICULTY: ●●●●●●○○○○○
REQUIRED: ◉ ✎
COMPLETION: ☐ TIME: _____

AREA EQUAL TO THE PERIMETER

A five-by-five square has a perimeter of 20 units and an area of 25 units. A four-by-five rectangle has a perimeter of 18 units and an area of 20 units. Can you find a square and a rectangle that have perimeters equal to their areas?

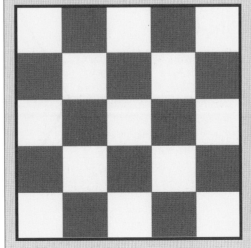

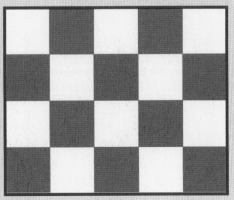

PLAYTHINK 300

DIFFICULTY: ●●●●●●●●○○
REQUIRED: ◉
COMPLETION: ☐ TIME: _____

INSCRIBED POLYGONS

The outermost circle has a radius of 1 unit. In that circle, inscribe an equilateral triangle. In the triangle, inscribe a circle. Inside the circle, a square, then another circle, then a regular pentagon and so on. At each step the number of sides of the regular polygon will become larger, and the size of the circle will become smaller. Can you make a rough guess as to how small the circle eventually will become?

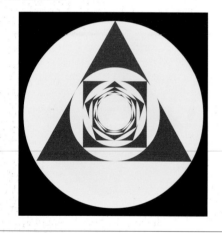

PLAYTHINK 301

DIFFICULTY: ●●●●●●●○○○
REQUIRED: ◉ ✎
COMPLETION: ☐ TIME: _____

OVERLAPPING TRIANGLES

Eight smaller equilateral triangles in three sizes (with sides of 1, 2 or 3 units) partly overlap a larger triangle with sides 5 units long. Can you tell which is greater, the red area of the big triangle or the blue area of the small triangles?

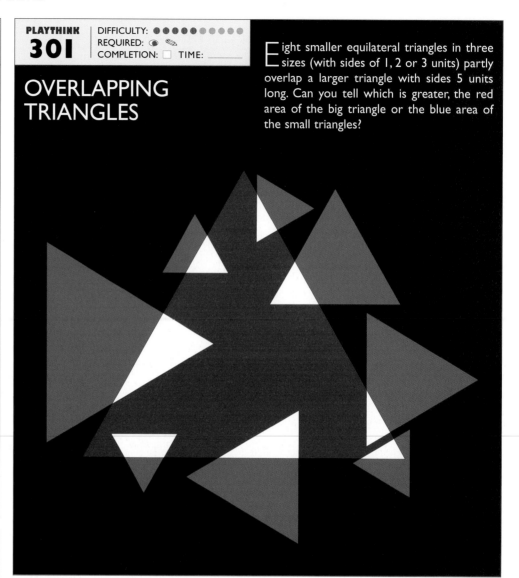

PLAYTHINK 302

DIFFICULTY: ●●●●●●●●●●
REQUIRED: ◉
COMPLETION: ☐ TIME: _____

PEG-BOARD AREA

The Peg-Board shown below has a rubber band stretched around the four red pegs. Can you calculate the area enclosed by the rubber band without measuring anything?

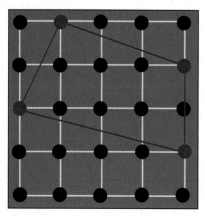

PLAYTHINK 303

DIFFICULTY: ●●●●●●●●○○
REQUIRED: ◉ ✎
COMPLETION: ☐ TIME: _____

HEXAGON IN-OUT

A regular hexagon circumscribes a circle, which circumscribes another regular hexagon. The inner hexagon has an area of 3 square units. What is the area of the outer hexagon?

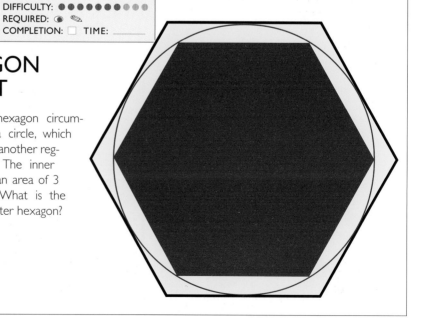

PLAYTHINK
304

DIFFICULTY: ●●●●●○○○○○
REQUIRED: ◉
COMPLETION: ☐ TIME: _____

TRIANGLE COUNT

A mask of unknown shape has been placed over this collection of triangles. Based on what you can see, how many triangles were there to begin with?

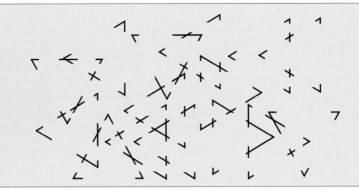

PLAYTHINK
305

DIFFICULTY: ●●●●●●●○○○
REQUIRED: ◉ ✎ 📄 ✂
COMPLETION: ☐ TIME: _____

POLYGO

Polygo is a game based on the creation and recognition of complex shapes built up from four simple polygons: triangles, squares, pentagons and hexagons. By assembling these basic shapes, it is possible to construct a great variety of new polygons.

Each tile possesses polygons filled in with four different colors—red, yellow, green and blue. In a two-person game, each player chooses to be represented by two of those colors. The object is to create complex shapes of solid colors by joining four tiles side by side. Each polygon so created has a value, which is the sum of the four tiles from which it was built: one point for each triangle, two for each square, three for each pentagon and four for each hexagon. The player with the most points at the end wins.

To play a game of solitaire, fit the twenty-four square tiles into the grid, matching the colors at each corner.

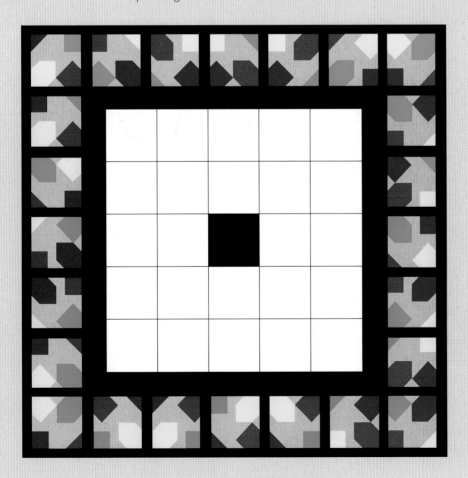

PLAYTHINK
306

DIFFICULTY: ●●●●●●●○○○
REQUIRED: ◉ ✎ ✂
COMPLETION: ☐ TIME: _____

WHIRLING POLYGONS

A blue triangle, a red square, a green pentagon and a pink hexagon are inscribed in the same circle and are revolving within it. (Imagine that the four circles shown below are actually one circle.) Can you envision what you would see as the circle turns?

To double-check your answer, make a paper wheel inscribed with the four shapes. Make a small hole in the center of the wheel and spin it on the point of a pencil.

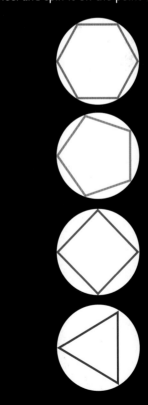

The Island Problem

As any primary school-teacher knows, area and volume are difficult ideas to grasp. Water will be spilled all over the classroom floor long before most children begin to understand the basic concept of conservation: that the amount of liquid inside a container does not depend on the container's shape.

Children are not the only ones who are confused by area and volume. Clever packaging fools many adults into thinking that they are buying more than they really are. Areas and volumes are easy to estimate for rectangular plots and boxes; estimating is more difficult for other shapes, especially ones with curved sides.

The ancient Greeks knew all about the significance of perimeter in terms of area enclosed—indeed, the word *meter* is derived from the Greek word for "measure around." Since many Greeks lived on islands, they had good reason to be aware of the pitfalls of measurement. After all, it is easy to see that the area of an island cannot be assessed using the time it takes to walk around it; a long coastline might simply mean that the shape of the island is irregular rather than that the island is large. Nevertheless, the custom was for landowners to base real estate values on the perimeter of their holdings, not the area.

One ancient story tells of Dido, the princess of Tyre, who fled to a spot on the North African coast. There she was given a grant of land that was terribly small—equal to what could be covered by the hide of an ox. Undaunted, Dido had the hide cut into strips and sewn together to make one ribbon about a mile in length. Then, using the shoreline as one boundary, she had her supporters stretch the ribbon of hide in as big a semicircle as was possible. In this way one ordinary ox hide encompassed about 25 acres of land. On that spot Dido founded the famous and powerful city of Carthage.

HIDDEN TRIANGLE

Trisect the angles of a triangle, as shown. Note that three points within the triangle form an equilateral triangle.

Does such an equilateral triangle appear in every trisected triangle?

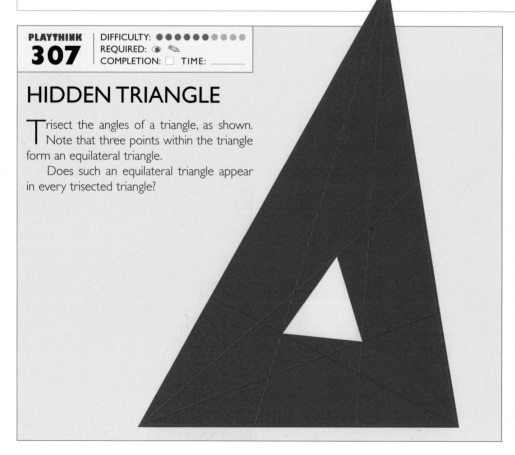

CONVEX QUADRILATERAL

Begin with five randomly placed points on a plane. Will it always be possible to connect four of those points to create a convex quadrilateral?

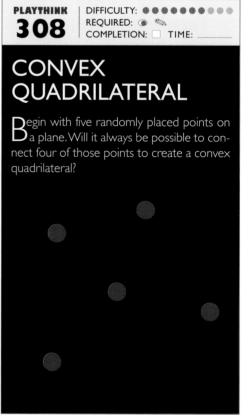

PLAYTHINK
309

DIFFICULTY: ● ● ● ● ● ● ● ○ ○ ○
REQUIRED: ◉ ✏
COMPLETION: ☐ TIME: _____

GOATS AND PEG-BOARDS

The blue pegs in the Peg-Board represent goats grazing in the fenced-off part of an orchard. Each goat needs an area equal to 1 square unit of the grid to graze on. Within the fenced-in areas (the fences are the black lines), how many goats can graze?

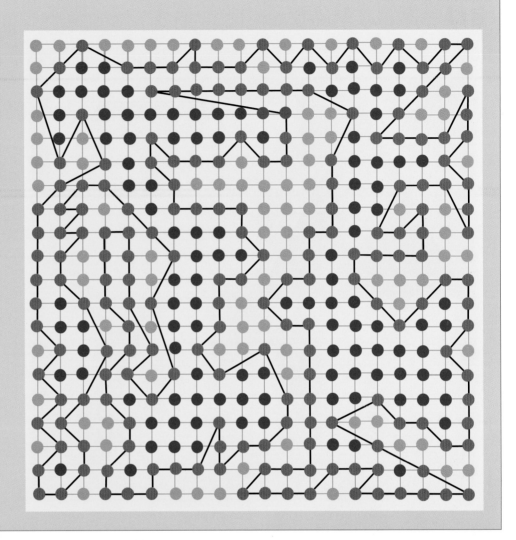

PLAYTHINK
310

DIFFICULTY: ● ● ● ● ● ● ● ○ ○ ○
REQUIRED: ◉ ✏
COMPLETION: ☐ TIME: _____

HOW MANY POLYGONS?

1. How many triangles?

2. How many triangles?

3. How many triangles and squares?

4. How many squares?

5. How many triangles?

6. How many triangles and squares?

7. How many regular hexagons?

8. How many squares?

9. How many squares?

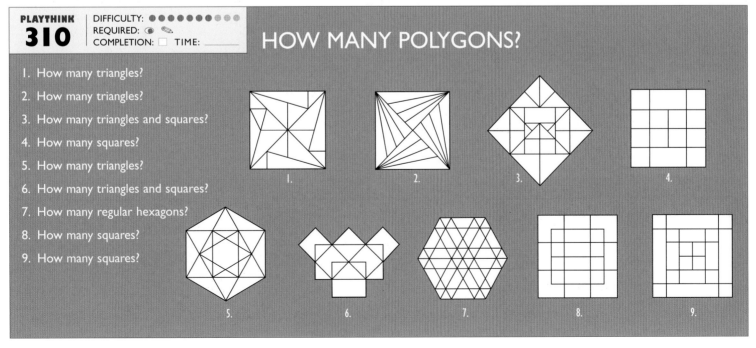

PLAYTHINK 311

DIFFICULTY: ●●●●●○○○○○
REQUIRED: 👁 ✎
COMPLETION: ☐ TIME: _____

POLYGON AREAS

These two regular polygons—a regular hexagon and an equilateral triangle—have equal perimeters. What is the ratio of their areas?

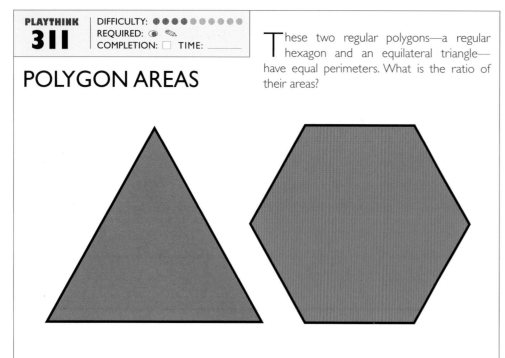

PLAYTHINK 312

DIFFICULTY: ●●●●●●○○○○
REQUIRED: 👁 ✎
COMPLETION: ☐ TIME: _____

TRIANGLES IN QUADRILATERALS

A straight line divides this quadrilateral into two triangles. Can you find a quadrilateral (which is simply a polygon with four sides) that can be divided with a straight line into three triangles?

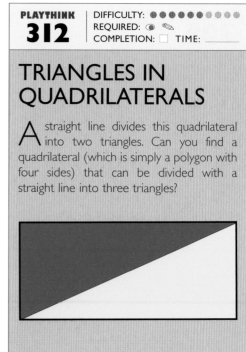

PLAYTHINK 313

DIFFICULTY: ●●●●●○○○○○
REQUIRED: 👁
COMPLETION: ☐ TIME: _____

HOW MANY TRIANGLES?

How many triangles of different sizes can you find in this pattern?

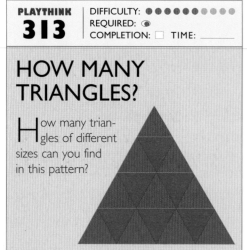

PLAYTHINK 314

DIFFICULTY: ●●●●●●●○○○
REQUIRED: 👁 ✎
COMPLETION: ☐ TIME: _____

HINGED SCREEN

A hinged screen made of two identical panels is placed in the corner of a room, as shown. At what angle should the panels be opened to enclose—with the walls—the largest possible area?

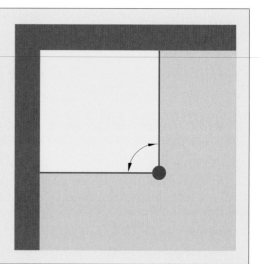

PLAYTHINK 315

DIFFICULTY: ●●●●●●○○○○
REQUIRED: 👁 ✎
COMPLETION: ☐ TIME: _____

BUILDING CAGES

Six cages, built of nineteen panels of equal lengths, hold six different animals. Disaster strikes, and seven of those panels become unusable. With just the twelve remaining panels, can you construct six new cages to hold the animals? Each animal must be completely surrounded by panels and must not share its cage.

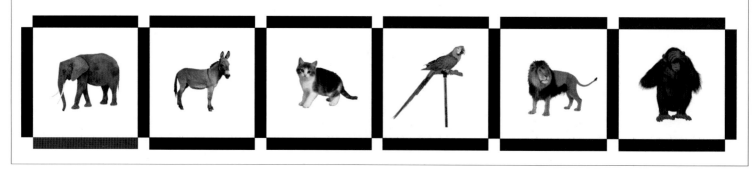

PLAYTHINK 316

DIFFICULTY: ●●●●●●●○○○
REQUIRED: 👁 ✎
COMPLETION: ☐ TIME: _____

FOUR SQUARES

There were four squares on this page before they were erased. The only evidence that remains is dots that marked the midpoints of the sides of the squares.

From this evidence, can you reconstruct the four squares?

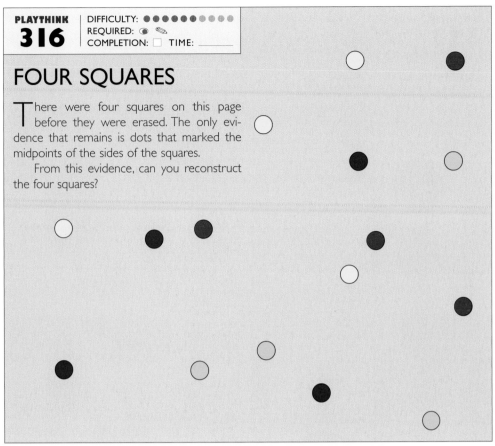

PLAYTHINK 317

DIFFICULTY: ●●●●●○○○○○
REQUIRED: 👁
COMPLETION: ☐ TIME: _____

HEXAPATTERNS

All but one of the smaller patterns are composed of the same twenty-four colored pieces that make up the large hexagon. Which hexagon is the odd one out?

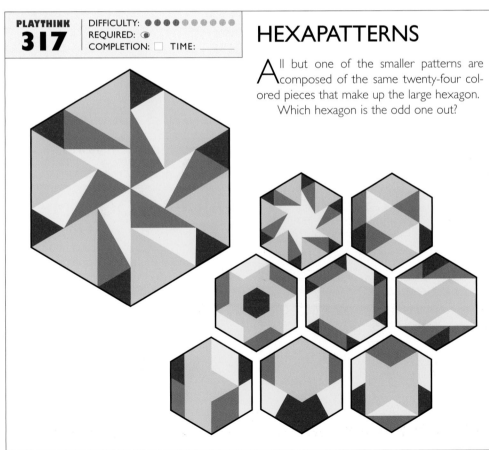

PLAYTHINK 318

DIFFICULTY: ●●●●●●○○○○
REQUIRED: 👁 ✎
COMPLETION: ☐ TIME: _____

TRIANGLES INSCRIBED 1

How many triangles can you draw from the vertices of a heptagon that don't possess sides that are also sides of the heptagon?

In a square and a pentagon, for instance, you can't draw such a triangle; in a regular hexagon you can draw two, as shown below.

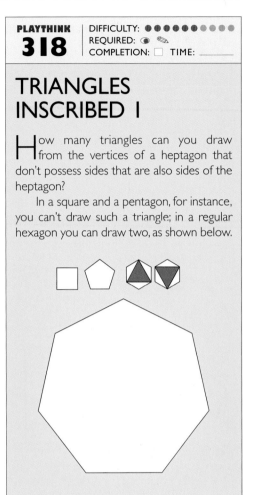

PLAYTHINK 319

DIFFICULTY: ●●●●●●○○○○
REQUIRED: 👁 ✎
COMPLETION: ☐ TIME: _____

TRIANGLES INSCRIBED 2

How many triangles can you draw from the vertices of an octagon that don't possess sides that are also sides of the octagon?

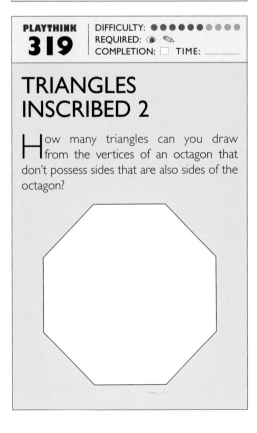

PLAYTHINK 320

DIFFICULTY: ●●●●●○○○○○
REQUIRED: 👁 ✏️
COMPLETION: ☐ TIME: _____

EQUAL PERIMETERS

All four shapes—circle, square, triangle and pentagon—are equal in perimeter. Rank the shapes in order of area, from largest to smallest. You may use logic, calculations or the superimposed grid to find your answer.

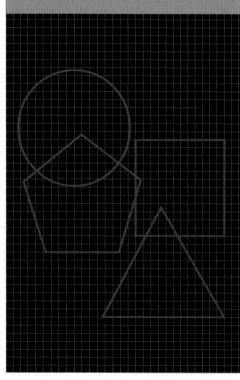

PLAYTHINK 322

DIFFICULTY: ●●●●●●●●○○
REQUIRED: 👁
COMPLETION: ☐ TIME: _____

HIDDEN SHAPES

Shapes can often hide in patterns; that is one reason why camouflage works. Pattern recognition is also one of the intelligent activities at which computers fail and humans excel. Below are six patterns and twelve shapes.

Each pattern hides more than one shape. The shapes contained in the patterns are the same size and in the same orientation as the examples around the perimeter. Can you match each shape to the right pattern?

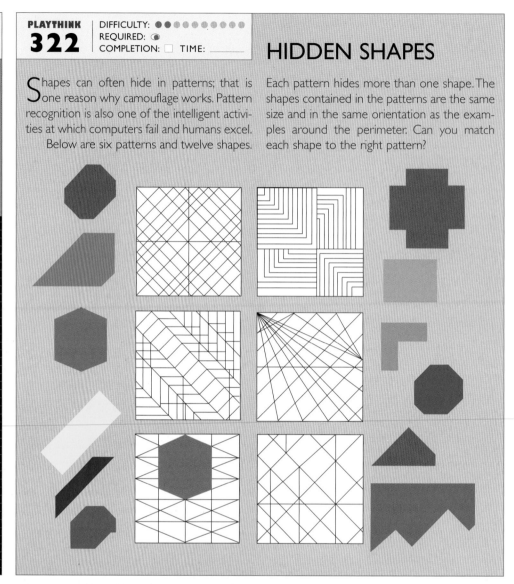

PLAYTHINK 321

DIFFICULTY: ●●●●●●○○○○
REQUIRED: 👁 ✏️
COMPLETION: ☐ TIME: _____

EQUAL AREA

All four shapes—circle, square, triangle and pentagon—are equal in area. Can you sort them in order of perimeter, from longest to shortest?

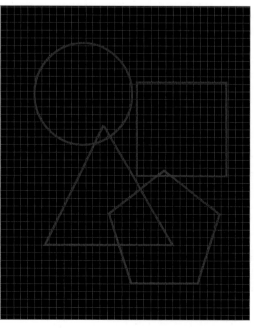

PLAYTHINK 323

DIFFICULTY: ●●●●○○○○○○
REQUIRED: 👁
COMPLETION: ☐ TIME: _____

PARALLELOGRAM CUT

How many straight cuts does it take to turn this parallelogram into a rectangle?

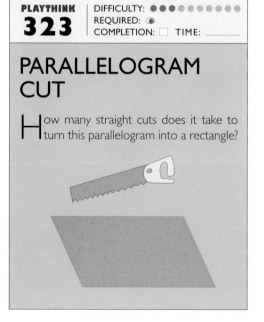

PLAYTHINK
324

DIFFICULTY: ●●●●●●●○○○
REQUIRED: 👁 ✎
COMPLETION: ☐ TIME: _____

FIND THE POLYGONS

At first glance the designs shown at right may seem like just squares crisscrossed with lines. But look again: you will spot regularities and symmetries—squares, triangles, rhombuses, kites and so on. In fact, there is an even more remarkable property in this pattern. It is composed simply of four equilateral triangles of the largest size that will fit within the square. A vertex of one of the triangles is at each corner of the square.

The object of this puzzle is to find the items listed below. To make things easier for you, I have provided a design that shows the shapes you are looking for. A pencil or pen may come in handy for marking the shapes you find.

1. First, find the four large equilateral triangles that create the pattern in each square.

2. Then find four squares. They are not all the same size.

3. Find four medium-sized equilateral triangles.

4. Find eight small equilateral triangles.

5. Find four halves of regular hexagons. (A regular hexagon has six sides of equal length.)

6. Find two large identical but irregular six-sided polygons.

7. Find two medium-sized identical but irregular six-sided polygons.

8. Find two small identical but irregular six-sided polygons.

9. Find an irregular eight-sided polygon.

10. Find four large right-angled isosceles triangles (that is, a right triangle with two equal legs).

11. Find four medium-sized right-angled isosceles triangles.

12. Find the eight largest right triangles that do not have sides of equal length.

13. Find eight medium-sized right triangles that do not have sides of equal length.

14. Find the eight smallest right triangles that do not have sides of equal length.

15. Find two large rhombuses of equal area.

16. Find four large parallelograms.

17. Find four medium-sized parallelograms.

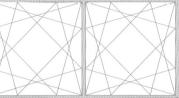
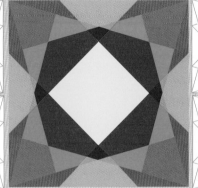
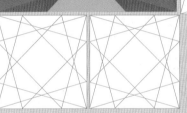
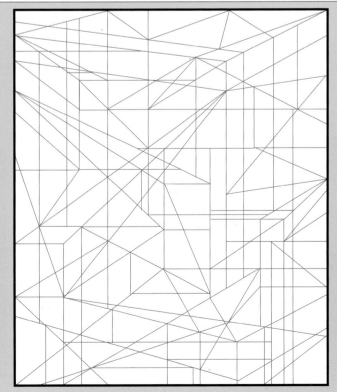

PLAYTHINK
325

DIFFICULTY: ●●●●●●○○○○
REQUIRED: 👁
COMPLETION: ☐ TIME: _____

HOW MANY CUBES?

Can you find six cubes portrayed in perspective in the pattern at right?

The Square

The square is the simplest, most symmetrical and most perfect quadrilateral. Its sides are all equal, and its angles are all right angles. But its simplicity is deceptive: the square conceals within its austere geometry untold intellectual depths. From the Pythagorean theorem to Einstein's theory of general relativity, from the flat geometry of Euclid to the curvature of space, there are only three or four short steps, and the square is their common thread.

The square is found in the crystals of many minerals, including common salt. It played a role in the structure of the Hebrew alphabet and gave birth to the ancient games of chess, go, solitaire and dominoes. The square has provided the proportions of famous ancient structures, as well as daring modern buildings. The endless tracts of the American Midwest are laid out in squares one mile on a side.

The square is everywhere.

> " IT'S A SQUARE:
> BEAUTIFUL,
> EQUILATERAL AND
> RECTANGULAR. "
>
> —LEWIS CARROLL

PLAYTHINK 326

DIFFICULTY: ●●●●●●○○○○
REQUIRED: ◉ ✎ 📄 ✂
COMPLETION: ☐ TIME: _____

THREE SQUARES INTO A BIG RECTANGLE

Three small squares are dissected into five parts, as shown. Can you rearrange the pieces to form one large rectangle?

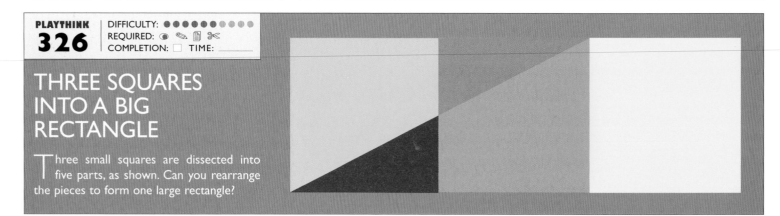

PLAYTHINK 327

DIFFICULTY: ●●●●○○○○○○
REQUIRED: ◉ ✎
COMPLETION: ☐ TIME: _____

TRIANGULATION

How many diagonals are needed to divide a heptagon, a nonagon and an undecagon into triangles? How many triangles will result from the divisions?

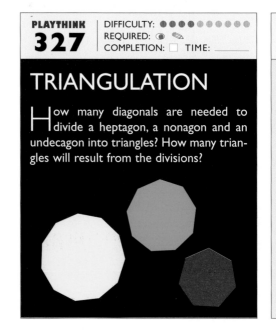

PLAYTHINK 328

DIFFICULTY: ●●●●●●●○○○
REQUIRED: ◉ ✎
COMPLETION: ☐ TIME: _____

INSCRIBED SQUARE

Can you inscribe a square on this seven-by-seven square matrix so that the sides of the inscribed square are of an integer length, in units of the grid? The vertices of the new square must lie on grid-line intersections.

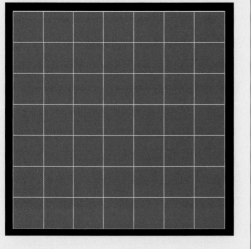

PLAYTHINK
329

DIFFICULTY: ●●●●●●○○○○
REQUIRED: ◉ ✎
COMPLETION: ☐ TIME: _____

CONDITION TRIANGLE

Four sets of strips of different lengths are shown. The sets are of lengths 3, 4 and 6; 3, 5 and 7; 4, 5 and 9 and 3, 5 and 9. Are there any sets of strips that cannot form a triangle when joined together?

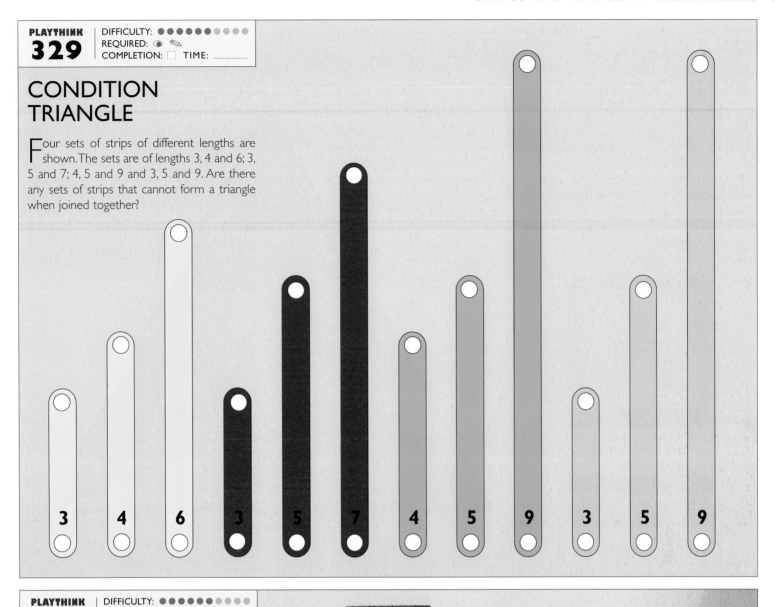

PLAYTHINK
330

DIFFICULTY: ●●●●●●●○○○
REQUIRED: ◉ ✎
COMPLETION: ☐ TIME: _____

ART GALLERY

An art gallery has fourteen walls of identical length. Several revolving security cameras keep a watch on the walls. The gallery owner would like to redesign the space so that the total number and length of walls stay the same and yet every square inch of wall can be watched with just one revolving camera. What design accomplishes this goal?

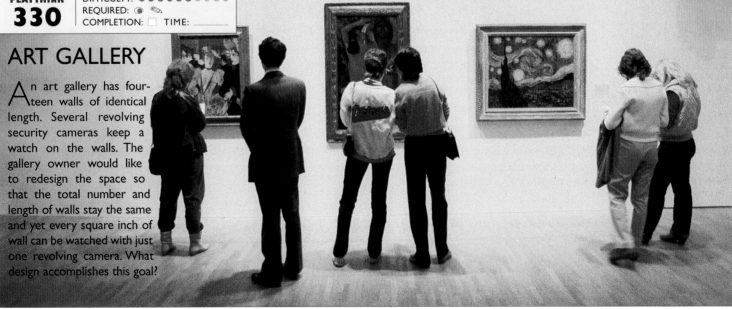

PLAYTHINK
331
DIFFICULTY: ●●●●●●●●●○
REQUIRED: ◉ ✎ 📄 ✂
COMPLETION: ☐ TIME: _____

RIGID SQUARE

Construct a square from four identical linkages hinged at the corners, as shown. Such a figure is capable of moving on its hinges to become a rhombus. How many linkages of the same length must be added in the same plane to make the square rigid? The linkages must be in the same plane as the square, and each one can be connected only at the hinges.

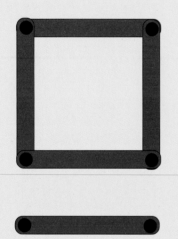

PLAYTHINK
332
DIFFICULTY: ●●●●●●●●○○
REQUIRED: ◉ ✎
COMPLETION: ☐ TIME: _____

TRISECTING TRIANGLE

A line connects each vertex of this triangle to a trisection point on the opposite side. (Such lines are called cevians, for Giovanni Ceva, an Italian mathematician who lived from 1648 to 1734.) The three lines divide the triangle into seven regions, with the area of each region a multiple of $\frac{1}{21}$ of the total area.

Can you work out the proportional area of all seven regions?

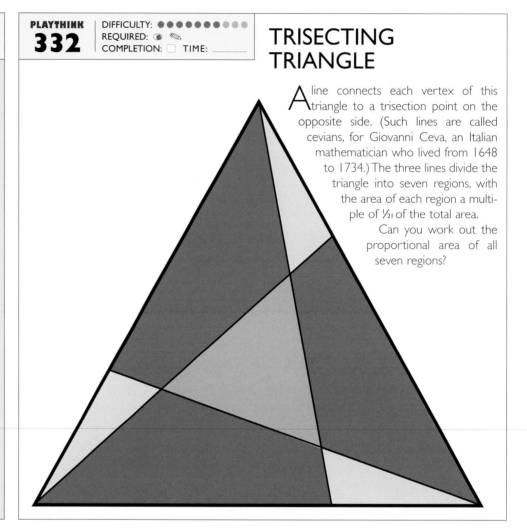

PLAYTHINK
333
DIFFICULTY: ●●●●●○○○○○
REQUIRED: ◉
COMPLETION: ☐ TIME: _____

PEG-BOARD TRIANGLES

Not counting rotationally symmetrical variations and translations, there are exactly eleven different triangles that can be formed by connecting three points on a three-by-three Peg-Board. Ten are shown here. Can you find the eleventh?

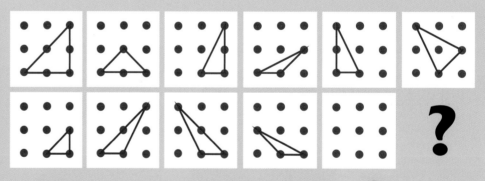

PLAYTHINK
334
DIFFICULTY: ●●●●●●○○○○
REQUIRED: ◉ ✎
COMPLETION: ☐ TIME: _____

MINIMAL TRIANGLES

Three villages would like to be connected by a set of paths but want to do this in the most economical way. Can you find a general way of determining how this can be done?

To make it easier to solve this problem, examine the two triangles at right. Can you find the point in each triangle that is at a minimum total distance from the three vertices?

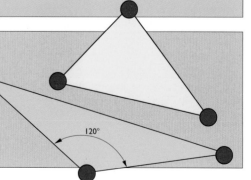

PLAYTHINK 335
DIFFICULTY: ●●●●●●●○○○
REQUIRED: 👁 ✎
COMPLETION: ☐ TIME: _____

NAPOLEON'S THEOREM

Draw a triangle as shown here in blue. Construct an equilateral triangle on each of its faces. Then, from the center of those new triangles, form another equilateral triangle.

Will this work every time? What if the triangles are constricted inward?

This theorem has been attributed to Napoleon, an enthusiastic amateur mathematician.

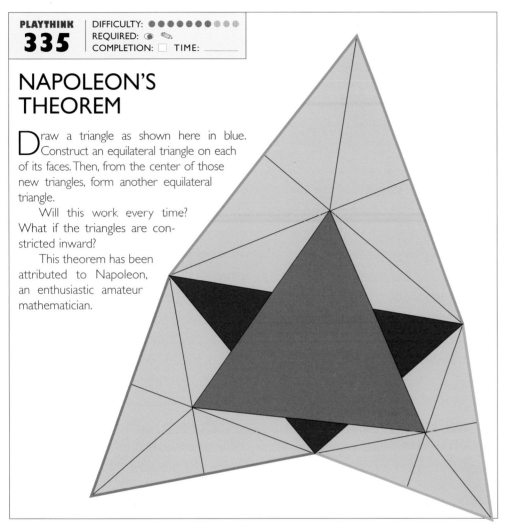

PLAYTHINK 336
DIFFICULTY: ●●●●●●●○○○
REQUIRED: 👁 ✎
COMPLETION: ☐ TIME: _____

MEDIANS OF A TRIANGLE

A median joins a vertex of a triangle to the midpoint of the opposite side. The point where all three medians meet is called the centroid and divides each median in a 2:1 ratio.

The centroid is the center of gravity of the triangle; it's the point at which it can be balanced.

A line from a vertex that bisects the median will divide the opposite side of the triangle by a certain proportion. What's the proportion?

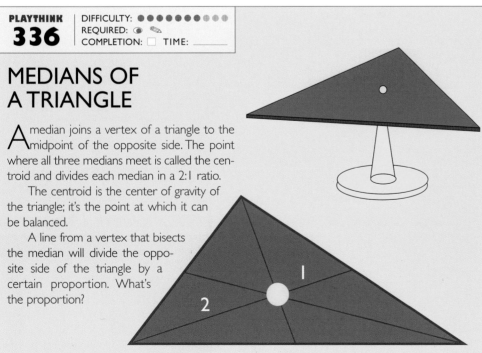

PLAYTHINK 337
DIFFICULTY: ●●●●●●○○○○
REQUIRED: 👁 ✎
COMPLETION: ☐ TIME: _____

SCANNING ART

In a strangely shaped modern art gallery, every square inch of floor space can be watched by the six revolving security cameras (red dots) mounted in the corners. Can you find the minimum number of cameras needed to do the same job? Where must they be placed?

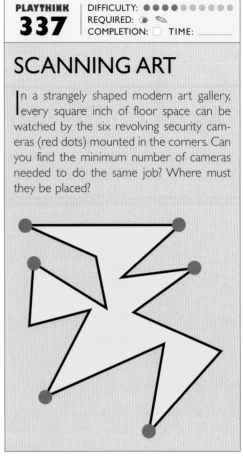

PLAYTHINK 338
DIFFICULTY: ●●●●●●●●○○
REQUIRED: 👁 ✎
COMPLETION: ☐ TIME: _____

SCANNING BANK

Five revolving security cameras (red dots) are installed in the corners of a bank. The cameras can cover every square inch of floor area. Where would you mount just three cameras so that they can cover the same area?

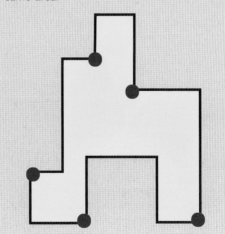

Polygons

Of all the possible polygons—closed figures bordered by straight lines—the triangle is the simplest. (If you don't believe it, try enclosing a figure with just two straight lines.) And as the engineer and architect Buckminster Fuller so aptly explained it, the triangle is also the only inherently stable form. What Fuller meant was that triangles are hard to deform. (And if you don't believe that, just try to push a triangular cardboard tube flat.)

Engineers take advantage of the stiffness of triangles by inserting them within structural forms; even rectangular girders are generally composed of triangular parts. But actually every polygon can be divided into triangles, or triangulated. The number of possible triangles is two less than the number of sides: a square can be divided into two triangles, and a heptagon into five. The number of diagonals from any vertex is three less than the number of sides. And the sum of the internal angles of a polygon is similarly related—two less than the number of sides, times 180.

Regular polygons are a special subset of polygons: all their sides are equal and all their angles are equal. (These qualities are not necessarily related; both the rhombus and the rectangle are instances in which only one of the equalities is present.) Regular polygons are an essential building block of regular solids, called polyhedrons. Indeed, the faces of regular polyhedrons—as well as other, irregular solids—are made up of just three basic shapes: the regular pentagon, the square and the equilateral triangle.

When ancient stargazers looked at the night sky, they combined the points of polygons—squares, triangles, rectangles, other shapes—into more elaborate figures, such as monsters, warriors and gods. The ancients assumed that such figures must have been placed there by some guiding hand. Modern mathematicians now know that whenever a collection of random points is great enough, they will inevitably begin to show signs of shapes and patterns.

PLAYTHINK 339 | DIFFICULTY: ●●●●●●●●●○ | REQUIRED: ◉ ✏ | COMPLETION: ☐ TIME: _____

JAPANESE TEMPLE PROBLEM FROM 1844

Five squares are arranged as shown. Can you demonstrate that the area of the green square is equal to that of the green triangle?

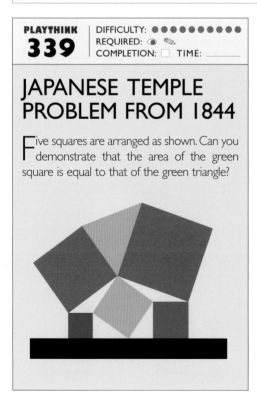

PLAYTHINK 340 | DIFFICULTY: ●●●●●●●○○○ | REQUIRED: ◉ | COMPLETION: ☐ TIME: _____

HIDDEN PICTURE

Can you find the picture hidden in the pattern? It is composed of the colored pieces shown below.

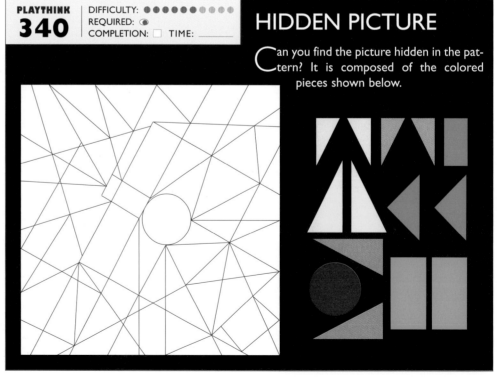

PLAYTHINK
341
DIFFICULTY: ●●●●●●○○○○
REQUIRED: ◉
COMPLETION: ☐ TIME: _____

STAINED GLASS WINDOW

There are four regular stars in this window: a three-pointed, a four-pointed, a five-pointed and a six-pointed star. Can you find all four?

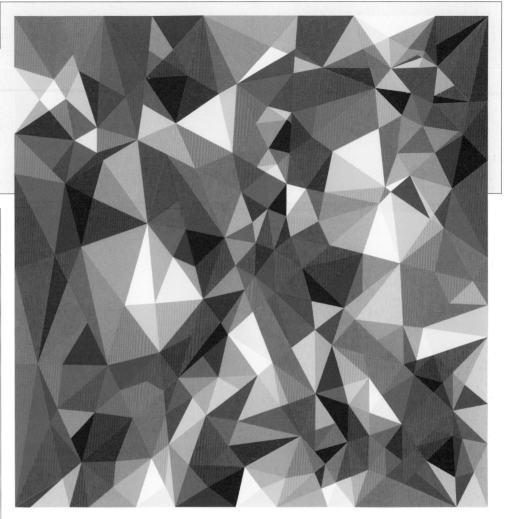

PLAYTHINK
342
DIFFICULTY: ●●●●●●●●○○
REQUIRED: ◉ ✎
COMPLETION: ☐ TIME: _____

SHARING CAKES

At a birthday party three cakes are cut as shown and divided between two groups. One group gets the red pieces, while the other gets the yellow.

Cake 1 is cut through the center three times, making six 60° angles.

Cake 2 is also cut three times, but through an off-center point. Again, the cuts make six 60° angles.

Cake 3 is cut through the same off-center point, but now four times, making eight 45° angles.

Did each group get identical shares of the three cakes?

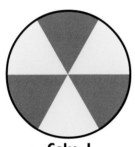

Cake 1

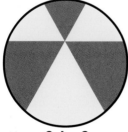

Cake 2

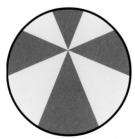

Cake 3

PLAYTHINK
343
DIFFICULTY: ●●●○○○○○○○
REQUIRED: ◉
COMPLETION: ☐ TIME: _____

PICK-UP POLYGONS

Ten regular polygons lie in a heap. Each polygon can be picked up, but only when no other figure lies on top of it Can you tell in what order the polygons may be removed?

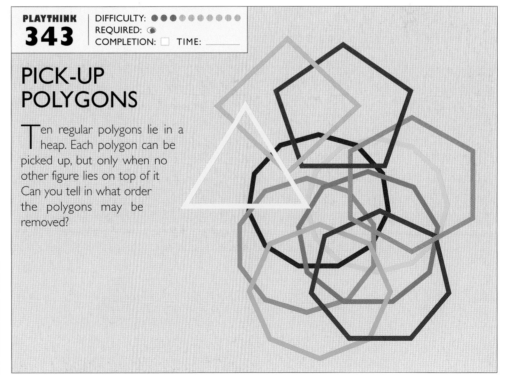

PLAYTHINK
344

DIFFICULTY: ●●●●●●○○○○
REQUIRED: 👁 ✎
COMPLETION: ☐ TIME: _____

QUADRILATERALS GAME

The object of this game is to form quadrilaterals. Players choose a color and take turns filling in the triangular fields along the grid lines with their colors. Each newly colored field must touch a field that has already been filled in. Points are scored when a quadrilateral is formed, one point per triangle within its boundaries, regardless of color. Certain conditions, however, must first be met:

• More than half of the triangles forming the quadrilateral must be of the color of the player who formed it.

• The perimeter of the quadrilateral cannot pass between two triangles of the same color.

• The quadrilateral cannot have any empty spaces.

• The quadrilateral must be symmetrical.

• Each triangle can be part of only one quadrilateral.

The game ends when all the triangles have been filled. The unfinished sample game demonstrates the above rules.

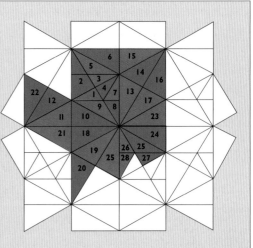

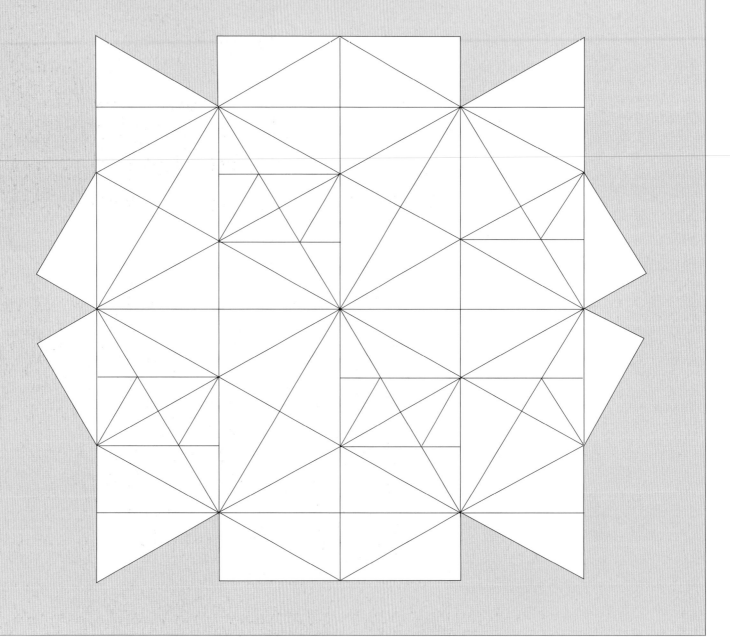

PLAYTHINK
345
DIFFICULTY: ●●●●○○○○○○○
REQUIRED: ◉ ✐
COMPLETION: ☐ TIME: _____

SQUARES ON A QUADRILATERAL

In the drawing below, squares are drawn on the sides of the red quadrilateral. The centers of the squares on opposite sides are joined, and not only do the two lines intersect at 90 degrees, but they are of equal length as well.

Will every quadrilateral—no matter its shape—lead to the same result?

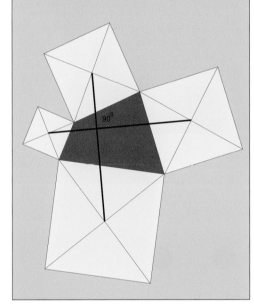

PLAYTHINK
346
DIFFICULTY: ●●●●○○○○○○○
REQUIRED: ◉ ✐
COMPLETION: ☐ TIME: _____

CONDITIONAL QUADRILATERAL

Four sets of strips are shown. Which set of strips cannot be joined to form a quadrilateral?

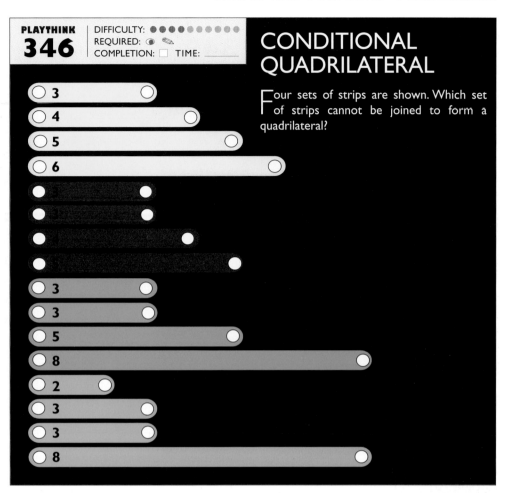

PLAYTHINK
347
DIFFICULTY: ●●●●●●●●○○
REQUIRED: ◉ ✐
COMPLETION: ☐ TIME: _____

INVISIBLE SQUARE

A square has disappeared except for four points, which lie in the exact positions they occupied on the four sides of the square. Can you re-create the position of the square?

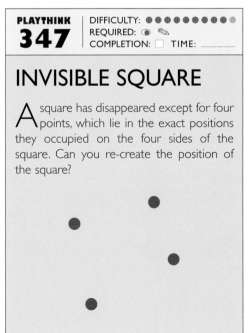

PLAYTHINK
348
DIFFICULTY: ●●●●●●○○○○
REQUIRED: ◉ ✐ 📄 ✂
COMPLETION: ☐ TIME: _____

FITTING SHAPES

Can you fit the six shapes into the board without overlap?

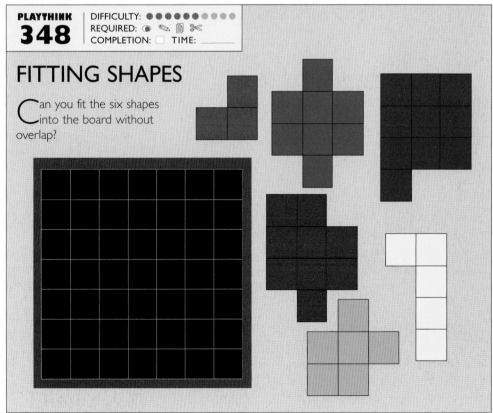

Quadrilateral Definitions

Square—
a quadrilateral with four equal sides and four right angles

Rectangle—
a quadrilateral with opposite sides parallel and four right angles

Rhombus—
a quadrilateral with opposite sides equal and parallel

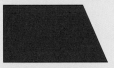

Parallelogram—
a quadrilateral with opposite sides parallel

Right-angle trapezoid —a quadrilateral with two parallel sides and a right angle

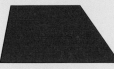

Isosceles trapezoid—
a quadrilateral with two parallel sides and two sloping sides equal

Scalene trapezoid—
a quadrilateral with two parallel sides

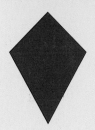

Deltoid—
a quadrilateral with two pairs of adjacent sides of equal length

---

SQUARE IN PENTAGON

What is the largest square that will fit in a regular pentagon? Is it bigger than the one shown here?

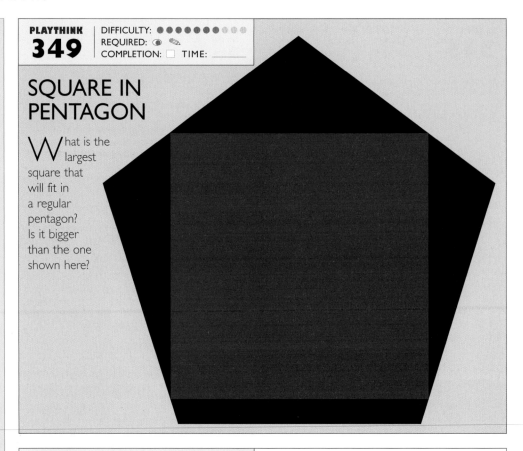

CROSSED PEG-BOARD

Peg-Boards are found in many games and educational activities. Almost all of them consist of a matrix of holes arranged in squares and squares-within-squares. On the board shown here, the pegs or holes are represented as dots.

Other boards may be arranged differently—say, in triangular matrices—but the same principles will apply.

How many squares of any size can you create by connecting four pegs on the board shown? Hint: The squares do not need to have horizontal bases.

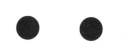
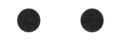
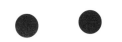
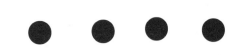
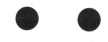
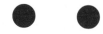

PLAYTHINK
351

DIFFICULTY: ●●●●●○○○○○
REQUIRED: 👁 ✏
COMPLETION: ☐ TIME: _____

PEG-BOARD POLYGONS

If the small square between four pegs represents 1 square unit, how much area is enclosed by each of the Peg-Board polygons, numbered 1 through 16?

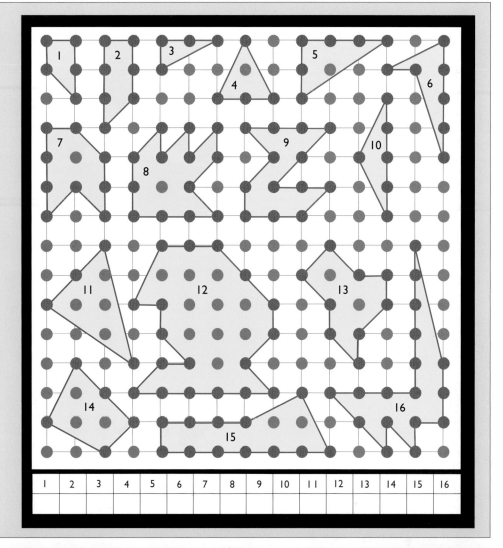

1	2	3	4	5	6	7	8	9	10	11	12	13	14	15	16

PLAYTHINK
352

DIFFICULTY: ●●●●●●○○○○
REQUIRED: 👁 ✏
COMPLETION: ☐ TIME: _____

CHESSBOARD SQUARES

How many squares of different sizes can you find along the grid of a chessboard? One place to start on this problem is with the sixty-four individual squares that make up the chessboard. But there are other squares that are composites, made up of several square units. Can you find them all?

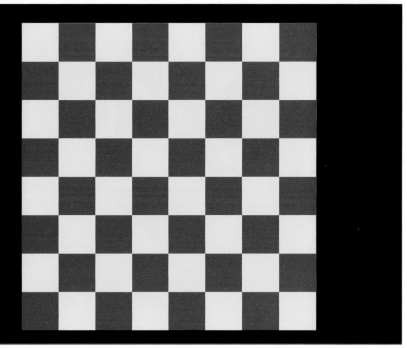

**PLAYTHINK
353**

DIFFICULTY: ●●●●●●○○○○
REQUIRED: 👁 ✏️
COMPLETION: ☐ TIME: _____

SQUARES AROUND

In the illustration here, five identical squares are arranged symmetrically around a circle so that their corners touch one another and each square touches the circle.

Given a circle with a radius equal to the sides of the squares, how many squares would it take to be similarly arranged?

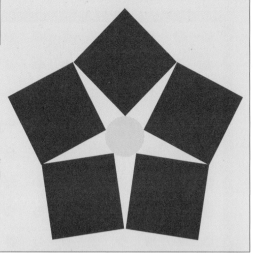

**PLAYTHINK
354**

DIFFICULTY: ●●●●●○○○○○
REQUIRED: ✏️ 📄 ✂️
COMPLETION: ☐ TIME: _____

SQUARE DISSECTIONS

Trace the colored shapes and join them to form nine identical squares.

Hint: The nine dissection puzzles here have all been created by bisection and trisection of the sides of the squares.

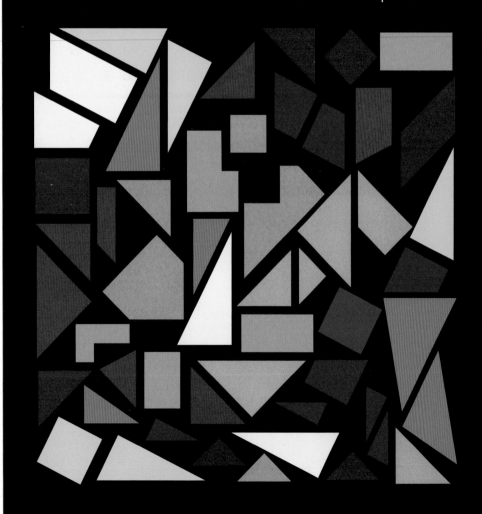

**PLAYTHINK
355**

DIFFICULTY: ●●●●●●○○○○
REQUIRED: 👁 ✏️
COMPLETION: ☐ TIME: _____

TRIANGLE—CIRCUMCENTER—INCENTER

Can you discover how to find both the center of a circle inscribing the triangle—touching the three sides—and the center of a circle circumscribing the triangle—that is, passing through the three vertices?

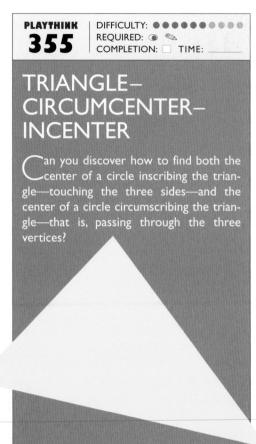

**PLAYTHINK
356**

DIFFICULTY: ●●●●●●●●○○
REQUIRED: 👁
COMPLETION: ☐ TIME: _____

SQUARE CUT

Just by looking at the figure below, can you figure out the area of the red square?

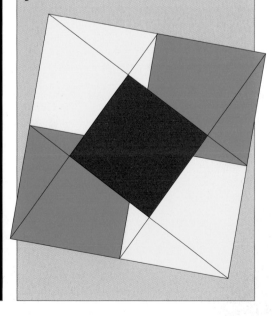

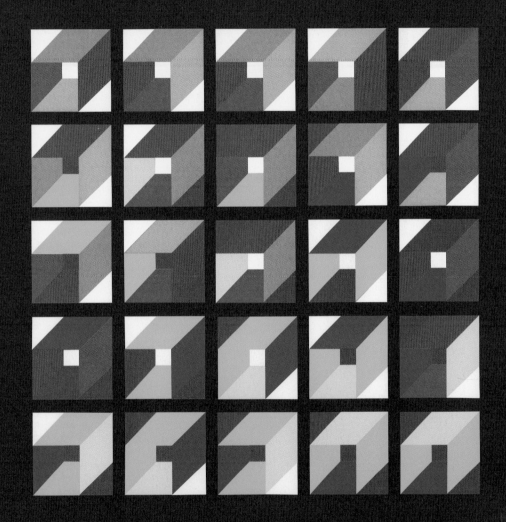

Patterns

PLAYTHINK
357

DIFFICULTY: ●●●●○○○○○○
REQUIRED: 👁 ✎
COMPLETION: ☐ TIME: _____

FACTORIALS

How many different words can you make from the letters *O*, *N* and *W*, using each one only once?

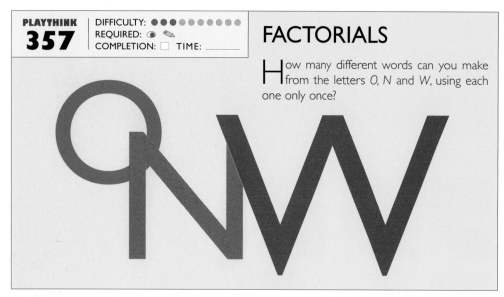

PLAYTHINK
358

DIFFICULTY: ●●●●●●○○○○
REQUIRED: 👁 ✎
COMPLETION: ☐ TIME: _____

COLOR DIADEM

How many different diadems can you make using seven different precious stones? Configurations that differ only through rotation are not considered different.

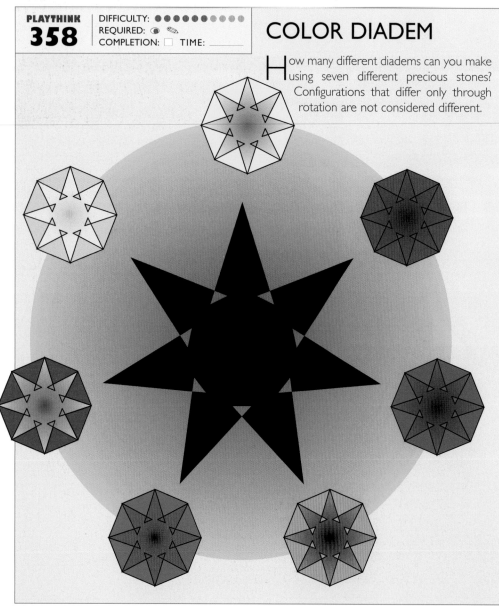

PLAYTHINK
359

DIFFICULTY: ●●●●●○○○○○
REQUIRED: 👁 ✎
COMPLETION: ☐ TIME: _____

MAGIC CUBE I

The three-by-three cube shown below can be divided into twenty-seven one-by-one cubes. Can you fill each of the smaller cubes with one of three colors (red, green or yellow) in such a way that each vertical column and each horizontal row contains all three colors? Each color will appear exactly nine times.

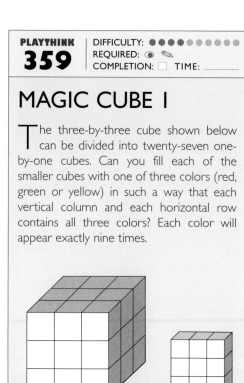

unit cubes

PLAYTHINK
360

DIFFICULTY: ●●●●●●●○○○
REQUIRED: 👁 ✎
COMPLETION: ☐ TIME: _____

BOYS AND GIRLS

Elementary schoolchildren on a field trip sit in groups of four, so that every girl sits next to at least one other girl. How many permutations are possible?

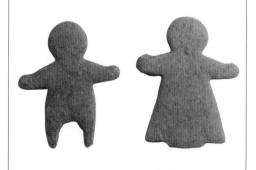

Pattern Recognition

Patterns are inescapable. Found in fantastic variety in the natural world, they show up in everything from atomic structures to snowflakes to spiral galaxies. Patterns are the basis of art as varied as Egyptian tomb painting and contemporary minimalism. And because patterns are everywhere— and so exquisitely beautiful—they make us curious. Children call their curiosity play; mathematicians name theirs research.

And what have we learned through all this research and play? That lines drawn on a flat surface divide the area into smaller bits. That if the lines are drawn so that the groups of smaller areas look the same, or at least similar, and those areas are aligned in a ordered manner, a pattern is formed. And that an area that is divided according to precise measurements to make a pattern that can then be applied to measuring or further drawing makes a grid.

The human talent for pattern recognition is simply the understanding that there is a systematic relationship between the elements in a group. These patterns, like the ones found in nature, indicate an underlying system of order. When this order is sought out, found and expressed, we are speaking the language of mathematics.

> "THE MATHEMATICIAN'S PATTERN, LIKE THE PAINTER'S OR THE POET'S, MUST BE BEAUTIFUL. . . . THERE IS NO PERMANENT PLACE IN THE WORLD FOR UGLY MATHEMATICS."
> —GODFREY H. HARDY

PLAYTHINK 361

DIFFICULTY: ●●●●●●○○○○
REQUIRED: 👁 ✎ 📄 ✂
COMPLETION: ☐ TIME: _____

SILHOUETTE

The six pieces fit together on the black background to form a silhouette of a familiar figure. Can you work out what that figure is?

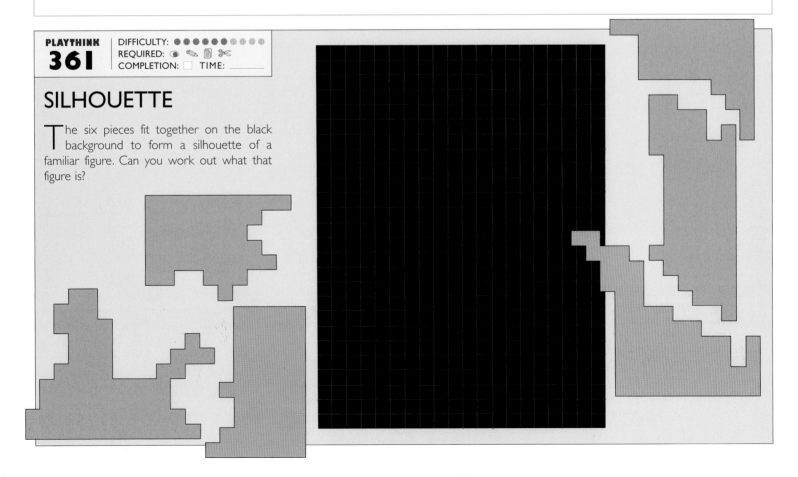

Combinations and Permutations

Probability, computer theory and many everyday situations depend on the principles of combination and permutations The number of possible arrangements in a system may seem small at first, but possibilities rise quickly with the number of elements and soon become impossibly large.

The basic instance is simplicity itself: one object by itself can be arranged in just one way and come in just one order.

Two objects, call them *a* and *b*, can be arranged as *ab* or *ba* for a total of two permutations. Three objects— *a*, *b* and *c*—can be arranged in six ways: *abc, acb, bac, bca, cab, cba*.

For the general case with *n* number of objects, the way to work out the permutations is to take the objects one at a time. The first object can fall at any of the *n* possible positions; for each of those possibilities, the second object can fall at one of *n* − 1 possible places (since it can't occupy the place the first object takes up); for every one of those n(n − 1) permutations, the third object can fall in one of n − 2 places; and so on.

In general, for *n* objects there are *n* times as many more permutations as there are in systems with only n − 1 objects. For example, there are four times as many possible permutations in a system with four objects than there are in a system with three — in other words, 24 permutations. There are 5 × 24, or 120, different ways to arrange five things and 6 × 120, or 720, ways to arrange six things. These numbers are called factorials and are designated with a *!*, as in 6!, or six factorial, to stand in for 720.

Therefore, the general formula is

$$n! = n \times (n - 1) \times (n - 2) \times (n - 3) \times \ldots \frac{}{3 \times 2 \times 1}$$

What about cases that deal not simply with ordering one group but with finding the permutations of *n* things taken *k* at a time? The mathematics here is only a bit trickier. Say you wanted to know how many ordered groups of three can be made from five different elements (such as colors or letters). You would calculate:

$$n!/(n - k)! = 5!/(5 - 3)! = 120/2 = 60$$

That means there are ten different possible groups of three elements (out of five), and each group has six possible permutations, for a total of 60. In the general formula, as you can see, *n* stands for the number of elements, and *k* stands for the size of the group.

Of course, the order of the elements does not always matter. Often it is only the raw constitution of the group that matters, such as the selection of a team from a group of athletes. A combination is a set of things chosen from a given group when no significance is attached to the order of the thing within the set. The number of combinations can be found by:

$$n!/k!(n - k)!$$

And, of course, sometimes there are objects within the group that are identical, so that picking one or the other doesn't change the set at all. In a case where the group is made up of *a* number of one thing, *b* number of another and *c* of a third, the number of different combinations can be found by:

$$n!/(a! \times b! \times c!)$$

PLAYTHINK	DIFFICULTY: ●●●●●●●○○○○
362	REQUIRED: ◉ ✎
	COMPLETION: ☐ TIME: _____

MAGIC STAR 1

Can you place the numbers from 1 to 10 on the blank circles so that the sum along any straight line equals 30?

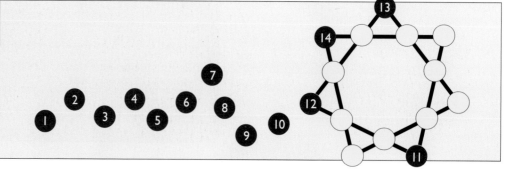

MATRIX PATTERN

Can you find the logic of this matrix and complete the pattern?

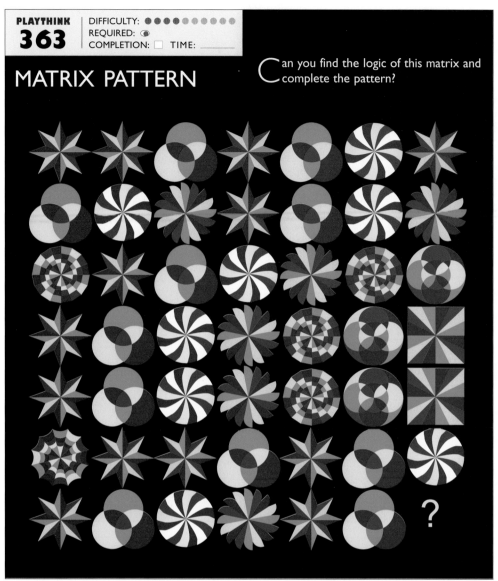

COLOR PAIRS

Sixteen pairs of circles are shown below. Using just yellow, red, green and blue, can you fill up each pair with a different combination of colors?

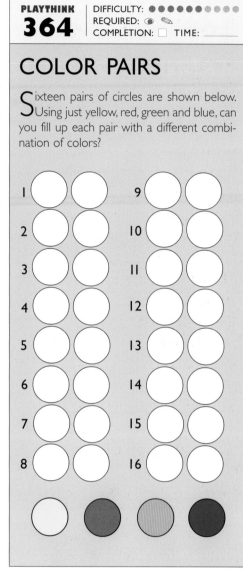

PERMUTATIONS

Line up the three fruits in as many different arrangements as possible. How many did you find?

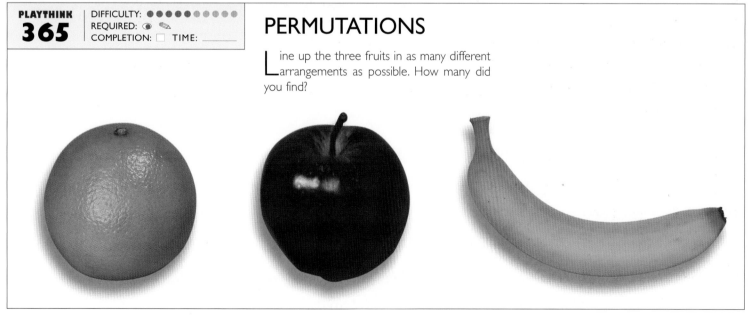

PLAYTHINK 366

DIFFICULTY: ●●●●●●○○○○
REQUIRED: 👁 ✎
COMPLETION: ☐ TIME: _____

SEATING PROBLEM

In how many different ways (ignoring rotations) can eight family members seat themselves around an octagonal dinner table?

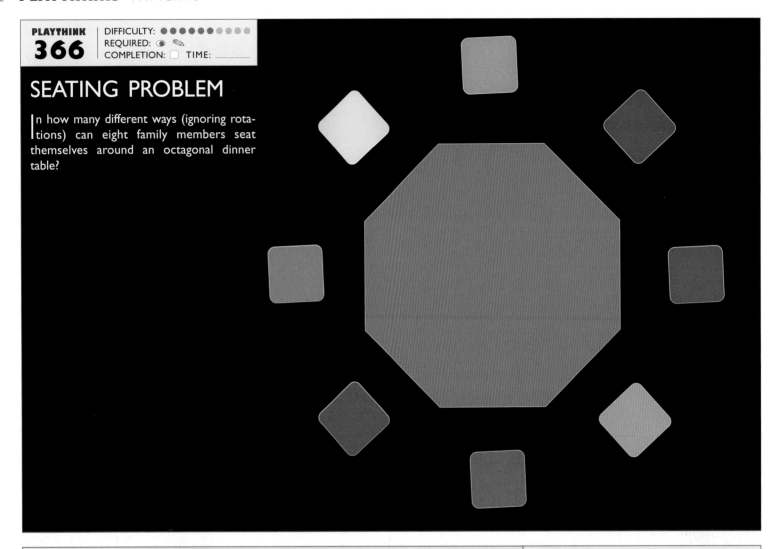

PLAYTHINK 367

DIFFICULTY: ●●●●●●●○○○
REQUIRED: 👁 ✎
COMPLETION: ☐ TIME: _____

MAGIC PENTAGRAM

Can you place the numbers 1 to 12 (except for 7 and 11) on the circles so that the sum of the numbers on any straight line equals 24? The numbers 3, 6 and 9 have been placed to guide you.

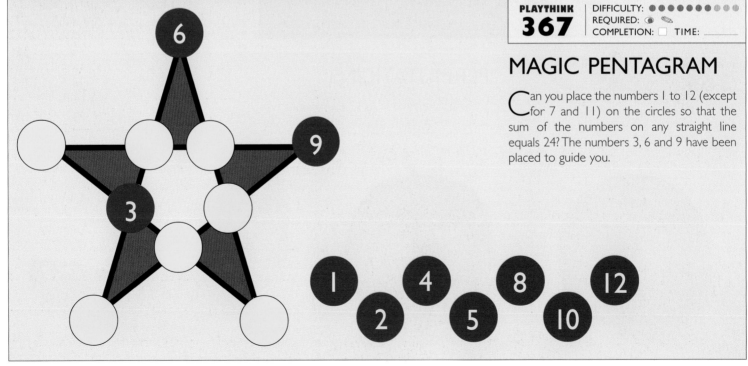

PLAYTHINK **368** | DIFFICULTY: ●●●●●●●○○○
REQUIRED: ◉ ✎ ▤ ✂
COMPLETION: ☐ TIME: _____

PERMUTINO

The strips here are made from the possible permutations of four blocks of color. One of the strips is missing. Can you figure out what its sequence should be?

Copying and cutting out the set of strips offers the possibility of playing many puzzles and games, including the "Permutino Game" (PlayThink 370).

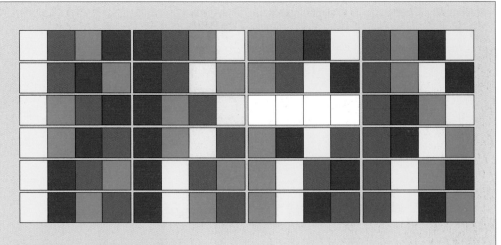

PLAYTHINK **369** | DIFFICULTY: ●●●●●●○○○○
REQUIRED: ◉ ✎
COMPLETION: ☐ TIME: _____

COLOR NECKLACE

With red, yellow, green and blue beads, can you design a necklace in which the sixteen possible color pairs occur only once in each direction?

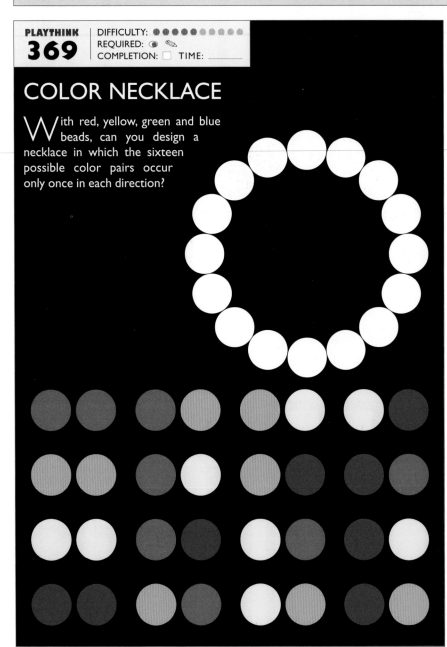

PLAYTHINK **370** | DIFFICULTY: ●●●●●●○○○○
REQUIRED: ◉ ✎
COMPLETION: ☐ TIME: _____

PERMUTINO GAME

The twenty-four four-color bands representing the twenty-four possible permutations of red, yellow, blue and green were placed on this ten-by-ten grid. The color for each block was recorded; the four empty spaces were marked black.

How long will it take you to fill in the outlines with the twenty-four strips from "Permutino" (PlayThink 368)?

This puzzle can be played as a two-person game, with players taking turns putting down strips that match the pattern on the game board. The last player to successfully place a strip on the game board wins.

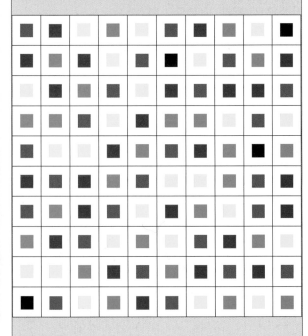

PLAYTHINK 371

DIFFICULTY: ●●●●●●○○○○○
REQUIRED: 👁 ✏
COMPLETION: ☐ TIME: _____

MAGIC SQUARE 1

Can you distribute the numbers 1 through 9 in such a way that when the central number in any horizontal, vertical or diagonal line of three is subtracted from the outer two, the sum is always the same?

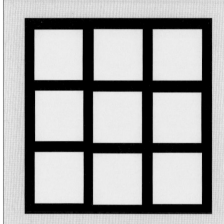

PLAYTHINK 372

DIFFICULTY: ●●●●●●●○○○○
REQUIRED: 👁 ✏
COMPLETION: ☐ TIME: _____

MAGIC SQUARE 2

Can you distribute the numbers 1, 2, 3, 4, 6, 9, 12, 18 and 36 in such a way that when multiplied, each horizontal, vertical and diagonal line has the same result?

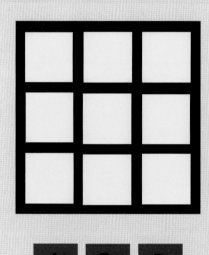

PLAYTHINK 373

DIFFICULTY: ●●●●●●●○○○○
REQUIRED: 👁 ✏
COMPLETION: ☐ TIME: _____

MAGIC SQUARE 3

Can you distribute the numbers 1, 2, 3, 4, 6, 9, 12, 18 and 36 in such a way that when the central number of any horizontal, vertical or diagonal line is divided into the product of the outer two numbers of the line, the result is always the same?

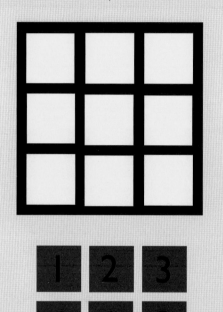

PLAYTHINK 374

DIFFICULTY: ●●●●●●●●○○○
REQUIRED: 👁 ✏
COMPLETION: ☐ TIME: _____

MAGIC SQUARE 4

Can you distribute the numbers 1 through 8 and −1 through −8 so that the sum of every horizontal, vertical and main diagonal line equals zero?

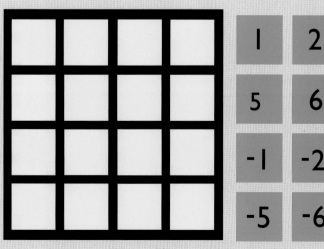

Magic Squares

The Rubik's Cube wasn't the first popular pastime that involved squares. As early as 4,500 years ago, people spent hours putting numbers in little boxes in hopes that the results would lead to mathematical beauty. What they were playing with was an ancient form of a puzzle called the magic square.

The writing of numbers in patterns started in ancient China, where numbers were often represented by circles or dots in a regular pattern, such as a triangle or a square. Since they were already thinking about numbers as forms unto themselves, Chinese mathematicians needed just a short step to create

the Lo-Shu (PlayThink 378), which was the first magic square. A magic square is a group of cells, each filled with one of a set of natural numbers, generally a series that runs in order from 1 to a number equaling the number of cells. A five-by-five magic square, for instance, would contain the numbers from 1 to 25. What's more, the numbers must be entered into the cells in a very specific way—the sum of any row or column (and often either diagonal) of numbers must be the same. That total is called the magic constant.

Magic squares are described by their order—that is, the number of cells on one side. It turns out that there are no order 2 magic squares

and only one of order 3: the Lo-Shu. Past order 3, the number of possible magic squares grows quickly. There are exactly 880 different types of order 4 magic squares, many of which are more "magic" than required by the definition of the magic square (see "Magic Square of Dürer," PlayThink 377), and there are millions of order 5 magic squares.

Magic squares have been widely popular throughout the ages, and some people have ascribed a different kind of magic to them. By A.D. 900, for instance, one Arab treatise recommended that pregnant women wear a charm marked with a magic square for a favorable birth.

PLAYTHINK 375

DIFFICULTY: ●●●●●○○○○○
REQUIRED: ◉ ✎
COMPLETION: ☐ TIME: _____

MAGIC SQUARE 5

Fill in the squares with the numbers 1 through 12 so that no two consecutive numbers appear either vertically, horizontally or diagonally.

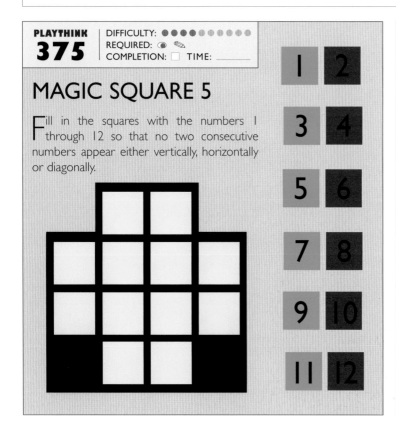

PLAYTHINK 376

DIFFICULTY: ●●●●●●●●●○
REQUIRED: ◉ ✎
COMPLETION: ☐ TIME: _____

MAGIC SQUARE 6

Some of the squares of the grid for this five-by-five magic square are highlighted. Can you distribute the numbers 1 through 25 so that the sum of every horizontal, vertical and main diagonal line is equal—and only odd numbers appear in the highlighted squares?

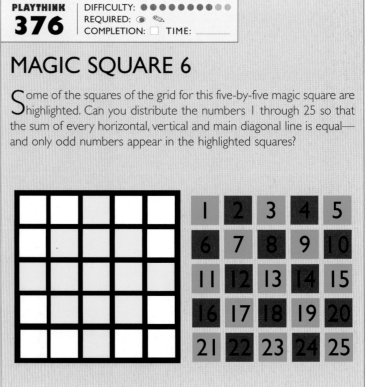

PLAYTHINK
377
DIFFICULTY: ●●●●●●○○○○
REQUIRED: 👁 ✎
COMPLETION: ☐ TIME: _____

MAGIC SQUARE OF DÜRER

The German artist Albrecht Dürer engraved this magic square of order 4 in his 1514 etching *Melancholia*. It is one of many magic squares that is magic in more ways than the simple definition requires.

First, can you fill in the missing numbers (see inset) so that the sum of every horizontal, vertical and main diagonal line totals 34?

Then can you find other ways in which this square is magic?

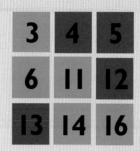

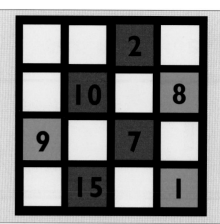

PLAYTHINK
378
DIFFICULTY: ●●●●●○○○○○
REQUIRED: 👁 ✎
COMPLETION: ☐ TIME: _____

THE LO-SHU

According to Chinese legend, the Lo-Shu dates back to at least the fifth century B.C. It is the oldest and simplest magic square.

The object of the Lo-Shu is to arrange the tiles numbered from 1 to 9 in the cells of the board so that the sum of every row, column and diagonal is the same. Not counting reflections and rotations, there is one answer.

Can you determine the sum without even solving the puzzle?

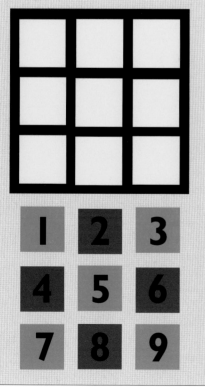

PLAYTHINK
379
DIFFICULTY: ●●●●●○○○○○
REQUIRED: 👁 ✎ 📄 ✂
COMPLETION: ☐ TIME: _____

MAGIC 15 GAME

This original game was inspired by the ancient magic square. Players take turns placing their numbered markers on the game board. (You'll find it easy to make your own on a large piece of paper.) After all the markers have been placed, players take turns moving their pieces along the grid lines to adjacent empty cells; jumps are allowed, as in checkers, but a marker may jump only an opponent's marker—and only if that marker is of a lower value.

The object is to form a row of three markers that add up to 15; at least two of the three markers should be the player's color. Once a row that adds up to 15 has been made, those pieces are frozen for the rest of the game and cannot be moved. The player who makes the most rows wins.

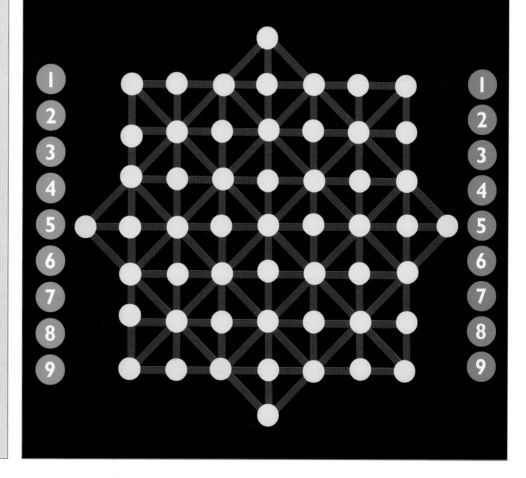

PLAYTHINK
380
DIFFICULTY: ●●●●●○○○○○
REQUIRED: 👁 ✎
COMPLETION: ☐ TIME: ___

HINGED MAGIC SQUARE

Flipping the numbered tiles along their hinges covers some numbers and reveals others that were hidden. The back of each tile has the same number as the front; behind the tile is a number that is twice as big as the original.

Can you flip just three numbered tiles so that the sum of every vertical, horizontal and main diagonal line equals the magic constant of 34?

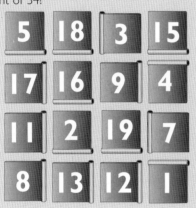

PLAYTHINK
381
DIFFICULTY: ●●●●●●○○○○
REQUIRED: 👁 ✎
COMPLETION: ☐ TIME: ___

COLOR LATIN SQUARES

Color the nine-by-nine square using nine different colors so that each row, each column and each three-by-three composite square contains each color exactly once. Since the colors are numbered, you can use the numbers to help solve the puzzles.

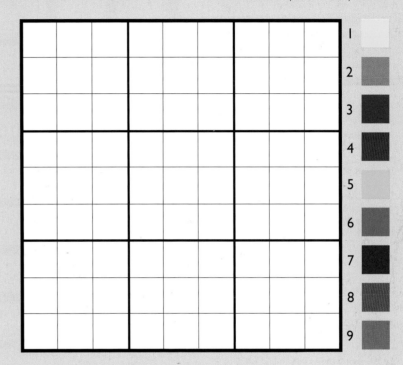

1
2
3
4
5
6
7
8
9

PLAYTHINK
382
DIFFICULTY: ●●●●●●●○○○
REQUIRED: 👁 ✎
COMPLETION: ☐ TIME: ___

MONKEYS AND DONKEYS

Five monkeys and three donkeys live in a zoo. If you had to select one monkey and one donkey, how many different combinations could you choose from?

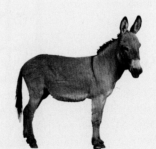
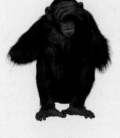
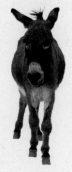
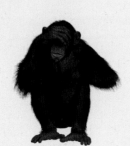
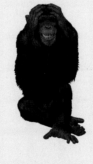
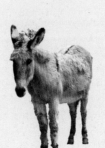
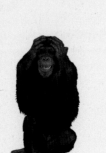
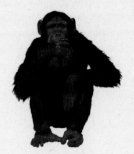

PLAYTHINK
383
DIFFICULTY: ●●●○○○○○○○
REQUIRED: ◉ ✎
COMPLETION: ☐ TIME: _____

MAGIC COLOR SQUARE OF ORDER 3

Can you distribute the colored tiles across the grid so that each color appears just once in every row and column?

Can you extend the rules to account for both main diagonals? What about every diagonal?

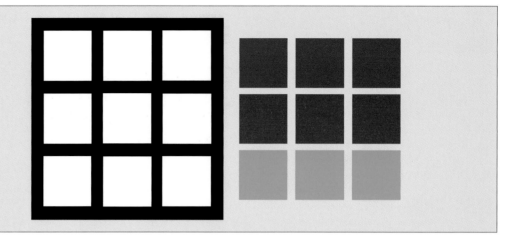

PLAYTHINK
384
DIFFICULTY: ●●●●●○○○○○
REQUIRED: ◉ ✎
COMPLETION: ☐ TIME: _____

MAGIC COLOR SQUARE OF ORDER 4

Can you distribute the colored tiles so that each color appears only once in every row and column?

Can the rule be extended to the main diagonals in this instance? To all diagonals?

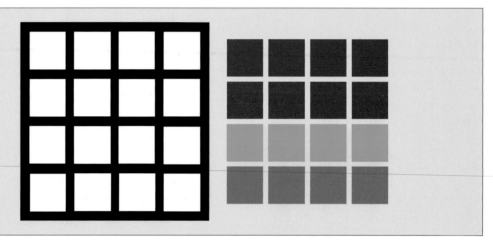

PLAYTHINK
385
DIFFICULTY: ●●●●●●○○○○
REQUIRED: ◉ ✎
COMPLETION: ☐ TIME: _____

MAGIC COLOR SQUARE OF ORDER 6

Can you distribute the thirty-six tiles so that each color appears only once in every row and column? Can you extend the rule to the two main diagonals?

This puzzle can become a two-player game. Players take turns placing tiles on the board so that no two tiles of the same color appear in any given row or column. The last player to make a legal move wins.

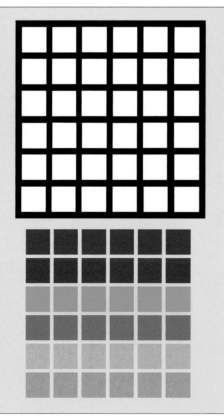

PLAYTHINK
386
DIFFICULTY: ●●●●●●●○○○
REQUIRED: ◉ ✎
COMPLETION: ☐ TIME: _____

MATHEMAGIC

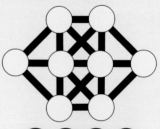

Can you place the numbers from 1 to 8 in the circles so that no adjacent numbers are connected by the black lines?

The inset shows an example of a puzzle that doesn't work.

Latin Squares

Near the end of his life, the great mathematician Leonhard Euler devised a new type of magic square, the Latin square. In a Latin square a number of symbols (numbers, letters, colors, etc.) are placed in a square of the same order so that each row or column contains each symbol only once. For example, a five-by-five square might contain five letters (*a, b, c, d, e*) five times each in such a way that no two *a*'s appear in the same row or column. There are also magic diagonal Latin squares, in which the same rules apply also across the two main diagonals or even across all smaller diagonals.

A further complication is found in the Greco-Latin magic square. This square consists of two Latin squares that have been superimposed so that each cell contains one element of each square, each element of one square is combined with an element of the second square only once, and each row and column contain every element from both squares. One simple illustration of such a square would be

$$1a, \quad 2b, \quad 3c$$
$$2c, \quad 3a, \quad 1b$$
$$3b, \quad 1c, \quad 2a$$

It is easy to see that no Greco-Latin magic square of order 2 can exist. The "Magic Color Shapes" puzzle-game (PlayThink 400) is a Greco-Latin square of order 4.

Latin and Greco-Latin magic squares are not mere diversions— they have valuable applications in experimental science. Suppose an agricultural researcher wished to test the effect of seven types of fungicides on wheat plants. He might divide an experimental field into seven parallel strips and treat each strip with a different fungicide. But such a test might be biased because of a favorable field condition in one of the plots—say, in the easternmost or southernmost strip. The best way to control for such biases is to divide the field into forty-nine plots in a seven-by-seven matrix and apply the chemicals according to the prescriptions of a Latin square. That way each fungicide is tested in every field condition. If the experiment needed to test the seven fungicides on seven different strains of wheat, then a Greco-Latin square could be applied.

In this way Euler's recreational problem has become a widely experimental design, not only in agriculture but also in biology, sociology, medicine and even marketing. The "cell" need not, of course, be a piece of land. It might be a cow, a patient, a leaf, a cage of animals, a city, a period of time and so on. The square is simply a way to combine variable elements in unique ways.

MAGIC COLOR SQUARE OF ORDER 5

Can you place the twenty-five tiles on the grid so that each color appears only once in each row and column? Again, can this be extended to the two main diagonals? What about every diagonal?

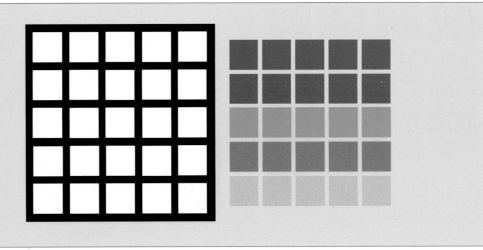

PLAYTHINK
388
DIFFICULTY: ●●●●●●●●●○○
REQUIRED: ◉ ✎ 📄 ✂
COMPLETION: ☐ TIME: _____

SPECTRIX

The colored tiles below can be placed one by one on the grid, but only if the following rules are observed:

• No tile can be placed on a square of the same color or horizontally, vertically or diagonally next to a square of the same color.

• Once a tile is placed on the board, that square takes on the color of the tile.

• No tile can be placed on another tile.

Can you place all sixteen tiles on the board?

The puzzle can be played as a two-person game. Players take turns placing tiles on the board in accordance with the rules above. The last person able to place a tile is the winner.

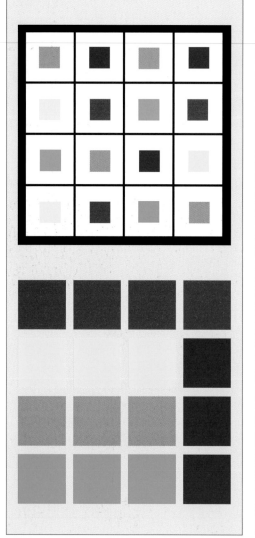

PLAYTHINK
389
DIFFICULTY: ●●●●●●●●○○○
REQUIRED: ◉ ✎ 📄 ✂
COMPLETION: ☐ TIME: _____

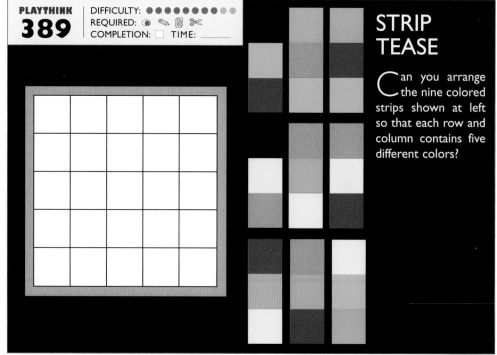

STRIP TEASE

Can you arrange the nine colored strips shown at left so that each row and column contains five different colors?

PLAYTHINK
390
DIFFICULTY: ●●●●●●○○○○○
REQUIRED: ◉ ✎
COMPLETION: ☐ TIME: _____

FOUR-COLOR SQUARES GAME

The object of this simple but rewarding game is to create rows or columns made up of four squares of different colors. Each player controls two colors, either red and yellow or blue and green.

At each turn players place two squares, one of each color, on the board. Squares of the same color may not share a side, and no more than four squares can make a contiguous row or column.

Players receive one point for each four-color line they create; if one tile completes both a row and a column, the points are doubled. For example, in the sample game shown below, the player placing the blue square would receive four points, double the points for creating a row and a column simultaneously.

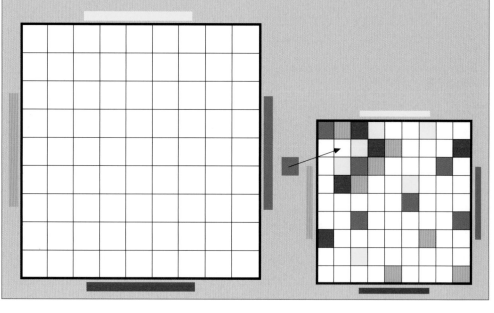

PLAYTHINK
391
DIFFICULTY: ●●●○○○○○○○
REQUIRED: ◉ 📄 ✂
COMPLETION: ☐ TIME: _____

CLOWN FUN

How many different clowns can you find in this four-by-four configuration of sixteen square tiles? Are all the clowns equally represented, or do some clowns appear more often than others? How many complete clowns are there? And how many can be shown completely in any given four-by-four arrangement?

These tiles may be copied and cut out to create tiles for many solitaire and party games. Simply use the game rules you'll find with PlayThink 123 and PlayThink 104.

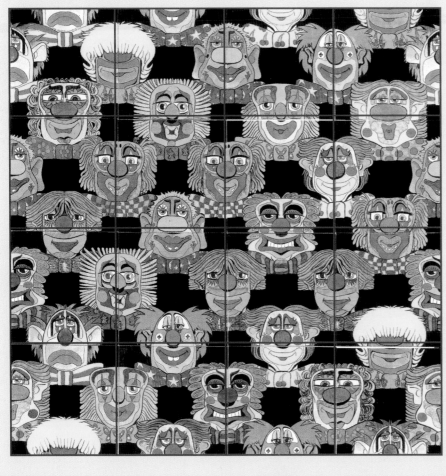

PLAYTHINK
392
DIFFICULTY: ●●●●●○○○○○
REQUIRED: ◉ ✎ 📄 ✂
COMPLETION: ☐ TIME: _____

RADIANT SQUARES

This grid could be configured so that every edge touches an edge of the same color if only four are rotated. Can you work out which four must be turned?

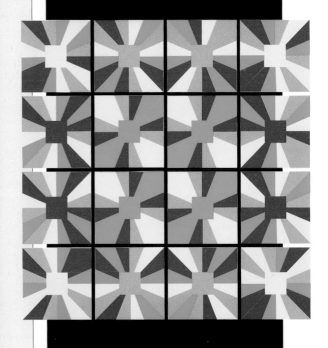

PLAYTHINK
393
DIFFICULTY: ●●●●○○○○○○
REQUIRED: ◉
COMPLETION: ☐ TIME: _____

BALANCING ACROBATS

What stunt will the acrobats do next?

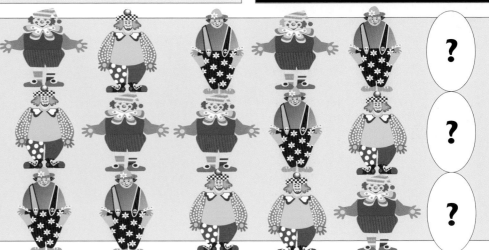

PLAYTHINK 394

DIFFICULTY: ●●●●●●●●○○○○
REQUIRED: 👁 ✏
COMPLETION: ☐   TIME: _____

MAGIC CIRCLES 2

At each point of intersection for the four circles is a spot for a number.

Can you add the numbers shown below to the empty spots so that the set of numbers along each circle adds up to 39?

PLAYTHINK 395

DIFFICULTY: ●●●●●●●●●○○○
REQUIRED: 👁 ✏ 📄 ✂
COMPLETION: ☐   TIME: _____

T-JUNCTIONS

Can you place the T shapes on the colored grid in such a way that, in the resultant pattern, no color appears more than once in any given row or column?

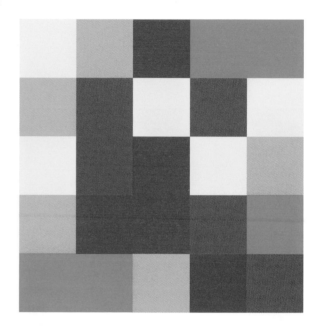

PLAYTHINK 396

DIFFICULTY: ●●●●●●●●○○○○
REQUIRED: 👁 ✏
COMPLETION: ☐   TIME: _____

SQUARE NUMBERS SQUARE

Can you place four different numbers in the circles here so that the sum of the two numbers along any given side is a square of another number?

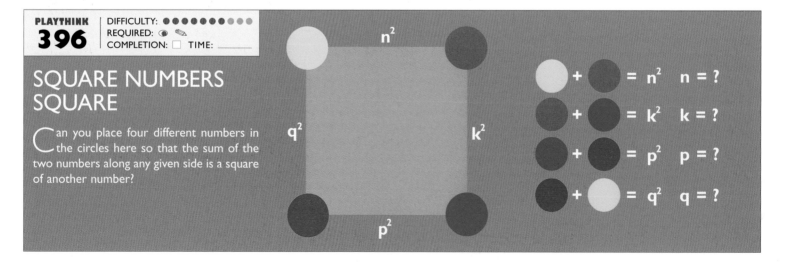

$$+ \quad = n^2 \quad n = ?$$
$$+ \quad = k^2 \quad k = ?$$
$$+ \quad = p^2 \quad p = ?$$
$$+ \quad = q^2 \quad q = ?$$

MAGIC TRIANGLE 1

Can you place the numbers from 1 to 6 in the circles along the sides of the triangle so that three numbers on each line of circles add up to the same total? How many different solutions can you find?

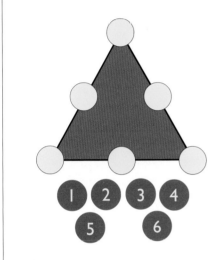

MAGIC TRIANGLE 2

Can you place the numbers 1 through 9 in the circles along the sides of the triangles so that the four numbers in each line of circles add up to the same total? How many different solutions can you find?

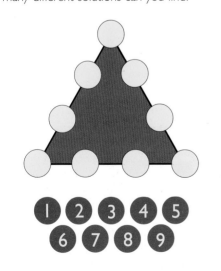

MAGIC HEXAGON 1

Can you add the missing numbers to the seven blank circles so that the sum of the numbers along any straight line is 21?

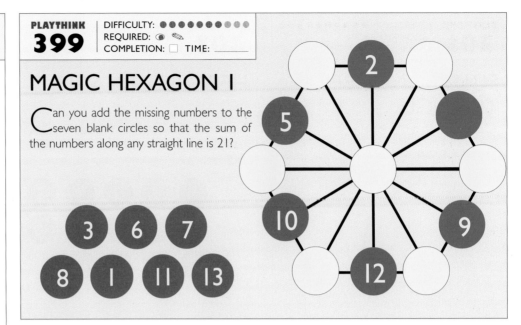

 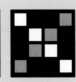

  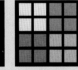

MAGIC COLOR SHAPES

Can you arrange the sixteen colored shapes in such a way that they form more than simply a magic color square, but instead the sixteen perfect four-color, four-shape configurations illustrated in the patterns below? In other words, your answer should include four different colors and four different shapes in each of these categories:

1. Four vertical columns

2. Four horizontal rows

3. Two main diagonals

4. Four corner squares

5. Four center squares

6. Four squares in each quadrant

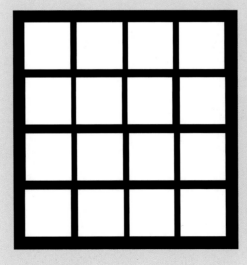

PLAYTHINK 401

DIFFICULTY: ●●●●●●●○○○○
REQUIRED: 👁 ✏
COMPLETION: ☐ TIME: _____

SQUARE NUMBER TRIANGLE

Can you place three different numbers in the circles below so that the sum of the two numbers along any given side is equal to the square of another number?

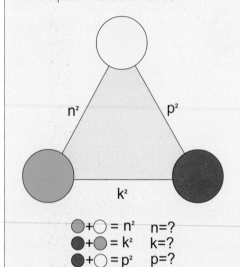

$\bigcirc + \bigcirc = n^2 \quad n=?$
$\bigcirc + \bigcirc = k^2 \quad k=?$
$\bigcirc + \bigcirc = p^2 \quad p=?$

PLAYTHINK 402

DIFFICULTY: ●●●●●●●●○○○
REQUIRED: 👁 ✏
COMPLETION: ☐ TIME: _____

MAGIC CIRCLE I

Can you distribute the numbers from 1 to 9 so that every line across the wheel adds up to 15?

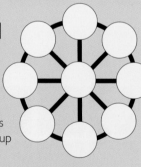

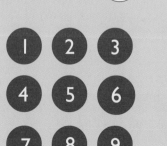

1 2 3
4 5 6
7 8 9

PLAYTHINK 403

DIFFICULTY: ●●●●●●●○○○○
REQUIRED: 👁 ✏
COMPLETION: ☐ TIME: _____

HEPTAGON MAGIC 2

Can you arrange the numbers from 1 to 14 along the sides of a heptagon in such a way that the three numbers on each side add up to 26?

1 2 3 4 5
6 7 8 9 10
11 12 13 14

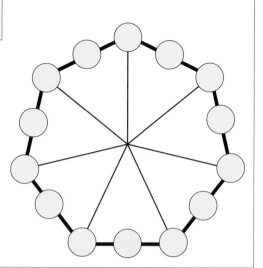

PLAYTHINK 404

DIFFICULTY: ●●○○○○○○○○○
REQUIRED: 👁
COMPLETION: ☐ TIME: _____

MAGIC ALIENS SQUARE

Which of the five aliens at the left will complete the magic square?

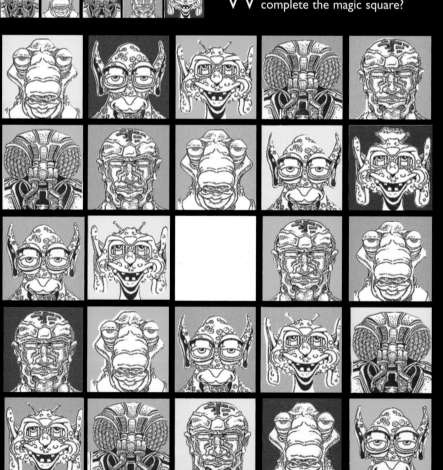

Greco-Latin Magic Square of Order 10

For many years it was thought that an order 10 Greco-Latin square was impossible. And it remained an unsolved problem even after the first computer search for an answer was conducted in 1959; after 100 hours, no solution was found. The programmers believed that a full search would take more than 100 years, but the failure reinforced the idea that no solution would ever be found.

Researchers discovered a new approach in 1960, one that found a wealth of solutions not only for squares of order 10 but for squares of order 14, order 18 and greater. Illustrated here is one solution for an order 10 Greco-Latin magic square, with colors substituted for the numbers from 1 to 10.

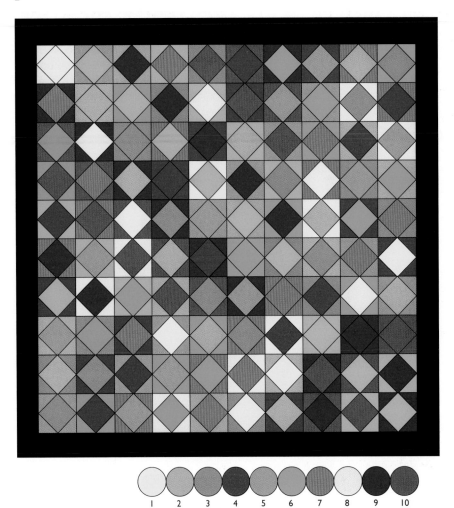

1 2 3 4 5 6 7 8 9 10

PLAYTHINK 405

DIFFICULTY: ●●●●●●○○○○○
REQUIRED: ◉ ✎
COMPLETION: ☐ TIME: _____

MAGIC CUBE 2

Can you distribute the numbers from 1 to 12 on the edges of the cube in such a way that the sum of the four edges on each face equals 26?

1 2 3 4
5 6 7 8
9 10 11 12

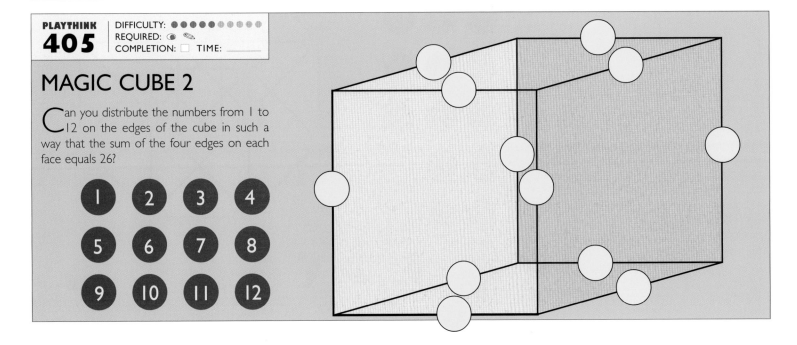

PLAYTHINK
406

DIFFICULTY: ●●●●●●●○○○
REQUIRED: ◉ ✎
COMPLETION: ☐ TIME: _____

MAGIC CIRCLES 3

Can you distribute the numbers from 1 to 6 on the intersections of the three circles so that the sum of the numbers on each circle is identical to the other two?

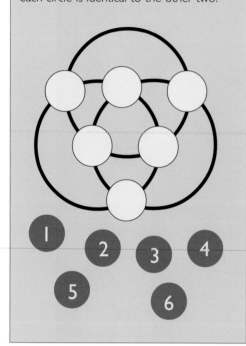

PLAYTHINK
407

DIFFICULTY: ●●●○○○○○○○
REQUIRED: ◉ ✎
COMPLETION: ☐ TIME: _____

SQUARE CASCADES

The object of this game is to arrange a set of numbers so that no square possesses a value smaller than its neighbor to the right or immediately below. The solution for a square with four fields is shown. Can you place the numbers 1 to 9 on the middle game board and 1 to 16 on the game board below it according to these rules?

When completed, the effect is like water cascading down from the top left to the lower right.

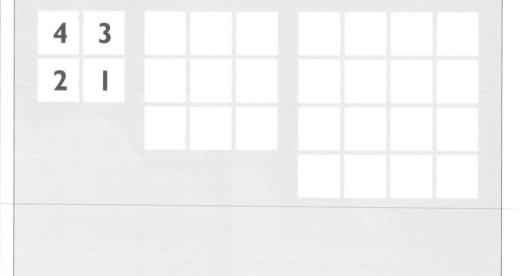

PLAYTHINK
408

DIFFICULTY: ●●●●●●●○○○
REQUIRED: ◉ ✎
COMPLETION: ☐ TIME: _____

HYPERCUBE

Islamic mystics first constructed the figure in this puzzle, called a tesseract. Modern mathematicians now consider it to be the two-dimensional representation of a four-dimensional hypercube.

Can the human brain really visualize four-dimensional space? Although humans are confined to three dimensions of space, it is conceivable that with the proper mathematical training, a person could develop the ability to fully visualize the tesseract.

For our puzzle, can you place the numbers from 0 to 15 on the circles of the hypercube in such a way that the numbers at the corners of the "square face" of the eight cubes shown at right in perspective add up to 30?

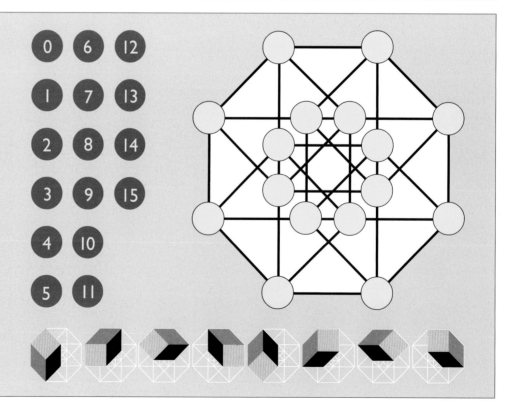

PLAYTHINK 409

DIFFICULTY: ●●●●●●●○○○
REQUIRED: 👁 ✏️
COMPLETION: ☐ TIME: _____

MAGIC CIRCLES 4

Arrange the numbers from 1 to 18 so that the sum of any two symmetrical pairs of numbers is 19. Three pairs have already been placed. Can you place the rest?

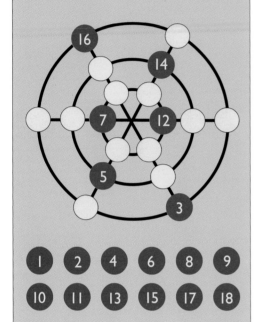

PLAYTHINK 410

DIFFICULTY: ●●●●●●●○○○
REQUIRED: 👁 ✏️
COMPLETION: ☐ TIME: _____

MAGIC HEXAGON 2

Volumes have been written about magic squares, but the "magic" can be embodied by other polygons, such as triangles, circles and hexagons. For example, can you distribute the numbers from 1 to 19 in the hexagonal game board illustrated below so that the sum of every straight line is identical? Can you work out what the magic constant must be?

To keep the puzzle from being too difficult, we've seeded some of the hexagons with numbers. You need to place only the remaining numbers.

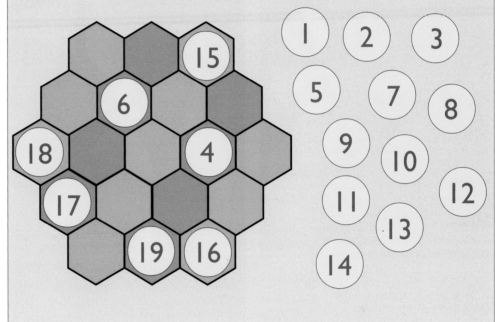

PLAYTHINK 411

DIFFICULTY: ●●●●●●○○○○
REQUIRED: 👁 ✏️ 📄 ✂️
COMPLETION: ☐ TIME: _____

MAGISTRIPS

The thirteen strips can be arranged into a seven-by-seven square in such a way that each horizontal row contains a single solid color.

Can you rearrange the strips so that no color appears more than once in any horizontal row? This is an easy problem with many solutions.

But can you then rearrange the strips again so that no color appears more than once in any row, column or diagonal line (including the small diagonals)? This puzzle can be played as a two-person game. Players take turns placing the strips on the board; the last player who can place a strip without violating the rules wins.

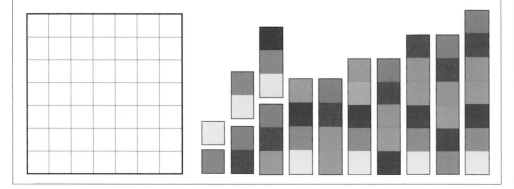

PLAYTHINK 412

DIFFICULTY: ●●●●●●○○○○
REQUIRED: 👁 ✏️
COMPLETION: ☐ TIME: _____

MAGIC STAR 2

Can you add the missing numbers to the nine blank circles so that the sum of the numbers along any straight line equals 26?

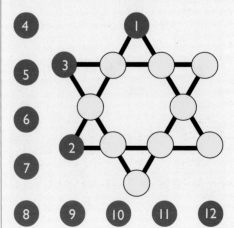

PLAYTHINK
413
DIFFICULTY: ●●●●●●●○○○
REQUIRED: 👁 ✏️ 📄 ✂️
COMPLETION: ☐   TIME: _____

OCTOPUZZLE 1

The octagons can be rotated so that at every point of contact, the edges are the same color. Can you meet that goal in the fewest possible rotations?

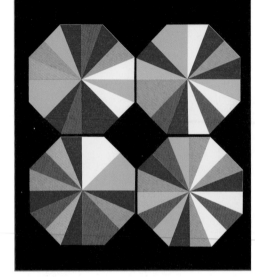

PLAYTHINK
415
DIFFICULTY: ●●●●●●○○○○
REQUIRED: 👁 ✏️
COMPLETION: ☐   TIME: _____

SQUARE DANCE

Each row is a sequence of predictable motions for five black squares, with one pattern missing from each sequence. By studying the three patterns given in each row, can you complete all four sequences?

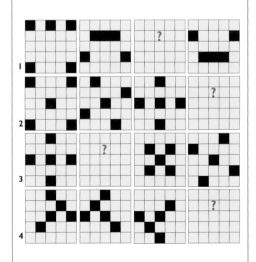

PLAYTHINK
414
DIFFICULTY: ●●●●●●●●○○
REQUIRED: 👁 📄 ✂️
COMPLETION: ☐   TIME: _____

OCTOPUZZLE 2

Can you rotate the nine octagons so that the edges that face each other share the same color? There are two possible solutions.

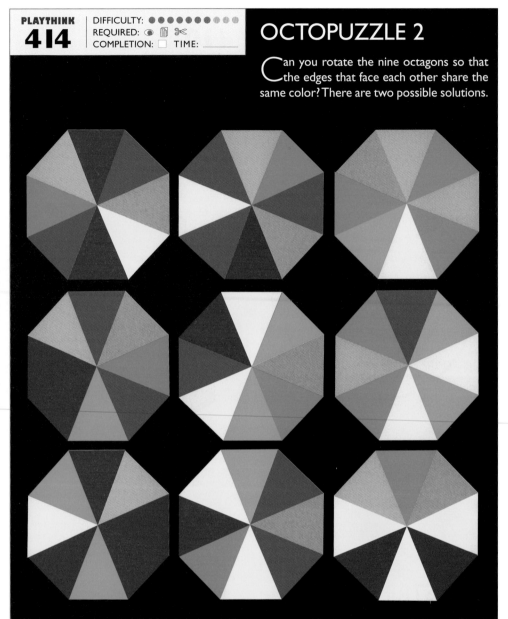

PLAYTHINK
416
DIFFICULTY: ●●●●●●●●○○
REQUIRED: 👁 ✏️
COMPLETION: ☐   TIME: _____

GRIDS AND ARROWS

The yellow squares around the square grid must be filled with one arrow each, drawn so that the arrow points vertically, horizontally or diagonally along the grid. Can you fill in the arrows in such a way that the number of arrows pointing to each square in the grid equals the number shown in that square?

	↓	↙				
	3	2	1	2	2	↙
↗	2	1	3	1	4	
	2	4	2	5	2	
	4	2	5	2	3	
→	3	4	2	3	3	
	↗	↑				

PLAYTHINK 417 | DIFFICULTY: ●●●●●●●●●○
REQUIRED: ◉ 📄 ✂
COMPLETION: ☐ TIME: _____

CUBES IN PERSPECTIVE 2

When a solid melts or a liquid boils, the object being heated suddenly loses much of its internal order. What was rigid becomes fluid; what was well defined is now vaporous. Such events, called phase transitions, can occur in art as well as nature.

In this puzzle the domino principle achieves a similar effect. Matching the colors leads to merging the patterns of the tiles. The foreground optical illusion and three-dimensional visual reversal add a dynamic dimension to the puzzle. Indeed, among the art puzzles I've included in this book, this is one of the toughest to crack.

First, copy and cut out the twenty-five tiles and reassemble them to form a five-by-five matrix that conforms to the domino principle—colors must match along all touching sides.

The number of possible configurations is staggering: $2^{25} \times 25!$

The four compositions shown in the inset form a sequence in which the degree of order present in the pattern becomes less and less. It is, in fact, hard to believe that all these compositions are made up from the same basic elements. But one of the insets shows one solution to the puzzle. Can you spot it?

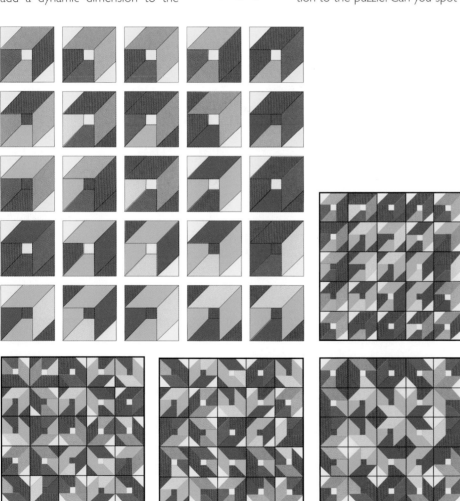

PLAYTHINK 418 | DIFFICULTY: ●●●●●○○○○○
REQUIRED: ◉ ✏
COMPLETION: ☐ TIME: _____

PIECE OF CAKE

The cakes below are sliced in such a way that they have the same number of concentric pieces as they have radial cuts. For example, one cake is divided into two pieces concentrically and two pieces radially, for a total of four pieces. Three radial cuts and three concentric pieces make for nine pieces.

For each cake, each slice should be filled in so that two pieces of the same color never contact each other—even across touching corners. The number of colors that can be used is equal to the number of concentric pieces: a two-cut cake can use only two colors; a three-cut cake, three colors.

As shown in the examples here, the task is impossible for a two-cut or three-cut cake. Can you make it work for a five-cut, five-color cake? How about a six-cut, six-color cake?

2-piece cake
2 colors

3-piece cake
3 colors

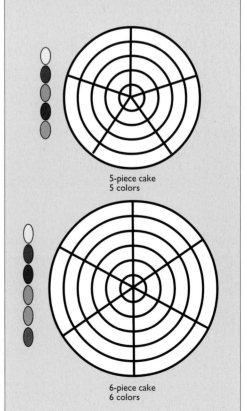

5-piece cake
5 colors

6-piece cake
6 colors

Dominoes and Combinatorial Games

Ordinary dominoes are two-by-one rectangular tiles with a different number on each end. The standard rule for playing dominoes is simple—the numbers on the adjacent ends of tiles must always match. The game of dominoes is the best-known example of a game that follows the so-called domino principle, but it is far from the only one.

The English mathematician Percy Alexander MacMahon devised a number of ingenious generalized domino games using colored polygonal dominoes that tile the plane. The set of tiles is not arbitrary: the same basic shapes or patterns are colored in all possible ways to form a complete set of tiles, no two of which are alike. (The reflections of a tile are considered to be different, but rotations are considered to be the same. This is a natural assumption because the tiles are usually colored on one side only and so cannot be turned over, but can be rotated in the plane without difficulty). The object of the games is to arrange the complete set of tiles according to the domino principle in some predetermined and pleasing pattern.

MacMahon's mathematical work was based on the theory of symmetrical functions—algebraic expressions that remain unchanged if the letters in them are permuted. For example, both $a + b + c$ and $ab + bc + ca$ are symmetrical functions of a, b and c. If the colors of a complete set of MacMahon's dominoes are permuted, we end up with exactly the same set of tiles as before. These tiles, in a sense, have a permutational symmetry.

PLAYTHINK 419

DIFFICULTY: ●●●●●●○○○○
REQUIRED: ◉ ✎ 📄 ✂
COMPLETION: ☐   TIME: _____

COLOR DOMINOES I

The fifteen dominoes shown here are made up of two squares, each of which is painted in one of five colors. With that color domino set can you re-create the five-by-six pattern shown below?

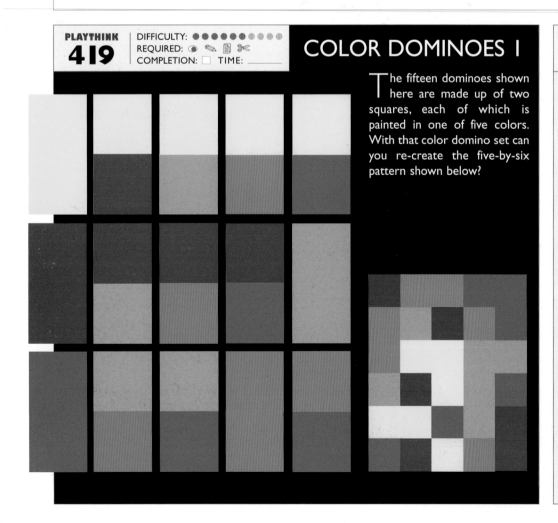

PLAYTHINK 420

DIFFICULTY: ●●●●●●●○○○
REQUIRED: ◉
COMPLETION: ☐   TIME: _____

DOMINO CHESSBOARD

This chessboard has been truncated so that it possesses sixty-two squares. Using red-yellow domino pieces, is it possible to replicate the pattern with thirty-one dominos?

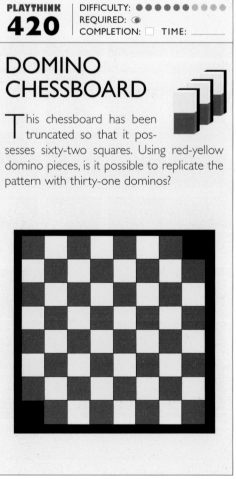

PLAYTHINK
421

DIFFICULTY: ●●●●●●○○○○
REQUIRED: 👁 ✎
COMPLETION: ☐ TIME: _____

TWO DESSERTS AND TWO PLATES

How many different ways can you serve two desserts with two plates?

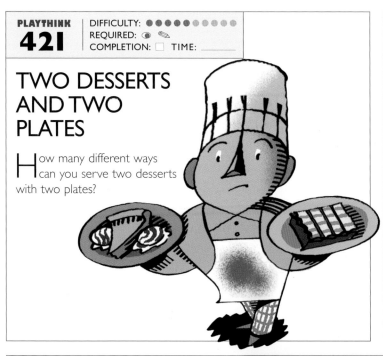

PLAYTHINK
422

DIFFICULTY: ●●●●●●○○○○
REQUIRED: 👁 ✎
COMPLETION: ☐ TIME: _____

TWO FRUITS IN THREE BOWLS

How many different ways can you serve two pieces of fruit with three bowls?

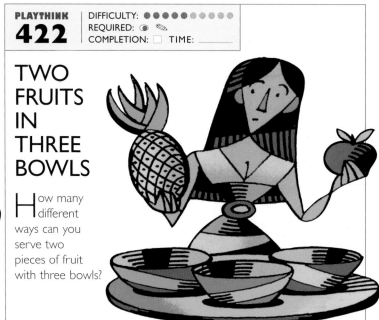

PLAYTHINK
423

DIFFICULTY: ●●●●●●●○○○
REQUIRED: 👁 ✎ 📄 ✂
COMPLETION: ☐ TIME: _____

COLOR DOMINOES 2

The twenty-eight dominoes shown here are made up of two squares, each painted in one of seven colors. Using that set of dominoes, can you re-create the pattern shown in the grid at top?

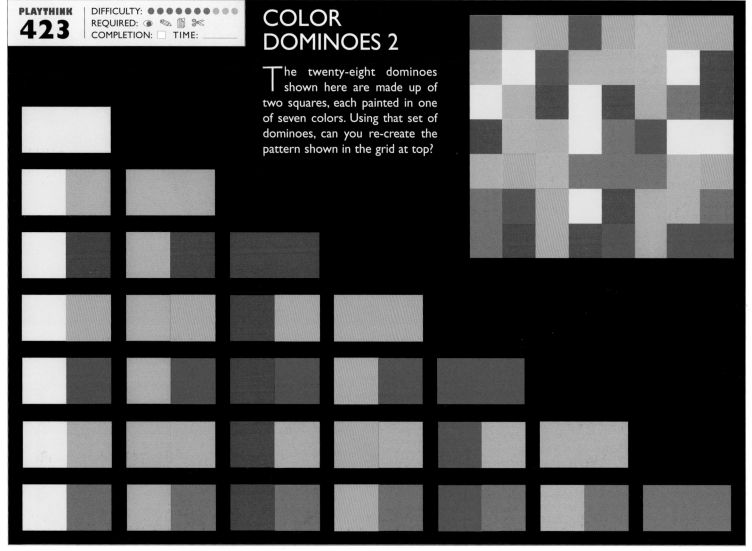

PLAYTHINK 424

DIFFICULTY: ●●●●●●●○○○
REQUIRED: ◉ ✎ 📄 ✂
COMPLETION: ☐ TIME: _____

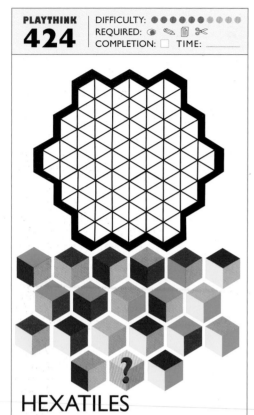

HEXATILES

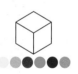

Each of the hexagons shown here is divided into three fields. The fields are filled in with one of six colors, and no hexagon may have any two fields that are the same color. Following those rules, there are twenty possible hexagons (rotations and reflections don't count as being different).

Nineteen hexagons are shown. What are the colors of the missing hexagon?

Can you fit the twenty hexagons into the grid at top so that every pair of touching sides is the same color?

PLAYTHINK 425

DIFFICULTY: ●●●●●●●○○○
REQUIRED: ◉ ✎ 📄 ✂
COMPLETION: ☐ TIME: _____

COLOR TRIANGLES 1

For three-segmented triangles there are twenty-four permutations of four possible colors. Twenty-three are shown. Can you find the missing permutation?

Then can you set all twenty-four triangles into the hexagon so that the colored edges of every triangle touch another edge that is the same color?

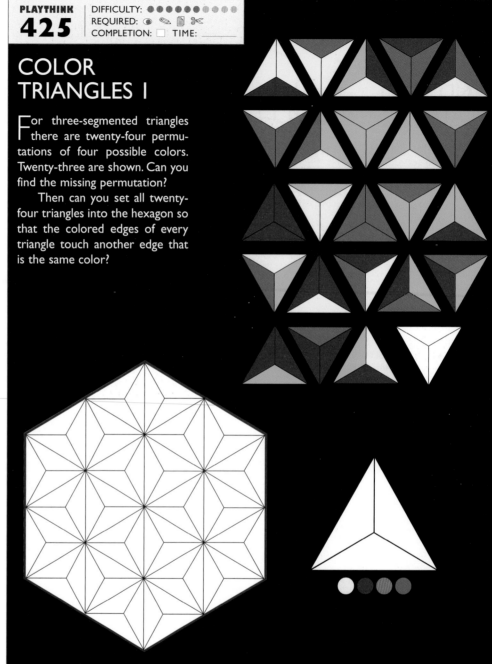

PLAYTHINK 426

DIFFICULTY: ●●●●●●○○○○
REQUIRED: ◉ ✎
COMPLETION: ☐ TIME: _____

TROMINOES AND MONOMINO

Can you cover a full chessboard with the twenty-one trominoes (dominoes made up of three squares) and one monomino shown here?

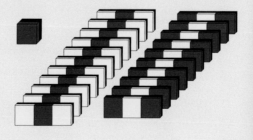

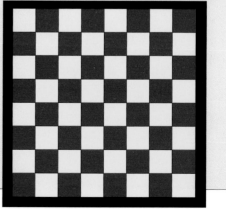

PLAYTHINK 427

DIFFICULTY: ●●●●●●○○○○
REQUIRED: ◉ ✎ 📄 ✂️
COMPLETION: ☐ TIME: _____

COLOR TRIANGLES 2

Each of the triangles shown has three segments, each of which can be filled by one of four permitted colors. There are twenty-four permutations of four colors possible; one permutation is missing. What are the colors of the blank triangle?

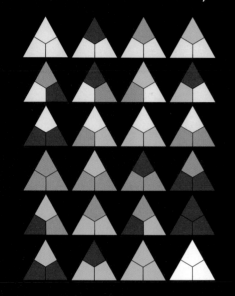

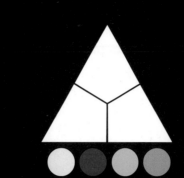

PLAYTHINK 429

DIFFICULTY: ●●●●●●●○○○
REQUIRED: ◉ ✎ 📄 ✂️
COMPLETION: ☐ TIME: _____

COLOR CONNECTION

Each side of each square is divided into six different colors. Can you place the squares side by side in the manner shown in the inset so that one color forms a continuous zigzag through the four squares? Can you do it in less than one minute?

The puzzle will work for only one color. Which color completes the zigzag?

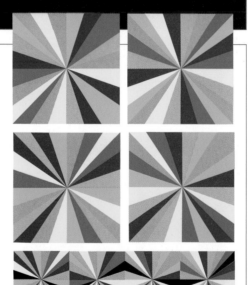

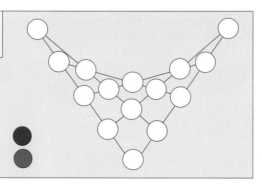

PLAYTHINK 430

DIFFICULTY: ●●●●●○○○○○
REQUIRED: ◉ ✎
COMPLETION: ☐ TIME: _____

ROWS OF COLOR

Using only red or blue, color the points of intersection one by one. Can you fill in the whole pattern without allowing any single line to have four points of the same color?

PLAYTHINK 428

DIFFICULTY: ●●●●●●●○○○
REQUIRED: ◉ ✎ 📄 ✂️
COMPLETION: ☐ TIME: _____

COLOR SQUARES

Each square is divided by its diagonals into four fields, each of which can be filled by one of three permitted colors. There are twenty-four permutations of three colors possible. Twenty-three are shown. What are the colors of the blank square?

Those twenty-four squares fit into a four-by-six board, shown below. Can you arrange the squares so that the outer border is all one color and the edge of each square comes into contact only with an edge of the same color?

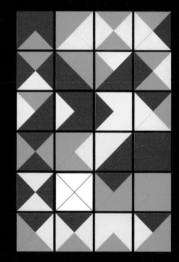

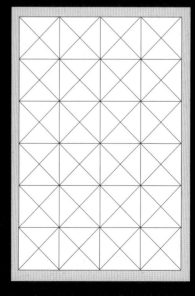

PLAYTHINK
431

DIFFICULTY: ●●●●●○○○○○
REQUIRED: ◉ 📄 ✂
COMPLETION: ☐ TIME: _____

SPACE RESCUE: THE GAME

This matching game requires concentration, powers of association and lightning-quick reflexes. Three or more persons can play.

First, copy and cut out the sixty decoder strips on the opposite page and place them in a box. Players take turns drawing a slip out of the box and placing it in view of the others. The player who draws the slip then acts as umpire as the rest try to find the alien that matches the description on the decoder strip.

When a player spots the correct alien, he or she zooms a "space module" (also known as a finger) to the picture. If first to select the matching alien, that player receives a point.

The first player to collect five points wins the game.

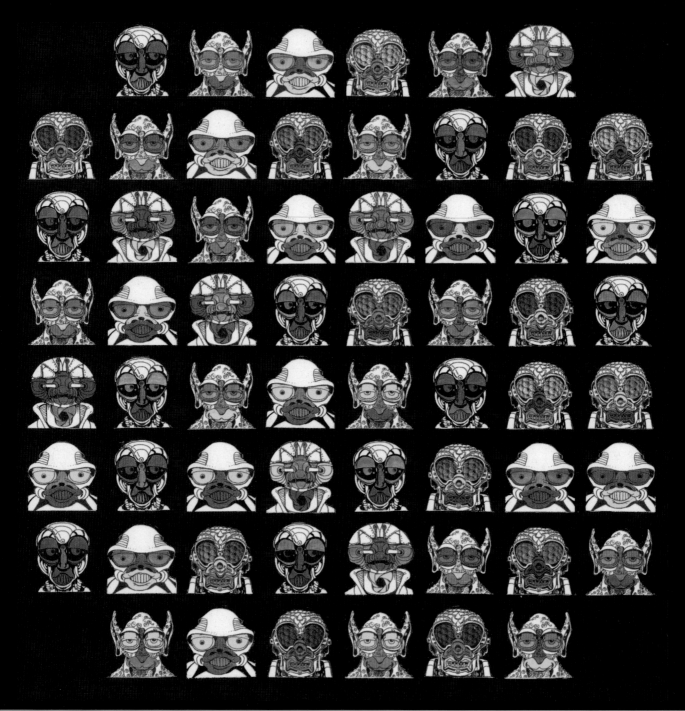

ALIEN	EYES	NOSE	MOUTH	ALIEN	EYES	NOSE	MOUTH	ALIEN	EYES	NOSE	MOUTH	ALIEN	EYES	NOSE	MOUTH
1				16				31				46			
2				17				32				47			
3				18				33				48			
4				19				34				49			
5				20				35				50			
6				21				36				51			
7				22				37				52			
8				23				38				53			
9				24				39				54			
10				25				40				55			
11				26				41				56			
12				27				42				57			
13				28				43				58			
14				29				44				59			
15				30				45				60			

PLAYTHINK
432

DIFFICULTY: ●●●●●●●●○○
REQUIRED: ◉ ✏ 📄 ✂
COMPLETION: ☐ TIME: _____

HEXAGONS I

Can you arrange the six hexagons shown here into the honeycomb so that each colored edge touches another edge of the same color?

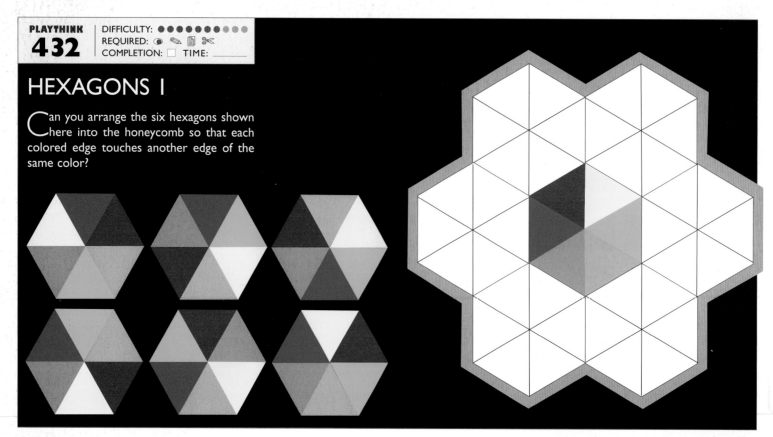

PLAYTHINK
433

DIFFICULTY: ●●●●●●●●○○
REQUIRED: ◉ 📄 ✂
COMPLETION: ☐ TIME: _____

HEXAGONS 2

Can you rearrange the six hexagons so that each edge comes into contact only with edges that have the same color pattern?

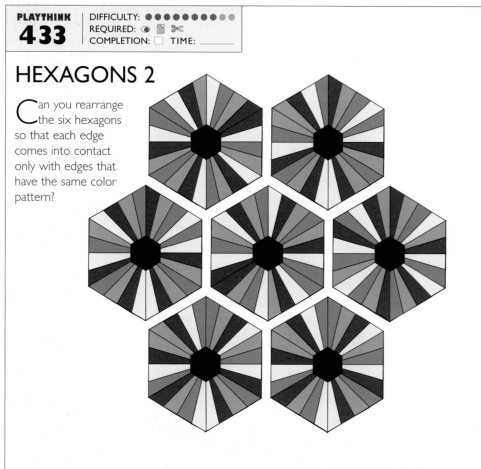

PLAYTHINK
434

DIFFICULTY: ●●●●●●●●○○
REQUIRED: ◉ ✏
COMPLETION: ☐ TIME: _____

COLOR CARDS 2

One of the three numbered cards cannot be found in the grid pattern. Can you see which one is missing?

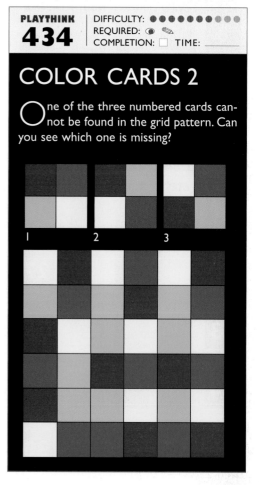

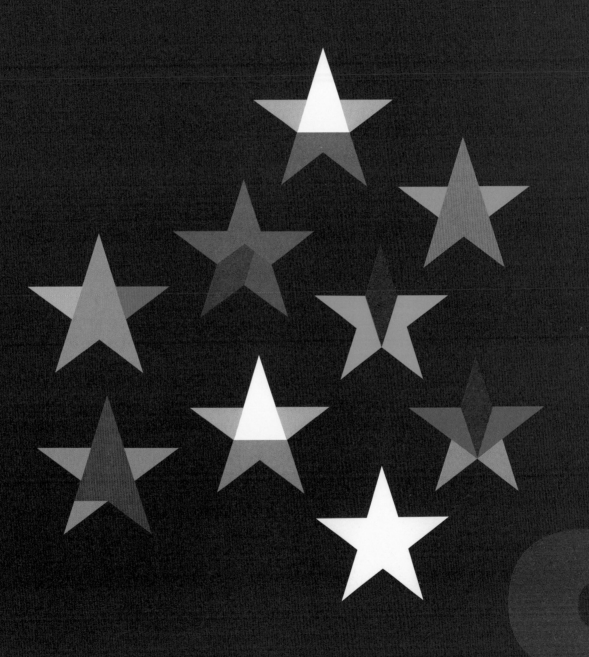

8

Dissections

Polygon Transformations

An easy way to learn about shapes is to cut them apart and reassemble the pieces to form new shapes according to simple rules. For example, if two different shapes with straight-line edges—polygons, in other words—can be assembled from the same set of pieces, then both shapes must have the same area. Conversely, any two polygons of equal area can be dissected into a finite number of pieces that can then be assembled to form either of the two original polygons. Rules like that, while simple, are useful for making calculations and predicting other relationships. The Pythagorean theorem is based on an observation of this kind.

There are many ways to divide a given shape into parts, and some of those divisions—called dissections—are particularly interesting. Although problems of dissections must have confronted humans many thousands of years ago, the earliest known systematic treatise on the subject was written by the tenth-century Persian astronomer Abdul Wefa. Only fragments of his book survive, but it contains some fascinating dissections, one of which is included below as PlayThink 435.

Dissections are found in lots of games. Jigsaw puzzles, in which the required assembly is unique, are one kind of dissection problem. Tangrams, which call for the creative reassembly of pieces, is another. Some dissection problems appear at first to do the impossible: the "Mystrix" puzzle problem (PlayThink 503) involves cutting a shape into a number of pieces, removing one of the pieces, and reassembling the remaining parts to form the original shape. It takes a keen eye to solve this paradox. But the most common use of dissections in recreational math is to find how to dissect one figure to make another in the fewest number of pieces.

In the nineteenth century mathematicians did not take problems of dissections seriously. But now there is a branch of mathematics, called dissection theory, that provides valuable insights into the solutions of many practical problems in plane and solid geometry.

In 1900 the famous mathematician David Hilbert gave an address in Paris in which he listed twenty-three unsolved mathematical problems. Many of those so-called Hilbert problems still tax our ingenuity, but the mathematician Max Dehn solved one within a year. Hilbert asked whether two polyhedral solids of equal volume can always be dissected into a system of identical pieces. Dehn proved that, unlike dissections of equal area, identical dissections of volume are not always possible. It turns out that volume is subtler than area.

PLAYTHINK **435** DIFFICULTY: ●●●●●●●●○○
REQUIRED: ◉ ✎
COMPLETION: ☐ TIME: _____

WEFA'S DISSECTION

The tenth-century mathematician Abdul Wefa posed one of the oldest and most beautiful dissection problems: Can you dissect three identical squares into pieces that can be reassembled into one large square? Wefa's solution involved creating nine pieces. Can you reproduce it?

PLAYTHINK
436
DIFFICULTY: ●●●●●○○○○○
REQUIRED: ◉
COMPLETION: ☐ TIME: _____

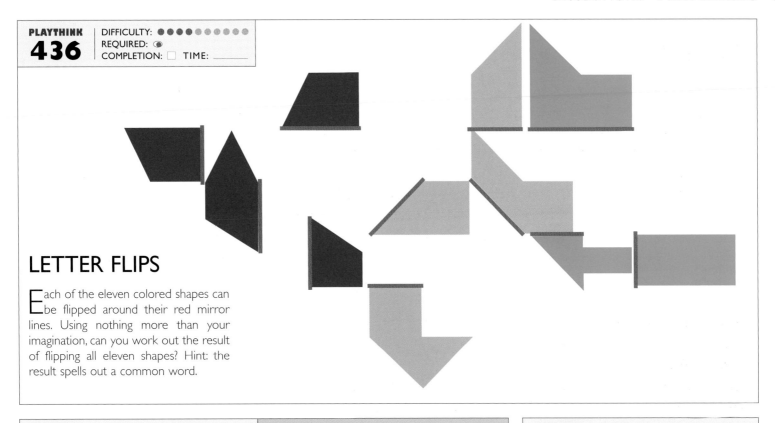

LETTER FLIPS

Each of the eleven colored shapes can be flipped around their red mirror lines. Using nothing more than your imagination, can you work out the result of flipping all eleven shapes? Hint: the result spells out a common word.

PLAYTHINK
437
DIFFICULTY: ●●●●●○○○○○
REQUIRED: ◉ ✎ 📄 ✂
COMPLETION: ☐ TIME: _____

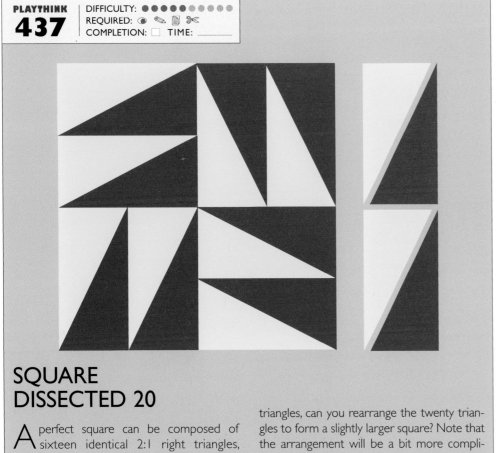

SQUARE
DISSECTED 20

A perfect square can be composed of sixteen identical 2:1 right triangles, as shown. If you add four more identical triangles, can you rearrange the twenty triangles to form a slightly larger square? Note that the arrangement will be a bit more complicated than it is in the sixteen-triangle square.

PLAYTHINK
438
DIFFICULTY: ●●●●○○○○○○
REQUIRED: ◉
COMPLETION: ☐ TIME: _____

MIRROR FLIPS

Each of the multicolored pieces can be flipped around the red mirror lines. Using only your visual imagination, can you work out what shape is produced when all four pieces are flipped?

PLAYTHINK
439

DIFFICULTY: ●●●●●●●○○○
REQUIRED: ◉ ✎ 📄 ✂
COMPLETION: ☐ TIME: _____

THREE SQUARES INTO ONE

Two of the three identical squares shown here have been dissected—one into two pieces, the other into three. Can you rearrange the six pieces to form a larger, perfect square?

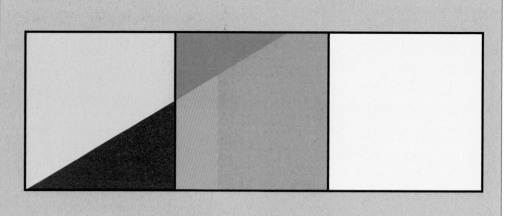

PLAYTHINK
440

DIFFICULTY: ●●●●●●●○○○
REQUIRED: ◉
COMPLETION: ☐ TIME: _____

HALVING SQUARE

Following the grid lines provided, there are only six ways that a square can be dissected into two congruent parts, not counting rotations and reflections. One of the six is shown. Can you find the other five?

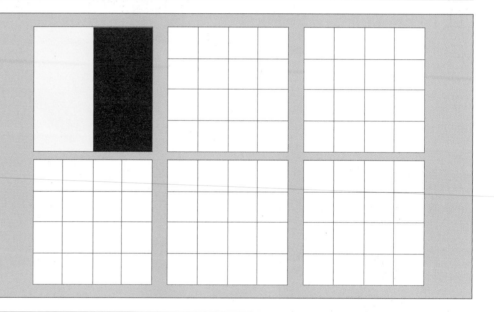

Tangrams

Cut a plane or solid figure into pieces, then fit the pieces together to form the original shape or completely new ones. That's a dissection puzzle—one of the oldest forms of recreational math. And one of the oldest dissection puzzles is the Chinese tangram. In its classic form— a square divided into seven sections— the tangram is one of the most beautiful puzzles ever constructed. From it a nearly limitless variety of

pictures, both abstract and figurative, can be created. Indeed, the subtlety and richness of the tangram's combinatorial possibilities can be revealed and appreciated only after playing with the puzzle for a while. But be forewarned: The challenge can prove as addictive as it is rewarding.

Although the earliest reference to a tangram is in a Chinese book published in 1826, many believe its origins date much earlier than that. We do know that Edgar Allan Poe

and Lewis Carroll were devotees; Napoleon spent endless hours in exile inventing and solving tangram problems.

There are dozens of variations of the tangram involving dissections of rectangles, circles, eggs, hearts and other shapes. After you have solved all the problems suggested here, you should try to create your own designs and figures. It is a meaningful artistic pastime that will strengthen your powers of abstract visualization.

PLAYTHINK 441

DIFFICULTY: ●●●●●●○○○○
REQUIRED: 👁 ✏️ 📄 ✂️
COMPLETION: ☐ TIME: _____

TANGRAM

In the classic tangram a square is divided into seven pieces. Can you rearrange the pieces to form the six shapes shown in silhouette?

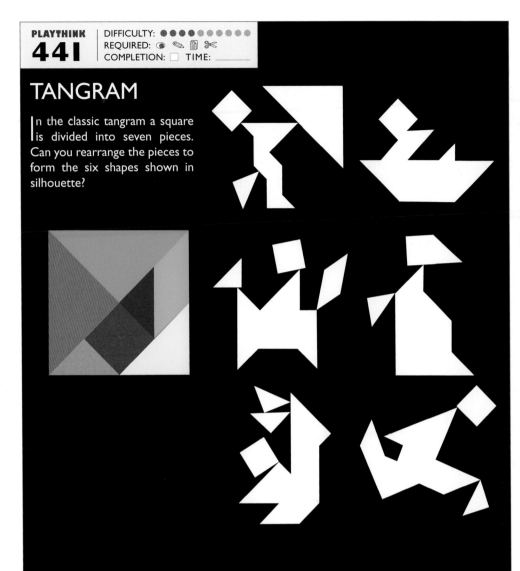

PLAYTHINK 442

DIFFICULTY: ●●●●●○○○○○
REQUIRED: 👁 ✏️ 📄 ✂️
COMPLETION: ☐ TIME: _____

TANGRAM PARADOX

Both silhouettes were made by carefully arranging all seven tangram pieces, but the one on the right seems to have an extra piece. Can you show how each shape was made?

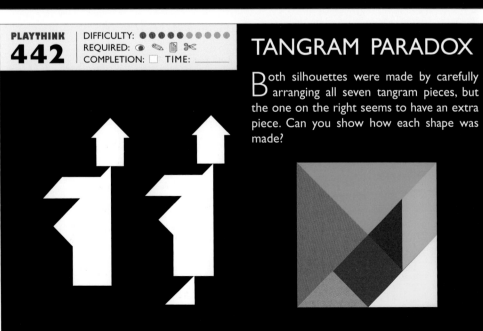

PLAYTHINK 443

DIFFICULTY: ●●●●●●●○○○
REQUIRED: 👁 ✏️ 📄 ✂️
COMPLETION: ☐ TIME: _____

DOUBLE TANGRAM

Copy and cut out the two identical tangram sets. Can you combine all fourteen pieces to form one large square?

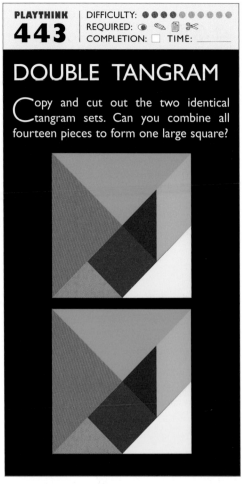

PLAYTHINK 444

DIFFICULTY: ●●●●●●○○○○
REQUIRED: 👁 ✏️
COMPLETION: ☐ TIME: _____

LUCKY CUTS

Can you dissect this horseshoe into six pieces with only two straight cuts?

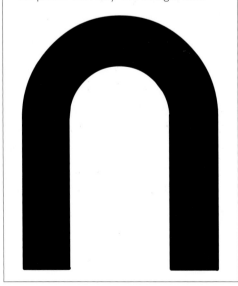

PLAYTHINK 445

DIFFICULTY: ●●●●●●●○○○
REQUIRED: ◉ ✎
COMPLETION: ☐ TIME: _____

SEPARATING MONKEYS

Each of the four monkeys needs an identical compartment that is fenced off from the other monkeys. Following the grid lines on the six-by-six square, can you find two possible ways of separating the monkeys?

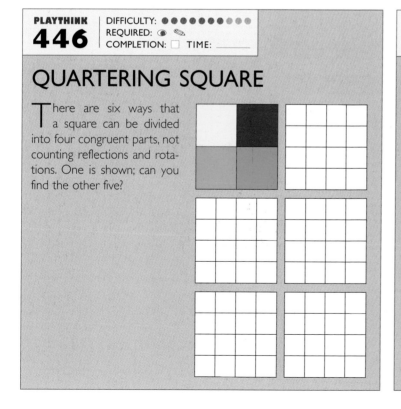

PLAYTHINK 446

DIFFICULTY: ●●●●●●●○○○
REQUIRED: ◉ ✎
COMPLETION: ☐ TIME: _____

QUARTERING SQUARE

There are six ways that a square can be divided into four congruent parts, not counting reflections and rotations. One is shown; can you find the other five?

PLAYTHINK 447

DIFFICULTY: ●●●●●○○○○○
REQUIRED: ◉ ✎
COMPLETION: ☐ TIME: _____

QUARTERING SQUARE 5

A five-by-five square with a unit square missing from the center can be cut along the grid lines into four congruent parts. (Removing the center square allows each quarter to have an area of six square units.) There are seven ways to accomplish this; one solution is shown. Can you find the other six?

PLAYTHINK 448

DIFFICULTY: ●●●●○○○○○○
REQUIRED: ◉ ✎
COMPLETION: ☐ TIME: _____

FENCES

Can you erect fences along the grid lines so that each of the four types of animals has a pen that is identical in size and shape?

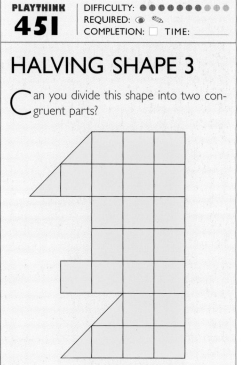

PLAYTHINK 449

DIFFICULTY: ●●●●●●○○○○
REQUIRED: ◉ ✎
COMPLETION: ☐ TIME: _____

HALVING SHAPE 1

Can you divide this irregular shape into two congruent parts? Then can you dissect the shape again to make four congruent parts? There are two possible quartering solutions, one of which does not follow the grid lines.

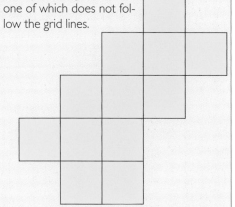

PLAYTHINK 450

DIFFICULTY: ●●●●●●○○○○
REQUIRED: ◉ ✎
COMPLETION: ☐ TIME: _____

HALVING SHAPE 2

Can you dissect this irregular shape into two congruent parts?

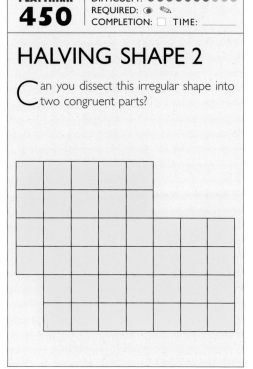

PLAYTHINK 451

DIFFICULTY: ●●●●●●●○○○
REQUIRED: ◉ ✎
COMPLETION: ☐ TIME: _____

HALVING SHAPE 3

Can you divide this shape into two congruent parts?

Not So Simple

A popular type of puzzle involves dividing a given shape into two, three, four or even more equal parts. In some cases *equal* means simply of equal area; in other cases the pieces must be congruent—that is, exactly identical in size and shape. One might think such problems would be easy to solve, but they often prove challenging in spite of their underlying simplicity.

PLAYTHINK 452

DIFFICULTY: ●●●●●●●○○○
REQUIRED: ◉ ✎
COMPLETION: ☐ TIME: _____

HALVING SHAPE 4

Can you divide this shape into two congruent parts?

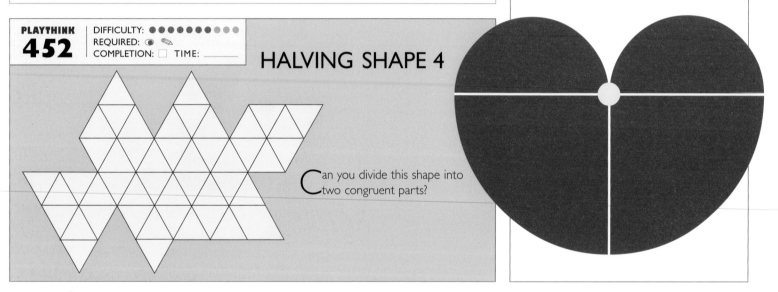

PLAYTHINK 453

DIFFICULTY: ●●●●●●●●○○
REQUIRED: ◉ ✎
COMPLETION: ☐ TIME: _____

HALVING HEART

Examine the diagram of the heart-shaped figure below. Can you work out which line through the yellow point divides the perimeter of the shape into two equal parts?

PLAYTHINK 454

DIFFICULTY: ●●●●●●○○○○
REQUIRED: ◉ ✎
COMPLETION: ☐ TIME: _____

QUARTERING SHAPE 1

Can you help Simon divide his L-shaped carpet into four congruent parts?

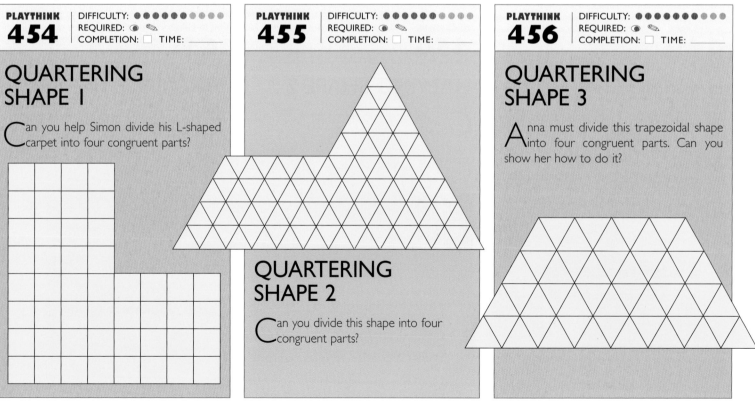

PLAYTHINK 455

DIFFICULTY: ●●●●●●●○○○
REQUIRED: ◉ ✎
COMPLETION: ☐ TIME: _____

QUARTERING SHAPE 2

Can you divide this shape into four congruent parts?

PLAYTHINK 456

DIFFICULTY: ●●●●●●●○○○
REQUIRED: ◉ ✎
COMPLETION: ☐ TIME: _____

QUARTERING SHAPE 3

Anna must divide this trapezoidal shape into four congruent parts. Can you show her how to do it?

PLAYTHINK
457 | DIFFICULTY: ●●●●●●○○○○
REQUIRED: ◉ ✎
COMPLETION: ☐ TIME: _____

CONNECTED SHAPES 1

Some shapes comprise two sections connected by a single point. Can you divide this polygon into two identical connected shapes?

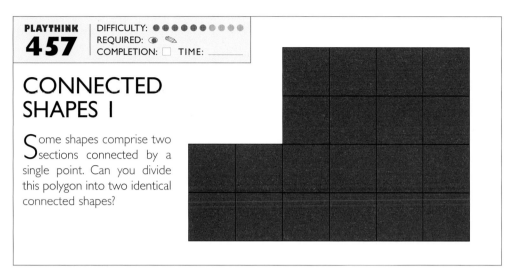

PLAYTHINK
458 | DIFFICULTY: ●●●●●○○○○○
REQUIRED: ◉ ✎
COMPLETION: ☐ TIME: _____

CONNECTED SHAPES 2

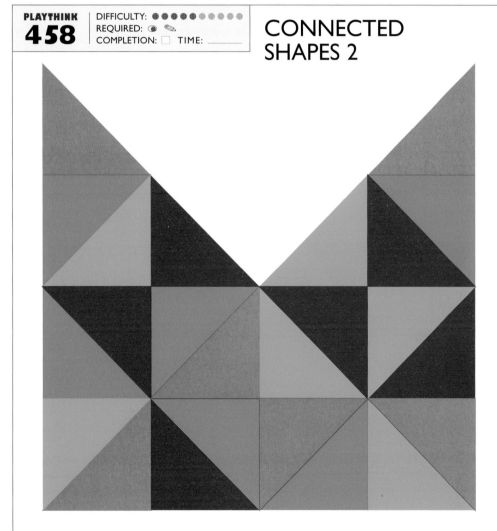

This nonconvex polygon is divided into twenty-four identical triangles, each of which is filled in with one of four colors. Can you rearrange the triangles within the boundary of the polygon to make four identical connected shapes? Each of the shapes should be of one color, and the shapes can be counted as identical even if they are reflections or rotations of one another.

PLAYTHINK
459 | DIFFICULTY: ●●●●●●●○○○
REQUIRED: ◉ ✎
COMPLETION: ☐ TIME: _____

LADYBUG SEPARATION

When ladybugs are hungry, they begin to fight. Can you place three straight fences in such a way that each ladybug is separated into its own compartment?

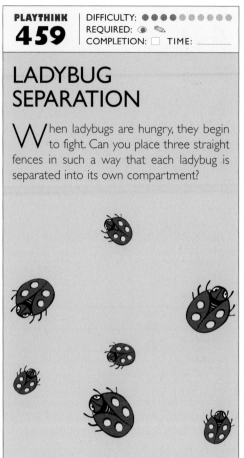

PLAYTHINK
460 | DIFFICULTY: ●●●●●●●○○○
REQUIRED: ◉ ✎ ▤ ✂
COMPLETION: ☐ TIME: _____

GREEK CROSS CUT

This figure can be divided into two identical parts in such a way that when the pieces are rearranged, they form a perfect Greek cross. Can you work out how this can be done?

PLAYTHINK 461

DIFFICULTY: ●●●●●●●○○○
REQUIRED: 👁 ✏️
COMPLETION: ☐ TIME: _____

FLIES

As you can see in the diagram below, every one of the nine flies on the grid has its row, column and diagonal to itself. Can you move three of the flies just one space each—horizontally, vertically or diagonally—and still preserve their right to an exclusive row, column and diagonal?

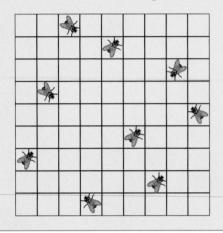

PLAYTHINK 462

DIFFICULTY: ●●●●●●●○○○
REQUIRED: 👁 ✏️
COMPLETION: ☐ TIME: _____

GREEK CROSS INTO SQUARES

Can you dissect this Greek cross into nine pieces that can fit together to form either five small squares or one large one?

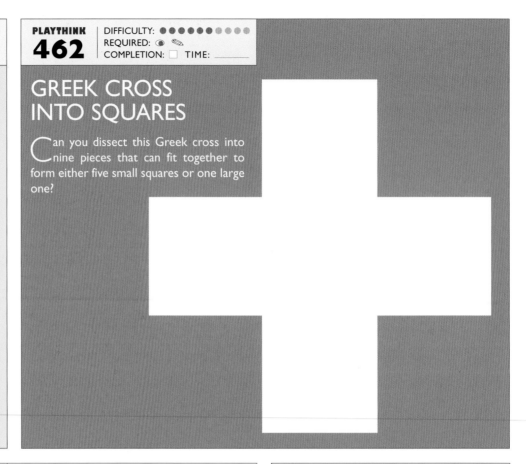

PLAYTHINK 463

DIFFICULTY: ●●●●●●●○○○
REQUIRED: 👁 📄 ✂️
COMPLETION: ☐ TIME: _____

STAR TO RECTANGLE

The six-pointed star has been dissected into six pieces. Can you reassemble the pieces to form a rectangle?

PLAYTHINK 464

DIFFICULTY: ●●●●●●●○○○
REQUIRED: 👁 ✏️
COMPLETION: ☐ TIME: _____

SQUARE INTO TWO SQUARES

Can you dissect the five-by-five square into the fewest number of pieces needed to make both a four-by-four square and a three-by-three square?

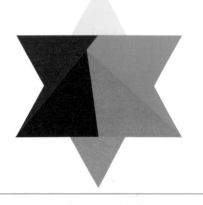

PLAYTHINK 465

DIFFICULTY: ●●●●●●●●○○
REQUIRED: 👁
COMPLETION: ☐ TIME: _____

HINGED TRIANGLE

This equilateral triangle has been dissected into four parts. Hinges, marked in red, connect the parts to each other. If you leave the blue piece fixed and swing the others around their hinges, you can rearrange the pieces to form a new shape. Can you work out what that new shape must be?

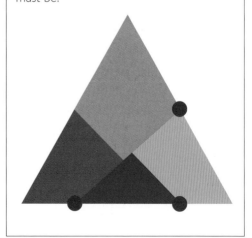

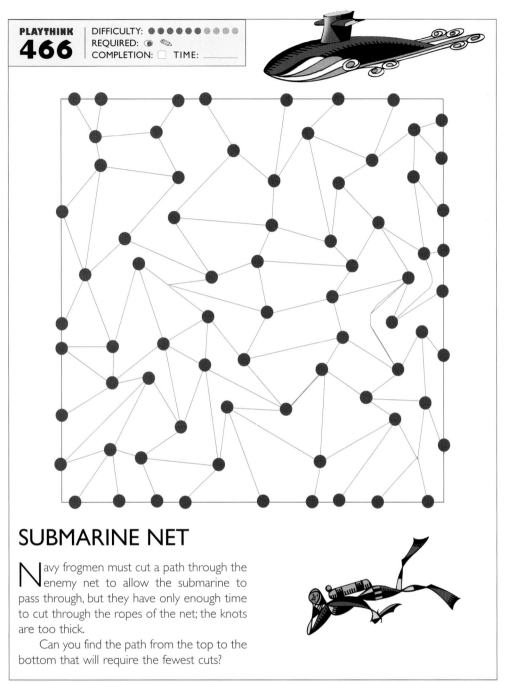

SUBMARINE NET

Navy frogmen must cut a path through the enemy net to allow the submarine to pass through, but they have only enough time to cut through the ropes of the net; the knots are too thick.

Can you find the path from the top to the bottom that will require the fewest cuts?

TRIANGLE TO HEXAGON

Can you find a way to arrange the six pieces to form an equilateral triangle? Then can you reassemble the pieces to make a hexagon?

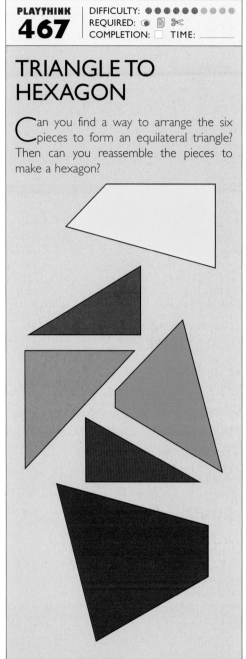

SQUARE INTO THREE SQUARES

Can you dissect this seven-by-seven square into the fewest pieces necessary to form three smaller squares: a six-by-six, a three-by-three and a two-by-two?

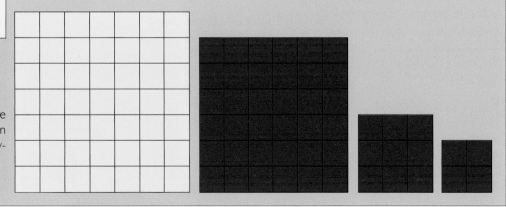

Pythagorean Theorem

The ancient geometric theorem attributed to Pythagoras is one of the few theorems that almost everybody has at least a nodding acquaintance with. It concerns the relationships between the two short sides of a right triangle and the long side, or hypotenuse.

It is as famous in words—the square of the hypotenuse of any right triangle is equal to the sum of the squares of the other two sides—as it is in symbols:

$$a^2 + b^2 = c^2$$

in which a and b are the lengths of the two short sides, and c is the length of the hypotenuse.

But what does this actually mean?

In numerical terms it means that we may construct right-angled triangles by using any three lengths a, b, c that satisfy the Pythagorean condition.

For example, since

$$3^2 + 4^2 = 5^2$$

a triangle with sides 3, 4 and 5 is necessarily right-angled. The surveyors of ancient Egypt, it is said, knew of this relationship and divided a rope into twelve equal parts by knots to form the so-called Egyptian triangle, which they used to construct nearly perfect right angles.

There are many other whole-number Pythagorean triplets: 5-12-13 and 8-15-17, to name two. The general rule for finding all Pythagorean triplets is known and was one of the first results to be obtained in the theory of Diophantine equations—that is, equations solved using only whole numbers. This is a surprising link between geometry and the theory of numbers.

Geometrically, the Pythagorean theorem asserts an equality of areas. A square whose side is laid against the hypotenuse of a right triangle has exactly the same area as two squares laid against the other two sides combined. One interesting problem (see PlayThink 469) demonstrates this directly, by finding a way to cut up the two smaller squares into pieces that can be reassembled to form the larger square. An alternative and very beautiful solution to this problem, known as Perigal's dissection (see PlayThink 470), leaves the smallest square intact and cuts the middle-sized square into four pieces of the same shape and size.

EGYPTIAN TRIANGLE

Surveyors in ancient Egypt had a simple tool for making near-perfect right triangles: a loop of rope divided by knots into twelve equal sections. When they stretched the rope to make a triangle whose sides were in the ratio 3:4:5, they knew the largest angle was a right angle.

Can you fit the five pieces at bottom into the two smaller squares above the right triangle? Then can you fit the same five pieces into the larger square below the right triangle? If you can do both, what have you done?

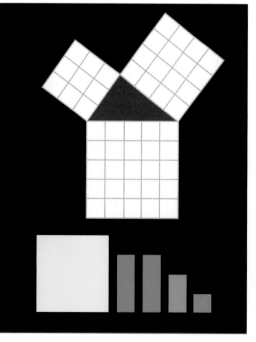

PERIGAL'S PUZZLE

Fill the medium-sized square with the red and pink trapezoids and cover the small square with the blue square. Can you then take the five parts and reassemble them to fill the large square?

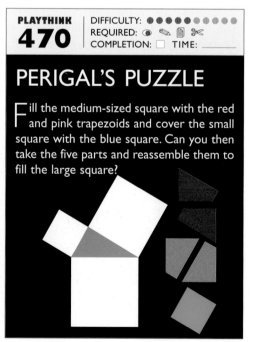

PLAYTHINK
471

DIFFICULTY: ●●●●●○○○○○
REQUIRED: 👁 ✎ 📄 ✂
COMPLETION: ☐ TIME: _____

PYTHAGORINO

This novel three-player domino game is based on a shape derived from the Pythagorean theorem: three squares arranged around an isosceles right triangle. The twenty-seven Pythagorean playing pieces come in various combinations of three colors—red, blue and yellow.

The pieces are placed one at a time on the grid so that the smaller squares align with the grid and the larger squares align with the diagonals. Players are assigned a color and take turns placing pieces on the grid in much the same way standard dominoes are played: adjacent squares—either small or large—must be the same color. See the example below for a demonstration of this. A player gets a point for every big square of his or her color that forms an unbroken strip consisting of at least two squares of that color. The play continues until no additional pieces can be placed. The player with the most points wins; in a tie, the win goes to the player whose points were made with the fewest number of strips.

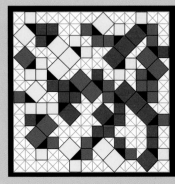

SAMPLE GAME OF PYTHAGORINO

The score of this game was red 6, blue 6 and yellow 5. Red wins the tie because the large red squares were linked using fewer strips (just two) than the blue ones. Notice that isolated large squares do not score points.

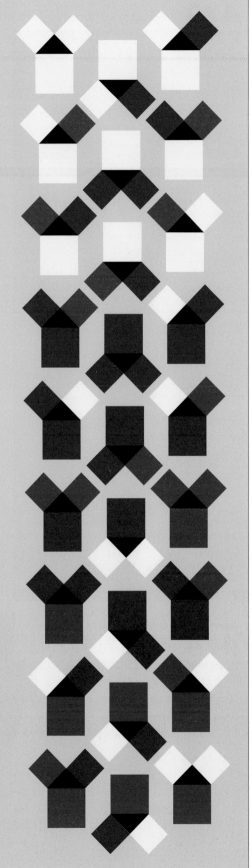

PLAYTHINK
472

DIFFICULTY: ❶●●●●●●●●●○○
REQUIRED: 👁 📄 ✂
COMPLETION: ☐ TIME: _____

FOUR PENTASTARS

The four pentagonal stars have been dissected into twelve pieces. Can you rearrange the pieces to form one large pentagonal star?

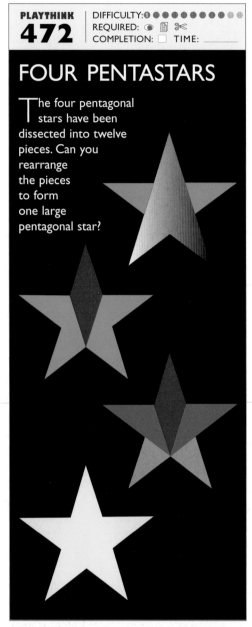

PLAYTHINK
473

DIFFICULTY: ●●●●●●●●○○○
REQUIRED: 👁
COMPLETION: ☐ TIME: _____

TRIANGLE TO STAR

This equilateral triangle is composed of twenty-four identical right triangles. Just by looking at it, can you work out how to rearrange the pieces to form a perfect six-pointed star?

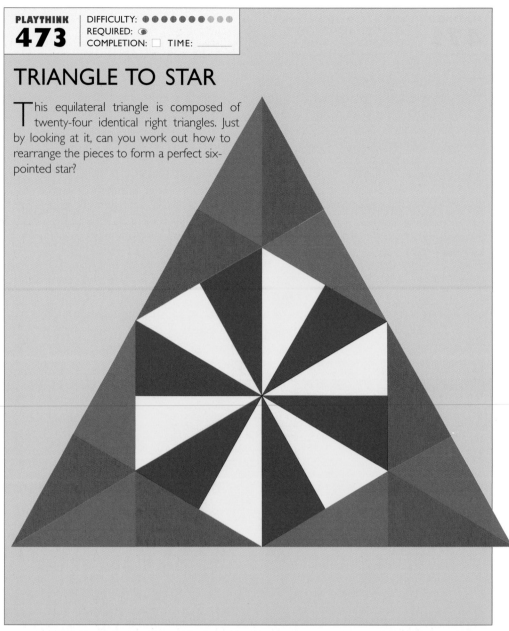

PLAYTHINK
474

DIFFICULTY: ●●●●●●●●○○○
REQUIRED: 👁 📄 ✂
COMPLETION: ☐ TIME: _____

PENTAGONAL STARS

These five pentagonal stars have been dissected into eighteen pieces. The pieces can be rearranged to form a large pentagonal star. Can you work out how that can be accomplished?

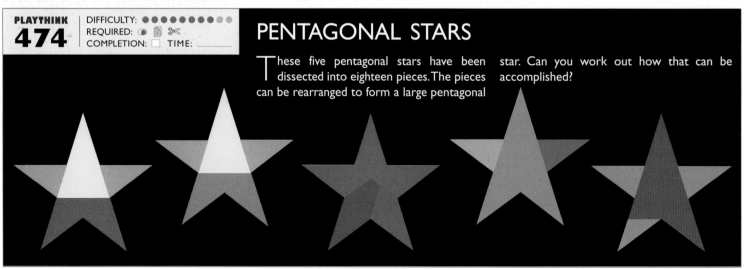

PLAYTHINK 475

DIFFICULTY: ●●●●●○○○○○
REQUIRED: ◉ 📄 ✂
COMPLETION: ☐ TIME: _____

T TO RECTANGLE

Can you reassemble the parts of the dissected *T* to form a rectangle?

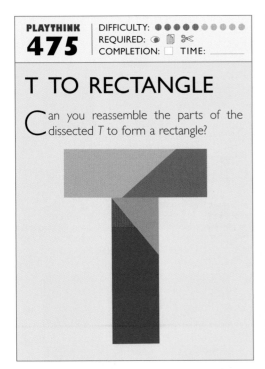

PLAYTHINK 476

DIFFICULTY: ●●●●●●○○○○
REQUIRED: ◉ 📄 ✂
COMPLETION: ☐ TIME: _____

GEOMETRIX

These five colored pieces fit together amazingly well. They can be assembled to form a square, a trapezoid, a triangle, a Greek cross or a parallelogram. Can you work out how to make all five shapes?

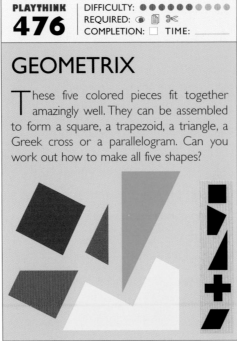

PLAYTHINK 477

DIFFICULTY: ●●●●●●●○○○
REQUIRED: ◉ ✏ 📄 ✂
COMPLETION: ☐ TIME: _____

RECTANGLING CIRCLE

This illustration was made with a compass set to a fixed radius. Can you dissect the circle with three straight cuts and then reassemble just the red pieces to form a rectangle?

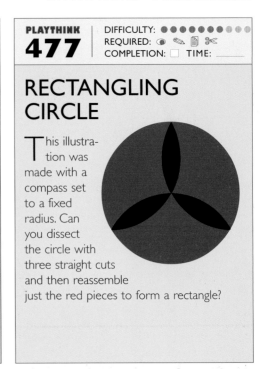

PLAYTHINK 478

DIFFICULTY: ●●●●●●●●○○
REQUIRED: ◉ 📄 ✂
COMPLETION: ☐ TIME: _____

NONAGON MAGIC

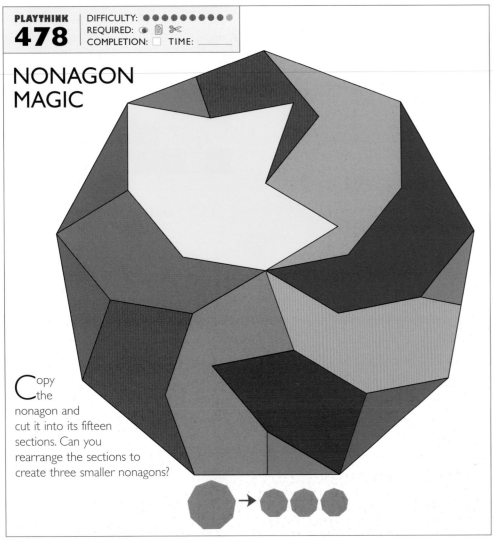

Copy the nonagon and cut it into its fifteen sections. Can you rearrange the sections to create three smaller nonagons?

PLAYTHINK 479

DIFFICULTY: ●●●●●●●●○○
REQUIRED: ◉ 📄 ✂
COMPLETION: ☐ TIME: _____

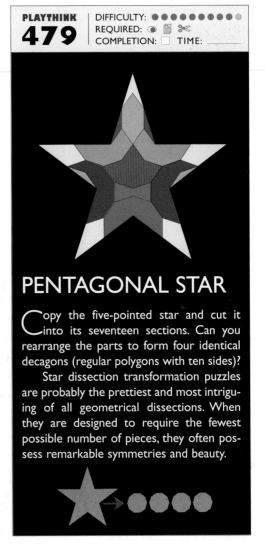

PENTAGONAL STAR

Copy the five-pointed star and cut it into its seventeen sections. Can you rearrange the parts to form four identical decagons (regular polygons with ten sides)?

Star dissection transformation puzzles are probably the prettiest and most intriguing of all geometrical dissections. When they are designed to require the fewest possible number of pieces, they often possess remarkable symmetries and beauty.

Packing Shapes

"Wheels within wheels" is a common phrase, but what about squares within squares? Suppose you have a number of identical squares to pack inside a larger square. What is the smallest size that the large box has to be to fit a given number of smaller squares without overlaps? If the smaller squares are not allowed to tilt, the problem is trivial. Allowing tilting adds to the difficulty, but it also allows more efficient solutions to emerge.

For one to four squares, tilting provides no advantage. But in order to pack five squares into a larger square without tilting, you must use a square with sides three times as large as the packed squares. Tilt the five squares into a cross, and the large square need be only 2.828 units on a side. A more efficient packing can be obtained if only the central square is tilted; then the larger square has side 2.707.

For n = 6, 7, 8 or 9, the untilted solutions are again as efficient as any other. But when you must pack ten squares, tilting provides a better solution, although no one yet knows if the solutions so far obtained are the best or whether some ingenious packing can be made to do it better.

As the number of squares becomes large, the task of proving that a given packing is minimal becomes increasingly difficult, except in cases in which the number of squares is itself a square—that is, 9, 16, 25 and so on. There are many other packing problems, most of which are equally baffling, especially those that allow irregular packing. An important example is the packing of circles in the plane. The analogous problem of spheres packed into space poses an even more severe problem. The densest regular packing is known, but whether any irregular packing would be better is still a mystery. Most mathematicians don't think they'll find a better solution, but that remains unproved.

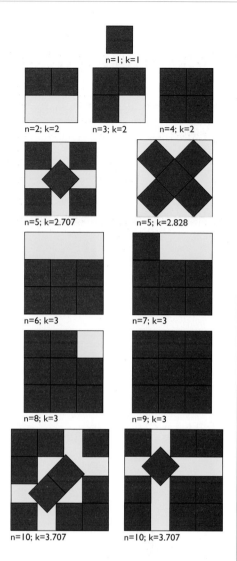

PACKING UNIT SQUARES

The best results for packing unit squares into a larger square are shown; the solutions range from one to ten squares.

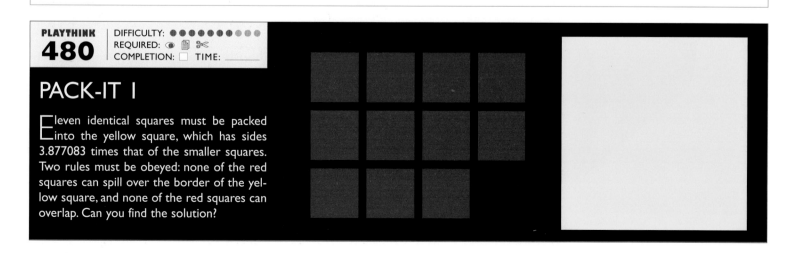

PACK-IT 1

Eleven identical squares must be packed into the yellow square, which has sides 3.877083 times that of the smaller squares. Two rules must be obeyed: none of the red squares can spill over the border of the yellow square, and none of the red squares can overlap. Can you find the solution?

PLAYTHINK 481

DIFFICULTY: ●●●●●○○○○○
REQUIRED: ◉ ✎ 📄 ✂
COMPLETION: ☐ TIME: _____

DISAPPEARING PENCIL

There are seven red pencils and six blue pencils in this drawing. Will cutting along the line and swapping the lower left and lower right parts of the figure have any effect on what you see?

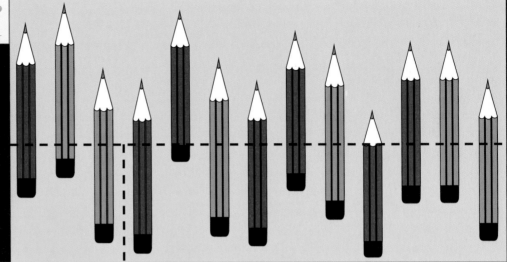

PLAYTHINK 482

DIFFICULTY: ●●●●●●●●○○
REQUIRED: ◉ 📄 ✂
COMPLETION: ☐ TIME: _____

STAR PUZZLE

This twelve-pointed star has been dissected into twenty-four sections. Can you rearrange the pieces to make three smaller twelve-pointed stars?

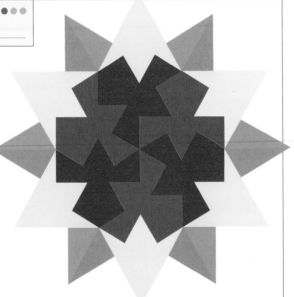

PLAYTHINK 483

DIFFICULTY: ●●●●●●●●○○
REQUIRED: ◉ 📄 ✂
COMPLETION: ☐ TIME: _____

TWELVE-POINTED STAR

Copy this twelve-pointed star and cut it into its twenty-four sections. Can you rearrange the parts to make three smaller twelve-pointed stars?

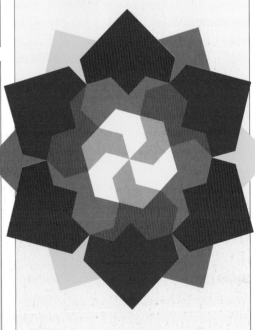

PLAYTHINK 484

DIFFICULTY: ●●●●●○○○○○
REQUIRED: ◉ 📄 ✂
COMPLETION: ☐ TIME: _____

DISSECTED PLOT

Just by looking at the dissected rectangular plot, can you tell the size of each region in terms of the unit squares of the grid? Which part of the plot is bigger: the large red triangle, or all the rest combined?

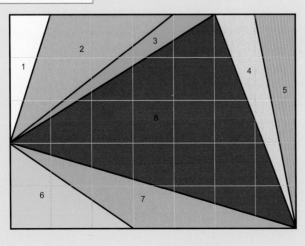

Squared Squares and Rectangles

Mathematicians look for order everywhere. And when they find it, they like to give expression to their enthusiasm by defining numbers, squares, rectangles, triangles and parallelograms as "perfect."

In 1934 the famous Hungarian mathematician Paul Erdös posed this dissection problem: *Can a square or rectangle be subdivided into smaller squares of which no two are alike?* Such squares or rectangles are called

perfect, or squared. (Squares or rectangles in which some of the element squares are identical are, not surprisingly, called imperfect.) Erdös concluded that such a square is impossible, probably influenced by the easily proved fact that one cannot dissect a cube into smaller cubes in which no two are identical. The best one could achieve, Erdös believed, was to dissect a rectangle into smaller squares no two of which are alike.

For many years Erdös appeared to be right. But then a team of mathematicians exploiting an analogy with the theory of electrical circuits found such a perfect square. Their square, which was made up of twenty-four different squares of consecutive sizes, was the longtime record holder for smallest perfect square. But in 1978 the Dutch mathematician A. J. W. Duijvestijn found a better solution— one that required only twenty-one element squares (see page 185).

PLAYTHINK **485**	DIFFICULTY: ●●●●●●●●○○
	REQUIRED: 👁 ✏️ 📄 ✂️
	COMPLETION: ☐ TIME: _____

SMALLEST SQUARED RECTANGLE

No rectangle has been found that can be divided into fewer than nine squares of different sizes—a so-called perfect rectangle. The smallest such rectangle is composed of

the squares, shown below, with sides of 1, 4, 7, 8, 9, 10, 14, 15 and 18 units. From those elements, can you form a perfect rectangle?

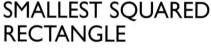

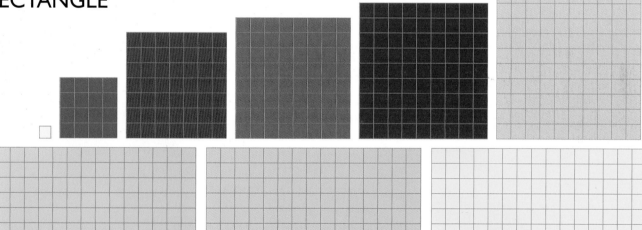

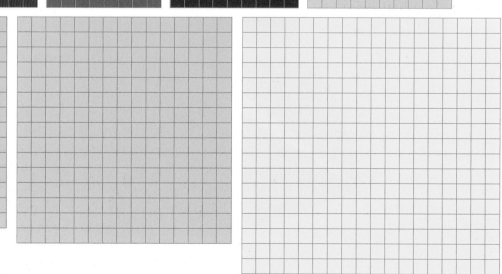

A Strange Coincidence

By now you have played with puzzles based on packing identical shapes, circles and squares. And you have begun to think about packing nonidentical squares. One possibility that springs to mind is to use consecutive squares of sides 1, 2, 3 ,4 . . . and so on, up to some particular limit. Is there a square that can be cut into such a system of smaller squares?

If the squares are to fill the large square completely, they cannot be placed at a tilt. So the outer square must have a side that is a whole number. Therefore, the total area of the system of small squares must itself be a square.

Summing the first few consecutive squares isn't very helpful.

$$1^2 + 2^2 + 3^2 + 4^2 + \ldots + 24^2 = 4{,}900 = 70^2$$

In fact, this is the only sum of consecutive squares that results in a square for the total. (The demonstration is a difficult exercise in the theory of numbers and was itself an unsolved problem for a considerable time.) That raises a geometrical problem that is one of the most beautiful puzzles in recreational geometry: Can one pack the first twenty-four

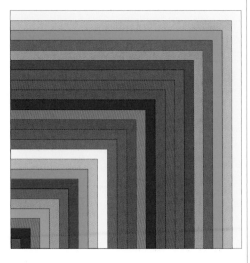

consecutive squares into a seventy-by-seventy square? If you want to try it, see PlayThink 486.

PLAYTHINK 486

DIFFICULTY: ●●●●●○○○○○
REQUIRED: 👁 ✏️ ✂️
COMPLETION: ☐ TIME: _____

SQUARE INFINITY

Twenty-four squares with sides ranging from 1 to 24 units have a total area of 4,900 square units. The seventy-by-seventy game board shown at right also has an area of 4,900 square units. Can you cover the board with the twenty-four squares without overlap? To give you a head start, the largest squares have been placed.

Is there a smaller number of consecutive squares that add up to a square number?

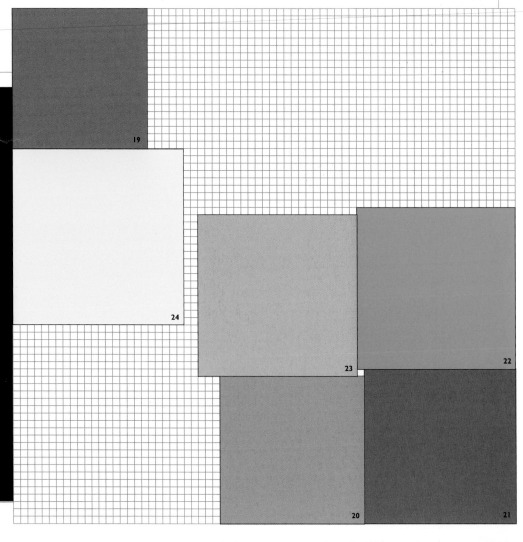

Squared Square

A square that is composed of smaller squares of different sizes is called a perfect square. (The smaller squares should all have sides that are whole numbers.) The smallest known perfect square is made up of twenty-one squares; those squares have sides of 2, 4, 6, 7, 8, 9, 11, 15, 16, 17, 18, 19, 24, 25, 27, 29, 33, 35, 37, 42 and 50 units. The diagram here shows how those squares are put together to make one larger square with sides of 112 units.

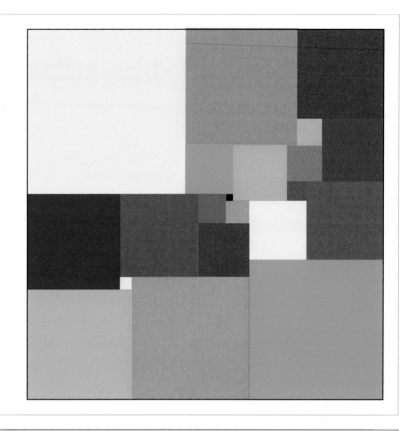

PLAYTHINK 487

DIFFICULTY: ●●●●●●○○○○○
REQUIRED: ◉ ✎
COMPLETION: ☐   TIME: _____

IMPERFECT SQUARE

Squares that have been divided into smaller squares, with two or more squares being of identical size, are called imperfect squares. For example, a three-by-three square can be dissected into one two-by-two square and five one-by-one squares—a total of six pieces. You might try dividing a four-by-four square into one three-by-three square and seven one-by-one squares, but the minimal solution will involve just four two-by-two squares.

In general, squares with sides that are of even-numbered lengths are easy to form as imperfect squares; those with sides that are of odd-numbered lengths are more complicated. To see how this is so, dissect these squares, with sides of 11, 12, 13 and 14 units, into imperfect squares with the least number of pieces.

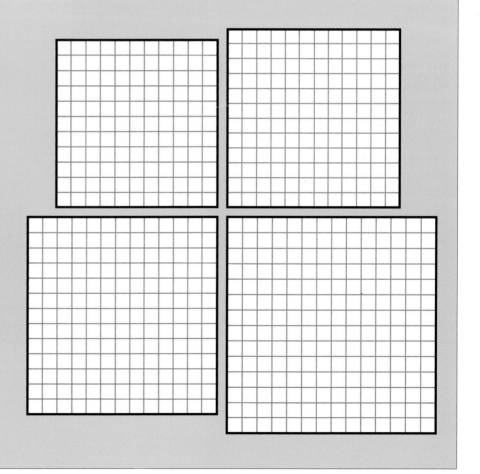

PLAYTHINK 488 | DIFFICULTY: ●●●●●●○○○○ REQUIRED: ◉ ✎ COMPLETION: ☐ TIME: ____

UNCOVERED SQUARE

If you try to fit the five chevron shapes onto the four-by-four board, one square will always be uncovered. After all, the five chevrons each cover an area of three units, and the board has an area of sixteen units. But can that uncovered square be anywhere on the board?

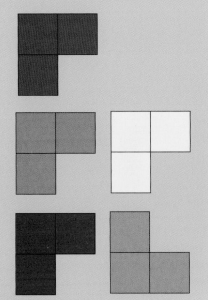

PLAYTHINK 489 | DIFFICULTY: ●●●●●●○○○○ REQUIRED: ◉ ✎ COMPLETION: ☐ TIME: ____

IMPERFECT SQUARE SPLIT

Fifteen squares can form an imperfect thirteen-by-thirteen square, as shown here. If you remove one of the five-by-five squares, can you reassemble the remaining squares to form a twelve-by-twelve perfect square?

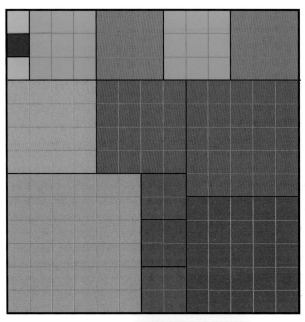

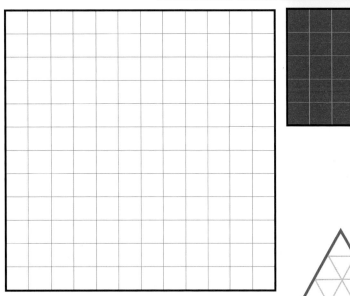

PLAYTHINK 490 | DIFFICULTY: ●●●●●●○○○○ REQUIRED: ◉ ✎ COMPLETION: ☐ TIME: ____

IMPERFECT TRIANGLE

Using the triangular grid as a guide, divide this equilateral triangle with sides 11 units long into smaller-integer triangles. What is the smallest number of such triangles that will completely cover the figure?

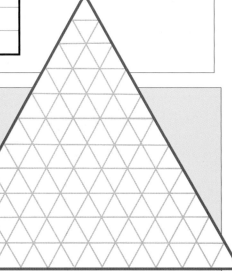

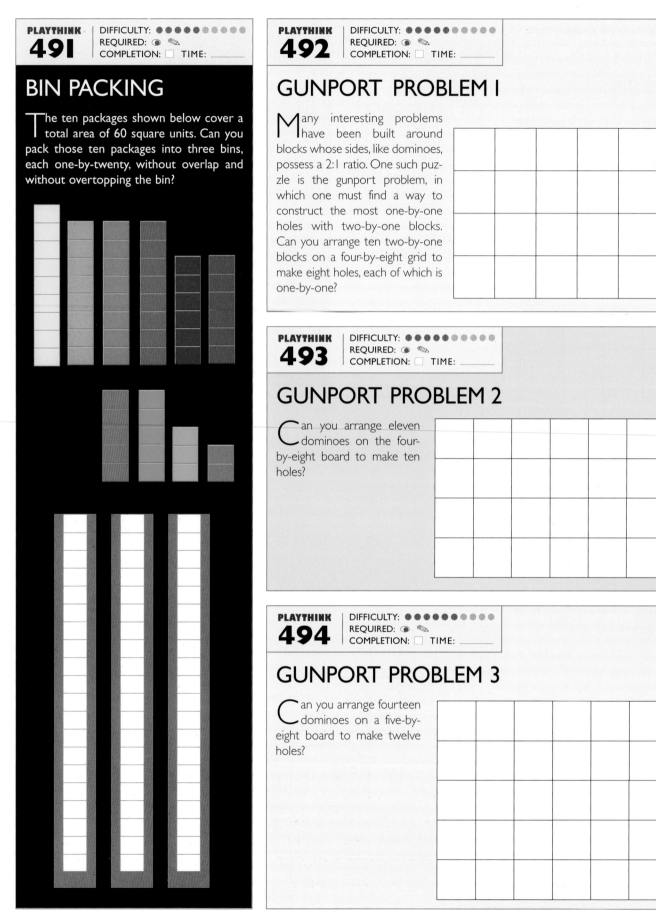

BIN PACKING

The ten packages shown below cover a total area of 60 square units. Can you pack those ten packages into three bins, each one-by-twenty, without overlap and without overtopping the bin?

GUNPORT PROBLEM 1

Many interesting problems have been built around blocks whose sides, like dominoes, possess a 2:1 ratio. One such puzzle is the gunport problem, in which one must find a way to construct the most one-by-one holes with two-by-one blocks. Can you arrange ten two-by-one blocks on a four-by-eight grid to make eight holes, each of which is one-by-one?

GUNPORT PROBLEM 2

Can you arrange eleven dominoes on the four-by-eight board to make ten holes?

GUNPORT PROBLEM 3

Can you arrange fourteen dominoes on a five-by-eight board to make twelve holes?

PLAYTHINK
495
DIFFICULTY: ●●●●●●○○○○
REQUIRED: 👁 ✏
COMPLETION: ☐ TIME: _____

GUNPORT PROBLEM 4

Can you arrange twenty-seven dominoes on an eight-by-ten board to make twenty-six holes?

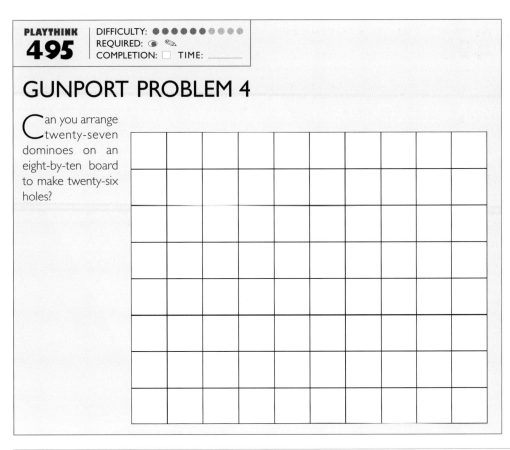

PLAYTHINK
496
DIFFICULTY: ●●●●●●●○○○
REQUIRED: 👁 ✏ 📄 ✂
COMPLETION: ☐ TIME: _____

HEXAGON PACKING

Can you fill a regular hexagon using six copies of the two shapes shown at left?

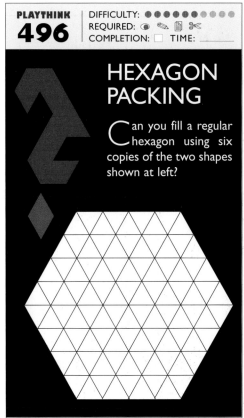

Vanishing Pieces

Most optical tricks and perceptual illusions fail to hold our attention because the secret of their trickery becomes obvious fairly quickly. But a remarkable group of images known as "geometrical paradoxes" are so subtle that they continue to intrigue and surprise even after their workings have been explained.

Geometrical paradoxes involve separating and rearranging parts of a total length or area. After reassembling the figure in what seems to be its entirety, a portion of the original figure is left over.

The explanation lies in what the

great American puzzle genius Martin Gardner calls the principle of concealed distribution. The eye has a great tolerance for subtle alterations in the rearranged version. Tiny increases in the gaps between the parts or in the lengths of the reassembled pieces go unnoticed, so people believe both must have the same area or length.

Sam Loyd, the greatest American puzzle creator (and the inventor of Parcheesi), was the originator of the most famous puzzle in this group: "Get Off the Earth" (a variation of which you can try; see PlayThink 481). Invented in 1896, it involves two disks attached at their common center. In one orientation the disks show parts

of thirteen warriors standing on the planet. But when the top disk is rotated a bit, one of the warriors disappears. The puzzle caused such a sensation that it was used as part of a publicity campaign for William McKinley's presidential bid.

Over the years the Canadian illusionist Melville Stover and many others have perfected the art, creating subtle variations of the principle and loads of exciting puzzles. Some crooks also used the method of concealed distribution—to convert fourteen $100 bills into fifteen by cutting each into two parts and gluing one part to the next. Although the effect was subtle, it was noticeable—and quite illegal.

PLAYTHINK
497
DIFFICULTY: ●●●●●●●○○○
REQUIRED: ◉
COMPLETION: ☐   TIME: _____

RECTANGLES IN TRIANGLE

Four examples of right isosceles triangles partially filled with squares or rectangles are shown below. Just by looking at them, can you tell in which examples the shapes cover the greatest proportion of the triangle?

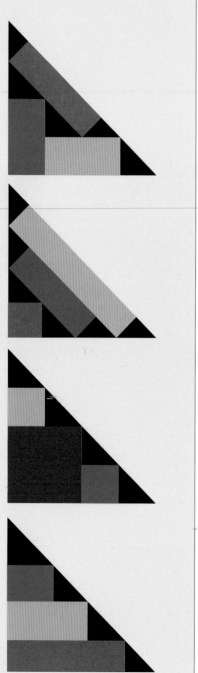

PLAYTHINK
498
DIFFICULTY: ●●●●●●●○○○
REQUIRED: ◉ ✎
COMPLETION: ☐   TIME: _____

IMPERFECT PARALLELOGRAM

This nineteen-by-twenty parallelogram has been covered with a triangular grid. Following that grid, can you divide the parallelogram into thirteen equilateral triangles, two or more of which may be the same size?

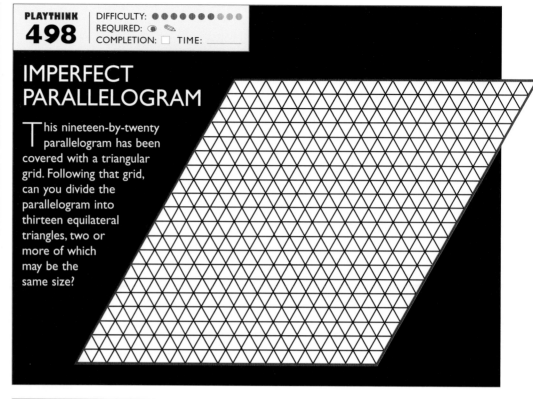

PLAYTHINK
499
DIFFICULTY: ●●●●●●●○○○
REQUIRED: ◉ ✎ 📄 ✂
COMPLETION: ☐   TIME: _____

INCOMPARABLE RECTANGLES

These seven rectangles are incomparable: none can be placed inside the other if the corresponding sides are parallel. What's more, these seven rectangles make up the smallest possible rectangle composed entirely of incomparable rectangles.

Can you assemble the seven rectangles into one larger rectangle?

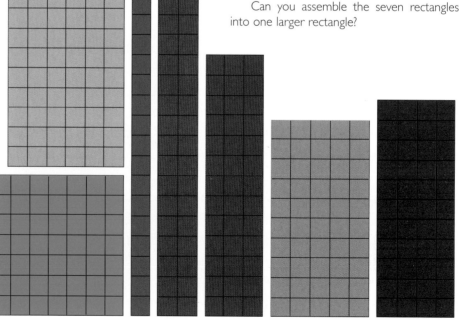

Polyominoes

Dominoes are the playing pieces, or tiles, of a centuries-old game. The tiles are made up of two unit squares joined along a common edge, and each square is marked with an independent number of dots. But mathematicians—recreational and otherwise—have elaborated on the basic domino shape by adding successively more unit squares. The results—three-square trominoes, four-square tetrominoes, five-square pentominoes and the like—are

collectively known as polyominoes.

The first polyomino problem appeared in 1907. Now no mention of [combinatorics] and puzzles can be made without a reference to polyominoes, and especially to pentominoes, on which volumes have been written.

The popularity of these shapes, both as a form of mathematical recreation and as educational tools, owes much to two men: Solomon Golomb, who invented them in 1953, and Martin Gardner, who

has introduced beautiful puzzles, games and problems based on them to wide audiences.

It's fun to think about the different polyominoes that can be constructed from a certain number of unit squares. For instance, the domino has but one possible shape, and the tromino just two. But there are 5 tetrominoes, 12 pentominoes and 12 hexominoes (six-squared polyominoes). After that, the numbers rise steeply: 108 heptominoes and 369 octominoes.

PLAYTHINK **500**	DIFFICULTY: ●●●●●○○○○○ REQUIRED: ◉ ✎ COMPLETION: ☐ TIME: _____

POLYOMINOES

Illustrated below are the nine different ways to join up to four identical squares so that their sides meet perfectly.

Can you find all the different ways to join the sides of five identical squares?

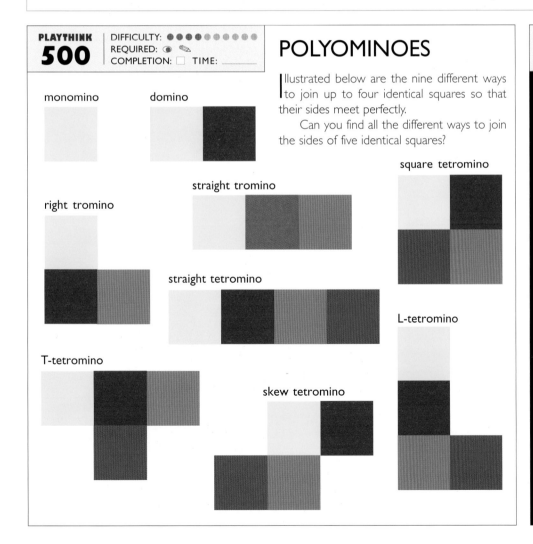

monomino

domino

right tromino

straight tromino

square tetromino

straight tetromino

L-tetromino

T-tetromino

skew tetromino

PLAYTHINK **501**	DIFFICULTY: ●●●●●○○○○○ REQUIRED: ◉ ✎ 📄 ✂ COMPLETION: ☐ TIME: _____

TETROMINOES

The five possible tetrominoes are shown. In how many different ways can you place each of them on a four-by-four square? (Rotations and reflections do not count as different.)

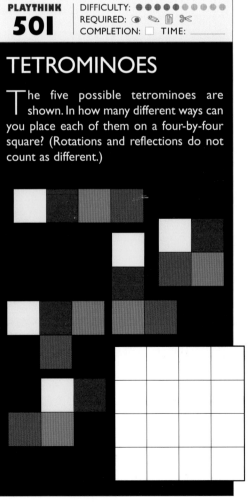

PLAYTHINK 502

DIFFICULTY: ●●●●●○○○○○
REQUIRED: ◉ ✎
COMPLETION: ☐ TIME: _____

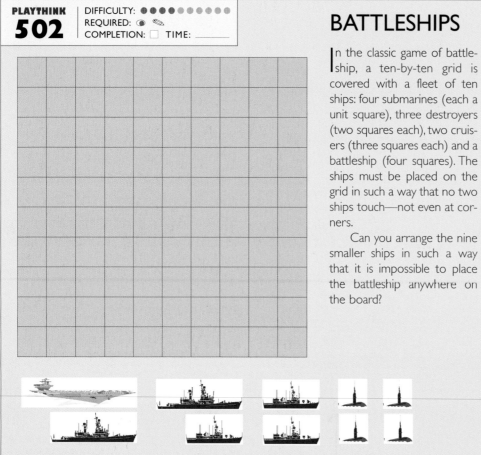

BATTLESHIPS

In the classic game of battleship, a ten-by-ten grid is covered with a fleet of ten ships: four submarines (each a unit square), three destroyers (two squares each), two cruisers (three squares each) and a battleship (four squares). The ships must be placed on the grid in such a way that no two ships touch—not even at corners.

Can you arrange the nine smaller ships in such a way that it is impossible to place the battleship anywhere on the board?

PLAYTHINK 504

DIFFICULTY: ●●●●●○○○○○
REQUIRED: ◉ ✎
COMPLETION: ☐ TIME: _____

TRIANGLE FITTING

How many of the small figures can you place in the larger one without overlap?

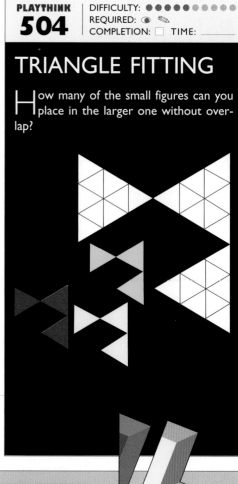

PLAYTHINK 503

DIFFICULTY: ●●●●●●●●○○
REQUIRED: ◉ 📄 ✂
COMPLETION: ☐ TIME: _____

MYSTRIX: THE DISAPPEARING SQUARE PUZZLE

Ever thought you were the center of attention, only to find that no one noticed when you were missing? This puzzle offers the same weird effect in geometric form: you can remove a central piece from a dissection and never notice it's gone.

No sleight of hand or hypnosis is necessary to pull off this feat of geometric magic. Simply copy and cut out all seventeen pieces. Use all the parts to completely cover the white square at right. Then remove the small green and yellow square and reassemble the remaining pieces on the white square. You'll find that you can cover the area again with virtually the same pattern!

Why doesn't the extra square make a difference?

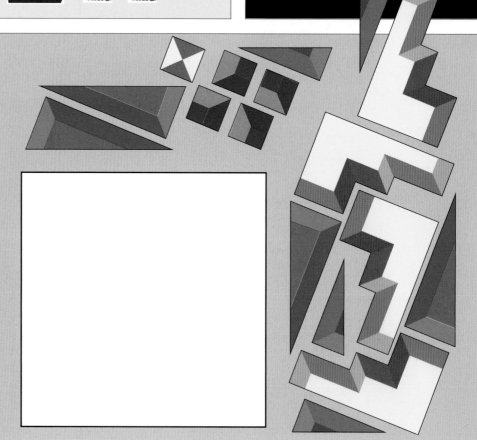

PLAYTHINK 505

DIFFICULTY: ●●●●●●○○○○
REQUIRED: ◉ ✎ 📄 ✂
COMPLETION: ☐ TIME: _____

PENTOMINO PUZZLES 1–6

Using the set of color pentominoes you can find with PlayThink 508, can you find all twelve pentominoes in each eight-by-eight grid? (The squares that are not covered are shown in black.) Note that reflections of the pieces are allowed. Once you've found all the positions, draw an outline around each pentomino.

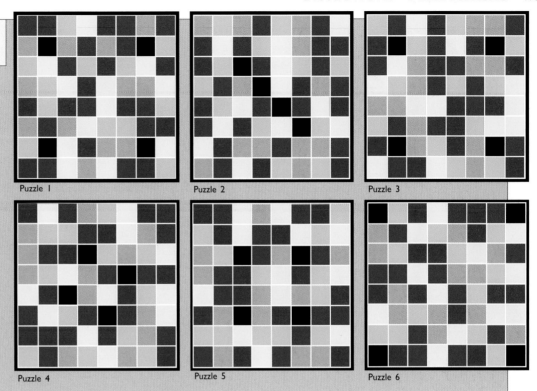

Puzzle 1 Puzzle 2 Puzzle 3

Puzzle 4 Puzzle 5 Puzzle 6

PLAYTHINK 506

DIFFICULTY: ●●●●●●●○○○
REQUIRED: ◉ ✎ 📄 ✂
COMPLETION: ☐ TIME: _____

T-TILES

A T-tile is a symmetrical shape composed of unit squares joined side by side. The smallest has four squares—one joined to three of the sides of a central square. Larger ones are built up in three directions from that junction: by adding a square to each end of the crossbar or by adding a square to the perpendicular arm.

The first twelve nonidentical T-tiles are shown. Can you fit them all onto a fifteen-by-fifteen grid without overlap? A sample attempt that failed to fit the thirteen-square tile is shown here.

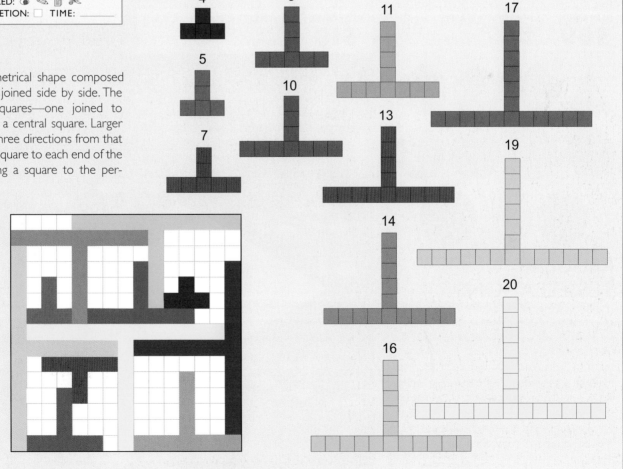

PLAYTHINK
507
DIFFICULTY: ●●●○○○○○○○
REQUIRED: ◉ ✎
COMPLETION: ☐ TIME: _____

REPLI-POLYGON

Can you work out how many of the smaller four-square T-tiles it takes to completely fill its larger replica? How would they fit?

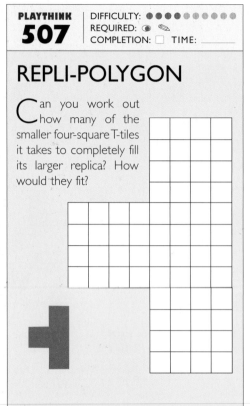

PLAYTHINK
508
DIFFICULTY: ●●●●●●○○○○
REQUIRED: ◉ ✎ ▤ ✂
COMPLETION: ☐ TIME: _____

PENTOMINO COLOR GAME

Adding a color pattern to the classic pentomino shapes opens up new puzzle and game possibilities, such as a color game played by two people. The colored pentominoes are placed in turn on a chessboard that has the four middle squares blocked off. Each pentomino played must be placed so that at least one side touches a side of a square of a matching color. The last player able to place a piece according to the rules wins the game. A variation could have players placing pieces in such a way that adjacent pieces create a pentomino of a solid color.

As an exercise, can you place all twelve pentominoes on the board?

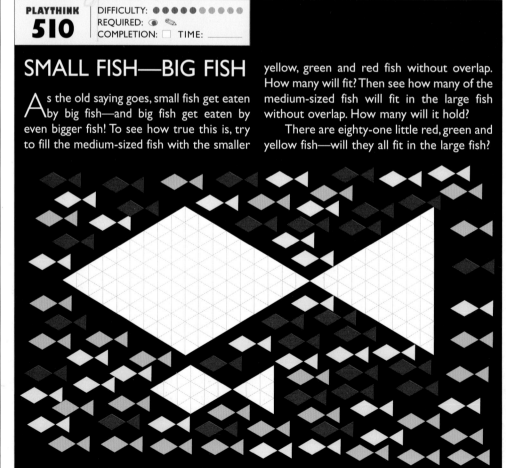

PLAYTHINK
509
DIFFICULTY: ●●●●●●○○○○
REQUIRED: ◉
COMPLETION: ☐ TIME: _____

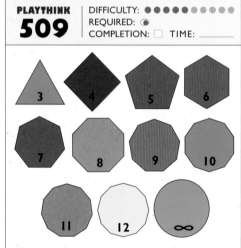

REGULAR TESSELLATIONS

A regular tessellation is a mosaic made up of identical regular polygons that completely fill a plane. There is an infinite number of regular polygons—from the equilateral triangle and the square up to the circle, which may be considered a regular polygon with an infinite number of sides. Can you work out how many of those regular polygons are capable of tessellating a plane?

PLAYTHINK
510
DIFFICULTY: ●●●●●●●○○○
REQUIRED: ◉ ✎
COMPLETION: ☐ TIME: _____

SMALL FISH—BIG FISH

As the old saying goes, small fish get eaten by big fish—and big fish get eaten by even bigger fish! To see how true this is, try to fill the medium-sized fish with the smaller yellow, green and red fish without overlap. How many will fit? Then see how many of the medium-sized fish will fit in the large fish without overlap. How many will it hold?

There are eighty-one little red, green and yellow fish—will they all fit in the large fish?

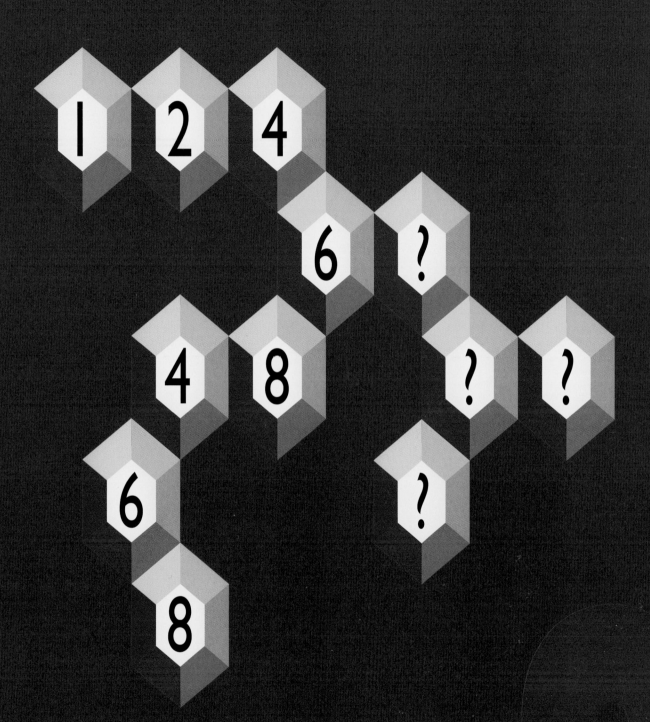

Numbers

Numbers and Sequences

Throughout history people have held that numbers, especially certain numbers, possess special powers. Some mystics used the numbers they found in names and words to weave ingenious patterns to explain everything. Others believed numbers helped them conjure spirits, perform witchcraft and predict the end of the world. Even today some people believe that certain telephone numbers are lucky or that the combination 666 is a symbol of great evil.

Numbers revealed the patterns of the universe to the ancients. And they still do: the British astronomer Martin Rees titled his masterful book describing the quest for a final theory of physics *Six Numbers*.

Nature is mathematics. Look at spirals and the golden ratio, at fractals and the periodic table of elements.

Nature can almost always be described with a simple formula—not because man has invented mathematics to do so but because of some hidden mathematical aspect of nature itself.

Numbers are also symbols—a quick way of writing or talking about objects. Instead of showing a handful of fingers and saying, "I want this many," early humans found it easier to say, "I want five"—especially when they wanted to indicate more things than could be counted on fingers and toes.

Furthermore, like the objects they can be imagined to represent, numbers can also form patterns. Indeed, though numbers are often considered individual entries, they can be presented as a sequence, enabling us to observe the tendencies of a pattern as a whole. Over the centuries number sequences have

helped mathematicians and scientists to interpret patterns found in nature, like the famous Fibonacci sequence (see PlayThink 551), a purely mathematical creation that was later found to match the growth of many natural forms.

Similarly, though mathematics was originally thought of as the study of numbers, it is now defined as the science of patterns, whether they are made with numbers, colors, shapes or anything else. The simplest kind of a pattern, a sequence, is just a list of numbers following a certain order; a more advanced pattern, called a series, is the sum of the numbers in a sequence. Recognizing the pattern behind a sequence or a series enables you to predict every other member in the group. But to see the pattern, you must first understand how things are organized.

PLAYTHINK 511

DIFFICULTY: ●●●●●○○○○○
REQUIRED: ◉ ✏
COMPLETION: ☐ TIME: _____

TETRAKTYS

Number the ten objects that make up the tetraktys from 0 to 9, as shown. Can you find how many different ways those objects can be arranged, not counting reflections and rotations?

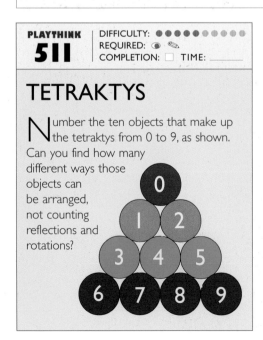

PLAYTHINK 512

DIFFICULTY: ●●●●●●○○○○
REQUIRED: ◉ ✏
COMPLETION: ☐ TIME: _____

TRIANGULAR NUMBERS

Triangular numbers can be found by stacking a group of objects in equilateral fashion—two objects are placed under one, three objects are placed under the two that are under the one and so on.

The fourth triangular number—10—was called the tetraktys by Pythagoras and his followers. They considered it sacred and revered it.

What is so special about the triangular pattern? Can you work out how many objects there are in the eighteenth triangular number?

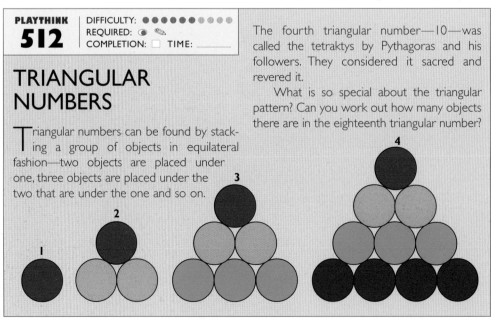

PLAYTHINK 513

DIFFICULTY: ●●●●●●○○○○
REQUIRED: ◉ ✎
COMPLETION: ☐ TIME: _____

NINES

Can you find a way to express the number 100 using six 9s?

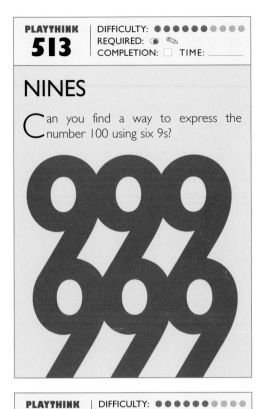

PLAYTHINK 514

DIFFICULTY: ●●●●●●●○○○
REQUIRED: ◉ ✎
COMPLETION: ☐ TIME: _____

HEX NUMBERS

The first four hexagonal numbers are illustrated here. The series runs 1, 7, 19 and 37. By examining the differences between successive hexagonal numbers, can you work out what the next hexagonal number must be?

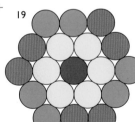
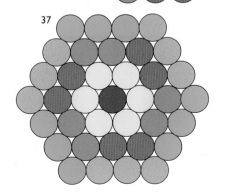

PLAYTHINK 515

DIFFICULTY: ●●●●○○○○○○
REQUIRED: ◉ ✎
COMPLETION: ☐ TIME: _____

SQUARE NUMBERS

A number that is multiplied by itself is called a square. The first six square numbers are illustrated below in figurate form. Can you continue the sequence by examining the difference in value between successive squares? What is the seventh square?

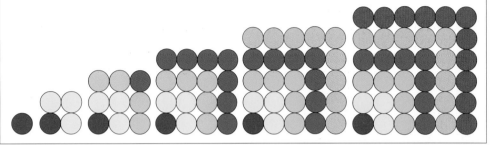

PLAYTHINK 516

DIFFICULTY: ●●●●○○○○○○
REQUIRED: ◉ ✎
COMPLETION: ☐ TIME: _____

TRIANGULAR-SQUARE NUMBERS

The seventh square number, 49, is illustrated by the circles at the right of the diagram. If each square number is the sum of two successive triangular numbers, can you work out what two triangular numbers make up 49?

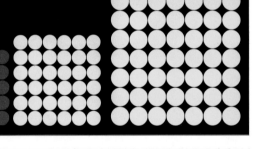

PLAYTHINK 517

DIFFICULTY: ●●●●●●○○○○
REQUIRED: ◉ ✎
COMPLETION: ☐ TIME: _____

TRIANGULAR NUMBERS— ODD SQUARES

The study of figurate numbers belongs to a branch of number theory called Diophantine analysis, a field that specializes in finding integral solutions of equations. The following puzzle is derived from that field of study.

The eleventh square number can be depicted as 121 objects in an eleven-by-eleven array. Diophantine analysis has shown that every odd square number is equal to eight times a triangular number, plus one. Can you work out the triangular number that plugs into that equation to make 121?

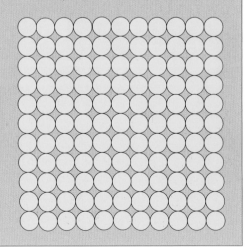

PLAYTHINK **518** | DIFFICULTY: ●●●●●●●○○○
REQUIRED: ◉ ✎
COMPLETION: ☐ TIME: _____

THREE-DIMENSIONAL FIGURATE NUMBERS

There are three-dimensional analogues to the plane figurate numbers. Such numbers can be found by packing spheres in three-dimensional pyramids: three-sided pyramids give tetrahedral numbers; four-sided pyramids give square pyramidal numbers.

The first three tetrahedral numbers are 1, 4, 10.

The first three square pyramidal numbers are 1, 5, 14.

Examine the differences in both series. Can you continue them both?

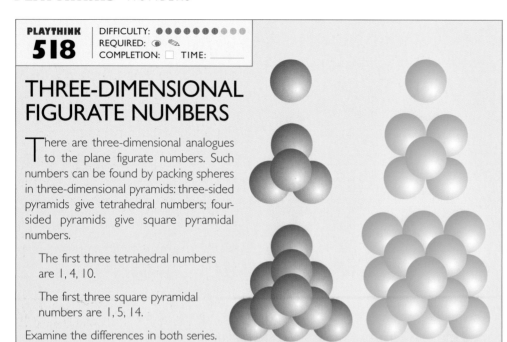

TETRAHEDRAL NUMBERS

SQUARE PYRAMIDAL NUMBERS

PLAYTHINK **519** | DIFFICULTY: ●●●○○○○○○○
REQUIRED: ◉
COMPLETION: ☐ TIME: _____

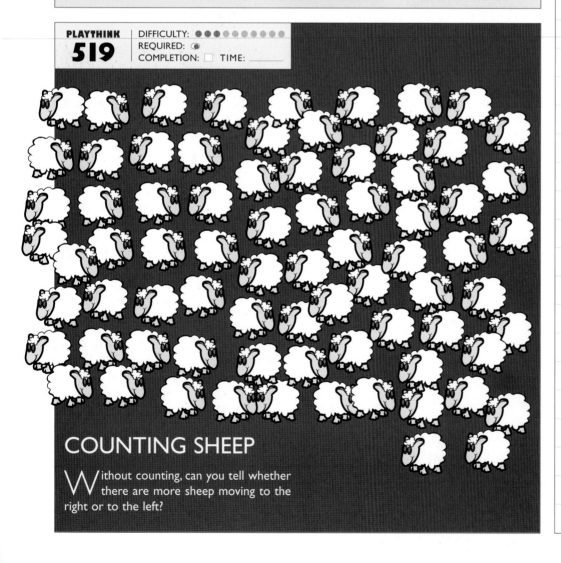

COUNTING SHEEP

Without counting, can you tell whether there are more sheep moving to the right or to the left?

PLAYTHINK **520** | DIFFICULTY: ●●●●●○○○○○
REQUIRED: ◉ ✎
COMPLETION: ☐ TIME: _____

FORTY TOTAL

Consider the numbers from 1 to 40, inclusive. Imagine trying to express each of those numbers as a combination of other numbers that are added or subtracted together—for example, 3 can be 1 + 2 or it can be 4 − 1.

Can you find four numbers that, either singly or combined with some or all of the other three numbers, can express every number from 1 to 40? In each combination, however, any given number can appear only once—for example, 5 + 5 is not allowed. To check your answer, fill in the table below with the various combinations.

=	1			=	21
=	2			=	22
=	3			=	23
=	4			=	24
=	5			=	25
=	6			=	26
=	7			=	27
=	8			=	28
=	9			=	29
=	10			=	30
=	11			=	31
=	12			=	32
=	13			=	33
=	14			=	34
=	15			=	35
=	16			=	36
=	17			=	37
=	18			=	38
=	19			=	39
=	20			=	40

PLAYTHINK 521

DIFFICULTY: ●●●●●●●○○○
REQUIRED: ◉
COMPLETION: ☐ TIME: _____

COUNTING GAUSS

When Carl Friedrich Gauss was six years old (back in 1783), his schoolteacher asked the students to add up all the numbers from 1 to 100.

Unfortunately for the teacher, who was hoping to keep the class occupied, it took young Gauss only a few seconds to work out the answer. He had spotted a pattern in the sequence and could provide the answer via a simple operation that he performed in his head. Of course, with a mind like that, it didn't take very long for Gauss to become one of Germany's most celebrated mathematicians and scientists.

Can you figure out what Gauss did to come up with the answer?

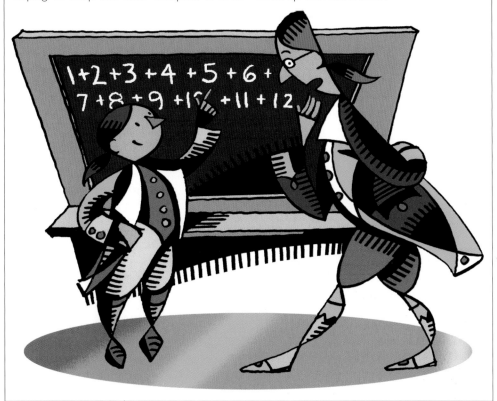

PLAYTHINK 522

DIFFICULTY: ●●●●●○○○○○
REQUIRED: ◉ ✎
COMPLETION: ☐ TIME: _____

SUM FIFTEEN

In this game each player selects a color (red or green) and then takes turns coloring one number at a time with it. The player who is first to color in three numbers that add up to exactly 15 wins.

Can you work out the best strategy for this game?

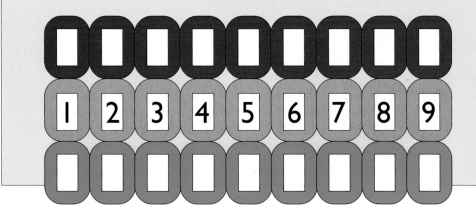

PLAYTHINK 523

DIFFICULTY: ●●●●○○○○○○
REQUIRED: ◉ ✎
COMPLETION: ☐ TIME: _____

LAGRANGE'S THEOREM

A famous theory of numbers states that every whole number can be expressed as the sum of, at most, four squares. This can be demonstrated graphically: Examine these two rectangles, one with 12 square units and one with 15 square units. Can you show how those rectangles are each composed of four smaller squares?

12

15

PLAYTHINK 524

DIFFICULTY: ●●●●●○○○○○
REQUIRED: ◉ ✎
COMPLETION: ☐ TIME: _____

IRRATIONAL

The ancient Greeks believed that any length or area could be expressed as the fraction of two whole numbers. Even a number as unusual as 1.000390625 could be written simply as the fraction 2,561/2,560. Such fractions are called rational numbers.

Pythagoras and his followers were preoccupied with right triangles, and their deep study led them to attempt to measure the hypotenuse of the simplest right triangle of them all: one in which both legs are of equal length. That research, however, resulted in an unexpected and disturbing answer.

Can you determine the length of a right triangle in which both legs are 1 unit long? Was it possible for the Pythagoreans to measure this length exactly?

?

1

1

PLAYTHINK 525 | DIFFICULTY: ●●●○○○○○○○
REQUIRED: ◉
COMPLETION: ☐ TIME: _____

HORSE COUNT

Each horse has a numerical value from 1 to 5, and most of the pairs of horses are connected by a line accompanied by an arithmetic operator: +, –, ×, or ÷.

Can you connect the horses in such a way that the mathematical operation of its path provides the maximum total? One possibility, 2 × 3 + 5 ÷ 1 – 4, gives a total of 7, which is not the maximum.

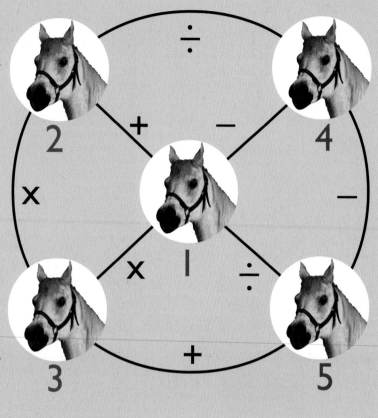

PLAYTHINK 528 | DIFFICULTY: ●●●●●●○○○○
REQUIRED: ◉
COMPLETION: ☐ TIME: _____

PERFECT NUMBERS

A perfect number is the sum of all the factors that divide evenly into it—including 1 but excluding the number itself. The first perfect number is 6, which is divisible by 3, 2 and 1 and is the sum of 1, 2 and 3.

So far, thirty-eight perfect numbers have been found. Can you work out what the second perfect number is?

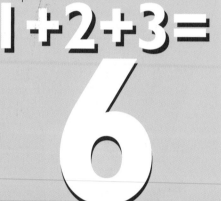

$$1 + 2 + 3 = 6$$

PLAYTHINK 529 | DIFFICULTY: ●●●●●○○○○○
REQUIRED: ◉ ✏
COMPLETION: ☐ TIME: _____

STACKING ORDER

You are asked to stack these eight blocks according to four simple rules:

1. Just one block must lie between the two red blocks.

2. Two blocks must lie between the pair of blue blocks.

3. Three blocks must separate the pair of green blocks.

4. Four blocks must separate the pair of yellow blocks.

Can you figure out how to do it?

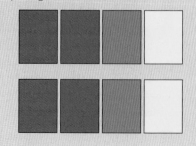

PLAYTHINK 526 | DIFFICULTY: ●●●●○○○○○○
REQUIRED: ◉ ✏
COMPLETION: ☐ TIME: _____

ODD SUM

Can you find five odd numbers that add up to 100?

What about six odd numbers that add up to 100?

	?		?
	?	+	?
+	?	+	?
+	?	+	?
+	?	+	?
+	?	+	?
100		**100**	

PLAYTHINK 527 | DIFFICULTY: ●●●●○○○○○○
REQUIRED: ◉
COMPLETION: ☐ TIME: _____

APPLE PICKERS

If five apple pickers can pick five apples in five seconds, how many apple pickers would it take to pick sixty apples a minute?

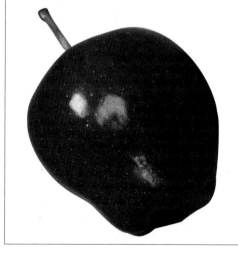

PLAYTHINK
530

DIFFICULTY: ●●●●●●●○○○
REQUIRED: ◉ 📄 ✂
COMPLETION: ☐ TIME: _____

NUMBER STRIP

■ *A Two-Player Memory Game*

Here's a simple game to test your memory for numbers.

Distribute the thirteen tiles face down in random order on the upper part of the game board. The game begins with the search for the number 1 and continues consecutively. Players choose to be red or green, and then take turns picking up one tile at a time. If the number on the tile matches the number being searched for (that is, 1 followed by 2, followed by 3, etc.), the tile is turned over and placed on the corresponding circle on that player's side of the strip. (In other words, place the tile on the small red circle if you're the red player or on the small green circle if you're the green player.) If the selected tile is not a match, then the tile is placed face down at the first blank space on the bottom row, starting at the right.

Each time a player makes a match, he or she gets to take another turn, picking tiles from either the top or bottom row—always searching for the next consecutive number. The player who matches the most numbers wins.

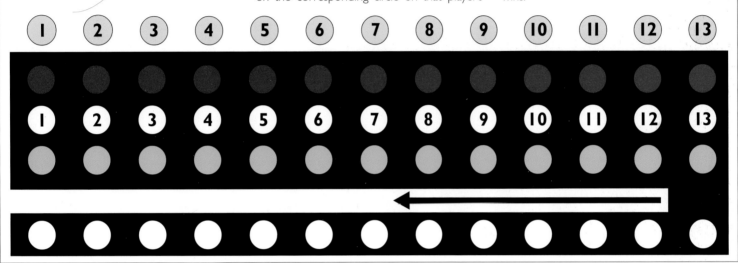

PLAYTHINK
531

DIFFICULTY: ●●●●●●○○○○
REQUIRED: ◉ ✏
COMPLETION: ☐ TIME: _____

PAIRING FIELDS GAME

The numbers from 1 to 8 must be distributed on the grid. Each number can appear only once in each column and row, and numbers can be entered only in the yellow and green cells. (The red cells must remain blank.) One additional rule: Each specific pair of numbers can appear only once on the grid; because the 1-8 pair was used in the top left-hand corner, neither the 1-8 pair nor the 8-1 pair can be used again.

The top row and left-hand column have been filled in for you. Can you complete the grid?

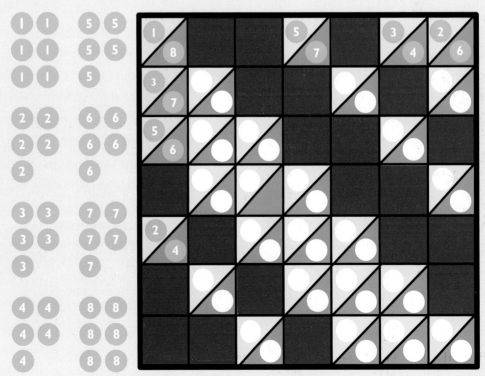

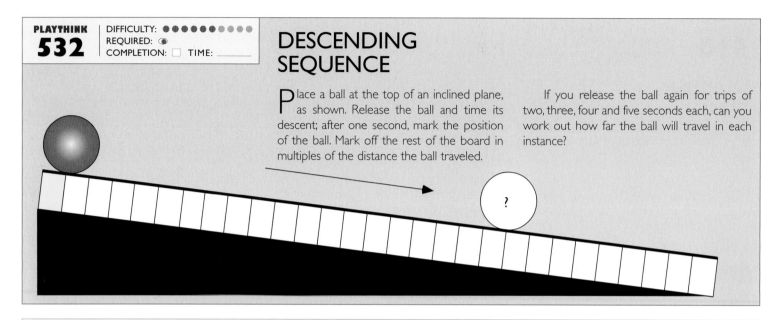

DESCENDING SEQUENCE

Place a ball at the top of an inclined plane, as shown. Release the ball and time its descent; after one second, mark the position of the ball. Mark off the rest of the board in multiples of the distance the ball traveled.

If you release the ball again for trips of two, three, four and five seconds each, can you work out how far the ball will travel in each instance?

Perfect Numbers

The Pythagoreans were obsessed with holding numbers to moral standards; to them a perfect number was the sum of all the smaller numbers that divided into it exactly, including 1 but excluding the number itself. The first perfect number was easy to find: the factors of 6 (excluding 6 itself) are 1, 2 and 3, which add up to 6.

Very few numbers have that characteristic. The factors for the number 12, for example, are 1, 2, 3, 4, 6 and 12. The sum of those numbers, excluding 12, is 16, so 12 is not a perfect number. In fact, the ancient Greeks discovered only the first four of those rare numbers: 6, 28, 496 and 8,128.

Over a millennium passed before the fifth perfect number—33,550,336—was discovered in 1460. Euler found another perfect number, one with nineteen digits, in 1782. The irony is that we know a great many perfect numbers today because of a formula discovered by Euclid.

In his book *Elements,* Euclid proved that if $2^n - 1$ is a prime number, then $2^{n-1}(2^n - 1)$ is a perfect number. Euclid's formula gives only even perfect numbers, and it is uncertain that any odd perfect numbers exist. Thus far none have been found up to 10^{200}.

Other curious properties of perfect numbers abound. All perfect numbers, for instance, are triangular. And the end digits of perfect numbers present a tantalizing mystery because every known perfect number ends in either 6 or 28, preceded by an odd number. The series of terminal digits for the twenty-three known perfect numbers is 6–8–6–8–6–6–8–8–6– 6–8–8–6–8–8–8–6–6–6–8–6–6–6.

The sequence contains infuriating hints of order. For example, if we partition the series into triplets, starting at the left, no triplet contains three of a kind. Are the digits trying to tell us something, or is this simply a coincidence waiting to be debunked?

Numbers whose divisors add up to less than themselves are called deficient; those numbers whose divisors add up to more than themselves are called abundant. The smallest abundant number is 12.

Numerologists have attributed special significance to perfect numbers; students of the Bible have noted that the first two perfect numbers are embedded in the structure of the universe. After all, God created the universe in six days, and the moon circles the earth every twenty-eight days.

PLAYTHINK 533

DIFFICULTY: ●●●●●●○○○○
REQUIRED: 👁 ✏️
COMPLETION: ☐ TIME: _____

DIFFERENCE TRIANGLES

Numbers must be inserted into the triangular array following two simple rules: Each number may appear only once, and each number must be the difference of the two numbers immediately above it. For example, if a 6 and a 4 appear on one line, the number immediately below must be a 2.

The smallest triangle has been filled in with the numbers from 1 to 3. Can you fill in the successive triangles with the numbers 1 to 6, 1 to 10 and 1 to 15?

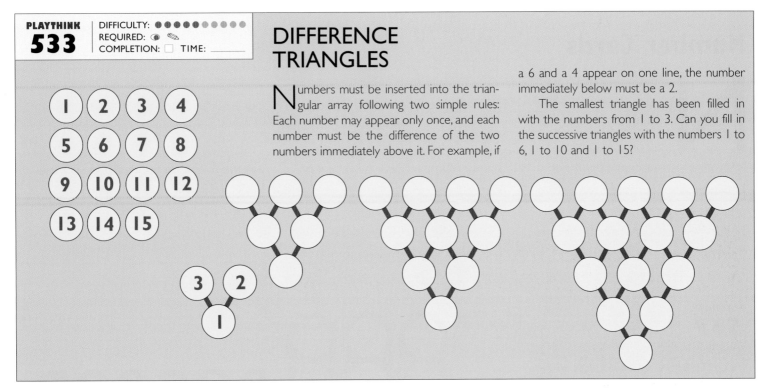

PLAYTHINK 534

DIFFICULTY: ●●●●●○○○○○
REQUIRED: 👁 ✏️
COMPLETION: ☐ TIME: _____

LADYBUG SPOTS

My daughter raises ladybugs. Her collection includes eight with red spots and one without any spots. If 55 percent of her ladybugs have yellow spots, what's the smallest possible size of her collection?

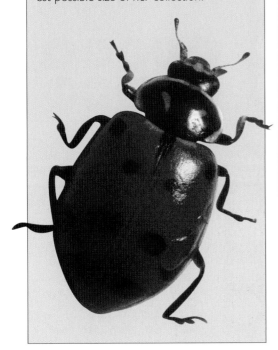

PLAYTHINK 535

DIFFICULTY: ●●●●●●○○○○
REQUIRED: 👁
COMPLETION: ☐ TIME: _____

EIGHT CARDS

Can you make the two columns of numbers add up to the same total by swapping just two cards?

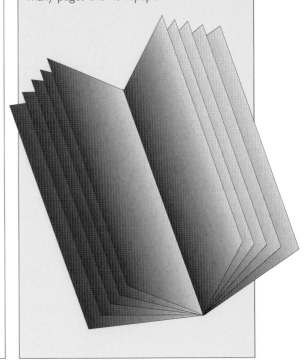

PLAYTHINK 536

DIFFICULTY: ●●●●●●●○○○
REQUIRED: 👁 ✏️
COMPLETION: ☐ TIME: _____

PAGE NUMBERS

You pull out a page from a newspaper and find that pages 8 and 21 are on the same sheet. From that, can you tell how many pages the newspaper has?

Number Cards

Number cards are a bit like families: every member is unique, yet each one has some feature that is strongly reminiscent of another. In every set of number cards, every number appears twice and no pair of numbers appears together more than once.

The simplest number card set has three cards, each with two numbers. The numbers are distributed 1-2, 1-3 and 2-3. Although each number appears only twice, every card possesses exactly one number in common with any other card. In a set of four number cards, then, each card has three numbers, so that the

numbers on one card are distributed one each to the other three.

Examine the numbers used in the four-, five- and six-card sets found in the following puzzles. Can you see why it takes forty-two numbers to make a seven-card set?

PLAYTHINK 537

DIFFICULTY: ●●○○○○○○○○○
REQUIRED: ◉ ✎
COMPLETION: ☐ TIME: _____

NUMBER CARDS 1

Can you fill in the three blanks on each of the four cards with numbers from 1 to 6 so that any given pair of cards has exactly one number in common?

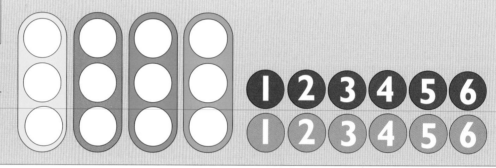

PLAYTHINK 538

DIFFICULTY: ●●●○○○○○○○○
REQUIRED: ◉ ✎
COMPLETION: ☐ TIME: _____

NUMBER CARDS 2

Can you fill in each of the four blanks on all five cards with a number from 1 to 10 in such a way that every number appears only twice and every pair of cards has exactly one number in common?

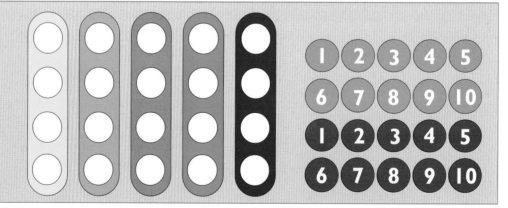

PLAYTHINK 539

DIFFICULTY: ●●●●○○○○○○○
REQUIRED: ◉ ✎
COMPLETION: ☐ TIME: _____

NUMBER CARDS 3

Can you fill in each of the spaces on the six cards with a number from 1 to 15 in such a way that each number appears only twice and every pair of cards has exactly one number in common?

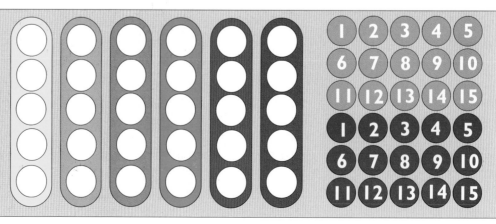

PLAYTHINK 540

DIFFICULTY: ●●●●●○○○○○
REQUIRED: 👁 ✎
COMPLETION: ☐ TIME: ___

SUM SQUARES

The first nine digits are arranged in a square, as shown below, so that the number formed on the first line can be added to the number on the second line to make the number on the third line. Can you make another square that adds up in that way?

```
    2  1  8
 +  4  3  9
 ─────────
 =  6  5  7
```

PLAYTHINK 541

DIFFICULTY: ●●●●●●●○○○
REQUIRED: 👁 ✎
COMPLETION: ☐ TIME: ___

TEN-DIGIT NUMBERS

How many different ten-digit numbers can be written with the digits 0 to 9? (Starting a number with 0 is not allowed.)

1,234,567,890

PLAYTHINK 542

DIFFICULTY: ●●●●●○○○○○
REQUIRED: 👁 ✎
COMPLETION: ☐ TIME: ___

Look closely at the number pattern. Can you discover the simple rule that created the pattern? What number should fill the space outlined in red?

FRIEZE NUMBER PATTERN

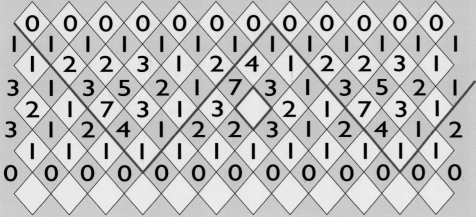

PLAYTHINK 543

DIFFICULTY: ●●●●●●●○○○
REQUIRED: 👁 ✎
COMPLETION: ☐ TIME: ___

PERSISTENCE OF NUMBERS

One property of numbers is their persistence. Take the number 723 as an illustration: if you multiply the digits 7, 2 and 3 together, the product is 42; multiply 4 and 2 together to get 8. Because this operation takes two steps to reach a single-digit number, the persistence of 723 is 2.

What is the smallest number of persistence? What are the smallest numbers that lead to persistences of 2, 3 and 4?

$$723$$
$$7 \times 2 \times 3 = 42$$
$$4 \times 2 = 8$$

PLAYTHINK 544

DIFFICULTY: ●●●●●●●●○○
REQUIRED: 👁 ✎
COMPLETION: ☐ TIME: ___

ARITHMAGIC SQUARE

Can you fill in the blanks with the numbers from 1 to 9 so that each mathematical equation is correct? (The operations read from left to right and from top to bottom.)

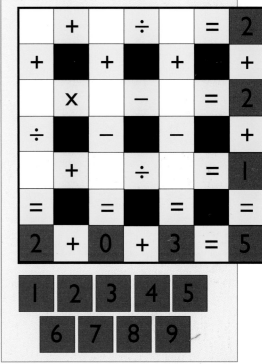

PLAYTHINK 545

DIFFICULTY: ●●●●●○○○○○
REQUIRED: 👁 ✎
COMPLETION: ☐ TIME: ___

NUMBER MATRIX

Examine the matrix. Can you fill in the missing number?

1	1	1	1
1	3	5	7
1	5	13	25
1	7	25	?

PLAYTHINK 546

DIFFICULTY: ●●●●●●○○○○
REQUIRED: 👁 ✎
COMPLETION: ☐ TIME: _____

NUMBER 4 MAGIC

This problem is more than 100 years old and has been revived in many different variations.

Can you express each number from 0 to 10 using only combinations of the number 4? You are allowed to use any of the basic mathematical operations (addition, subtraction, multiplication, division and grouping with parentheses), and you may employ as many fours as needed. But try to find the most compact expression for each number.

PLAYTHINK 548

DIFFICULTY: ●●●●●●○○○○
REQUIRED: 👁 ✎
COMPLETION: ☐ TIME: _____

TARGET PRACTICE

How many darts does it take to score exactly 100?

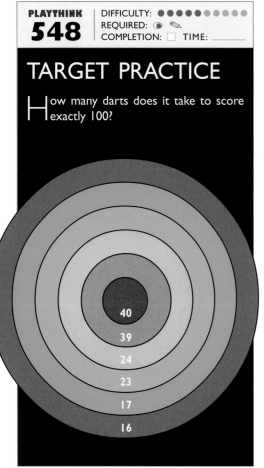

40	
39	
24	
23	
17	
16	

PLAYTHINK 547

DIFFICULTY: ●●●●●●○○○○
REQUIRED: 👁 ✎
COMPLETION: ☐ TIME: _____

SUM TWENTY

There are eleven different ways in which 20 can be written as the sum of eight odd numbers. Can you find them all?

	+		+		+		+		+		+		+		=	**20**
	+		+		+		+		+		+		=	**20**
	+		+		+		+		+		+		=	**20**
	+		+		+		+		+		+		=	**20**
	+		+		+		+		+		+		=	**20**
	+		+		+		+		+		+		=	**20**
	+		+		+		+		+		+		=	**20**
	+		+		+		+		+		+		=	**20**
	+		+		+		+		+		+		=	**20**
	+		+		+		+		+		+		=	**20**
	+		+		+		+		+		+		=	**20**

PLAYTHINK 549

DIFFICULTY: ●●●●●●○○○○
REQUIRED: 👁 ✎
COMPLETION: ☐ TIME: _____

Can you rearrange the order of the seven strips so that each row contains a correct mathematical statement? Note that the strips containing operators can be inverted if necessary.

NUMBER STRIPS

13	5	2	16	÷	+	−
10	15	3	2	+	÷	×
4	7	14	11	=	=	+
6	8	9	12	=	×	=

PLAYTHINK 550

DIFFICULTY: ●●●●●●●○○○
REQUIRED: ◉ ✎
COMPLETION: ☐ TIME: _____

SUM TOTAL

Both sums below are composed of the same number of digits from 1 to 9. Can you tell which sum is greater?

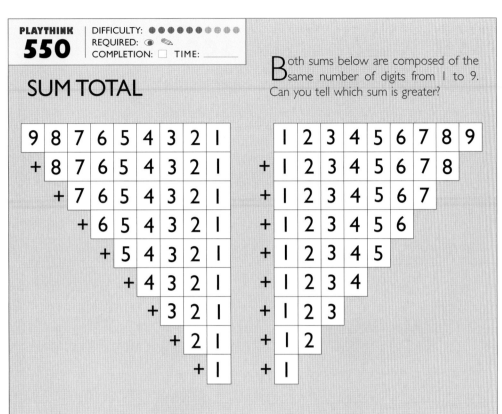

PLAYTHINK 551

DIFFICULTY: ●●●●○○○○○○
REQUIRED: ◉
COMPLETION: ☐ TIME: _____

FIBONACCI SEQUENCE

This series is the beginning of the famous Fibonacci number sequence. Discovered by the Italian mathematician Leonardo Fibonacci in the thirteenth century, the sequence appears throughout nature. The organic growth patterns in daisies, sunflowers and nautilus shells follow spirals described by the sequence.

Examine the sequence at right. Can you fill in the next number?

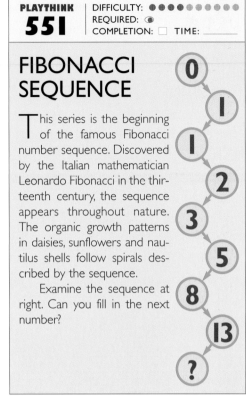

PLAYTHINK 552

DIFFICULTY: ●●●●●●○○○○
REQUIRED: ◉ ✎
COMPLETION: ☐ TIME: _____

NONCONSECUTIVE DIGITS

How many two-digit numbers possess no consecutive digits?

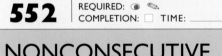

PLAYTHINK 553

DIFFICULTY: ●●●●●●●○○○
REQUIRED: ◉ ✎
COMPLETION: ☐ TIME: _____

MISSING LINKS

The numbers below are part of an equation in which all the plus or minus signs have been stripped out. What's more, two of the digits are actually part of a two-digit number. Can you work out the correct form of the equation?

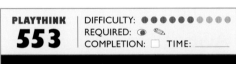

PLAYTHINK 554

DIFFICULTY: ●●●●●●●●○○
REQUIRED: ◉ ✎
COMPLETION: ☐ TIME: _____

DIVISION

What is the smallest number divisible by 1, 2, 3, 4, 5, 6, 7, 8 and 9?

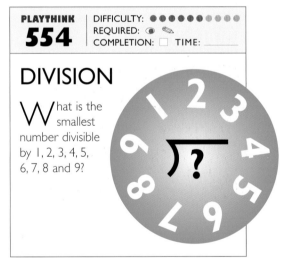

PLAYTHINK 555

DIFFICULTY: ●●●●●●●○○○
REQUIRED: ◉ ✎
COMPLETION: ☐ TIME: _____

NOB'S TRICKY SEQUENCE

Nob Yoshigahara discovered this beautiful number sequence, and there is no misprint: the last circle should contain a 7, not an 8. Can you work out the logic behind the sequence and fill in the missing number?

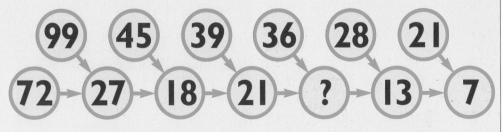

PLAYTHINK 556

DIFFICULTY: ●●●●●●●○○○
REQUIRED: ◉
COMPLETION: ☐ TIME: _____

NUMBER SEQUENCE 1

Examine the series of numbers. Can you work out the logic behind it and fill in the next number in the sequence?

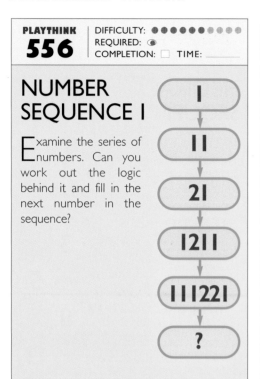

1
11
21
1211
111221
?

PLAYTHINK 557

DIFFICULTY: ●●●●●●○○○○
REQUIRED: ◉
COMPLETION: ☐ TIME: _____

NUMBER SEQUENCE 2

Can you uncover the logic behind this sequence and fill in the next number in the series?

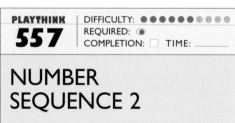

2 → 4 → 7 → 11 → 16 → ?

PLAYTHINK 558

DIFFICULTY: ●●●●●●○○○○
REQUIRED: ◉
COMPLETION: ☐ TIME: _____

PERSISTENCE SEQUENCE

Examine the sequence. Can you discover the underlying logic and fill in the final number?

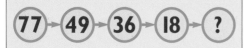

77 → 49 → 36 → 18 → ?

PLAYTHINK 559

DIFFICULTY: ●●●●●●●○○○
REQUIRED: ◉ ✎
COMPLETION: ☐ TIME: _____

BIRTHDAY CANDLES

On every birthday since I was born, I have had a cake decorated with the appropriate number of candles. I have blown out 210 candles so far. How old am I?

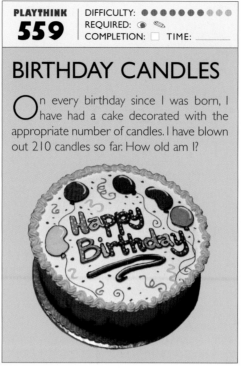

PLAYTHINK 561

DIFFICULTY: ●●●●●●○○○○
REQUIRED: ◉ ✎
COMPLETION: ☐ TIME: _____

AGE DIFFERENCE

I have a friend who became a professional magician more than 45 years ago, shortly after the birth of his son. He told me recently that his age and the age of his son are numerically reversed. If he is 27 years older than his son, how old are they?

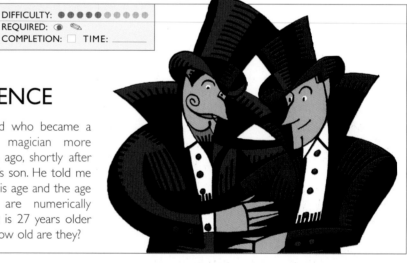

PLAYTHINK 562

DIFFICULTY: ●●●●●●●○○○
REQUIRED: ◉
COMPLETION: ☐ TIME: _____

TIME WISE

A very clever digital clock had a programming error and displayed the pattern shown below when the actual time was 9:50. Can you move the minus sign to a position where it can help display the correct time?

- 1 0 1 0 1 0

PLAYTHINK 560

DIFFICULTY: ●●●●●●●○○○
REQUIRED: ◉
COMPLETION: ☐ TIME: _____

HONEYCOMB COUNT

What are the four missing numbers in the honeycomb?

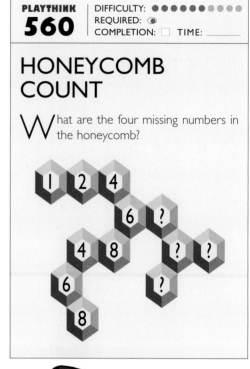

1 2 4
6 ?
4 8 ? ?
6 ?
8

PLAYTHINK 563

DIFFICULTY: ●●●●●●●●○○
REQUIRED: ◉ ✎
COMPLETION: ☐ TIME: _____

MISSING NUMBERS

The nine empty boxes must be filled with the digits from 1 to 9. Can you work out the way to place the numbers so that the mathematical operations are correct?

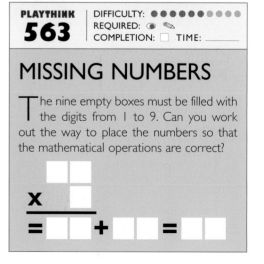

PLAYTHINK 564

DIFFICULTY: ●●●○○○○○○○
REQUIRED: 👁 ✏
COMPLETION: ☐ TIME: _____

ADD A NUMBER

Can you work out what number can be added to both 170 and 30 so that the resultant sums have a ratio of 3:1?

$$\frac{170}{+X} \quad \frac{30}{+X}$$

$$\frac{Y}{Z} \quad \frac{Y}{Z} = \frac{3}{1} \quad X = ?$$

PLAYTHINK 565

DIFFICULTY: ●●●●●●○○○○
REQUIRED: 👁
COMPLETION: ☐ TIME: _____

RIGHT EQUATION

Can you move one digit to a new position so that the equation below is correct? (Moving signs is not allowed.)

62−63 = 1

PLAYTHINK 566

DIFFICULTY: ●●●○○○○○○○
REQUIRED: 👁 ✏
COMPLETION: ☐ TIME: _____

JIGSAW

A jigsaw puzzle has 100 pieces. A move involves joining two clusters of pieces, or joining one piece to a cluster. Work out the fewest moves needed to complete the puzzle.

PLAYTHINK 567

DIFFICULTY: ●●●●●●●●○○
REQUIRED: 👁 ✏
COMPLETION: ☐ TIME: _____

MONASTERY PROBLEM

Place digits from 0 to 9 in the outer squares of the grid. Every red square must contain the same number; every yellow square should contain the same number; the sum of the numbers on each side should equal nine. How many different solutions can you find, not counting the one shown?

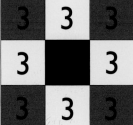

PLAYTHINK 568

DIFFICULTY: ●●●○○○○○○○
REQUIRED: 👁
COMPLETION: ☐ TIME: _____

WINE DIVISION

There are fourteen wineglasses on a table: seven are full, seven are half full. Without changing the amount of wine in any glass, can you divide the glasses into three groups so that each has the same total amount of wine?

PLAYTHINK 569

DIFFICULTY: ●●○○○○○○○○
REQUIRED: 👁 ✏
COMPLETION: ☐ TIME: _____

SOCCER ELIMINATION

Fifty-eight teams are entered in a single-elimination soccer tournament. How many matches must be scheduled?

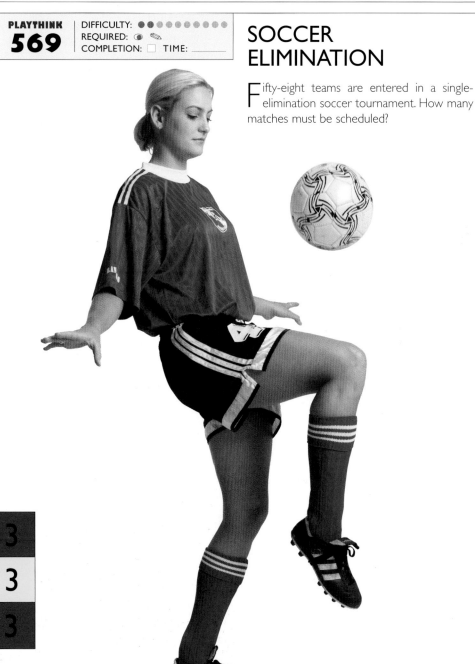

PLAYTHINK
570
DIFFICULTY: ●●○○○○○○○○○
REQUIRED: ◉
COMPLETION: ☐ TIME: _____

FLOWERS PURPLE AND RED

There are exactly forty flowers, red and purple, in a garden. And no matter which two flowers you pick, at least one will be purple. Can you work out how many red flowers there are?

PLAYTHINK
571
DIFFICULTY: ●●○○○○○○○○○
REQUIRED: ◉
COMPLETION: ☐ TIME: _____

FLOWERS PURPLE, RED AND YELLOW

There are purple, red and yellow flowers in a garden. Anytime you pick three flowers, at least one will be red and at least one will be purple. From that information, can you work out how many flowers there are?

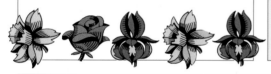

PLAYTHINK
572
DIFFICULTY: ●●●●●●○○○○○
REQUIRED: ◉ ✎
COMPLETION: ☐ TIME: _____

PRISON ESCAPE

A prison warden runs a two-story prison that has eight cells on each floor. To provide extra security, he has the cells occupied according to very specific rules:

1. There must always be twice as many prisoners on the top floor as on the ground floor.

2. No cell may be unoccupied.

3. There must always be exactly eleven prisoners in the six cells running along any given exterior wall (as marked by heavy red lines on diagrams of top and ground floors.)

One night nine prisoners escape. Yet the next morning when the warden makes his rounds, all the cells are occupied according to his rules. Can you work out how many prisoners there were to begin with and how they rearranged themselves to conceal their escape?

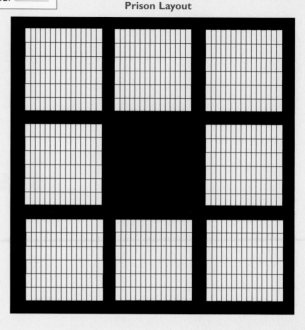

Prison Layout

Top Floor

Ground Floor

PLAYTHINK
573
DIFFICULTY: ●●○○○○○○○○○
REQUIRED: ◉ ✎
COMPLETION: ☐ TIME: _____

COUNTING ANIMALS

I went to the zoo and saw the camels and the emus. If, all told, I saw thirty-five heads and ninety-four feet, how many camels and emus did I see?

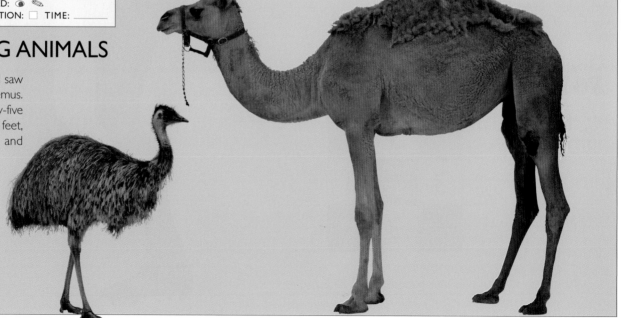

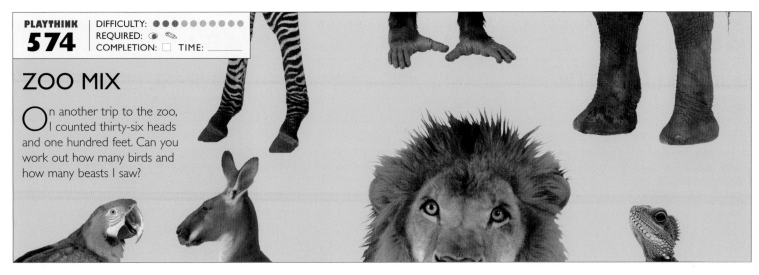

PLAYTHINK 574

DIFFICULTY: ●●●●○○○○○○○○
REQUIRED: ◉ ✎
COMPLETION: ☐ TIME: _____

ZOO MIX

On another trip to the zoo, I counted thirty-six heads and one hundred feet. Can you work out how many birds and how many beasts I saw?

PLAYTHINK 575

DIFFICULTY: ●●●●●●●●○○○○
REQUIRED: ◉ ✎
COMPLETION: ☐ TIME: _____

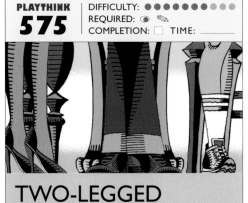

TWO-LEGGED THREE-LEGGED

In a reading room at a library, there are several three-legged stools and four-legged chairs, and they are all occupied. If you count thirty-nine legs in the room, is it possible to figure out how many stools, chairs and people there are?

PLAYTHINK 576

DIFFICULTY: ●●●●○○○○○○○○
REQUIRED: ◉ ✎
COMPLETION: ☐ TIME: _____

PUPPIES GALORE

A woman owns ten female dogs. Every one of the dogs has had a puppy, and none has had as many as ten. Does that mean that at least two of the dogs have had the same number of puppies?

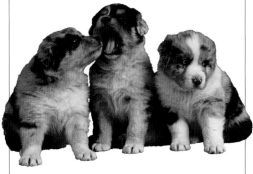

PLAYTHINK 577

DIFFICULTY: ●●●●●●●●○○○○
REQUIRED: ◉ ✎
COMPLETION: ☐ TIME: _____

THREE'S COMPANY

There are nine people in your circle of friends, and you want to invite them to dinner, three at a time, over the next twelve Saturdays. Is there a way to arrange the invitations in such a way that pairs of friends meet each other at your dinners just once?

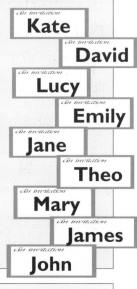

Kate
David
Lucy
Emily
Jane
Theo
Mary
James
John

PLAYTHINK 578

DIFFICULTY: ●●●●●●●○○○○○
REQUIRED: ◉ ✎
COMPLETION: ☐ TIME: _____

CAT LIVES

The following is derived from an ancient Egyptian puzzle.

A mother cat has spent seven of her nine lives. Some of her kittens have spent six, and some have spent only four.

Together, the mother and her kittens have a total of twenty-five lives left.

Can you tell with certainty how many kittens there are?

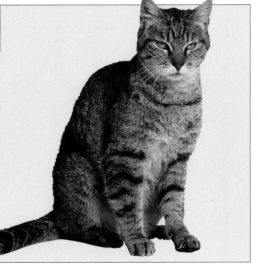

PLAYTHINK 579

DIFFICULTY: ●●●●●●●○○○○○
REQUIRED: ◉ ✎
COMPLETION: ☐ TIME: _____

NUMERATOR

Over the course of numbering every page in a book, a mechanical numerator stamped 2,929 individual digits. Can you work out how many pages the book must have?

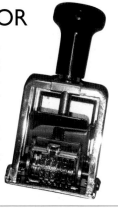

PLAYTHINK 580

DIFFICULTY: ●●●●○○○○○○
REQUIRED: ◉ ✎
COMPLETION: ☐ TIME: _____

MINIMAL LENGTH CIRCLE 1

The circumference of a circle, shown below, is divided into seven equal distances. Can you place three points on the circumference so that every number from 1 to 6 corresponds to an arc distance between two of the three placed points?

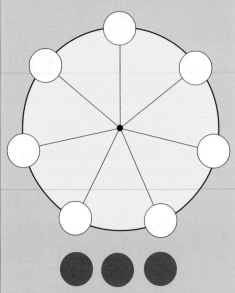

PLAYTHINK 581

DIFFICULTY: ●●●●●●○○○○
REQUIRED: ◉ ✎
COMPLETION: ☐ TIME: _____

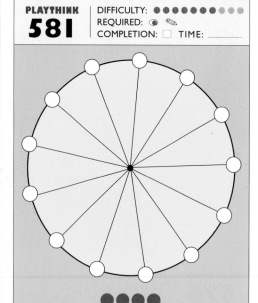

MINIMAL LENGTH CIRCLE 2

The circumference of this circle is divided into thirteen segments of equal length. Can you place four points along the circumference so that every number from 1 to 12 will correspond to an arc distance between two of the four points?

PLAYTHINK 582

DIFFICULTY: ●●●●●●●○○○
REQUIRED: ◉ ✎
COMPLETION: ☐ TIME: _____

MINIMAL LENGTH CIRCLE 3

The circumference of this circle has been divided into twenty-one segments of equal length. Can you find a way to represent every number from 1 to 20 as an arc distance between two points on the circle? Is it possible to do this while marking only five points on the circumference?

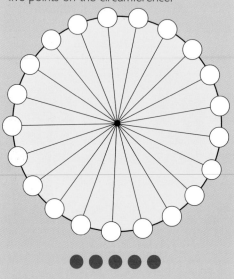

PLAYTHINK 583

DIFFICULTY: ●●●●●●○○○○
REQUIRED: ◉ ✎
COMPLETION: ☐ TIME: _____

PERSISTO

Here is a challenging paper-and-pencil number game. Two players take turns entering numbers in the cells of a square grid. The first player may enter a 1 anywhere on the grid. Subsequent numbers must be entered in the same column or row as the previously played number, with the restriction that the new number must have a clear "line of sight" with the old number. In other words, no player may "jump" a previously played number.

Whoever plays the last number scores that number of points. Play continues until one side tops 100.

A sample round with a score of 18 is shown at bottom.

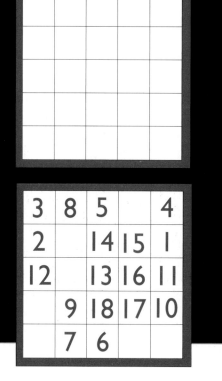

PLAYTHINK 584

DIFFICULTY: ●●●●●●●○○○
REQUIRED: ◉ ✎
COMPLETION: ☐ TIME: _____

JAILHOUSE WALK

Nine prisoners are handcuffed in groups of three for their daily exercise. If the warden wants to arrange the men so that no two individuals are chained side by side more than once over the course of a six-day period, how might he handcuff them?

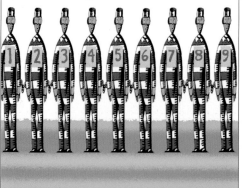

PLAYTHINK
585
DIFFICULTY: ●●●●●●●●○○
REQUIRED: ◉
COMPLETION: ☐ TIME: _____

JEKYLL AND HYDE

Sixteen coins are distributed randomly on a four-by-four game board. On one side of each coin is Jekyll; on the other, Hyde.

The object of the game is to turn over the coins until all show Jekylls or all show Hydes. The coins are flipped according to one simple rule: At each turn you must flip all the coins in a single row, column or diagonal. (A diagonal may be a short one—even the corner counts as a diagonal of just one coin.)

Two random starting configurations are shown below. Can you work out whether every starting configuration will lead to an all-Jekyll or all-Hyde outcome?

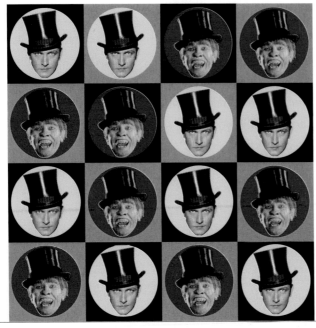

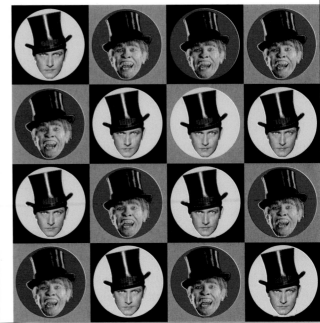

PLAYTHINK
586
DIFFICULTY: ●●●●●●●○○○
REQUIRED: ◉ ✎
COMPLETION: ☐ TIME:

MINIMAL LENGTH RULER

Four marks have been placed on the ruler at the top so that you can use it to measure every whole number of distance units from 1 to 6. Can you place five marks on the lower ruler so that you can measure the ten possible whole distances between 1 and 11 units? The two end marks have been made, so you need place only the middle three.

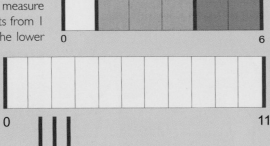

PLAYTHINK
587
DIFFICULTY: ●●●●●●●○○○
REQUIRED: ◉ ✎
COMPLETION: ☐ TIME:

LADYBUG FAMILY

One-fifth of the ladybug family flew to the garden with the yellow roses. One-third of the family flew to the violets, and three times the difference between these two numbers flew to the red poppies far away. And the mother of the ladybug family went to the river to do laundry. When all the ladybugs met up back home, how many were there?

PLAYTHINK
588
DIFFICULTY: ●●●●●●●●○○
REQUIRED: ◉ ✎
COMPLETION: ☐ TIME:

HINGED RULER 1

Five unmarked rulers have been hinged at two points, as shown. What lengths should each of the rulers have so that one or a combination of rulers can measure every distance from 1 to 15 units?

PLAYTHINK
589
DIFFICULTY: ●●●●●●●●○○
REQUIRED: ◉ ✎
COMPLETION: ☐ TIME:

HINGED RULER 2

Three unmarked rulers are hinged at one point, as shown. What three lengths should the rulers have so that, singly or in combination, they can measure every length from 1 to 8 units?

It can't be done? Try including measurements in which the rulers are folded back against one another.

The Principle of Similitude

In *Gulliver's Travels,* Jonathan Swift described Brobdingnag, a land of giants where every person was twelve times taller than normal. But could a 70-foot-tall man even support his own weight? Actually, no: such people are physical impossibilities. When scaling objects linearly, you have to keep in mind that their cross-sectional area goes up by the square of the linear factor, and the volume goes up by the cube. A person who was twelve times larger in every dimension would weigh 12^3, or 1,728 times more than a normal human. What's more, because the strength of a bone scales according to its cross-sectional area, the bones would be only 144 times as strong. Any Brobdingnagian who tried to stand would snap his leg bones.

This sort of problem faces anyone who tries to scale an object up or down. A thirty-story office building cannot be constructed in the same manner as a three-story house. A model airplane and a modern jetliner are built with different types of materials. Many would-be inventors have been disappointed through ignorance of the effects of change in scale.

Galileo, with his law of similitude, explained why large bodies suffer relatively greater deformation from the force of their own weight than do smaller objects. The stability of objects of identical shape, the law

states, decreases directly with increased height because the distorting force of gravity increases with volume while the magnitude of supporting ability, because it depends upon cross-sectional area, cannot exhibit a comparable increase. A body that increases in linear dimensions by a factor of 10 increases in volume by a factor of 1,000.

Also, surface area per unit of volume is greater for the smaller object than for the larger one; small animals are particularly vulnerable to the loss of water by evaporation due to their comparatively large surface area. The law of similitude, then, helps explain why elephants and mice not only look different but act different. And why you are unlikely ever to meet a Brobdingnagian.

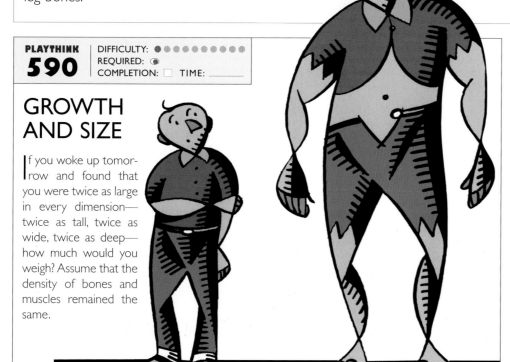

PLAYTHINK **590**	DIFFICULTY: ●●●●●●●●●●● REQUIRED: ◉ COMPLETION: ☐ TIME: _____

GROWTH AND SIZE

If you woke up tomorrow and found that you were twice as large in every dimension—twice as tall, twice as wide, twice as deep—how much would you weigh? Assume that the density of bones and muscles remained the same.

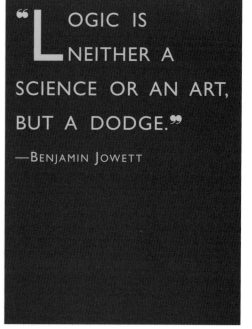

"LOGIC IS NEITHER A SCIENCE OR AN ART, BUT A DODGE."

—BENJAMIN JOWETT

PLAYTHINK 591

DIFFICULTY: ●●●●●●○○○
REQUIRED: ◉ ✎
COMPLETION: ☐ TIME: _____

PROGRESSION I

Examine this beautiful geometric progression. Can you work out the total area of the red triangles as a proportion of the area of the outer square?

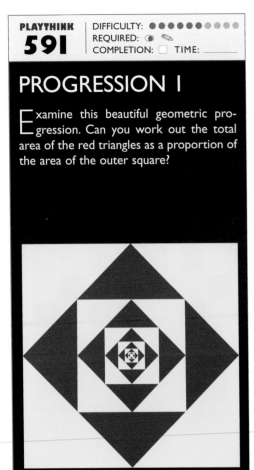

PLAYTHINK 592

DIFFICULTY: ●●●●●●●○○○
REQUIRED: ◉ ✎
COMPLETION: ☐ TIME: _____

PROGRESSION 2

What is the area of the red arm as a proportion of the entire square?

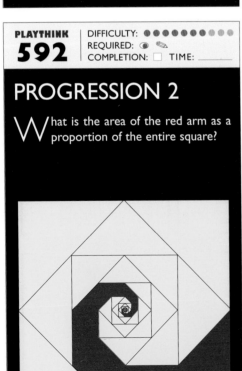

PLAYTHINK 593

DIFFICULTY: ●●●●●●●○○○
REQUIRED: ◉ ✎
COMPLETION: ☐ TIME: _____

ASCENT–DESCENT

Can you arrange the nine strips in a row so that you will be unable to find four that are either in ascending or descending order?

The strips in an ascending or descending sequence need not be next to each other. For example, 7, 5, 8, 1, 9, 4, 6, 2, 3 fails because 7, 5, 4, 2 is a descending sequence, in spite of the fact that other numbers come between them.

Can you find at least one sequence that follows the rule?

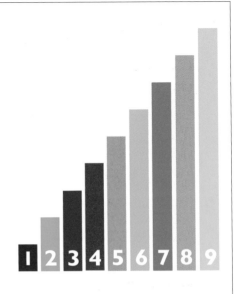

PLAYTHINK 594

DIFFICULTY: ●●●●●●●○○○
REQUIRED: ◉ ✎
COMPLETION: ☐ TIME: _____

INCREASING–DECREASING

Is it possible to arrange ten strips of differing lengths so that there is no set of four in ascending or descending order? The four strips do not have to be next to each other to count as a sequence. For example, in the sequence 1, 2, 8, 0, 3, 6, 9, 4, 5, 7, the set 1, 2, 8, 9 is an ascending sequence, even though the 8 and the 9 are not side by side.

Can you find a sequence that works?

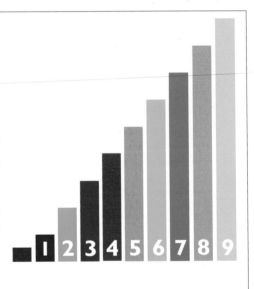

PLAYTHINK 595

DIFFICULTY: ●●○○○○○○○○
REQUIRED: ◉
COMPLETION: ☐ TIME: _____

AMOEBA SPLIT

A single amoeba in a beaker can divide into two in one minute. After another minute, each of those two amoebas split, leaving four amoebas. At the end of forty minutes, the beaker is full.

How many minutes did it take for the beaker to be half full of amoebas?

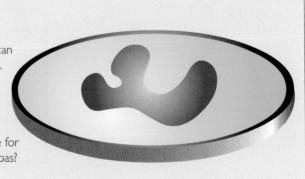

PLAYTHINK 596

DIFFICULTY: ●●●●●●○○○○
REQUIRED: ◉ ✎
COMPLETION: ☐ TIME: _____

CELLULAR AUTOMATON

The squares in grid 1 are randomly distributed between red and black. In every grid after that, the color of each square is determined by that of its neighbors in the generation before. For example, if a black square is surrounded by a majority of black squares, it will flip from black to red. A majority of red squares changes the color to black. (In case of a tie, the color remains the same.)

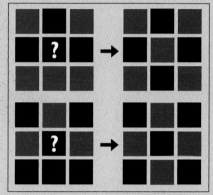

Six generations of the puzzle are shown. Can you complete the next three?

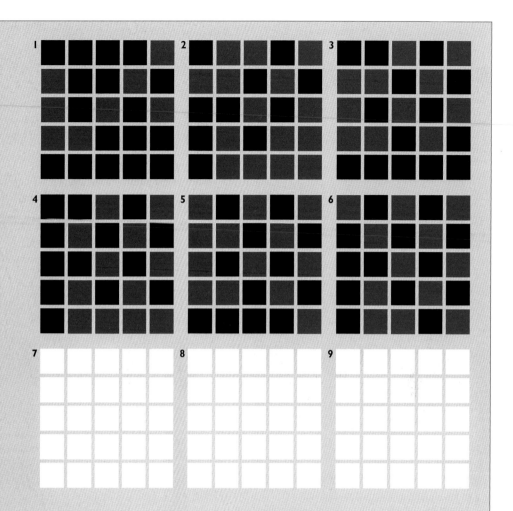

PLAYTHINK 597

DIFFICULTY: ●●●●●●○○○○
REQUIRED: ◉ ✎
COMPLETION: ☐ TIME: _____

FREDKIN'S CELLULAR AUTOMATON

■ *A Two-Dimensional Self-Generating Mechanism*

Five red cells sit in the middle of grid 1. Each successive grid holds a new generation of cells that have been added or subtracted according to a simple rule: If the number of red cells horizontally or vertically adjacent to the cell is even, then the cell is white in the next generation; if the number of adjacent red cells is odd, the cell is red in the next generation. (See the inset for a demonstration of the growth pattern.)

Can you carry out the growth pattern over five generations? If you do, you will see a surprising result.

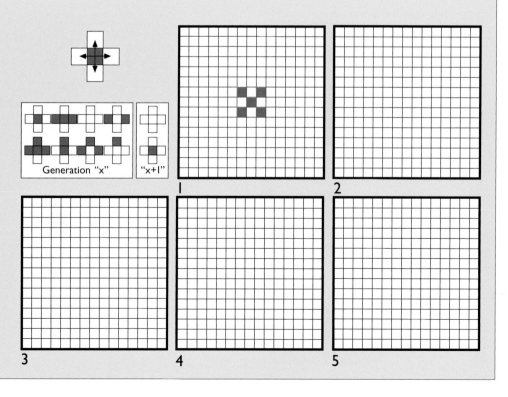

PLAYTHINK
598

DIFFICULTY: ●●●●●○○○○○
REQUIRED: 👁 ✏ 📄 ✂
COMPLETION: ☐ TIME: _____

GROWTH PATTERN TRIANGLES

Many items in nature—crystals, colonies of bacteria, even the clouds that form stars—show highly geometric patterns in their growth. This puzzle helps harness such a pattern for the purpose of art.

Begin with a single triangle in the center of a grid, as shown. Add triangles one generation at a time, following one simple rule: Each new triangle should touch one—and only one—side of a triangle from the previous generation. To make each wave of growth distinct, use the palette for the color of each generation of triangles. After fourteen generations you can recycle the colors.

How many triangles are there in each generation? Is there any regularity in the sequence of numbers?

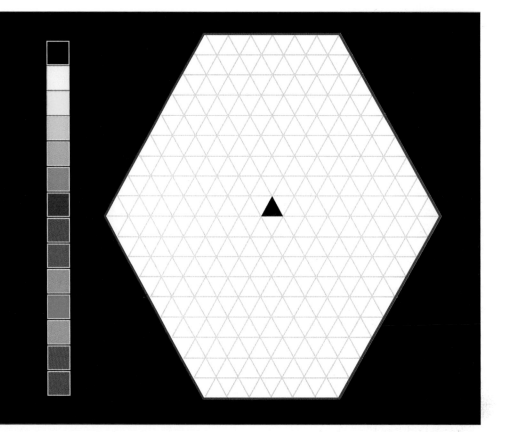

PLAYTHINK
599

DIFFICULTY: ●●●●○○○○○○
REQUIRED: 👁 ✏ 📄 ✂
COMPLETION: ☐ TIME: _____

GRADIENT PATTERN SQUARES

There is a single dark square at the center of the grid. Additional squares can be added to the grid following a simple growth rule: Squares are added one generation at a time so that each new square touches one—and only one—square from the previous generation.

To help show the patterns of growth, color each generation according to the palette at right. Can you work out how many squares will be added for each generation? Is there a pattern to the number of new squares in each generation?

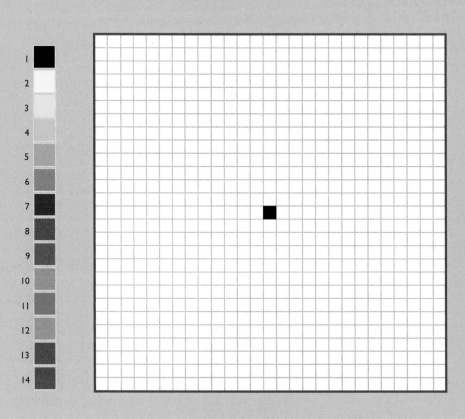

PLAYTHINK 600

DIFFICULTY: ●●●●●○○○○○
REQUIRED: ◉ ✎
COMPLETION: ☐ TIME: _____

LADYBUG WALKS

These five games build on a regular series of walks and turns. Imagine that five ladybugs follow the circuits described below. Will any of them return to their starting places?

Game 1—Starting at the yellow point, crawl a distance of 1 unit up, then turn right. Crawl 2 units, then turn right again. Crawl 3 units and so forth, up to a 5-unit crawl. After 5 units, turn right and start the sequence over again with a 1-unit crawl.

Game 2—The same as Game 1, except that the sequence builds to a 6-unit crawl before returning to 1 unit.

Game 3—As above, except that it is extended to 7 units.

Game 4—As above, except extended to 8 units.

Game 5—As above, except extended to 9 units.

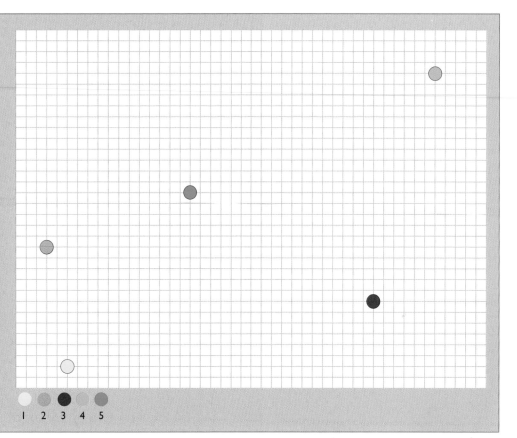

1 2 3 4 5

PLAYTHINK 601

DIFFICULTY: ●●●●●●○○○○
REQUIRED: ◉ ✎
COMPLETION: ☐ TIME: _____

GOLYGONS

■ *A Walk in a Square Matrix*

The mathematician Lee Sallows of the University of Nijmegen in The Netherlands conceived of the following problem.

Start at the yellow point on the grid. Pick a direction and "walk" one block. At the end of the block, turn left or right and walk two more blocks; turn left or right and then walk three blocks. Continue this way, walking one more block in each segment than before. If after a number of turns you return to the starting point, then the path you have traced is the boundary of a golygon.

The simplest golygon has eight sides, meaning it can be traced in eight segments. Can you find it?

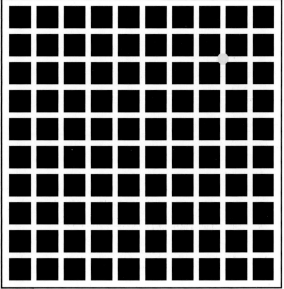

PLAYTHINK 602

DIFFICULTY: ●●●●●●●○○○
REQUIRED: ◉ ✎
COMPLETION: ☐ TIME: _____

PRIME DOUBLES

Can you always find a prime number somewhere between any number and its double (excluding 1, of course)?

4 5 6 7 8

PLAYTHINK 603

DIFFICULTY: ●●●●●●●●○○
REQUIRED: ◉ ✎
COMPLETION: ☐ TIME: _____

PRIME CHECK

There are exactly 9!, or 362,880, different nine-digit numbers in which all the digits from 1 to 9 appear. The number below is an obvious example. Of those 362,880 numbers, can you work out how many will be prime—divisible only by 1 and themselves?

123,456,789

Snowflake Curve

What kind of shape has an infinite length yet only a finite area?

It sounds impossible, but, surprisingly, such figures exist. One of them is the beautiful snowflake curve. This curve is essentially a growth pattern created as a sequence of polygons. The snowflake curve is built on the sides of an equilateral triangle according to a very simple progression principle. On the central third of each side, another equilateral triangle is added, and that progression is carried out generation after generation forever.

The snowflake curve is a good first introduction to the idea of limit and the concept of fractals. It is not possible to draw the limiting curve. We can create the polygons only for the next sequence, and the ultimate curve must be left to the imagination.

PLAYTHINK 604

DIFFICULTY: ●●●●●●●○○○
REQUIRED: 👁 ✏
COMPLETION: ☐ TIME: _____

SNOWFLAKE AND ANTI-SNOWFLAKE CURVES

The red figures at the bottom of this illustration show the first four stages of the famous snowflake pattern. As the fractal pattern continues indefinitely, can you work out the limit on the length of its perimeter and the area it will eventually enclose?

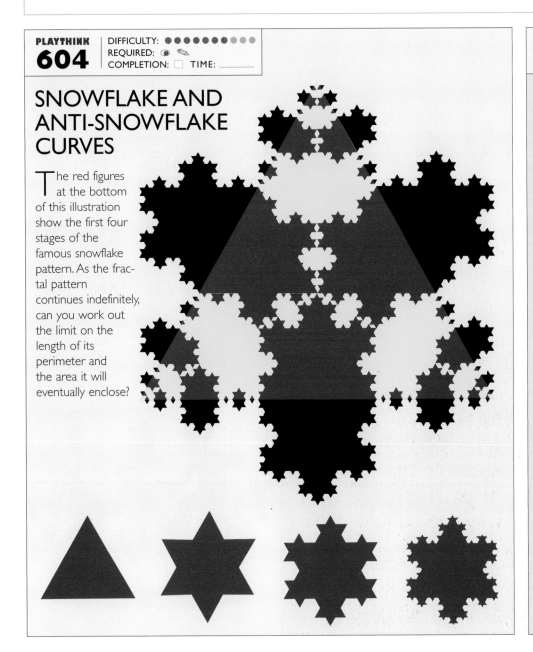

PLAYTHINK 605

DIFFICULTY: ●●●●●●●○○○
REQUIRED: 👁
COMPLETION: ☐ TIME: _____

INFINITY AND LIMIT

Each picture is half the height of the image it is set in. If this pattern continued, there would be an infinite number of pictures. Rather than setting them one inside another, imagine stacking them atop each other. How tall would the tower of pictures grow?

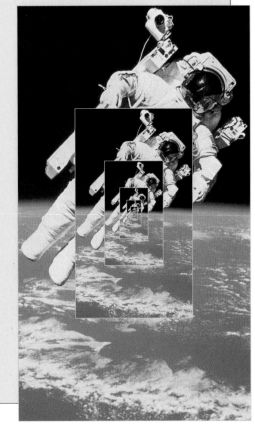

Fractal Geometry

Twentieth-century mathematicians revolted against the classical mathematics of previous centuries when they discovered that mathematical structures and curves did not fit the patterns laid down by Euclid. The new structures and curves were at first regarded as "pathological," because they seemed to upset established standards of the time. How ironic that term is, since the bizarre, abstract structures invented to break free of the Euclidean mold turned out to be present in many familiar objects.

Fractals are an example. Forests, coastlines, star clusters and atomic tracks may not seem to have much in common, but they are all linked by this extraordinary geometrical notion.

Fractals begin with the simple. Take the shortest distance between two points, a straight line. Add a few kinks and bumps, and it gets longer. The more convoluted it becomes, the longer it grows. If the line becomes irregular enough, it will become infinitely long. Then you have a fractal. A coastline is a perfect example. No matter how much you magnify the scale of a map, a coastline presents the same sort of jagged shape.

A set discovered by Polish mathematician Benoit Mandelbrot in 1977 is another example of the confluence of simplicity and complexity found in fractal geometry. His fractal set can be generated by just a few lines of computer code, but an infinite amount of information would be needed to create a full description of the shape of its outline. Fractals derived from Mandelbrot's work have been used by computer graphic artists to create imaginary landscapes that seem as natural as any found on earth.

Fractals delineate a whole new way of thinking about structure and form. They show that the world of pure mathematics contains a richness of possibilities that go far beyond the simple structures that earlier mathematicians saw in nature.

PLAYTHINK 606 | DIFFICULTY: ●●●●●●●●●○○ REQUIRED: ◉ ✎ | COMPLETION: ☐ TIME: ___

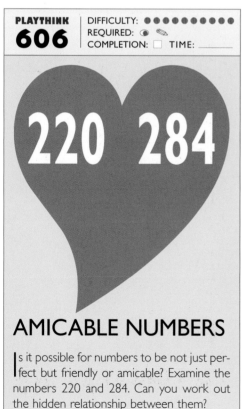

AMICABLE NUMBERS

Is it possible for numbers to be not just perfect but friendly or amicable? Examine the numbers 220 and 284. Can you work out the hidden relationship between them?

PLAYTHINK 607 | DIFFICULTY: ●●●●●○○○○○ REQUIRED: ◉ ✎ | COMPLETION: ☐ TIME: ___

FACTORING

Natural numbers can be either composite or prime. Prime numbers are like the bricks from which composite numbers are made. Indeed, any natural number can be uniquely represented as a product of prime numbers.

Can you find the prime numbers that are the factors of 420?

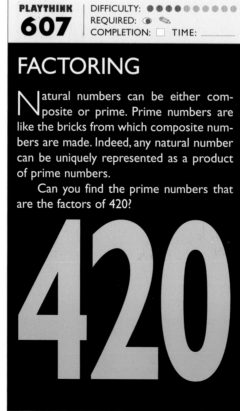

PLAYTHINK 608 | DIFFICULTY: ●●●●○○○○○○ REQUIRED: ◉ ✎ | COMPLETION: ☐ TIME: ___

CIRCLE OF DANCE

Anne and her friends are dancing in a circle. The circle is set up so that every dancer is next to two people who are both of the same gender.

How many girls are there if there are twelve boys in the circle?

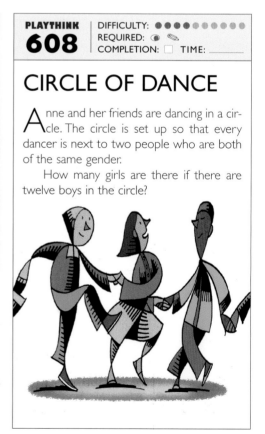

Big Numbers

What counts as a really large number? One Indian legend recounts a gift granted by King Shirhan to his vizier, who had just invented the game of chess. The vizier, thinking about the most he could ask for without being presumptuous, said, "Give me a gram of wheat to put on the first square of the chessboard, and two grams on the second square. Continue this doubling for each successive square for all sixty-four squares of the chessboard." The king agreed to the request at once, which was a big mistake. Although the first few squares could be covered easily, the power of doubling soon made the vizier's request impossible. The sequence, called a geometrical progression, runs:

$$1 + 2 + 2^2 + 2^3 + 2^4 + 2^5 + 2^6 \ldots$$
$$2^{62} + 2^{63} = 2^{64} - 1$$

The amount requested by his vizier, totaling more than 10 billion billion grams, turned out to be equal to the world's wheat production for a period of some 2,000 years. Although this is an almost unbelievably large number, it is still finite and, theoretically at least, given enough time, one could count it down to the last decimal.

Infinite numbers, on the other hand, are larger than any number you can possibly write down no matter how long you work. Many ideas related to infinite numbers are surprising and counterintuitive; for example, it is possible to compare two infinite sets and determine which set is larger.

The German mathematician Georg Cantor, known as the founder of the arithmetic of infinity, found the answer. Cantor concluded that if one can pair two objects of two infinite groups so that each object of one infinite collection pairs with each object of another infinite collection and no object in either group is left alone, the two infinities are equal. Otherwise, one infinite set is larger than the other.

Applying this rule leads to some surprising results. Compare, for example, the infinity of all even numbers to the infinity of all odd numbers. No problem here: your intuition tells you that there are as many even numbers as there are odd. But what about the infinite set of all whole numbers versus the set of just the even numbers? Surely the set of whole numbers is greater than the set of just the even numbers—after all, the even numbers are contained within the whole numbers. But when one begins to compare the two sets, one finds:

$$1\text{-}2, 2\text{-}4, 3\text{-}6, 4\text{-}8, 5\text{-}10,$$
$$6\text{-}12, 7\text{-}14, 8\text{-}16 \ldots$$

For every whole number there is an even number. The infinity of even numbers, therefore, is exactly as large as the infinity of all numbers. It is a paradox, but one of the bizarre things about dealing with infinities is that *a part may be equal to the whole.*

Not every infinity is the same. There are many more geometrical points on a line than there are integers or fractional numbers because it is impossible to establish a one-to-one correspondence between the points on a line and the integer numbers. But it also follows that the same number of points are in lines 1 inch, 1 foot, or 1 mile long. But the number of all geometrical points, though larger than the number of all integers and fractional numbers, is not the largest infinity known to mathematicians; the number of geometrical curves is greater than the collection of all geometrical points on a line.

Cantor denoted the different infinities by the Hebrew letter aleph ($\aleph$), and the complete sequence of all numbers today looks like:

$\aleph_1$ integers and fractional numbers

$\aleph_2$ points on a line

$\aleph_3$ different geometric curves

The Tower of Hanoi

The Babylon puzzle (PlayThink 609) is a variation of one of the most beautiful puzzles ever created: the Tower of Hanoi. Created by the French mathematician Edouard Lucas in 1883, the puzzle is framed within a legend. At a great temple at Benares, there is a brass plate into which three vertical pins are fixed. At the beginning of time, sixty-four golden disks were stacked on one pin in decreasing order of size, with the largest resting at the bottom of the brass plate. Day and night, so the legend goes, a priest transfers the disks from one pin to another at a constant rate, never allowing any disk to be placed on top of a smaller one. Once the tower is rebuilt on one of the other two pins, the universe will end.

Even if the legend were true, there would be no reason to worry. Allowing one second per move of a disk, the task would take about 600 billion years, or about sixty times longer than the lifetime of the sun.

The number of moves necessary to complete a Tower of Hanoi of a given number of disks can be calculated as $2^n - 1$. So two disks require three moves, three disks require seven and so on.

PLAYTHINK
609

DIFFICULTY: ●●●●●●●○○○
REQUIRED: 👁 ✎ 📄 ✂
COMPLETION: ☐ TIME: _____

BABYLON

This puzzle is a variation of the classic Tower of Hanoi. You can play it on several different levels of difficulty and with variant sets of rules.

The puzzle begins with a stack of disks in the left-hand column, as shown in the insets below. Your objective in each puzzle is to transfer the disks to the right-hand column, keeping the same numerical order.

The basic rule is, don't place a disk on another disk of smaller value. Otherwise, shuttle the disks, one at a time, among the three columns until you have the proper arrangement in the right-hand column.

Puzzles 1, 2, 3 and 4 (see first diagram below left)—Find the minimum number of moves to transfer 2, 3, 4 and 5 disks, respectively, to the right-hand column.

Puzzle 5 (second diagram below)— Find the minimum number of moves to transfer the four disks, observing an additional rule that a disk cannot be placed on another disk of the same color. That means that disk 1 cannot be placed on disk 4.

Puzzle 6 (third diagram below)— Find the minimum number of moves to transfer the four disks, observing an additional rule that a disk cannot be placed on another disk of the same color. That means that disk 1 cannot be placed on disk 3, and disk 2 cannot be placed on disk 4.

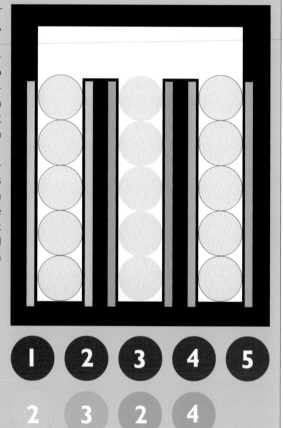

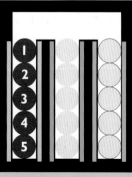

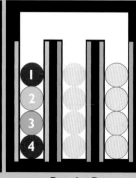

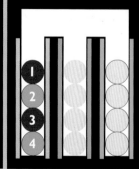

Puzzles 1 to 4   Puzzle 5   Puzzle 6

PLAYTHINK 610

DIFFICULTY: ●●●●●●●○○○
REQUIRED: ◉ ✎
COMPLETION: ☐ TIME: _____

HIGHLY COMPOSITE

Composite numbers are the product of two or more primes, but a "highly composite" number has more divisors than any number below it. For example, 12 is a highly composite number, since no number less than 12 has six distinct divisors. Twelve is composed of 1, 2, 3, 4, 6 and 12.

What is the next highly composite number? The answer, of course, has eight divisors.

$$1,2,3,4,6,12 \big) 12$$

PLAYTHINK 611

DIFFICULTY: ●●●●●○○○○○
REQUIRED: ◉ ✎
COMPLETION: ☐ TIME: _____

ADD AND MULTIPLY

What three numbers have a sum equal to their product?

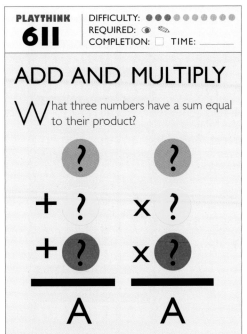

PLAYTHINK 613

DIFFICULTY: ●●●●●●●○○○
REQUIRED: ◉
COMPLETION: ☐ TIME: _____

HIDDEN MAGIC COIN

One of the most beautiful coin tricks is often explained as a feat of extrasensory perception. But it is really an example of the mathematical concept of parity.

Ask someone to toss a handful of coins on a table. After a quick peek at the result, turn your back and ask the person to turn over pairs of coins at random—as many pairs as he or she likes. Then ask the person to cover up one coin.

When you turn around, you can tell immediately whether the covered coin is showing heads or tails.

Can you work out the mathematical secret at the heart of this trick?

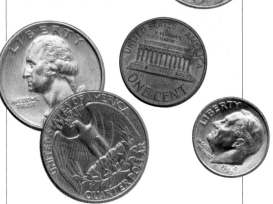

PLAYTHINK 612

DIFFICULTY: ●●●●●●●●○○
REQUIRED: ◉ ✎
COMPLETION: ☐ TIME: _____

BINARY ABACUS

Because at heart computers are simply a collection of electronic switches, the base 2—or binary—system of numbers is the language of the information age. Even though binary notation uses just 1s and 0s, it can represent any whole number.

The abacus illustrated here can represent numbers in binary form. Can you work out how you would use it to express 53? What about 63?

○ 0
● 1

2^5	2^4	2^3	2^2	2^1	1^0
32	16	8	4	2	1

Bits and Computers

For all their prowess at making calculations and controlling machinery, computers are essentially little more than a collection of switches. Each of the thousands of electronic circuits in a computer can switch on and off incredibly fast. When a pulse of electricity flows through a circuit, it is on; when no electricity flows, it is off. Circuits that are on have a value of 1; circuits that are off have a value of 0.

The digits 1 and 0 are the basis of the binary number system used in computers. Each number is called a bit, short for binary digit. Computers usually deal with strings of eight or sixteen bits at a time. (A group of eight bits is a byte.)

Four switches can be set in 2^4, or 16, different ways. Those four switches can be represented by the cells of a two-by-two square, with the "on" switches colored red and the "off" switches colored yellow. Running through all the binary possibilities will give you a set of sixteen tiles with which you can play games and puzzles.

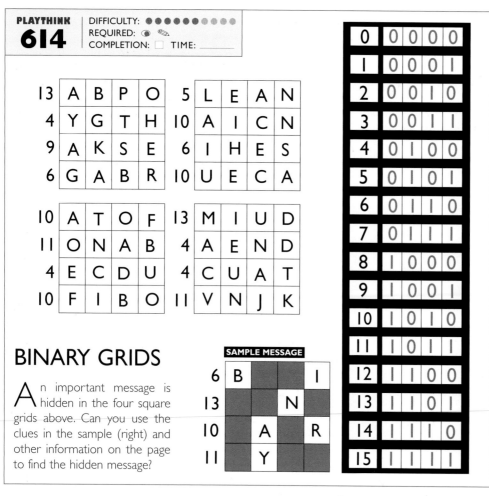

PLAYTHINK 614
DIFFICULTY: ●●●●●●○○○○
REQUIRED: ◉ ✎
COMPLETION: ☐ TIME: _____

13	A	B	P	O		5	L	E	A	N
4	Y	G	T	H		10	A	I	C	N
9	A	K	S	E		6	I	H	E	S
6	G	A	B	R		10	U	E	C	A

10	A	T	O	F		13	M	I	U	D
11	O	N	A	B		4	A	E	N	D
4	E	C	D	U		4	C	U	A	T
10	F	I	B	O		11	V	N	J	K

0	0	0	0	0
1	0	0	0	1
2	0	0	1	0
3	0	0	1	1
4	0	1	0	0
5	0	1	0	1
6	0	1	1	0
7	0	1	1	1
8	1	0	0	0
9	1	0	0	1
10	1	0	1	0
11	1	0	1	1
12	1	1	0	0
13	1	1	0	1
14	1	1	1	0
15	1	1	1	1

BINARY GRIDS

An important message is hidden in the four square grids above. Can you use the clues in the sample (right) and other information on the page to find the hidden message?

SAMPLE MESSAGE

6	B			I
13			N	
10		A		R
11		Y		

PLAYTHINK 615
DIFFICULTY: ●●○○○○○○○○
REQUIRED: ◉ ✎ 📄 ✂
COMPLETION: ☐ TIME: _____

BINARY BITS

If there is one square to color—and two possible colors to choose from—it is pretty easy to figure out how limited your possibilities are. With two squares and two colors, there are four possibilities, as shown below.

Can you work out the possibilities for a three-square strip? And how about a two-by-two square matrix?

Once you have properly colored in the two-by-two matrices, you will have the playing pieces for the Q-Bits game (PlayThink 616).

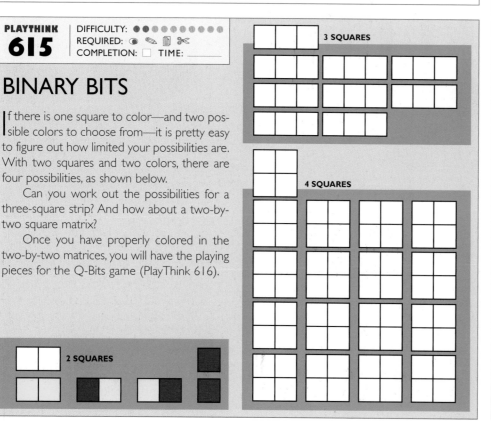

2 SQUARES

3 SQUARES

4 SQUARES

PLAYTHINK 616
DIFFICULTY: ●●●●●●●○○○
REQUIRED: ◉ ✎ 📄 ✂
COMPLETION: ☐ TIME: _____

Q-BITS

There are many different ways to arrange sixteen tiles on a four-by-four grid. But is it possible to do it in such a way that the colors of adjacent tiles will match along every edge?

That is the goal of this puzzle, which can be played as either a solitaire or competitive game.

To play as a solitaire game, cover the board with all sixteen tiles from PlayThinks 615 according to the domino principle: with all touching edges matching. How many different solutions can you find? If you copy your solutions onto grid paper, you will see that some of them have a strong aesthetic appeal.

To play as a two-person game, start by mixing the tiles face down. The players take turns selecting a tile and placing it on the board. As in the solitaire game, any tiles that touch must possess matching colors along their edges. The last player who can place a tile according to the rules wins.

The longest game is sixteen moves and will fill up the board. Can you find the shortest possible game, that is, the fewest tiles needed to block further moves?

PLAYTHINK
617
DIFFICULTY: ●●●●●●●○○○
REQUIRED: ◉ ✎
COMPLETION: ☐ TIME: _____

HEXABITS 1

If you divide a hexagon with lines drawn between its vertices, you can fill in the alternating regions with two different colors, as shown. Discounting rotations but accepting reflections as different, there are nineteen unique patterns that can be created in this manner. You have been given seventeen—can you find the other two?

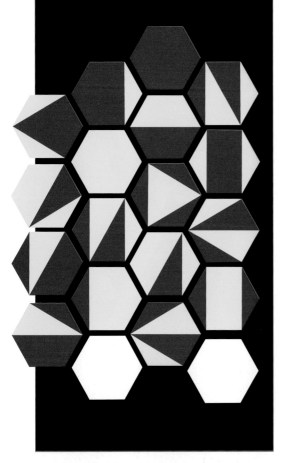

PLAYTHINK
618
DIFFICULTY: ●●●●●●●●○○
REQUIRED: ◉ ✎
COMPLETION: ☐ TIME: _____

POSI-NEGA Q-BITS

The fifty solutions to the Q-Bits puzzle are shown below, along with their color-reversed duplicates. The tiles are numbered 1 to 10 on the first row, 11 to 20 on the second row and so on. As you can see, tiles 1 and 100 are a color-reversed pair.

How long will it take you to match all fifty more pairs?

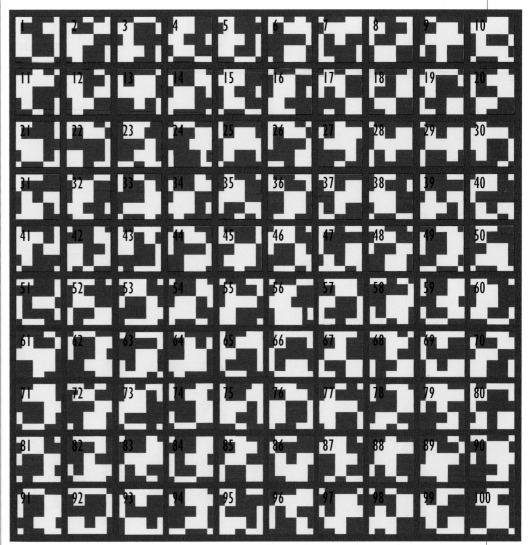

PLAYTHINK
619
DIFFICULTY: ●●●●●●●○○○
REQUIRED: ◉ ✎
COMPLETION: ☐ TIME: _____

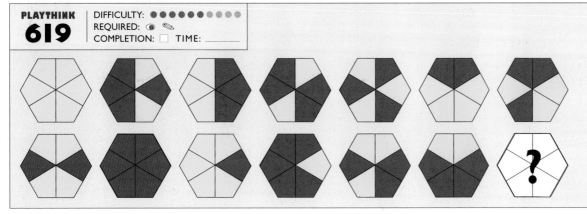

HEXABITS 2

If you divide a hexagon into six wedge-shaped pieces and fill in each section with one of two colors, you can get up to fourteen unique patterns.

Thirteen patterns are shown. Can you work out which one is missing?

PLAYTHINK 620

DIFFICULTY: ●●●●●○○○○○
REQUIRED: ◉
COMPLETION: ☐ TIME: _____

THREE GLASSES TRICK

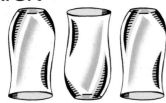

Place three glasses on a table, as shown above. Your goal is to bring all three glasses to the upright position in exactly three moves, turning over two glasses at a time. A quick examination will reveal that this is easy to do—in fact, it can be done after any number of moves.

Once you succeed, turn all three glasses over to the inverted position, as shown below. Then challenge your friends to duplicate your feat.

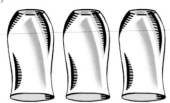

PLAYTHINK 622

DIFFICULTY: ●●●●●●○○○○
REQUIRED: ◉
COMPLETION: ☐ TIME: _____

POLICE CHASE

In this game the policeman (the green dot) chases the thief (the red dot). They alternate moves, going from circle to adjacent circle. The policeman catches the thief if, in his move, he can place his green dot on the red dot. Can the policeman catch the thief in fewer than ten moves?

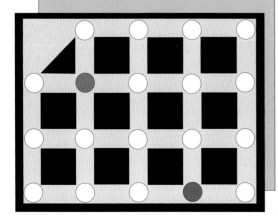

PLAYTHINK 621

DIFFICULTY: ●●●●●○○○○○
REQUIRED: ◉
COMPLETION: ☐ TIME: _____

SIX GLASSES PROBLEM

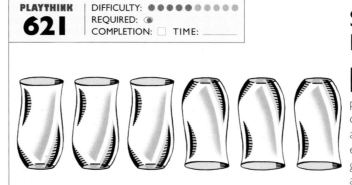

Place six glasses on a table, as shown. Take any pair and invert them. If you continue to invert pairs for as long as you like, will you ever end up with all six glasses upright? How about all six glasses upside-down?

PLAYTHINK 623

DIFFICULTY: ●●●●●○○○○○
REQUIRED: ◉
COMPLETION: ☐ TIME: _____

PAIRING HEXAGONS

There are twelve pairs of identical hexagons. Which hexagon is the odd one out?

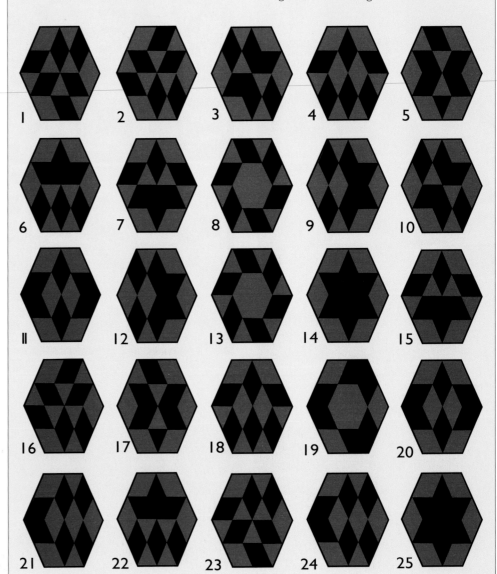

PLAYTHINK
624
DIFFICULTY: ●●●●●●○○○○○
REQUIRED: ◉
COMPLETION: ☐ TIME: _____

POKER CHIPS PATTERN

Sixteen chips lie on a table in an alternating pattern, as shown.

If you are allowed to slide only two chips into new positions, can you find a way to turn the pattern into horizontal rows of solid colors?

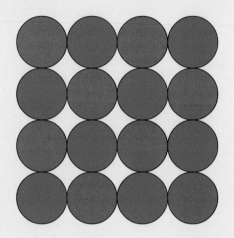

PLAYTHINK
625
DIFFICULTY: ●●○○○○○○○○○
REQUIRED: ◉
COMPLETION: ☐ TIME: _____

GEAR CHAIN

Nine gears are meshed in a closed loop, as shown. How should the red gear revolve so that the green gear turns clockwise?

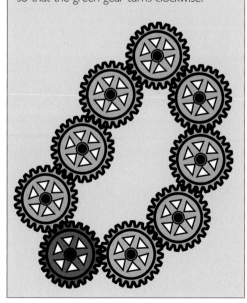

PLAYTHINK
626
DIFFICULTY: ●●●●●●●○○○○
REQUIRED: ◉
COMPLETION: ☐ TIME: _____

LAMP IN THE ATTIC

One of the three switches on the ground floor turns on the lamp in the attic. Your job is to find out which of the three switches activates the lamp, but you are allowed only one trip to the attic to check on the light.

Can you figure out how to tell which light switch works?

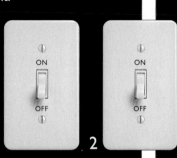

PLAYTHINK
627
DIFFICULTY: ●●●●●●●●○○○
REQUIRED: ◉ ✎
COMPLETION: ☐ TIME: _____

RANDOM SWITCHING

There are three unmarked light switches that have been randomly set to "on" and "off" positions. Each is connected to a lamp in another room, which will shine only when all three are in the "on" position.

If you were offered the chance to bet, for even money, that you could turn on the lamp with the flip of just one switch, should you take it?

PLAYTHINK
628
DIFFICULTY: ●●●●●●●○○○○
REQUIRED: ◉ ✎
COMPLETION: ☐ TIME: _____

HEPTAGON COLORING

Using just two colors, can you fill in the seven sides of a heptagon in eighteen different ways? Rotations and reflections are not counted as different in this problem.

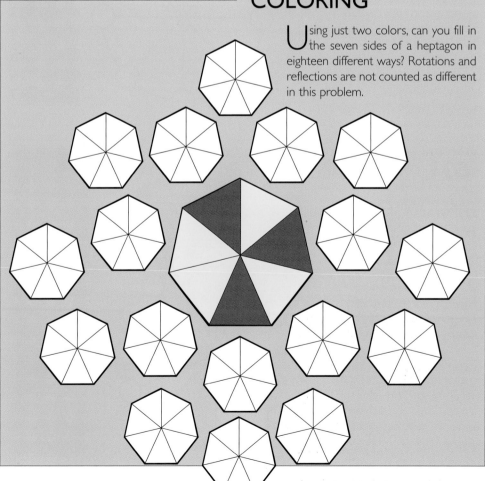

PLAYTHINK 629

DIFFICULTY: ●●●●●●●○○○
REQUIRED: ◉ ✎
COMPLETION: ☐ TIME: _____

TURNING GLASSES

You must turn all the glasses right side up, inverting three glasses at each move. How many moves will it take you?

PLAYTHINK 630

DIFFICULTY: ●●●●●●○○○○
REQUIRED: ◉ ✎
COMPLETION: ☐ TIME: _____

BINARY OR MEMORY WHEEL 1

All the possible triplets of digits 1 and 0 can be embodied in three switches, which may be in either the "on" or "off" position. These triplets represent the first eight numbers (including 0) of the binary numbering system. It is interesting to note that, altogether, twenty-four switches are needed to express the first eight digits simultaneously, as shown at right.

In the "binary" or "memory" wheel, the same amount of information can be condensed to just eight switches. To show how, examine the necklace outline. Can you find a way to use four red and four green beads in such a way that all eight triplets will be represented by consecutive beads as you go around the necklace clockwise? Although the beads in the triplet must be consecutive, each triplet need not be next to the other.

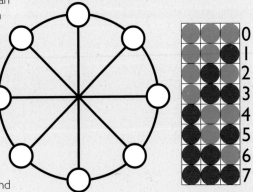

PLAYTHINK 631

DIFFICULTY: ●●●●●●●○○○
REQUIRED: ◉ ✎
COMPLETION: ☐ TIME: _____

BINARY OR MEMORY WHEEL 2

Can you make a necklace from eight red beads and eight green beads so that all the four-bead color sequences (embodying the first sixteen binary numbers, including 0) are represented by consecutive beads as you move clockwise around the necklace?

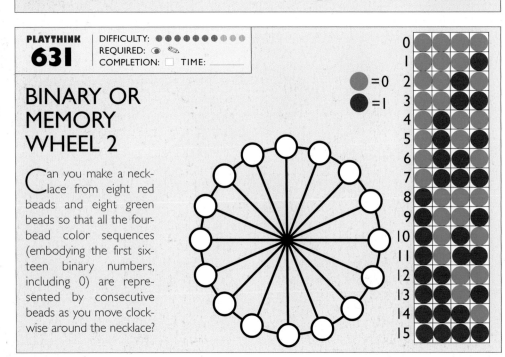

● =0
● =1

PLAYTHINK 632

DIFFICULTY: ●●●●●●●●○○
REQUIRED: ◉ ✎
COMPLETION: ☐ TIME: _____

NECKLACE COLORING

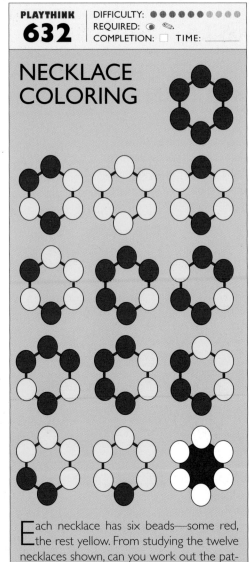

Each necklace has six beads—some red, the rest yellow. From studying the twelve necklaces shown, can you work out the pattern for the thirteenth?

PLAYTHINK 633

DIFFICULTY: ●●●●●○○○○○
REQUIRED: ◉ ✎
COMPLETION: ☐ TIME: _____

NECKLACE

Can you work out how many different necklaces can be made using five identical red beads and two identical green ones?

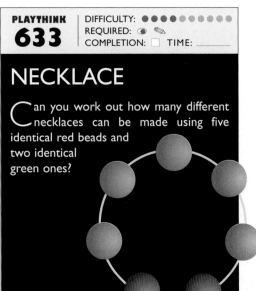

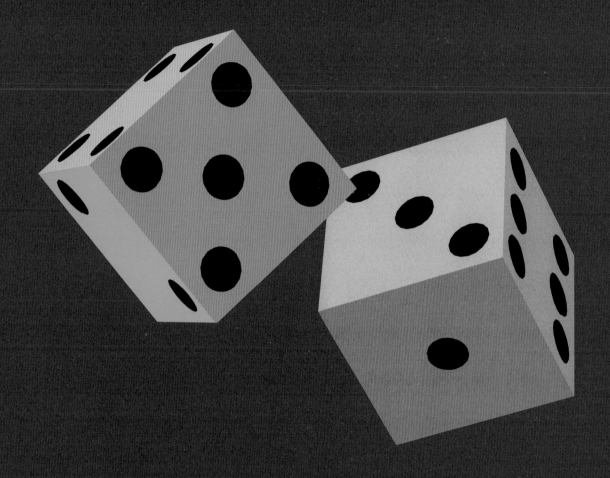

Logic and Probability

PLAYTHINK 634 | DIFFICULTY: ●●●●●○○○○○ REQUIRED: ◉ ✎ COMPLETION: ☐ TIME: _____

HIERARCHY

In logic the basic form of reasoning is deduction, in which a specific conclusion is reached based on one or more premises. The conclusion must be true if all the premises are true.

Here is a classic deduction problem that will show you how this works.

In a certain company the positions of chairman, director and secretary are held by Gerry, Anita and Rose—but not necessarily in that order. The secretary, who is an only child, earns the least. And Rose, who is married to Gerry's brother, earns more than the director.

From that information, can you work out who does what?

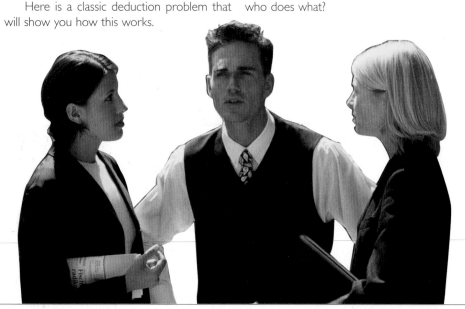

PLAYTHINK 635 | DIFFICULTY: ●●○○○○○○○○ REQUIRED: ◉ COMPLETION: ☐ TIME: _____

PARROT

Madame M. decided to buy a parrot to keep her company. But she wanted one that talked. "Does this parrot speak?" Madame M. asked the pet store clerk.

The clerk was unequivocal. "This parrot," he said, "repeats every word he hears."

That convinced Madame M. to buy the bird. But after months of trying to teach the parrot to speak, she never heard a word out of him.

Was the clerk lying? Or is there a piece of important information he left out?

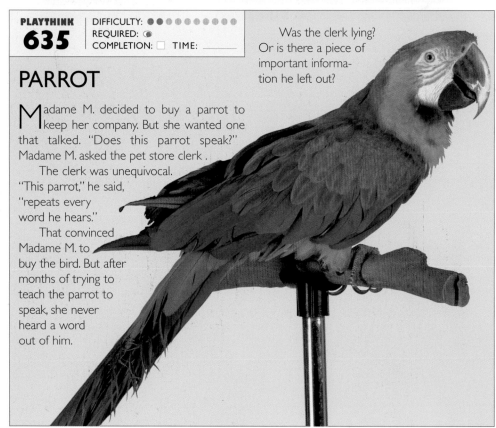

PLAYTHINK 636 | DIFFICULTY: ●●●●●●○○○○ REQUIRED: ◉ COMPLETION: ☐ TIME: _____

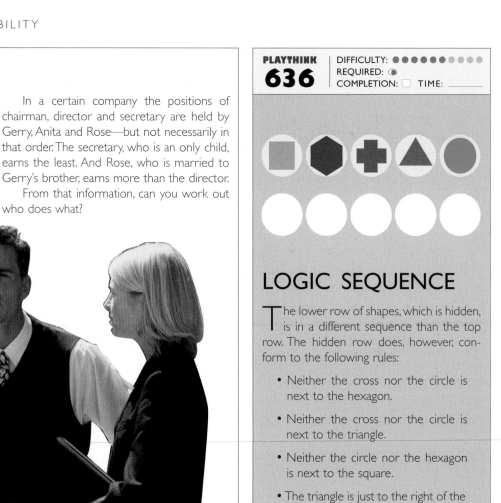

LOGIC SEQUENCE

The lower row of shapes, which is hidden, is in a different sequence than the top row. The hidden row does, however, conform to the following rules:

- Neither the cross nor the circle is next to the hexagon.

- Neither the cross nor the circle is next to the triangle.

- Neither the circle nor the hexagon is next to the square.

- The triangle is just to the right of the square.

Can you work out the hidden sequence?

PLAYTHINK 637 | DIFFICULTY: ●●●●●○○○○○ REQUIRED: ◉ ✎ COMPLETION: ☐ TIME: _____

GIRL-GIRL

Mr. and Mrs. Smith have two children, and they tell you that at least one of them is a girl. Assuming that boys and girls are equally likely, what is the probability that their other child is a girl?

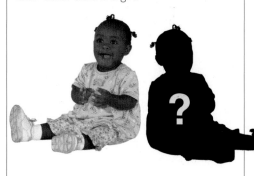

PLAYTHINK 638

DIFFICULTY: ●●●●○○○○○○
REQUIRED: ◉
COMPLETION: ☐ TIME: _____

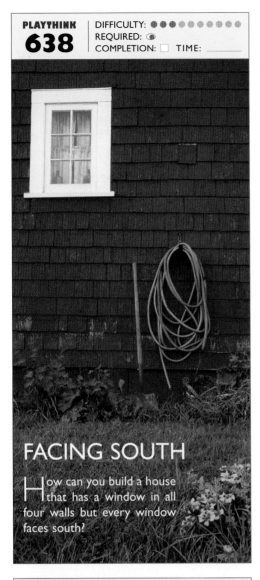

FACING SOUTH

How can you build a house that has a window in all four walls but every window faces south?

PLAYTHINK 639

DIFFICULTY: ●●○○○○○○○○
REQUIRED: ◉
COMPLETION: ☐ TIME: _____

GHOTI

The word below may seem odd, but it is pronounced just like a common English word. Pronounce the *gh* as in "tough," the *o* as in "women" and the *ti* as in "emotion."

What, then, is the common word that "ghoti" sounds like?

GHOTI

PLAYTHINK 640

DIFFICULTY: ●●●●●●○○○○
REQUIRED: ◉
COMPLETION: ☐ TIME: _____

COLOR DIE

The same die is shown in four different positions. From this information, can you work out the color of the bottom (or opposite) face of the bottom die?

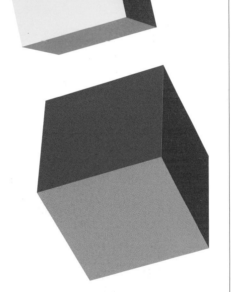

PLAYTHINK 641

DIFFICULTY: ●●●○○○○○○○
REQUIRED: ◉
COMPLETION: ☐ TIME: _____

MARRIAGE

Many years ago a man married the sister of his widow. How did he do it?

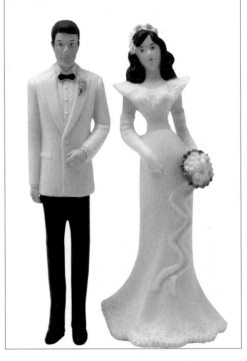

PLAYTHINK 642

DIFFICULTY: ●●●●●●●○○○
REQUIRED: ◉
COMPLETION: ☐ TIME: _____

SETTLING THE ACCOUNT

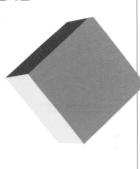

102004180

A man ordered dinner at an expensive restaurant. When the meal was brought to him, he looked at it, wrote the above note for the waiter and left the restaurant. The waiter took the note to the cashier, who understood its meaning and placed it in the cash register.

Can you work out what the note meant?

PLAYTHINK
643
DIFFICULTY: ●●●●●●●●●○
REQUIRED: ◉
COMPLETION: ☐ TIME: _____

WATCHING BIRDS

A great number of birds sit randomly spaced on a wire, each watching its nearest neighbor. Not counting the two birds on the end of the wire, what percentage of the birds sits unwatched?

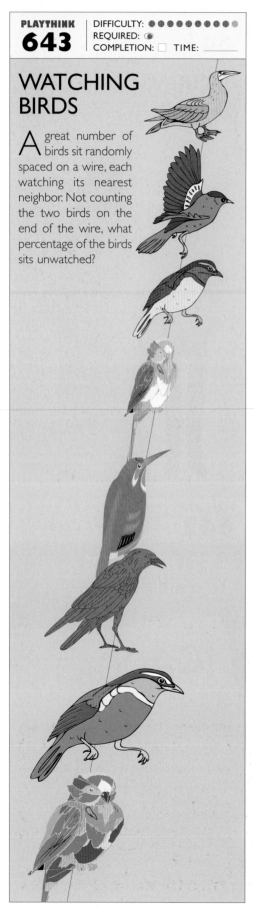

PLAYTHINK
644
DIFFICULTY: ●●●○○○○○○○
REQUIRED: ◉
COMPLETION: ☐ TIME: _____

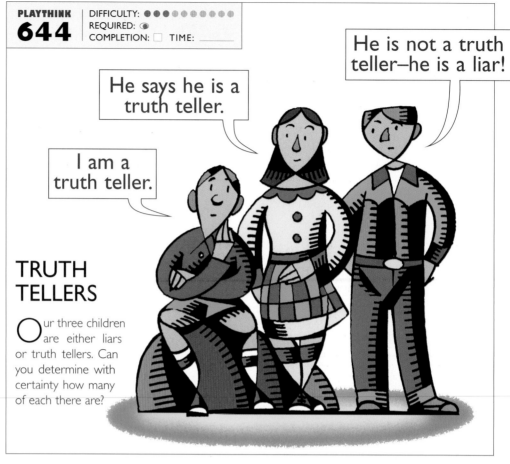

TRUTH TELLERS

Our three children are either liars or truth tellers. Can you determine with certainty how many of each there are?

PLAYTHINK
645
DIFFICULTY: ●●●●●●●●●○
REQUIRED: ◉
COMPLETION: ☐ TIME: _____

HORSE RACE

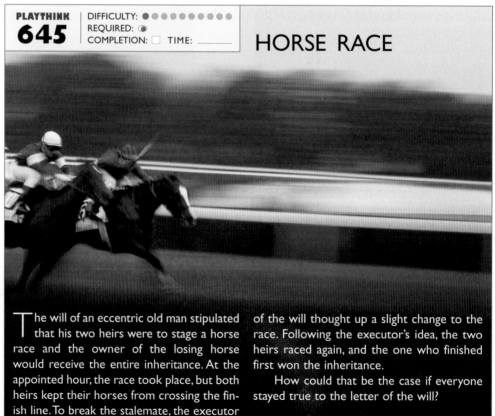

The will of an eccentric old man stipulated that his two heirs were to stage a horse race and the owner of the losing horse would receive the entire inheritance. At the appointed hour, the race took place, but both heirs kept their horses from crossing the finish line. To break the stalemate, the executor of the will thought up a slight change to the race. Following the executor's idea, the two heirs raced again, and the one who finished first won the inheritance.

How could that be the case if everyone stayed true to the letter of the will?

PLAYTHINK
646

DIFFICULTY: ●●●●○○○○○○
REQUIRED: ◉ ✎
COMPLETION: ☐ TIME: _____

HANGMAN

In this version of the classic word game, both players get a hangman. They both think of a word of up to six letters and enter a number of dashes on the opponent's board equal to the letters in the secret word.

Players alternate calling out one letter at a time. If the letter is part of the secret word, it is entered above the appropriate dash (and if the letter occurs more than once, it must be entered as often as it appears). If the guess is incorrect, the opponent starts to draw in the pieces of the illustration one at a time—first the gallows, then the six parts of the condemned man. If a player calls out seven incorrect letters, his man is hanged.

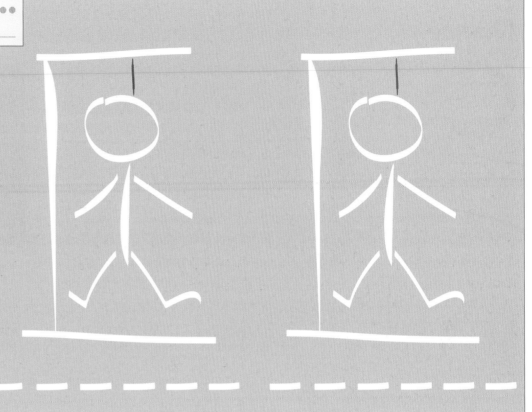

PLAYTHINK
647

DIFFICULTY: ●●●●●●○○○○
REQUIRED: ◉ ✎
COMPLETION: ☐ TIME: _____

DRAWING COLORED BALLS

A container holds twenty red balls and thirty blue balls. If you draw a ball without looking, what is the probability that it is a red ball?

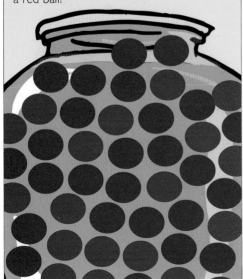

PLAYTHINK
648

DIFFICULTY: ●●●●●●●○○○
REQUIRED: ◉ ✎
COMPLETION: ☐ TIME: _____

SQUARE ALPHABET

The key at the bottom encoded the message at the top. Can you work out the encrypted message?

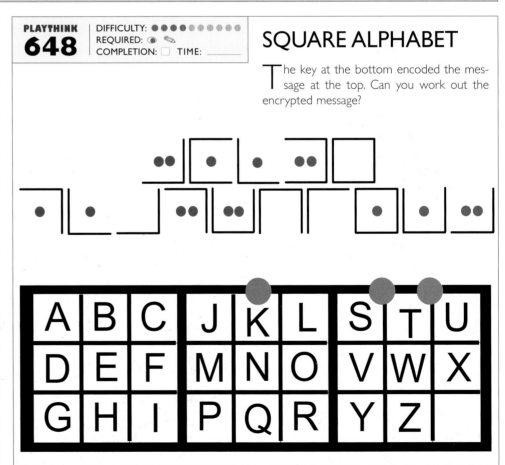

Chance

Classical logic and high school mathematics tend to operate in an unreal world of utter certainty. Every question can be answered by "yes" or "no," and every decision is either "right" or "wrong."

But the real world is quite a different place. Few answers and few decisions are wholly right or wholly wrong. The whole physical universe obeys the laws of chance. The seeming order of large-scale phenomena is sometimes simply the average outcome of millions of elementary random events.

That doesn't mean that any answer or decision is just as good as another. Most events follow the laws of probability, and if we know those laws, our chances of finding the most likely answers and the most promising decisions are greatly enhanced. There are varying degrees of plausibility or probability for every alternative. They can be compared, their reliability fixed, and useful estimates can be made of the comparative possibilities. This is the kind of logic that is developed in the theory of probability.

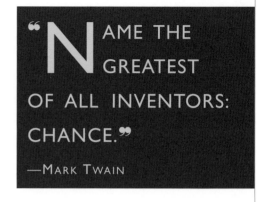

"NAME THE GREATEST OF ALL INVENTORS: CHANCE."

—MARK TWAIN

PLAYTHINK 649

DIFFICULTY: ●●●●●○○○○○
REQUIRED: ◉ ✎
COMPLETION: ☐ TIME: _____

HATCHECK

Six men check their hats at the theater. An inattentive attendant mixes up the claim checks, so when the men return after the show, the hats are essentially handed out at random.

If someone offered you even money to bet that at least one of the men got his own hat back, would you take the bet? In other words, do you believe the probability of one of the six men getting his own hat back is greater than 0.5?

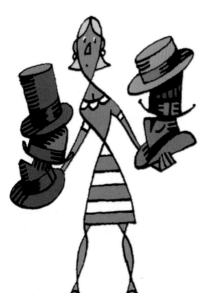

PLAYTHINK 650

DIFFICULTY: ●●●●○○○○○○
REQUIRED: ◉ ✎
COMPLETION: ☐ TIME: _____

DICE STACK

Can you add all the numbers on the unseen sides of the six dice?

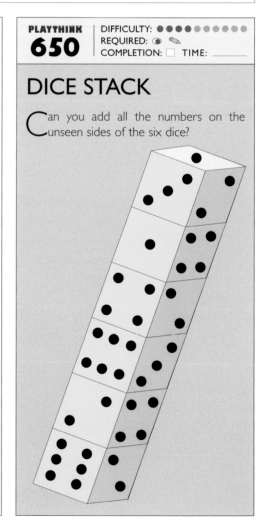

Probability

Probability is the likelihood that an event will occur. The study of probability deals with questions that are answered, in colloquial terms, with "possibly," "sometimes," "often" or "almost always."

Unlike the fuzziness of "maybe," however, probabilities can be measured, calculated or—when calculation is impossible—estimated. The result is a numerical value. A probability of 1 corresponds to absolute certainty; a value of 0 means the outcome is impossible. Values that fall in between give a sense of likelihood: 0.7 for something that is fairly likely, 0.1 for something that is rather rare, and 0.5 for an event that is purely random, such as the toss of a coin.

Like all numbers, probabilities can be compared. Researchers use past events to calculate the probability of similar events occurring in the future. Such calculations have an important role to play in preparations for natural disasters. In locations where the probability of a hurricane is high but that of an earthquake is low, local safety workers can be trained in rescue techniques that are different from those in areas where the dangers are reversed.

In general, the probability of an event is defined by the equation:

$$P = n/N$$

in which N is the total number of equally probable outcomes and n is the number of specified outcomes whose probability is being calculated.

In many games it is customary to talk about the odds for (or against) an outcome, rather than its probability. Odds are calculated as n to N − n, so for an event that has a ⅕ probability of occurring, the odds are 1 in 4.

PLAYTHINK 651

DIFFICULTY: ●●●●●○○○○○
REQUIRED: ◉ ✎
COMPLETION: ☐ TIME: _____

PROBABILITY MACHINE

If sixteen balls are released from the top of the hopper, how many on average will end up in each of the five compartments, according to the laws of probability?

This puzzle is based on the famous probability machine designed in the nineteenth century by Francis Galton. And though you won't be able to say how any individual ball may fall, you will be able to predict how a great many balls will be distributed. Although one random event is unpredictable, a great number of random events generally adhere to the laws of probability. Even the relatively few balls in this demonstration should give you a feel for how such a device works.

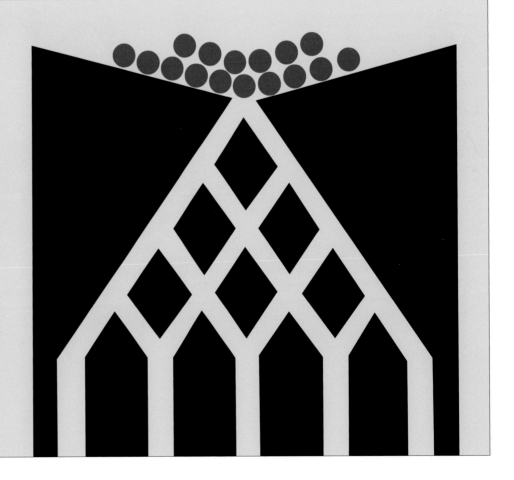

PLAYTHINK 652

DIFFICULTY: ●●●●●○○○○○○
REQUIRED: 👁 ✏
COMPLETION: ☐ TIME: _____

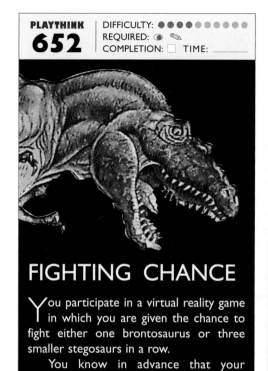

FIGHTING CHANCE

You participate in a virtual reality game in which you are given the chance to fight either one brontosaurus or three smaller stegosaurs in a row.

You know in advance that your chances of defeating the brontosaurus are one in seven, while the probability of defeating one of the stegosaurs is ½.

Which alternative should you choose?

PLAYTHINK 653

DIFFICULTY: ●●●●○○○○○○○
REQUIRED: 👁
COMPLETION: ☐ TIME: _____

SHELLS HAVEN

An old wartime story describes a sailor who, during a pitched battle, put his head through a hole made in the side of his ship by an enemy shell. His theory was that the odds of another shell landing in exactly the same spot should be exceedingly small.

Was his reasoning correct?

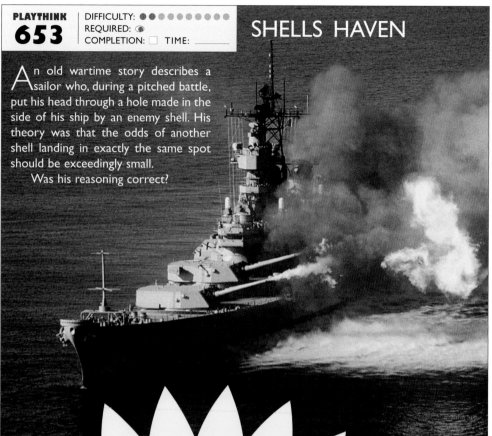

PLAYTHINK 654

DIFFICULTY: ●●●●●○○●○○○
REQUIRED: 👁
COMPLETION: ☐ TIME: _____

VORACIOUS LADYBUGS

A hungry ladybug will try to eat every thirteenth bug she comes across as she goes around the flower. If it is an aphid, she will be happy; if it is a bumblebee, she will be stung.

Can you work out which aphid she should start with so that she will eat all thirteen aphids and avoid the bumblebee?

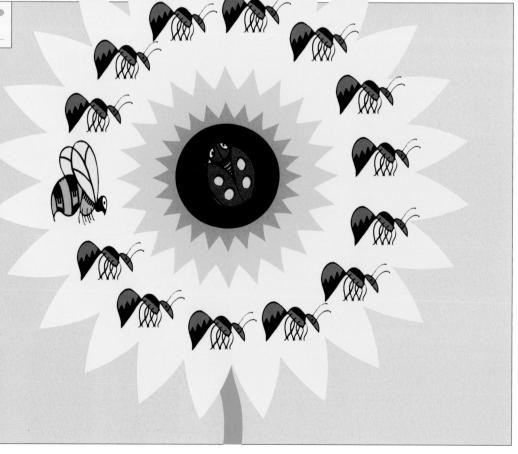

PLAYTHINK 655

DIFFICULTY: ●●●●●●●○○○
REQUIRED: 👁 ✎
COMPLETION: ☐ TIME: _____

INTERPLANETARY COURIER

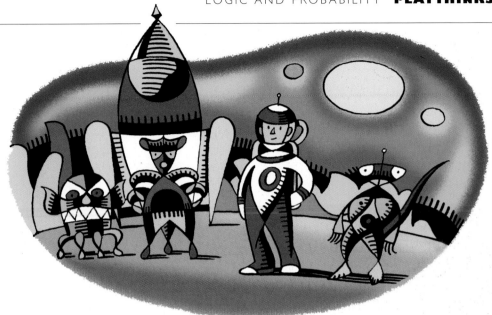

I have a job (in my dream) as an interplanetary courier at the Alpha Centauri spaceport, which means I am responsible for transporting passengers from the spaceport to the spaceliner in orbit many zerks above us. My shuttlecraft can hold just two people at a time—a passenger and me. Also, all the passengers must wait in the spaceliner's airlock until the last one has arrived.

Generally, the job is hassle-free, but on one recent occasion it was a real nightmare. There were three passengers waiting to be transported: a Rigellian, a Denebian and a weird-looking quadripedal creature called a Terrestrial. This caused all sorts of problems. First, the Denebians and the Rigellians were at war, so leaving them alone at the airlock could have caused an intergalactic incident. And unlike the vegetarian Rigellian, the Denebian was a voracious carnivore and, if left alone with the Terrestrial, would have devoured the hapless creature in a second.

It took me a minute, but I found a way to shuttle the passengers up to the spaceliner without any "accidents." One passenger may have had to accompany me more than once, but at the end all three were able to emerge safely from the airlock. Can you work out how I did it?

PLAYTHINK 656

DIFFICULTY: ●●●●●●○○○○
REQUIRED: 👁
COMPLETION: ☐ TIME: _____

LIKES AND DISLIKES

The picture below shows members of a group I belong to discussing their favorite food. Can you work out who is who and who likes what?

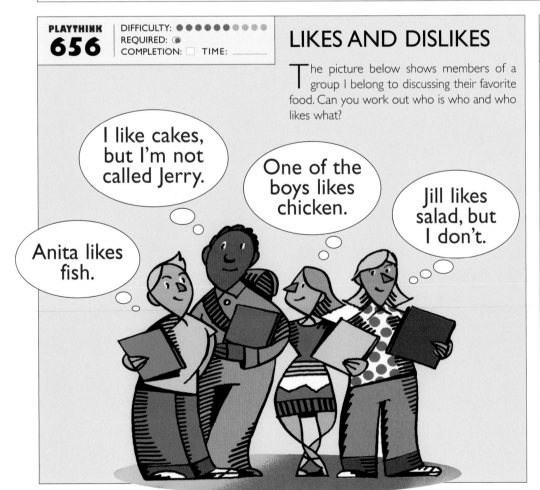

I like cakes, but I'm not called Jerry.

One of the boys likes chicken.

Jill likes salad, but I don't.

Anita likes fish.

1   2   3   4

PLAYTHINK 657

DIFFICULTY: ●●●●●●●○○○
REQUIRED: 👁 ✎
COMPLETION: ☐ TIME: _____

THREE COINS PARADOX

Suppose you have three coins—one with a head and a tail, one with two heads and one with two tails—that are dropped in a hat. If you draw one coin from the hat and lay it flat on a table without looking at it, what are the chances that the hidden side is the same as the visible side?

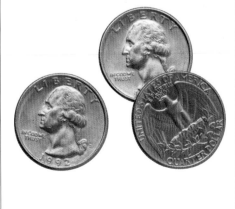

PLAYTHINK 658

DIFFICULTY: ●●●●●○○○○○○
REQUIRED: 👁 ✎
COMPLETION: ☐ TIME: ___

WORD SQUARE

Word squares are matrices in which the same set of words appears both horizontally and vertically.

Can you fit in the extra letters to form a four-by-four word square?

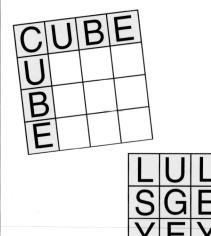

PLAYTHINK 659

DIFFICULTY: ●●●●●○○○○○○
REQUIRED: 👁
COMPLETION: ☐ TIME: ___

SPLIT GREETINGS

The two transparent disks are each one-half of a special greeting. If you superimpose one disk on the other, can you work out the hidden message?

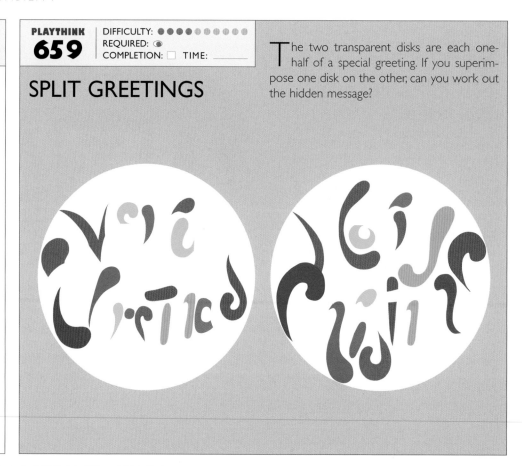

PLAYTHINK 660

DIFFICULTY: ●●●●●●●○○○
REQUIRED: 👁 ✎
COMPLETION: ☐ TIME: ___

HOLLOW CUBE I

Imagine you can peer into a hollow cube that has an eight-by-eight mosaic on the bottom. At any one time, however, only parts of the mosaic can be seen. The pattern involves a bit of bilateral symmetry, so it is possible to deduce the answer from the visual information given.

Can you construct or deduce the whole mosaic from the bits you see here?

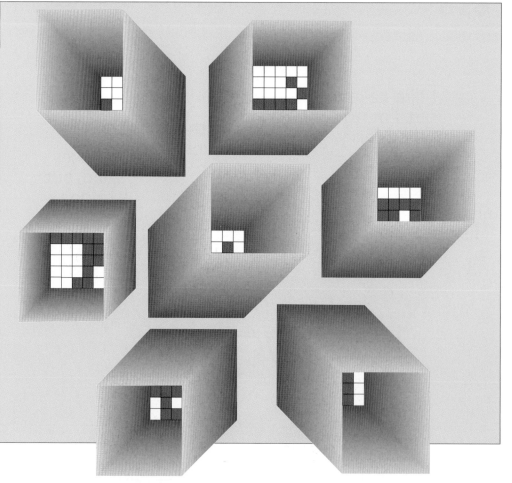

PLAYTHINK 661

DIFFICULTY: ●●●○○○○○○○○
REQUIRED: ◉
COMPLETION: ☐ TIME: _____

ROULETTE

What is the only sure way to win at roulette?

PLAYTHINK 662

DIFFICULTY: ●●●●○○○○○○○
REQUIRED: ◉
COMPLETION: ☐ TIME: _____

REBUSES

Can you solve the two rebus word problems illustrated below?

ME   JUST   YOU

TIMING TIM ING

PLAYTHINK 664

DIFFICULTY: ●●●●●○○○○○
REQUIRED: ◉ ✎
COMPLETION: ☐ TIME: _____

ROLLING MARBLES

Peter and Paul are equally good at marbles. If Peter has two marbles and Paul has one, can you work out the probability of Peter winning? To win, a marble must land closest to a fixed point.

PLAYTHINK 663

DIFFICULTY: ●●●●●●●○○○○
REQUIRED: ◉ ✎
COMPLETION: ☐ TIME: _____

HOLLOW CUBE 2

Imagine you are peering into the bottom of a hollow cube that contains a six-by-six mosaic at its base. Only bits of the pattern can be seen at any given time. Can you piece together your observations to construct or deduce the pattern of the mosaic?

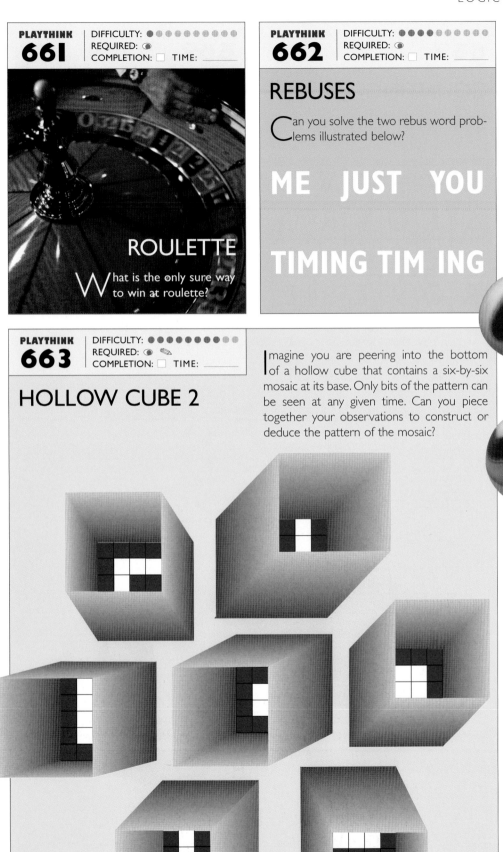

PLAYTHINK 665

DIFFICULTY: ●●●●●●○○○○
REQUIRED: ◉
COMPLETION: ☐ TIME: _____

THREE MISTAKES

There are three mistakes in the message below. Can you spot them all?

What are the tree mistake

in this sentence?

PLAYTHINK 666

DIFFICULTY: ●●●○○○○○○○
REQUIRED: 👁 ✐
COMPLETION: ☐ TIME: _____

ANAGRAM

In a different order the letters *N, A, G, R* and *E* can form a meaningful word. There are two possibilities; can you find them both?

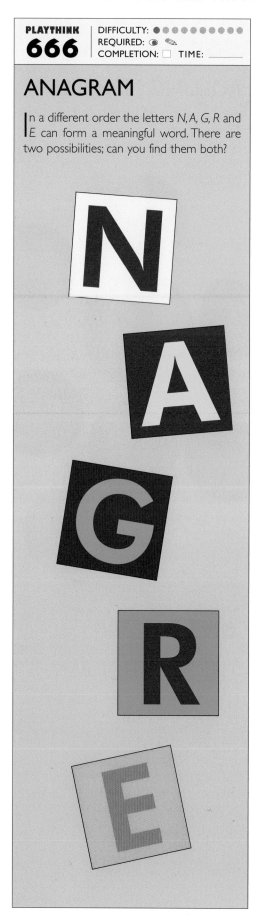

PLAYTHINK 667

DIFFICULTY: ●●●●●○○○○○
REQUIRED: 👁
COMPLETION: ☐ TIME: _____

COUNTING

There is a secret word hidden in this matrix of letters. Can you discover it?

R	V	E	O	V	C
S	I	O	V	R	D
V	E	R	C	V	O
R	O	V	E	S	E
E	R	S	C	R	I
C	E	R	E	O	R

PLAYTHINK 668

DIFFICULTY: ●●●●●●○○○○
REQUIRED: 👁 ✐
COMPLETION: ☐ TIME: _____

SMALL WORLD

Pick any two of the 284 million people living in the United States. If you wanted to link those two by a chain of acquaintances (a friend of a friend of a friend . . .) how many people (or "links") would you need on average?

PLAYTHINK 669

DIFFICULTY: ●●●●●●●○○○
REQUIRED: 👁 ✐
COMPLETION: ☐ TIME: _____

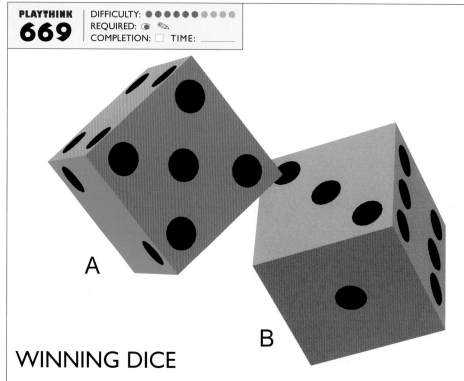

A

B

WINNING DICE

Two prisoners are spending their life sentences throwing dice. Each of them has just one old die so worn out that only three sides are legible. The three legible sides for each are shown above.

If their game awards the player who rolls the highest number, which player will win most often over the long run? (A game is not counted if either die lands with an illegible side face up.)

PLAYTHINK
670
DIFFICULTY: ●●●●●○○○○○
REQUIRED: ◉ ✏
COMPLETION: ☐ TIME: _____

BASIC SHAPES

Five overlapping compositions of a triangle, a rectangle and an oval are illustrated here. Can you find the odd one out?

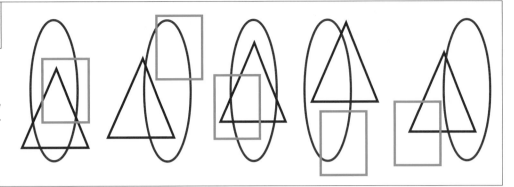

PLAYTHINK
671
DIFFICULTY: ●●●●●○○○○○
REQUIRED: ◉
COMPLETION: ☐ TIME: _____

ALIEN LANDING

Twenty-four aliens just landed on the earth. They look identical except for the color of their hair, eyes, noses and mouths, which come in four colors in different combinations.

The aliens all carry a letter or a space for a message in English, but they are not in the right order. Can you use the color key below to put the aliens in the correct order and spell out their important message?

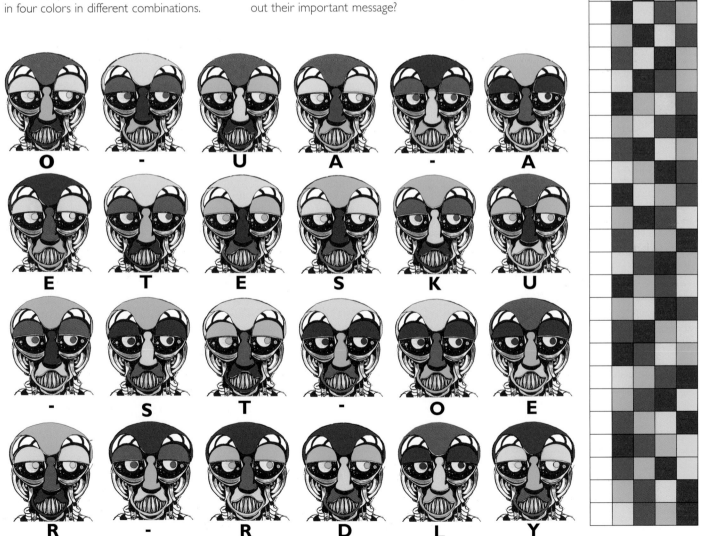

PLAYTHINK 672

DIFFICULTY: ●●○○○○○○○○
REQUIRED: ◉
COMPLETION: ☐ TIME: _____

SQUARE COUNT

A teacher held up a piece of paper and asked his students to tell him how many squares they saw. They replied, "Six," which was the right answer.

The teacher held up the paper again and asked his students how many squares they saw. "Eight," they replied, again correct. So how many squares were really on the sheet? Six? Eight?

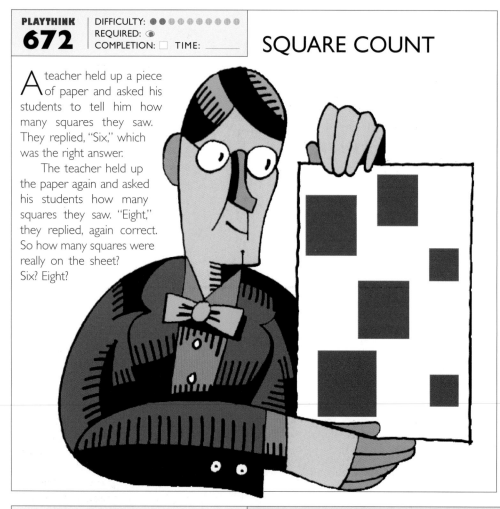

PLAYTHINK 673

DIFFICULTY: ●●●●○○○○○○
REQUIRED: ◉
COMPLETION: ☐ TIME: _____

TRUE STATEMENT

Which of the three statements is true?

1) One statement here is false.

2) Two statements here are false.

3) Three statements here are false.

PLAYTHINK 674

DIFFICULTY: ●●●●●○○○○○
REQUIRED: ◉
COMPLETION: ☐ TIME: _____

TUNNEL PASSAGE

Three men sat by open windows on a steam train that passed through a tunnel. All three of their faces became covered with soot. When the three passengers saw this, they started laughing at one another. Then one of them suddenly stopped because he realized that his face was also soiled.

What was his reasoning?

PLAYTHINK 675

DIFFICULTY: ●●○●●○○○○○
REQUIRED: ◉
COMPLETION: ☐ TIME: _____

LOGIC PATTERN

Each of the symbols in this matrix represents a number. The sum for each row and for three of the four columns is given. From that information, can you find the value of each symbol?

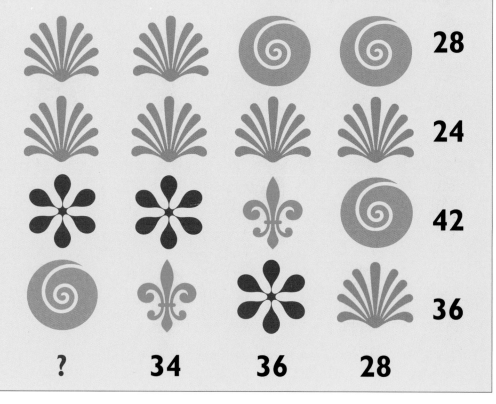

Coincidence

The improbable, Aristotle once said, is extremely probable. But when one looks at the bizarre coincidences that occur on a weekly or daily basis, it is easy to conclude that many coincidences are too improbable to be explained by known laws.

The parapsychologist Lewis Vaughn warned in *Skeptics* magazine of the dangers of trying to predict synchronistic events by telling the following tale.

A man was the seventh child of parents who were each the seventh child in their families. The man was born on the Sabbath—the seventh day—of the seventh month of 1907. Over the course of his life, a number of odd things occurred, all related to the number seven, which he soon took as his lucky number. On his twenty-seventh birthday, the man went to the racetrack and saw that a horse named Seventh Heaven was listed to run from the seventh gate in the seventh race. The odds were seven to one. The man borrowed all the money he could and bet on the horse. The horse, of course, came in seventh.

Like the man in the story, we can develop subjective concepts about probability that may lead us to wrong conclusions. In order to relate to chance intelligently, we must learn to understand the laws of chance, which often have a strongly counterintuitive aspect.

PLAYTHINK 676

DIFFICULTY: ●●●●●●●○○○
REQUIRED: ◉ ✎
COMPLETION: ☐ TIME: ____

DRAWING BALLS

A cloth bag contains either a red ball or a blue ball. A red ball is then dropped in the bag, so now the bag has two balls.

A drawing is held, and a red ball is drawn out of the bag. Can you work out the probability of the remaining ball also being red?

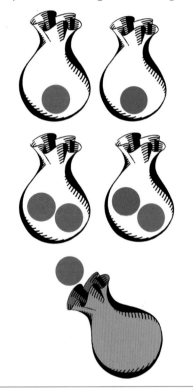

PLAYTHINK 677

DIFFICULTY: ●●●●●●●○○○
REQUIRED: ◉ ✎
COMPLETION: ☐ TIME: ____

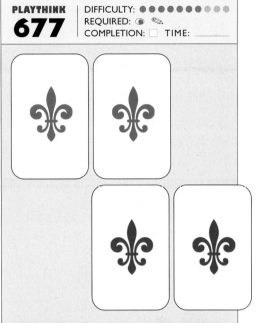

FOUR-CARD SHUFFLE

You begin a game with four cards. Two have a red pattern and two have a blue pattern, and all are blank on one side.

You shuffle the four cards and place them face down. If you pick two cards at random, what is the probability that the two cards will be the same color?

Your friend tries to convince you that the chances are ⅔ with this reasoning: there are three possibilities—two red, two blue or one of each—and since two of those are of the same color, the chances are two out of three.

Are you convinced?

PLAYTHINK 678

DIFFICULTY: ●●●●●●●●●○
REQUIRED: ◉ ✎
COMPLETION: ☐ TIME: ____

TRIPLE DUEL

Amos, Butch and Cody decide to settle their differences with a gunfight. The three cowboys draw lots for the shooting order and then take one shot each until only one is left standing.

Amos and Butch are sure shots and never miss, but Cody can hit the mark only 50 percent of the time. From that information, can you work out who has the best chance of survival?

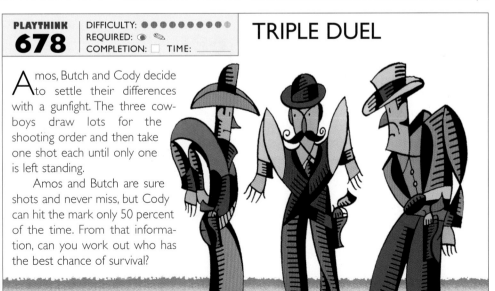

LAST ALIVE

Imagine you have just become the emperor of Rome. One of your first duties is to condemn thirty-six prisoners to be eaten by lions in the arena. The lions can eat only six victims a day, and there are six hated enemies you would like to dispatch right away, but you also want to appear impartial.

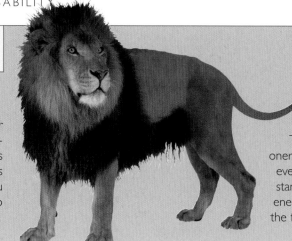

The traditional Roman way to select prisoners for execution is decimation—picking every tenth person. If you have the prisoners stand in a circle, is there a way to plant your enemies at specific positions so they will be the first six selected to die?

Coin Tossing

Although no one can say with certainty the outcome of a single toss of a coin, the result of a million tosses is easy to predict: half a million heads and half a million tails, or within a percent or two of each. This, in essence, is the basis of the theory of probability.

Two laws underlie probability: the "both-and" law, employed to calculate the probability of two events both happening, and the "either-or" law, used to calculate the probability of one or the other of two events happening. The both-and law states that the chance of two independent events both happening is equal to the probability of one happening multiplied by the probability of the other happening. For example, the chance of one flip of a coin turning up heads is ½. The chance of the coin turning up heads on both the first and second flips is ½ × ½, or only ¼.

The either-or law states that the chance of either one or the other of two mutually exclusive probabilities coming true equals the sum of the separate chance that each would occur individually. The chance of one flip of a coin turning up either heads or tails is equal to the chance of throwing heads plus the chance of throwing tails: ½ + ½, or 1—absolute certainty.

FLIP FRAUD

You ask a friend to flip a coin 200 times and record the outcome. When you are given the results, you want to know whether your friend really flipped the coin all those times or just faked it.

How can you check the results to see whether they are genuine?

COIN TOSSING

How many different outcomes are possible in one toss of two coins?

ONE WORD

Can you rearrange the letters to form one word in the space provided?

REARRANGE THE TWO WORDS

N	E	W		D	O	O	R

TO MAKE ONE WORD

PLAYTHINK 683

DIFFICULTY: ●●●●●●○○○○
REQUIRED: ◉ ✎
COMPLETION: ☐ TIME: _____

DICE—EVEN-ODD

Louis Pasteur once said, "Chance favors only the prepared mind." Let's see if you have been prepared for this puzzle.

When you throw a pair of dice, what are the chances that the number that comes up will be even?

PLAYTHINK 684

DIFFICULTY: ●●●●●●●○○○
REQUIRED: ◉ ✎
COMPLETION: ☐ TIME: _____

DICING FOR SIX

In many games you need a roll of 6 to start. One roll is generally not sufficient to get the 6. In fact, in some new games you are given a number of consecutive rolls to try to get at least one 6.

If the design of the game is to make the odds favor starting in the first round, what is the least number of rolls that players should be given?

PLAYTHINK 685

DIFFICULTY: ●●●●●●○○○○
REQUIRED: ◉ ✎
COMPLETION: ☐ TIME: _____

BIRTHDAY PARADOX

You want to have a party at which at least two people share the same birthday—same month and day but not necessarily the same year. If you don't know the birthdays of any of your guests, how many people do you have to invite so that the probability of two people sharing a birthday is more than 0.5? How many people do you need to invite for birthday sharing to be a practical certainty?

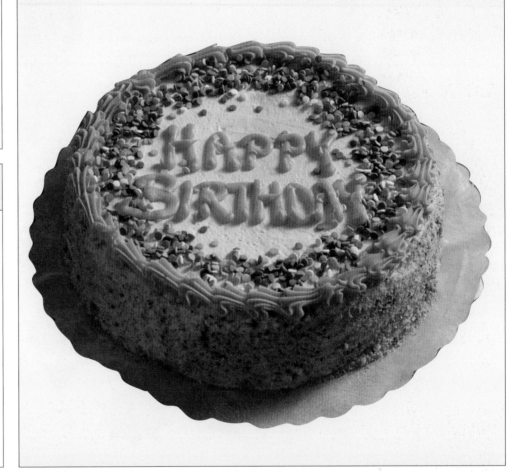

PLAYTHINK 686

DIFFICULTY: ●●●●●●●○○○
REQUIRED: ◉
COMPLETION: ☐ TIME: _____

COLOR WORDS

How strongly do words affect perception? Try reading the four lines of colored words at right—but instead of saying the words, say the color of each word.

Can you say more than five in a row without making a mistake?

RED YELLOW BLUE GREEN
YELLOW BLUE GREEN RED
GREEN RED YELLOW BLUE
BLUE GREEN RED YELLOW

PLAYTHINK 687 | DIFFICULTY: ●●●●●●●●○○ REQUIRED: ◉ ✎ COMPLETION: ☐ TIME: _____

DICING FOR DOUBLE SIX

You need to roll a double 6 in at least one of twenty-four throws. Are the odds in your favor?

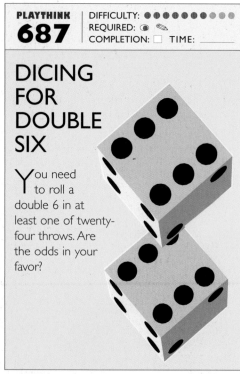

PLAYTHINK 688 | DIFFICULTY: ●●●●●●●○○○ REQUIRED: ◉ ✎ COMPLETION: ☐ TIME: _____

GAME SHOW

Imagine you have been selected for a game show that offers the chance to win an expensive new car. The car sits behind one of three doors; monkeys reside behind the other two.

You choose a door, and the host opens one of the remaining two, revealing a monkey. The host then offers you a choice: stick with your initial choice or switch to the other, still-unopened door. Do you stick with your door, or do you take the host up on the offer?

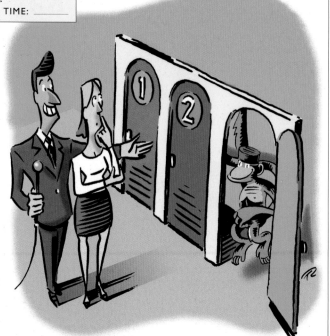

PLAYTHINK 689 | DIFFICULTY: ●●●●●○○○○○ REQUIRED: ◉ COMPLETION: ☐ TIME: _____

ARROWGRAM

This is an arrowgram. When you work out how it works, you'll discover the name of a famous Englishman.

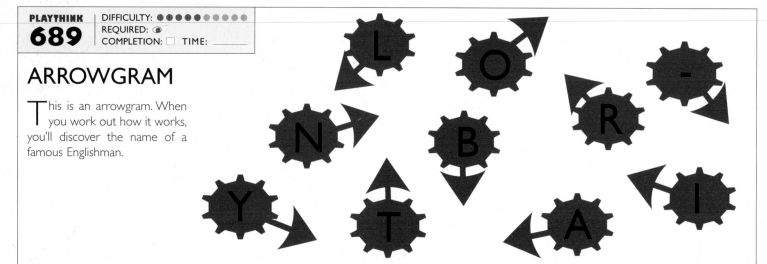

PLAYTHINK 690 | DIFFICULTY: ●●●●●●●○○○ REQUIRED: ◉ ✎ COMPLETION: ☐ TIME: _____

COIN TRIPLETS

There are eight possible coin triplets, as shown. I offer you a simple game with the following bet: Pick any triplet you want, and I'll pick a different triplet. Then we'll flip a fair coin until one of our triplets occurs.

If you have your doubts, let me sweeten the odds: when you win, you'll get three dollars; when I win, you'll give me only two.

Do you want to play? What are the chances that you will win?

HHH	HHT	HTH	THH	HTT	TTH	THT	TTT
1	2	3	4	5	6	7	8

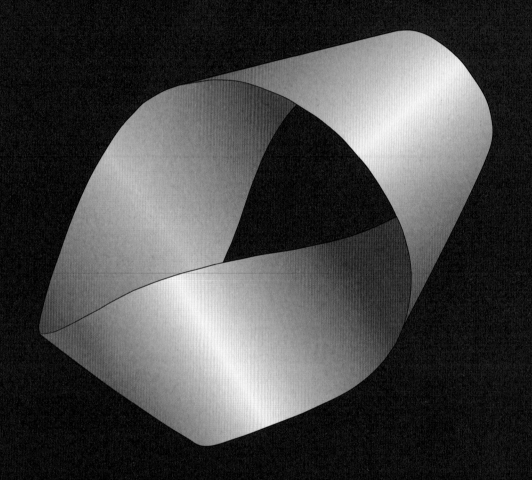

Topology

What is Topology?

Euclidean geometry is clear: A triangle is utterly different from a circle, which has little in common with a trapezoid. But not every type of mathematics ascribes to those boundaries. Take topology: the emphasis in topology isn't on angles or curves but on surfaces. It studies those properties of a figure that remain unchanged under deformation.

Little traditional geometry survives from the topological perspective. From the point of view of a topologist, the number of sides and angles of a triangle are unimportant. One can easily deform a triangle to make its angles change. The lengths of the sides are similarly uninteresting. Indeed, even being a triangle is not a topological property—by introducing a bend in one side of a triangle, the shape can be continuously deformed

into a rectangle. In fact, to topologists, a triangle is the same as a square, a parallelogram—even a circle.

The topologist studies surfaces, and topology looks at the continuity from one surface to another. The fact that a triangle has an inside and an outside and that it is impossible to pass from one to the other without crossing an edge of the triangle—those are topological properties. The fact that a car inner tube has a hole in the middle is a topological property. Whether a loop or string is knotted is a topological property.

Two figures are topologically equivalent if one can be continuously deformed into another. (Continuous deformation means a shape is bent, twisted, stretched or compressed.) So a sphere and a cube are topologically equivalent, as are the figure *8* and letter *B*. A fundamental problem in topology is to group objects into

classes of things that are topologically equivalent.

The basic concepts of topology include many ideas we learn in childhood: insideness and outsideness, right- and left-handedness, linking, knotting, connectedness and disconnectedness. Indeed, some of the concepts are so basic that topologists have been called mathematicians who don't know the difference between a coffee cup and a doughnut. But topology has become a cornerstone of modern mathematics. During the last forty years it has been applied to problems in practically all fields of science.

Because topology deals with space, surfaces, solids, regions and networks and because it is full of impossibilities and paradoxes, it is a rich topic for fun, games, puzzles and problem solving.

PLAYTHINK 691	DIFFICULTY: ●●●○○○○○○○
	REQUIRED: ◉ ✎
	COMPLETION: ☐ TIME:

DOT WIGGLING 1

Anyone can connect all nineteen points in a closed, continuous path. But can you find the path that possesses the most wiggles? The path shown in the diagram at the left has seventeen angles. Can you find another path that has seventeen angles?

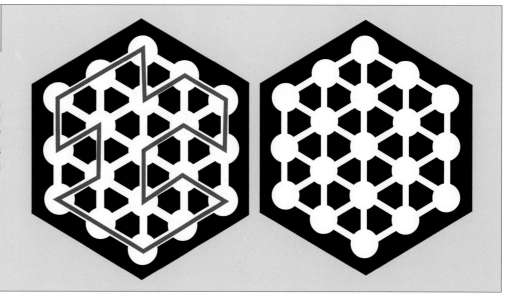

PLAYTHINK 692

DIFFICULTY: ●●●●●●●○○○
REQUIRED: ◉
COMPLETION: ☐ TIME:

TOPOLOGICAL EQUIVALENCE I

The figures marked *a*, *b* and *c* were each topologically deformed into one of nine numbered configurations. Can you find their topological equivalents?

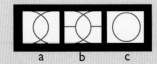

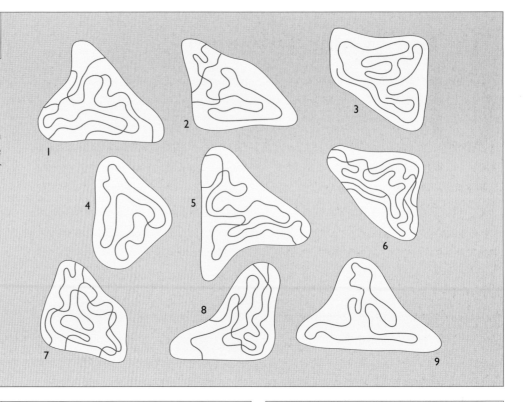

PLAYTHINK 693

DIFFICULTY: ●●●●○○○○○○
REQUIRED: ◉
COMPLETION: ☐ TIME:

PICK-UP STICKS 2

In this puzzle each stick can be picked up only when no other stick lies on top of it. Can you work out the sequence in which to pick up all twenty sticks? Also, how many different lengths are represented?

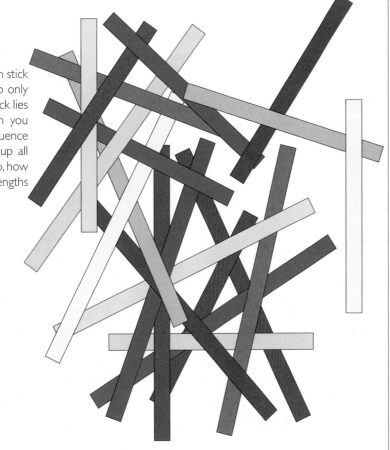

PLAYTHINK 694

DIFFICULTY: ●●●●●●●●●●
REQUIRED: ◉ ✎ 📄 ✂
COMPLETION: ☐ TIME:

HYPERCARD

■ *The Impossible flap*

With just three straight cuts and one fold, can you create this three-dimensional structure from an ordinary rectangular piece of cardboard?

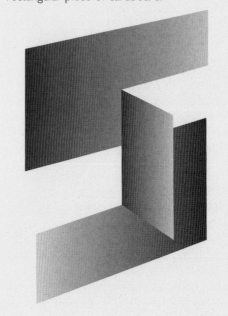

The Four-Color Theorem

Until recently a long-standing problem in topology dealt with the coloring of maps. In the mid-nineteenth century an Englishman named Francis Guthrie was filling in a map of England—coloring in the counties so that no two adjacent counties had the same color—and wondered how many colors were necessary to complete the job. That bit of puzzling set off a mathematical problem that stayed alive for more than a century.

Mathematicians streamlined the question considerably to make it more general. How many colors, they asked, are needed so that *any* map can be colored in such a way that no adjacent regions (which must touch along an edge, not just at a point) have the same color? It is easy to show that at least four colors are needed. In 1879, a few years after Guthrie posed the four-color problem, an English mathematician named Alfred Bray Kempe published a proof that no map needed five colors, but in 1890 a subtle but crucial mistake was found in his proof: it actually showed that no map requires *six* colors.

Mathematicians wrestled with the problem for almost a century. No one could find a map that actually needed five colors, but then no one could prove that no such map existed. The four-color problem became notorious as one of the simplest remaining unsolved mathematical problems. To make matters worse, in the efforts to answer such a simple question, analogous problems dealing with more complicated surfaces were solved conclusively. For example, a map on a doughnut can always be colored with seven colors. A strange, one-sided surface called the Klein bottle requires six or more colors to fill in all possible regions.

It took a pair of mathematicians using a supercomputer to finally crack the four-color problem. Wolfgang Haken and Kenneth Appel of the University of Illinois broke the problem into a set of subproblems, each of which could be solved by computer. By 1976 they had found a solution, and now the former "problem" is called the four-color theorem.

PLAYTHINK
695

DIFFICULTY: ●●●●●●●○○○
REQUIRED: ◉ ✎
COMPLETION: ☐ TIME: _____

COLOR CUL-DE-SAC

■ *Coloring Map of 210 Countries*

Can you fill in this map with just four colors? If you start filling in the regions, you may soon run into problems. The difficulty of avoiding color cul-de-sacs—regions that have been filled in to create areas where none of the four colors can be used—is what makes this two-player game so much fun.

The first player selects a region and fills it in with one of the four colors: ■ ■ ■ ■ The second player colors in an adjacent region, following the exact opposite of the domino principle—no two regions that touch can be the same color. The last player who can fill in a region while following the rules wins the game.

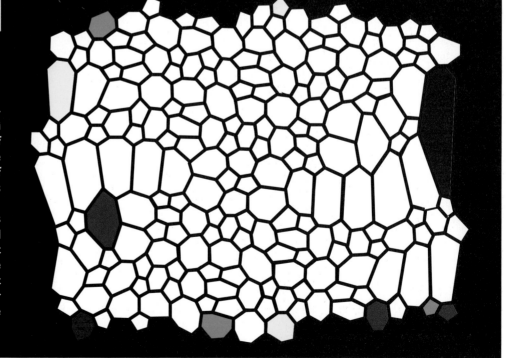

PLAYTHINK
696

DIFFICULTY: ●●●●●●○○○○
REQUIRED: ◉
COMPLETION: ☐ TIME:

TOPOLOGICAL EQUIVALENCE 2

Consider that these structures are made from rubber bands and beads. Can you work out which are topologically equivalent?

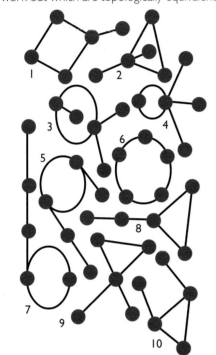

PLAYTHINK
697

DIFFICULTY: ●●●●○○○○○○
REQUIRED: ◉ ✎ 📄 ✂
COMPLETION: ☐ TIME:

FOUR-COLOR HONEYCOMB

■ *A Topological Game*

This two-person game tests your ability to anticipate so-called color cul-de-sacs.

Copy and cut out the sixteen colored hexagons and lay them face down on the table. The first player selects a hexagon and places it on any space on the board that does not share an edge with a boundary region of the same color. Players then alternate selecting and placing hexagons on spaces that do not border a boundary region or hexagon of the same color. The last player who can place a hexagon wins.

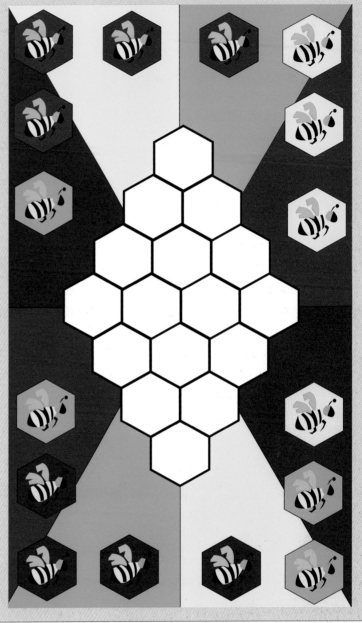

PLAYTHINK
698

DIFFICULTY: ●●●●●●●●○○
REQUIRED: ◉ ✎
COMPLETION: ☐ TIME:

COLORING PATTERN

Say you wanted to fill in this outlined pattern without using the same color in two adjacent areas. What is the minimum number of colors you would need?

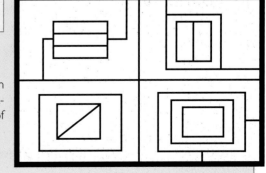

The Two-Color Theorem

Although four colors are needed for regular maps, maps drawn in a special way may not need even that many. One extreme case involves maps drawn using only straight lines. A little scratch-paper experimenting suggests that two colors might be sufficient. Is this true?

The proof that it is requires little effort to grasp. Simply add lines one by one to a map; as you add each line, interchange the two colors on all regions that lie on one side of the new line. The colored regions that remain the same still differ across old boundaries, while they differ across the new borders thanks to the interchange of colors.

The same proof can be generalized to apply to maps on which the boundaries are either single curves that run right across the whole plane or closed loops. Each of those two-color maps possesses an even number of edges that meet at any junction. That must be true of any map that can be colored with just two colors, because the regions around a junction or corner must be of alternate colors. Moreover, it can be proved that any map on a plane can be colored with just two colors if and only if all its junctions have an even number of edges. That's the two-color theorem.

PLAYTHINK 699

DIFFICULTY: ●●●●●○○○○○
REQUIRED: ◉ ✎
COMPLETION: ☐ TIME: _____

MAP COLORING I

Can you fill in the regions on these maps using the least number of colors? Regions of the same color can meet at a point, but they cannot share a border.

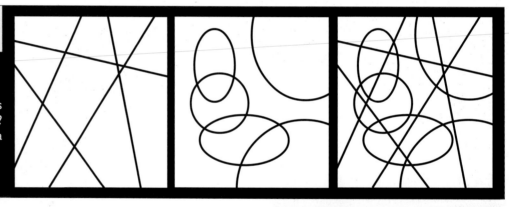

PLAYTHINK 700

DIFFICULTY: ●●●●○○○○○○
REQUIRED: ◉
COMPLETION: ☐ TIME: _____

POLYGONAL NECKLACE

This necklace is made up of eight links, each in the form of a regular polygon, from a triangle to a decagon. Can you tell in what order the polygons are linked?

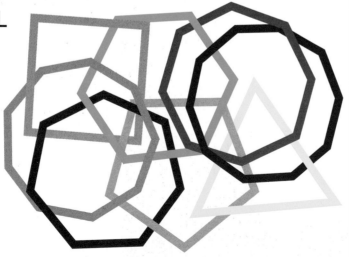

"A TOPOLOGIST IS ONE WHO DOESN'T KNOW THE DIFFERENCE BETWEEN A DOUGHNUT AND A COFFEE CUP."

—JOHN L. KELLEY

PLAYTHINK 701 | DIFFICULTY: ●●●●●●○○○○
REQUIRED: 👁 ✎
COMPLETION: ☐ TIME: _____

OVERLAPPING CARDS

Eight playing cards of different colors are stacked in two overlapping patterns, shown here. Can you work out the order the cards were laid down—from 8 for the bottom card to 1 for the top—for each pile?

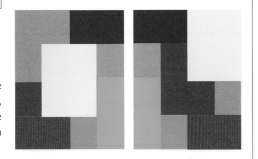

PLAYTHINK 702 | DIFFICULTY: ●●●●○○○○○○
REQUIRED: 👁 ✎
COMPLETION: ☐ TIME: _____

FOUR-IN-A-ROW GAME

Up to four can play this strategy game. Play begins with each player making ten counters in a color of his or her choice. Then players take turns placing one counter at a time on the board. After all the counters are on the board, each person in turn moves one counter from its circle to any adjacent circle connected by a line. If a move places a counter in a row in which the player has more counters than an opponent, the player may remove that opponent's piece.

Play continues until a player wins by moving four counters to the same line.

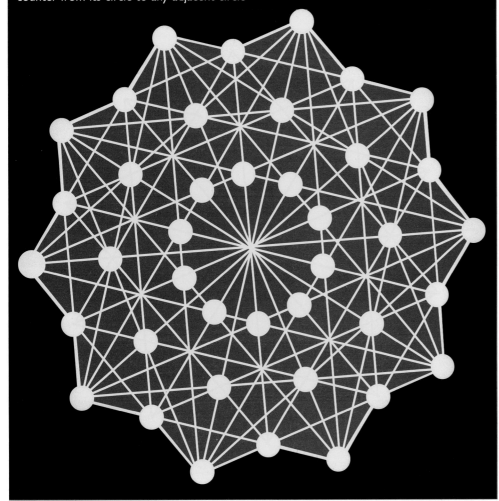

PLAYTHINK 703 | DIFFICULTY: ●●●●●●●●○○
REQUIRED: 👁 ✎
COMPLETION: ☐ TIME: _____

MARS COLONY

German mathematician Gerhard Ringel proposed this map problem in 1950.

Imagine that the eleven major nations on Earth have staked out territory on Mars for colonization. There is one region for each nation. To help keep the political distinctions clear, the nations insist that maps of Mars depict colonies in the same color used for mother countries on Earth maps.

Using the same color for regions that have the same number, can you fill in both maps so that no neighboring regions share a color? How many colors will you need?

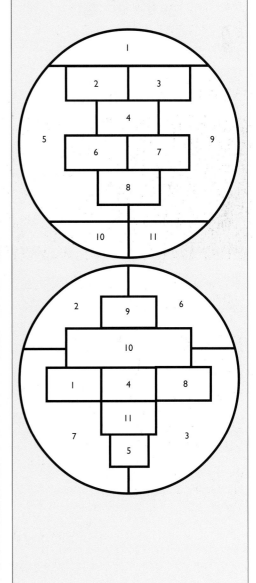

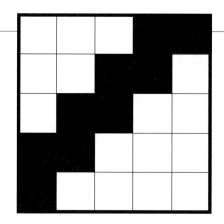

PLAYTHINK 704

DIFFICULTY: ●●●●●●●○○○
REQUIRED: 👁 ✎
COMPLETION: ☐ TIME: _____

QUEENS' STANDOFF

1. Can you place ten queens on a standard chessboard so that each queen can attack only one other queen?

2. Can you place fourteen queens so that each can attack exactly two other queens?

3. Can you place sixteen queens on a standard chessboard so that each can attack only three other queens?

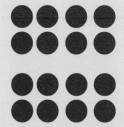

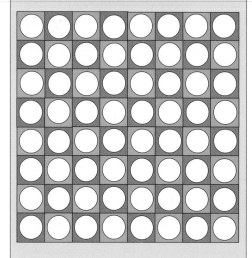

PLAYTHINK 705

DIFFICULTY: ●●●●●●○○○○
REQUIRED: 👁 ✎ 📄 ✂
COMPLETION: ☐ TIME: _____

ZIGZAG OVERLAP

Can you work out how to fit the eight strips into the five-by-five grid so that you will see the continuous black band running diagonally across the board, as shown?

What is the sequence in which the strips must be laid?

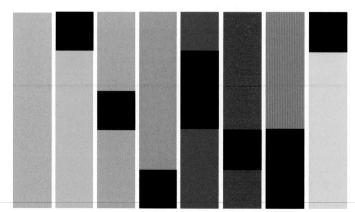

PLAYTHINK 706

DIFFICULTY: ●●●●●●○○○○
REQUIRED: 👁 ✎
COMPLETION: ☐ TIME: _____

OVERLAP

Three identical rectangular frames are placed one on top of the other, as shown. The result of their intersections is seven regions. Can you work out a way to obtain twenty-five regions from the intersection of the same overlapping rectangles?

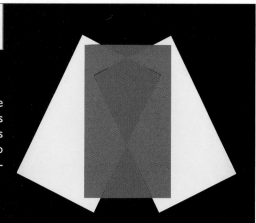

PLAYTHINK 707

DIFFICULTY: ●●●●●●●○○○
REQUIRED: 👁 ✎
COMPLETION: ☐ TIME: _____

SNAKE

Nine disks are arranged as shown, with the eye of the snake on the left. The object of this puzzle is to transfer the eye to the other end in the fewest possible number of moves. (In this puzzle a move counts as an instance in which you place a disk in one of the three spaces in the side of the snake.)

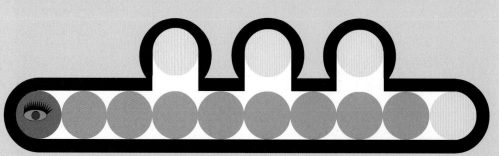

Möbius Strip

Bizarre shapes and strange connections make math interesting, and nothing is more strangely fascinating than the simplicity and topology of the Möbius strip. The nineteenth-century German mathematician A. F. Möbius discovered that it was possible to make a surface that has only one side and one edge.

Although such an object seems impossible to imagine, making a

Möbius strip is very simple: take a strip of ordinary paper and give one end a twist, then glue the two ends together. And there it is. If you begin drawing a line lengthwise down the strip, after one full revolution you will be at the point where you started— but on the opposite "side" of the strip! Drawing the line through another full revolution will find you back at the beginning.

Möbius strips are fun to play

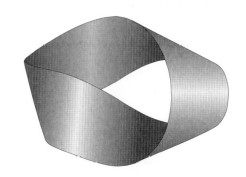

with, but industrial engineers have made good use of the shape as well. Conveyor belts are often designed as Möbius strips so that the surface wears out half as fast.

PLAYTHINK 708

DIFFICULTY: ●●●●○○○○○○○○
REQUIRED: ◉ ✂
COMPLETION: ☐ TIME:

MÖBIUS STRIP I

If you cut a Möbius strip lengthwise down the center until you wind up back at the beginning, can you work out what will happen to the strip?

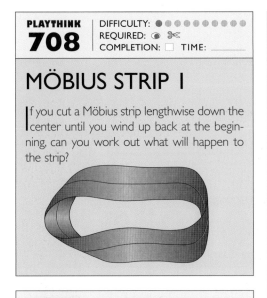

PLAYTHINK 709

DIFFICULTY: ●●●●●●●●○○○○
REQUIRED: ◉ ✂
COMPLETION: ☐ TIME:

MÖBIUS STRIP 2

If you cut a Möbius strip lengthwise into thirds, each one-third from an edge, can you work out what will happen to the strip?

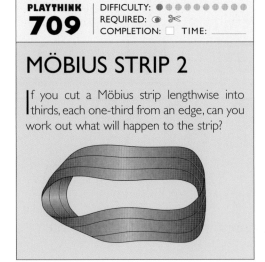

PLAYTHINK 710

DIFFICULTY: ●●●●○○○○○○○○
REQUIRED: ◉ ✎
COMPLETION: ☐ TIME:

MAP COLORING 2

Try your newly acquired map-coloring skills on these eight puzzles. Any two neighboring regions must be filled in with different colors. What is the smallest number of colors necessary to completely fill in each map?

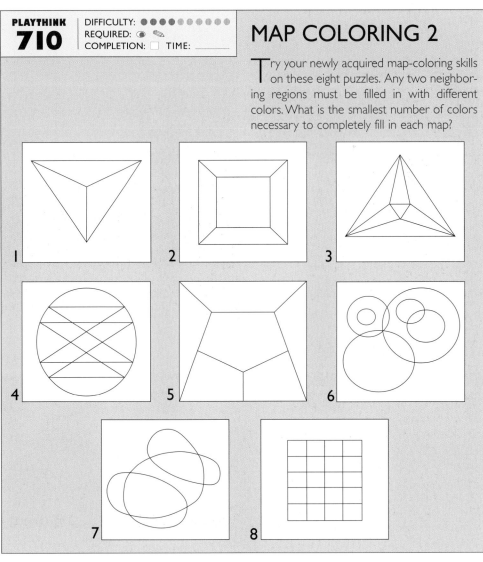

PLAYTHINK 711

DIFFICULTY: ●●●●○○○○○○
REQUIRED: ◉ ✄
COMPLETION: ☐ TIME: _____

HYPERCARD RING

This diagram shows a curious piece of furniture made from a single piece of bent plywood. As you can see, it is circular, with two benches on the inside of the ring and one bench on the outside.

Can you construct a model of the structure from a single strip of paper? Once you have made the model, can you see how to use it to show an opposite configuration for the benches—two on the outside and one on the inside?

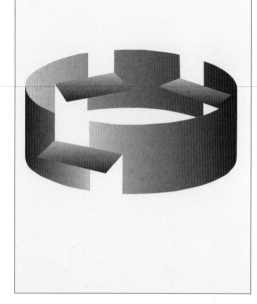

PLAYTHINK 712

DIFFICULTY: ●●●●●○○○○○
REQUIRED: ◉ ✎
COMPLETION: ☐ TIME: _____

LADYBUG GAME

■ *Three-in-a-Row Problem*

Twenty-one ladybugs must divide up a seven-by-seven flowerbed. Only three ladybugs may share a row, and any pair of adjacent rows or columns can have no more than one pair of bugs that share a common edge.

Can you find a way to distribute the ladybugs in that manner?

You can make this a two-person game. Players alternate placing ladybugs on the board according to the rules; the last player who can do so wins.

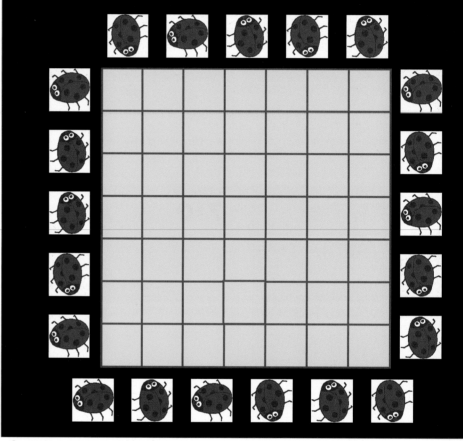

PLAYTHINK 713

DIFFICULTY: ●●●●●●○○○○
REQUIRED: ◉
COMPLETION: ☐ TIME: _____

TOPOLOGICAL EQUIVALENCE 3

These fourteen drawings include three quartets and one pair of topologically equivalent figures.

Can you identify the solitary pair amid the quartets?

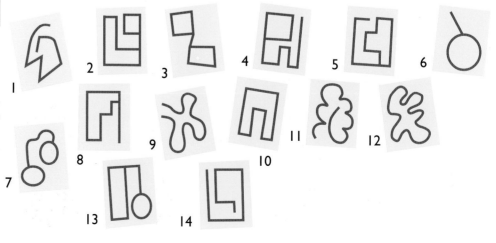

PLAYTHINK
714 | DIFFICULTY: ●●●●●●●●○○
REQUIRED: ◉ ✎
COMPLETION: ☐ TIME: _____

M-PIRE COLORING GAME

The four-color problem is the most famous map puzzle, but there's another, equally challenging puzzle that involves allowing different regions of the map to belong to the same "empire," which requires that they receive the same color. If each empire consists of exactly *M* regions this is called the "M-pire" problem.

The usual map-coloring question is a 1-pire problem. A 2-pire problem considers maps in which pairs of allied regions are considered—and the map must use the same color for both halves of the 2-pire, though different 2-pires can be different colors. And, of course, no two adjacent areas can be the same color.

Given that, can you work out the minimum number of colors needed to complete a 2-pire map?

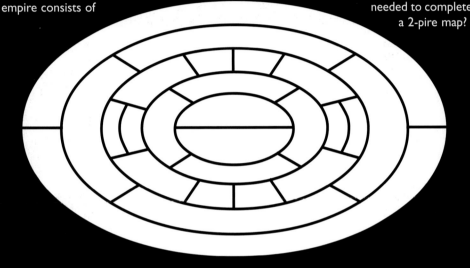

PLAYTHINK
715 | DIFFICULTY: ●●●●●●●○○○
REQUIRED: ◉
COMPLETION: ☐ TIME: _____

TOPOLOGY OF THE ALPHABET

Two figures are topologically equivalent if one can be continuously deformed into the other. A triangle, to the topologist's eye, is no different than a square or even a circle.

The letter *E*, in the font shown below, is topologically equivalent to five other letters. Can you work out which ones?

ABCDE
FGHIJ
KLMNO
PQRST
UVWXYZ

PLAYTHINK
716 | DIFFICULTY: ●●●●●●○○○○
REQUIRED: ◉ ✎
COMPLETION: ☐ TIME: _____

COLORING POLYHEDRONS

There are five regular solids, or polyhedrons: the tetrahedron (four faces), the cube (six faces), the octahedron (eight faces), the dodecahedron (twelve faces) and the icosahedron (twenty faces). To help you color in each face, you can think of each polyhedron as a map on a sphere, although it's a rather bent and bumpy sphere.

To aid in coloring, the five regular solids shown at right are covered with a rubber sheet. This allows us to "skin" the figures to create plane graphs that can easily be colored.

Using these graphs as a guide, can you work out how many colors are needed to fill in the faces of the five regular polyhedrons? Remember, the areas beyond the edges of the graph count as an additional side.

1

2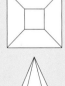

3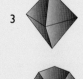

4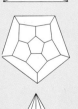

PLAYTHINK 717 | DIFFICULTY: ●●●●●●○○○○
REQUIRED: ◉ ✎
COMPLETION: ☐ TIME: _____

NO-TWO-IN-A-LINE 1

■ *Queens' Standoff*

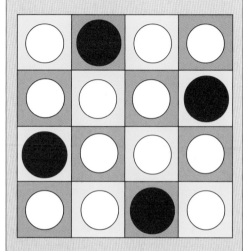

The four red counters in the top diagram are placed in a four-by-four matrix so that no two lie on the same vertical, horizontal or diagonal line. Can you place five counters on a five-by-five board under the same restrictions?

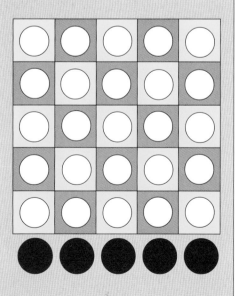

PLAYTHINK 718 | DIFFICULTY: ●●●●●●○○○○
REQUIRED: ◉ ✎
COMPLETION: ☐ TIME: _____

NO-TWO-IN-A-LINE 2

Can you place six counters on this six-by-six board so that no two lie on the same vertical, horizontal or diagonal line?

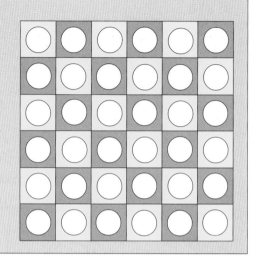

PLAYTHINK 719 | DIFFICULTY: ●●●●●●○○○○
REQUIRED: ◉ ✎
COMPLETION: ☐ TIME: _____

NO-TWO-IN-A-LINE 3

Can you place seven counters on the seven-by-seven board so that no two lie on the same vertical, horizontal or diagonal line?

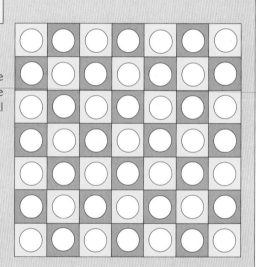

PLAYTHINK 720 | DIFFICULTY: ●●●●●●●○○○
REQUIRED: ◉ ✎
COMPLETION: ☐ TIME: _____

NO-TWO-IN-A-LINE 4

■ *The Eight Queens Puzzle*

Can you place eight counters on the eight-by-eight board so that no two are on the same vertical, horizontal or diagonal line?

This is essentially the same as asking how to place eight queens on a chessboard so that none can attack another. Can you find the twelve different solutions?

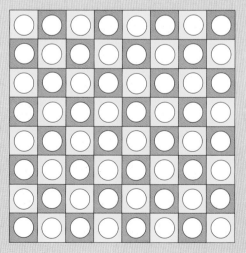

PLAYTHINK 721

DIFFICULTY: ●●●●●●●○○○
REQUIRED: ◉ ✎
COMPLETION: ☐ TIME: _____

NO-TWO-IN-A-LINE 5

■ *Triangular Grid*

Can you place seven counters on the circles so that no two will be on the same grid line in any direction?

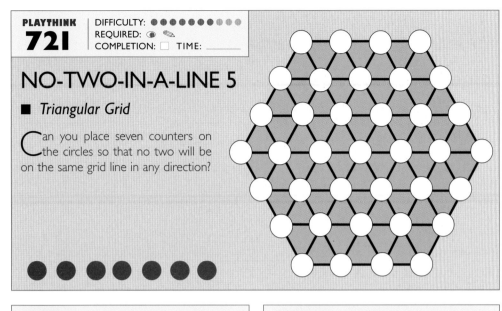

PLAYTHINK 722

DIFFICULTY: ●●●●●●●●○○
REQUIRED: ◉ ✎
COMPLETION: ☐ TIME: _____

QUEENS' COLOR STANDOFF 1

An interesting variation of the classic eight queens problem involves the placement of differently colored queens. The general question is, how many queens of two (or even more) colors can be placed on a given board so that no queen can be attacked by a piece of another color? That is, no two queens of differing colors may lie on the same vertical, horizontal or diagonal line.

Can you work out how to place five red queens and five blue queens on a six-by-six chessboard so that no queen can be attacked?

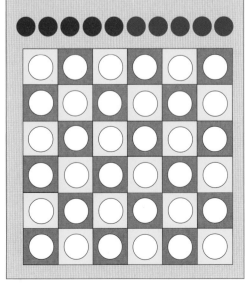

PLAYTHINK 723

DIFFICULTY: ●●●●●●●●○○
REQUIRED: ◉ ✎
COMPLETION: ☐ TIME: _____

QUEENS' COLOR STANDOFF 2

Can you put all twelve red queens and all twelve blue queens on a nine-by-nine chessboard so that no queen can attack a queen of another color?

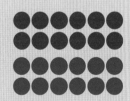

PLAYTHINK 724

DIFFICULTY: ●●●●●●●○○○
REQUIRED: ◉
COMPLETION: ☐ TIME: _____

CUTTING A CUBE

How many of the shapes shown below can be made with a single stroke of a sharp knife through a cube?

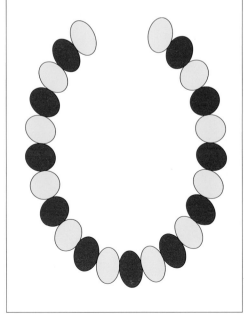

PLAYTHINK 725

DIFFICULTY: ●●●●●●○○○○
REQUIRED: ◉ ✎
COMPLETION: ☐ TIME: _____

MINIMAL NECKLACE

A twenty-three-bead necklace is shown here. You want to disconnect individual beads to break the necklace into smaller lengths that can then be rejoined to form every possible length from one to twenty-three beads.

Can you work out how many beads must be disconnected to accomplish this?

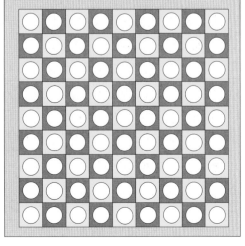

Knots

Everyone who can tie his shoes understands a little about knots. But mathematicians have turned knots into a field for deep topological study. Don't expect to untie a mathematical knot: both ends of the mathematician's knot are joined to form an endless loop. Such linear structures extending into three dimensions are the simplest representations of curves in three-dimensional space. (The more advanced topological concepts are surfaces and the multidimensional structures known as manifolds.)

This is the first question in knot theory: Can two closed strings made of extensible but impenetrable material be changed by continuous transformation into strings of congruent form? Although knots are one-dimensional, they are trickier than surfaces; untying them poses great problems, many of which are still unanswered. Even in the simplest cases, establishing the proof is a daunting task.

The topology of knots is not merely of interest to recreational and professional mathematicians. It has enormous importance in several other branches of science, particularly molecular biology. The structure of the DNA molecule and those of complexly folded proteins have been elucidated with the help of the mathematical answer to the question, How does one untangle very long three-dimensional knots?

PLAYTHINK 726

DIFFICULTY: ●●●●●●○○○○
REQUIRED: ◉
COMPLETION: ☐   TIME: _____

SHADOW KNOT

You see a length of rope on the floor before you. It is too dark to tell whether the strands pass over or under the loop at the three points of intersection. Depending on how the rope lies, pulling on the ends could tighten a knot in the rope.

Is that likely? Given that the way the rope lies is purely random, can you work out the probability that the rope is knotted rather than simply looped loosely?

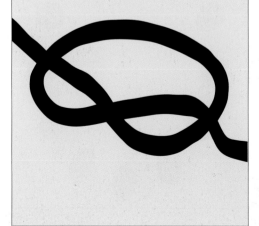

PLAYTHINK 727

DIFFICULTY: ●●●●●●○○○○
REQUIRED: ◉
COMPLETION: ☐   TIME: _____

WATER HOSE

This garden hose is a mess. If you pull it tight at both ends, how many knots will be formed?

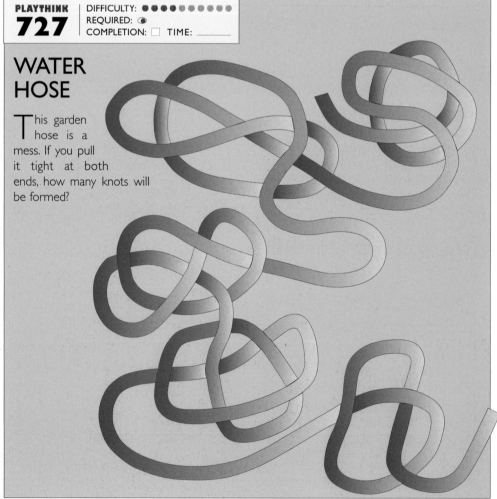

PLAYTHINK 728 | DIFFICULTY: ●●●●●○○○○○
REQUIRED: ◉ ✏
COMPLETION: ☐ TIME: _____

BEE ROOKS

The mathematician Herbert Taylor investigated the nonattacking principle found in the queens' standoff puzzles on hexagonal and triangular matrices. Here's a puzzle based on his findings.

Bees will attack one another if they share the same triangular row or column in the hexagonal grid. With that in mind, can you work out the greatest number of bees that can be placed on each of the four grids shown here?

Can you work out the minimum number of bees needed to guard the four grids, placed so that the addition of one more bee would trigger an attack?

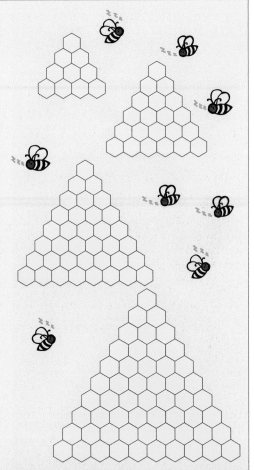

PLAYTHINK 729 | DIFFICULTY: ●●●●●●●○○○
REQUIRED: ◉
COMPLETION: ☐ TIME: _____

3-D KNOT

This figure shows a three-dimensional knot composed of the least possible number of unit cubes. Each cube is the same size, there are no loose ends, and the cubes are connected across their full faces.

Can you work out the number of cubes needed to make this figure?

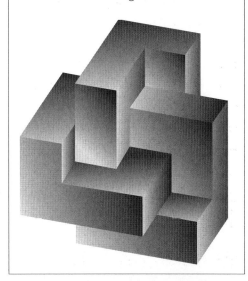

PLAYTHINK 730 | DIFFICULTY: ●●●●●●●○○○
REQUIRED: ◉
COMPLETION: ☐ TIME: _____

DIVORCEE'S BELT

A faded movie queen, recently divorced (for the third time) and down to her last mink coat, is stranded in a fashionable hotel in Cannes with no immediately available liquid assets. The hotel management has cut her credit line and put her on a cash-in-advance status. The ex-star is willing to make payments only one day at a time. She is expecting an alimony payment in just eleven days, but until then she has no cash on hand.

She has persuaded the hotel to accept a link of her gold belt for a day's rent, with the understanding that when the check arrives, she can buy it back. Her problem is that because she expects to have belt back soon, she does not want to cut it up any more than required.

Can you find the minimum number of cuts needed so that she can pay for one to eleven days, one day at a time?

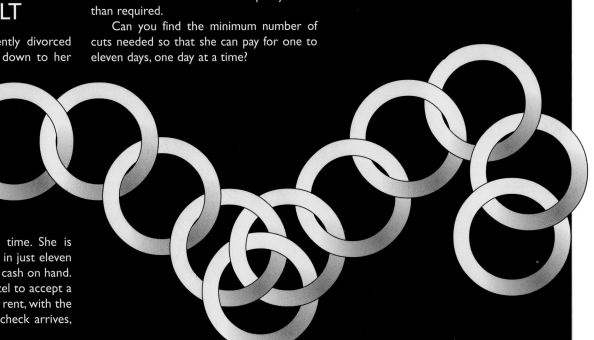

PLAYTHINK
731
DIFFICULTY: ●●●●●●○○○○
REQUIRED: 👁 ✎
COMPLETION: ☐ TIME: _____

TURNABOUT GAME

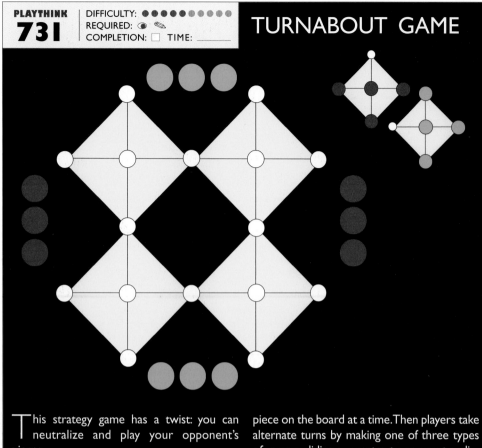

This strategy game has a twist: you can neutralize and play your opponent's pieces.

Each player gets six counters—either red or blue on one side and black on the other. When a piece is flipped over to its black side, it can be moved by either player.

Play begins with each person placing one piece on the board at a time. Then players take alternate turns by making one of three types of moves: sliding a counter to an empty adjacent space, jumping over another piece into an empty space or turning a counter over.

The first player who can maneuver four of his or her non-neutral pieces into the shape of a triangle, as shown in the inset diagram, wins.

PLAYTHINK
732
DIFFICULTY: ●●●●●●●●●○
REQUIRED: 👁
COMPLETION: ☐ TIME: _____

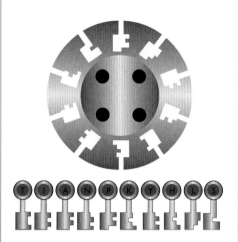

COMBINATION LOCK

A safe has ten locks requiring ten keys, each bearing a different letter. The safe opens only after all ten keys have been inserted in the locks.

There are 3.6 million possible combinations, but fortunately, you have a diagram of the interior of the locks that shows the shapes of the appropriate keys.

Can you work out the correct order for the keys? What word do the keys spell out?

PLAYTHINK
733
DIFFICULTY: ●●●●●●○○○○
REQUIRED: 👁
COMPLETION: ☐ TIME: _____

KEYS TO THE KEYS

A circular ring holds ten keys, each with a round handle. The keys are in an order that you have memorized, and each fits one of ten different locks. The trouble is that you work in the dark and you can't see the key ring—you have to feel the keys with your fingers. If you had a way to tell by touch which key was which, it wouldn't take you long to unlock the doors.

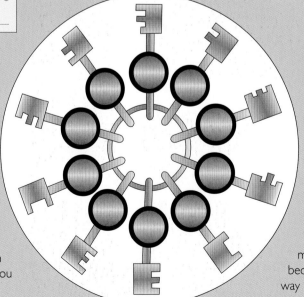

One solution is to give the keys differently shaped handles. But do you have to give all ten different handles?

Can you work out the smallest number of keys you need to mark so that you can identify where you are on the ring by touch alone? Is there a specific arrangement that the marked keys must have along the ring?

One clue: Remember that any symmetrical arrangement of keys will fail. That's because in the dark you won't know which way you are holding the ring.

PLAYTHINK 734

DIFFICULTY: ●●●●●●●●○○
REQUIRED: 👁 ✏
COMPLETION: ☐ TIME: _____

SUPERQUEENS

A superqueen is an imaginary chess piece that has the attacking range of a queen and a knight combined.

More than sixty years ago the mathematician George Polya discovered that with less than ten, it was impossible to place *n* superqueens on an *n*-by-*n* chessboard so that none would come under attack.

But what about ten superqueens? Can you work out how to place ten superqueens on a ten-by-ten board so that none of them can attack another?

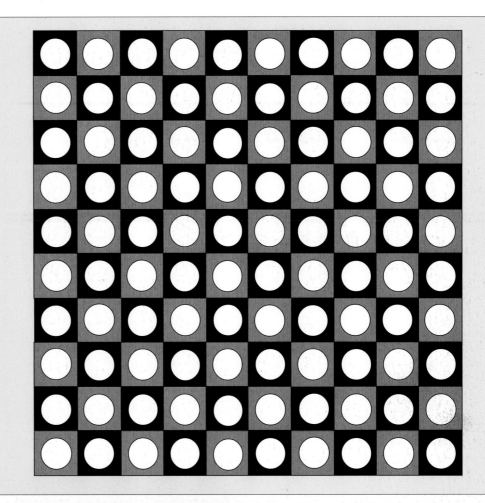

PLAYTHINK 735

DIFFICULTY: ●●●●●●●○○○
REQUIRED: 👁
COMPLETION: ☐ TIME: _____

SLIDING LOCK

The disk and colored blocks are embedded in a grooved plate. The blocks can slide in the grooves whenever another block isn't in the way. The disk can rotate freely and carries a square red block in its notch.

Given that information, can you find a way to slide the yellow piston from the bottom of the groove to the top of the groove? How many moves will be needed, and in what sequence?

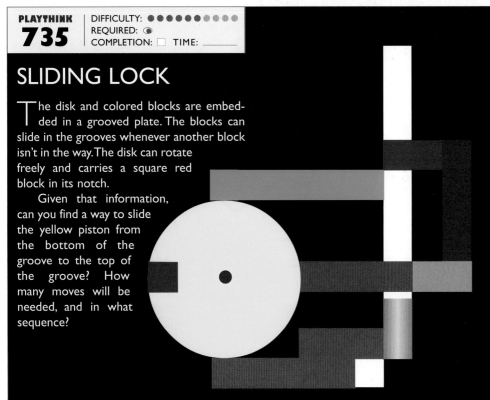

PLAYTHINK 736

DIFFICULTY: ●●●●●●●○○○
REQUIRED: 👁 ✏ 📄 ✂
COMPLETION: ☐ TIME: _____

POLYGON CYCLE

Set up the five disks with polygons as shown. Moving one disk at a time into an empty adjacent circle along the connecting lines, can you exchange the star with the hexagon? What is the smallest number of moves needed to do this?

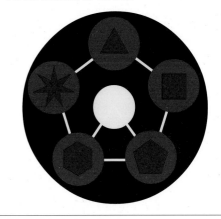

PLAYTHINK **737** | DIFFICULTY: ●●●●●●○○○○
REQUIRED: 👁 ✏ 📄 ✂
COMPLETION: ☐ TIME: _____

SLIDING ZOO

Ten animals have been distributed randomly into ten cages. Each cage has three doorsize — one to the cage on either side and one to the center enclosure.

Without putting two animals together in the same cage or in the central enclosure at the same time, can you work out a plan for moving all the animals to their proper cages (by matching the colors in the circles to the colors of the cages)? How many moves will it take?

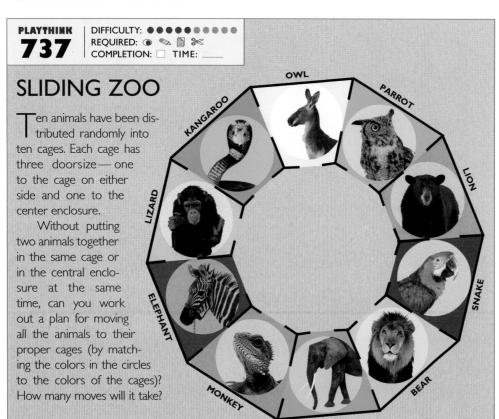

PLAYTHINK **738** | DIFFICULTY: ●●●●●○○○○○
REQUIRED: 👁
COMPLETION: ☐ TIME: _____

LOOP RELEASE

The man shown would like to release the loop, but he is unwilling to take his hand out of his pocket, take off his vest or stuff the rope into his pocket. Can you work out how he can do it?

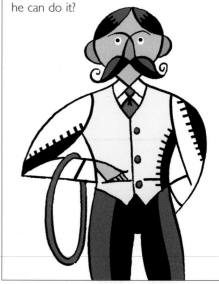

PLAYTHINK **739** | DIFFICULTY: ●●●●●●●●●●
REQUIRED: 👁 ✏
COMPLETION: ☐ TIME: _____

BRAMS'S COLORING GAME

This is a more advanced map-coloring game devised by New York University political scientist Steven J. Brams. Two players take turns filling in the map one region at a time so that no two adjacent regions have the same color. Each player has a selection of five colors to choose from.

This may sound like other map-coloring games, but here's where it differs: The two players have different roles. Player 1 is the minimizer, whose aim is to play so that by the end of the game the entire map has been filled in using five or fewer colors. Player 2 is the maximizer, whose aim is to play so that at some point none of the five colors will be sufficient to fill in an empty region. Whoever achieves his or her aim wins the game.

Can you work out a strategy for the maximizer so that he or she will always win?

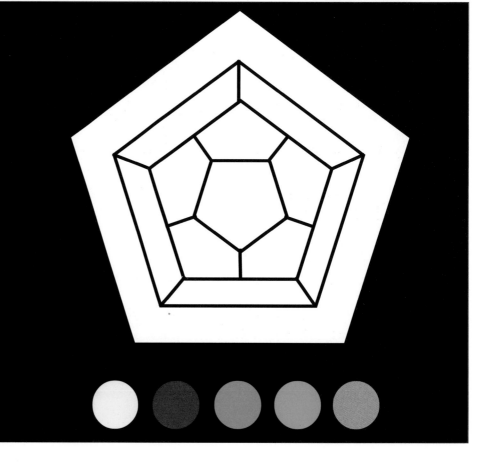

PLAYTHINK
740
DIFFICULTY: ●●●●●●○○○○
REQUIRED: ◉ ✎
COMPLETION: ☐ TIME: _____

NO-THREE-IN-A-LINE I

Minimal Problem

Can you place six counters on the five-by-five board so that placing a seventh counter on any vacant circle will make a vertical, horizontal or diagonal line contain three counters?

Maximal Problem

Can you place ten counters on the five-by-five board so that placing an eleventh counter on any vacant circle will make a vertical, horizontal *and* diagonal line contain three counters?

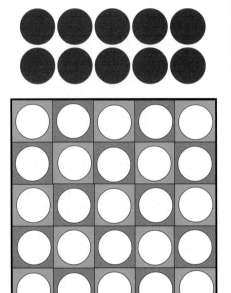

PLAYTHINK
741
DIFFICULTY: ●●●●●●○○○○
REQUIRED: ◉ ✎
COMPLETION: ☐ TIME: _____

NO-THREE-IN-A-LINE 2

Minimal Problem

Can you place six counters on the six-by-six board so that placing a seventh counter on any vacant circle will make a vertical, horizontal or diagonal line contain three counters?

Maximal Problem

Can you place twelve counters on the six-by-six board so that placing a thirteenth counter on any open circle will make a vertical, horizontal *and* diagonal line contain three counters?

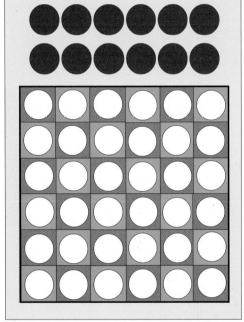

PLAYTHINK
742
DIFFICULTY: ●●●●●●●○○○
REQUIRED: ◉ ✎
COMPLETION: ☐ TIME: _____

NO-THREE-IN-A-LINE 3

Minimal Problem

Can you place eight counters on the seven-by-seven board so that placing a ninth counter on any open circle will make a vertical, horizontal or diagonal line contain three counters?

Maximal Problem

Can you place fourteen counters on the seven-by-seven board so that placing a fifteenth counter on any open circle will make a vertical, horizontal *and* diagonal line contain three counters?

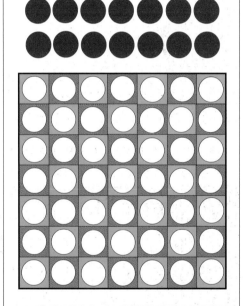

PLAYTHINK
743
DIFFICULTY: ●●●●●●●●○○
REQUIRED: ◉ ✎
COMPLETION: ☐ TIME: _____

NO-THREE-IN-A-LINE 4

Can you place sixteen counters on the eight-by-eight board so that placing a seventeenth counter on any open circle will make a vertical, horizontal or diagonal line contain three counters?

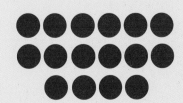

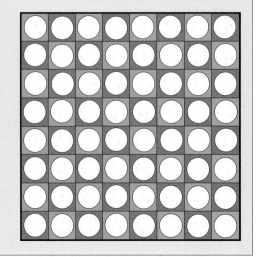

Map Folding

Ever since the twentieth-century Polish mathematician Stanislaw Ulam first posed the question of how many different ways a map can be folded, the problem has frustrated researchers in the field of modern combinatorial theory. Indeed, the general problem is still unsolved.

The difficulty arises from the fact that even the simplest map—or any rectangular piece of paper—has many possible ways of being folded. There is an old saying that you have no doubt come across: "The easiest way to fold a map is differently."

PLAYTHINK 744 | DIFFICULTY: ●●●●●○○○○○ | REQUIRED: ◉ ✂ | COMPLETION: ☐ TIME: _____

FOLDING A THREE-SQUARE STRIP

How many different ways can you find to fold a three-square paper strip?

The folds must be confined to creases between the squares, and the final product must be a stack with each square neatly under another.

The squares are the same color on both sides, so it doesn't matter which side is up on the final stack.

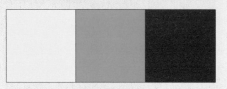

PLAYTHINK 745 | DIFFICULTY: ●●●●●●●○○○ | REQUIRED: ◉ ✂ | COMPLETION: ☐ TIME: _____

FOLDING A FOUR-SQUARE SQUARE

How many different ways can you find to fold a four-square paper square?

The folds must be confined to creases between the squares, and the final product must be a stack with each square neatly under another.

The squares are the same color on both sides, so it doesn't matter which side is up on the final stack.

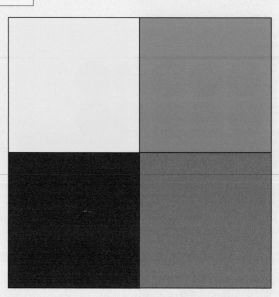

PLAYTHINK 746 | DIFFICULTY: ●●●●○○○○○○ | REQUIRED: ◉ | COMPLETION: ☐ TIME: _____

FOLDING A NEWSPAPER

Take a sheet of ordinary newspaper and fold it in half. Easy, right?

Do you think you can fold the newspaper on itself ten more times?

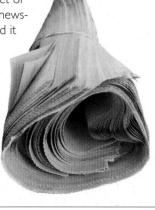

PLAYTHINK 747 | DIFFICULTY: ●●●●●○○○○○ | REQUIRED: ◉ ✂ | COMPLETION: ☐ TIME: _____

FOLDING A FOUR-SQUARE STRIP

How many different ways can you find to fold a four-square paper strip?

The folds must be confined to creases between the squares, and the final product must be a stack with each square neatly under another.

The squares are the same color on both sides, so it doesn't matter which side is up on the final stack.

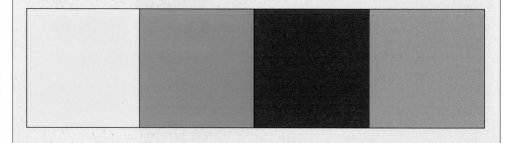

PLAYTHINK
748 | DIFFICULTY: ●●●●●●○○○○
REQUIRED: ◉
COMPLETION: ☐ TIME: _____

WORD CHAINS

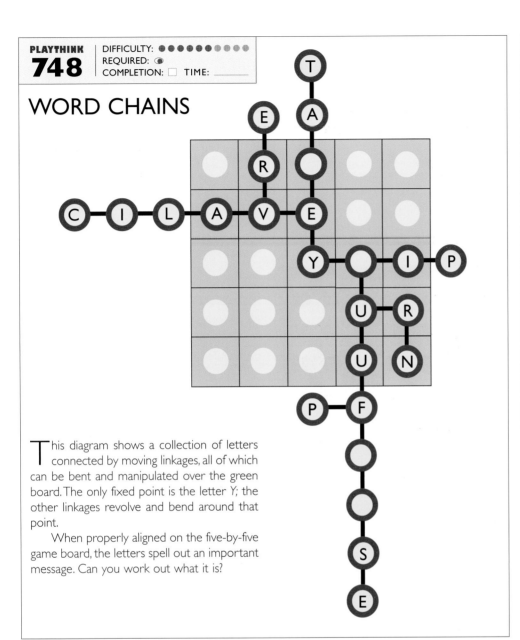

This diagram shows a collection of letters connected by moving linkages, all of which can be bent and manipulated over the green board. The only fixed point is the letter Y; the other linkages revolve and bend around that point.

When properly aligned on the five-by-five game board, the letters spell out an important message. Can you work out what it is?

PLAYTHINK
750 | DIFFICULTY: ●●●●●●○○○○
REQUIRED: ◉ ✎
COMPLETION: ☐ TIME: _____

DIFFERENT DISTANCE MATRIX 5

Can you work out how to place five counters on a five-by-five matrix so that the distance between any two counters is unique?

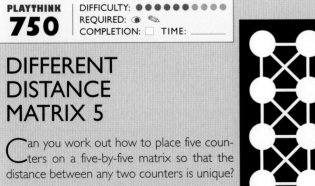

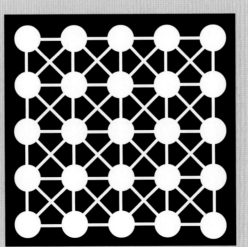

PLAYTHINK
749 | DIFFICULTY: ●●●●●●●○○○
REQUIRED: ◉ ✎
COMPLETION: ☐ TIME: _____

DIFFERENT DISTANCE MATRIX 4

The class of problems known as different distance matrices asks how to place counters on a square grid so that the distance between every two counters is unique. On a straight line the problem is very simple—three counters on a number line could be at points 0, 1 and 3 to ensure that the distance between every pair of counters is unique. In two dimensions the problem becomes much more complicated.

For the purposes of these puzzles, assume that each counter marks the center of the circle and that the distances are measured along a straight line joining the two centers.

Can you work out how to place four counters on a four-by-four matrix so that every pair of counters has a unique distance?

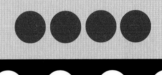

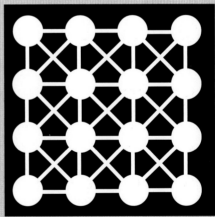

PLAYTHINK 751

DIFFICULTY: ●●●●●●●○○○
REQUIRED: ◉ ✎
COMPLETION: ☐ TIME: _____

DIFFERENT DISTANCE MATRIX 6

Can you work out how to place six counters on a six-by-six matrix so that the distance between any pair of counters is unique?

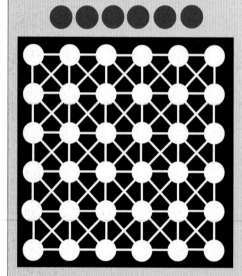

PLAYTHINK 752

DIFFICULTY: ●●●●●●●●○○
REQUIRED: ◉ ✎
COMPLETION: ☐ TIME: _____

DIFFERENT DISTANCE MATRIX 7

Can you work out how to place seven counters on a seven-by-seven matrix so that the distance between any pair of counters is unique?

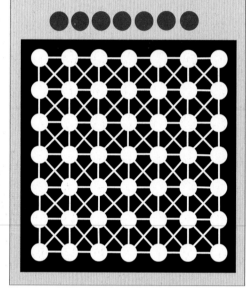

PLAYTHINK 753

DIFFICULTY: ●●●●●●○○○○
REQUIRED: ◉ ✎
COMPLETION: ☐ TIME: _____

CROSSROADS

The object of this puzzle is to place seven coins or counters on the eight points of the octagonal star. Coins are placed one at a time on any unoccupied circle. But every coin that is placed must be immediately transferred to one of two other points that are connected by a straight line to the initial circle. Once moved, a coin cannot be moved again.

Although the puzzle is complicated, a simple strategy will enable you to solve it every time. Can you work it out?

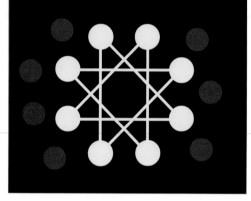

PLAYTHINK 754

DIFFICULTY: ●●●●●●●○○○
REQUIRED: ◉ ✎
COMPLETION: ☐ TIME: _____

TWO-COLOR CUBES

Can you work out all the distinct ways the faces of a cube may be filled in using just two colors?

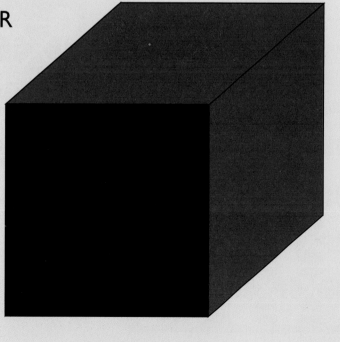

PLAYTHINK 755

DIFFICULTY: ●●●●●●●○○○
REQUIRED: ◉
COMPLETION: ☐ TIME: _____

SHORTEST CATCH

The ladybug wants to reach the aphid as quickly as possible. Is the path marked the shortest route possible?

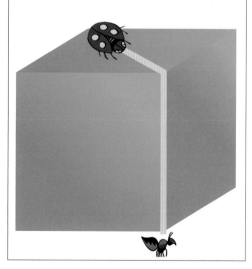

PLAYTHINK
756

DIFFICULTY: ●●●●○○○○○○○○
REQUIRED: ◉
COMPLETION: ☐ TIME: _____

LINK RINGS

A blacksmith has been asked to make one long chain from five three-link bits of chain. Can you find a way to do it so that he has to make just three welds?

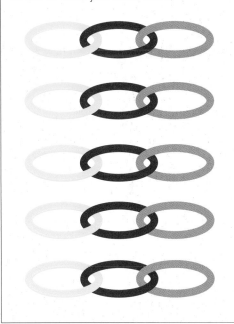

PLAYTHINK
757

DIFFICULTY: ●●●●●●○○○○○○
REQUIRED: ◉ ✎
COMPLETION: ☐ TIME: _____

CROSSING THE BRIDGE

Your job is to move all the blue cars to the right bank of the river and all the red cars to the left bank. You are allowed to move only one car at a time, and each continuous movement, no matter the distance, is considered one move.

Can you work out how to transfer the cars in the fewest possible moves?

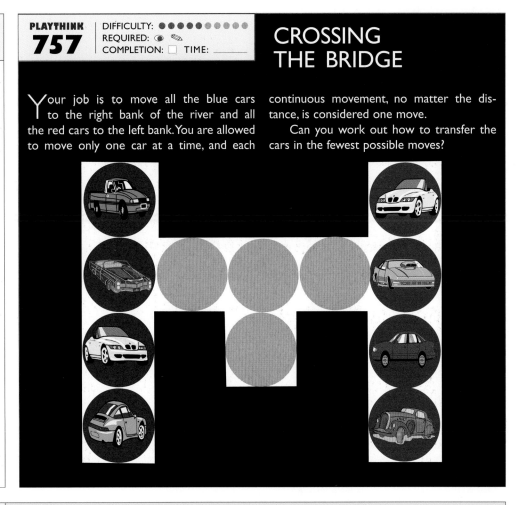

PLAYTHINK
758

DIFFICULTY: ●●●●●●●○○○○○
REQUIRED: ◉ ✎
COMPLETION: ☐ TIME: _____

JUMPING DISKS

The object of these two puzzles is to reverse the pattern by exchanging the two sets of disks. To do this, five rules must be observed:

1. Only one disk may be moved at a time.

2. A disk may move into an adjacent empty space.

3. A disk may jump over a disk of the opposite color into the space immediately beyond it.

4. A disk may not jump over a disk of the same color.

5. No backward moves are permitted.

Also, each move must involve landing in a numbered space (no jumping off the ends!), and no move may disturb another disk in the process (no pushing).

Can you solve the puzzles in fifteen and twenty-four moves, respectively?

For a hint, look at the numbers below the disks. If you find the key there, you can solve not only these puzzles but others that are much more complicated.

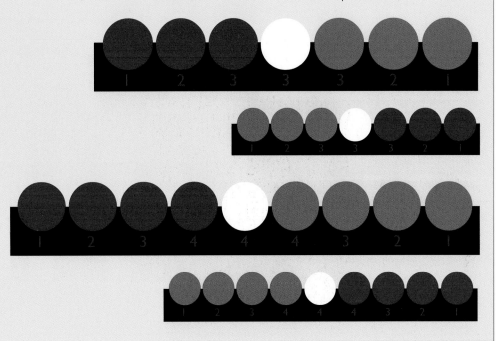

PLAYTHINK 759

DIFFICULTY: ●●●●●●●●●●
REQUIRED: 👁 ✏️
COMPLETION: ☐ TIME: _____

DISTORTRIX I

Can you tell what is the subject of this distorted image just by looking at it? If not, redraw the image using the empty grid at the bottom.

You can check your solution by placing a cylindrical mirror on the red circle. You will see the undistorted image in the mirror.

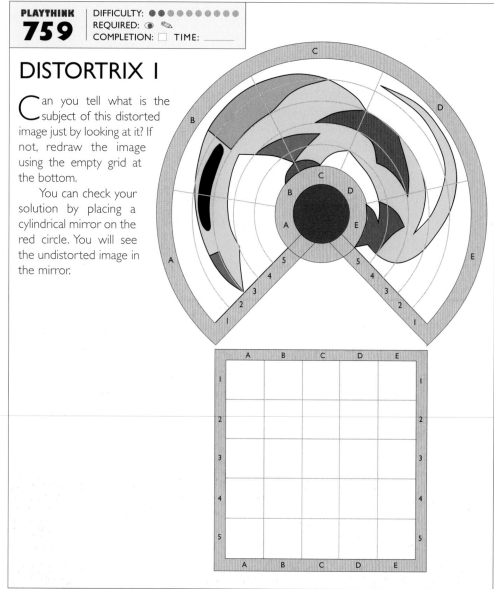

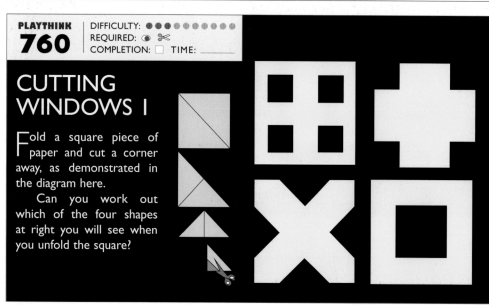

PLAYTHINK 760

DIFFICULTY: ●●●●●●●●●●
REQUIRED: 👁 ✂️
COMPLETION: ☐ TIME: _____

CUTTING WINDOWS I

Fold a square piece of paper and cut a corner away, as demonstrated in the diagram here.

Can you work out which of the four shapes at right you will see when you unfold the square?

PLAYTHINK 761

DIFFICULTY: ●●●●●●●●●●
REQUIRED: 👁
COMPLETION: ☐ TIME: _____

CUBE FOLD I

The pattern below can be folded along the creases between the squares to form a cube box. Can you work out which colors will be on opposite faces when the cube is folded?

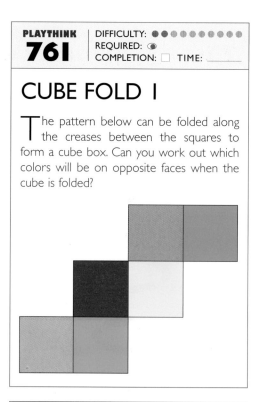

PLAYTHINK 762

DIFFICULTY: ●●●●●●●●●●
REQUIRED: 👁
COMPLETION: ☐ TIME: _____

ONE IN SEVEN

Which of the cubes cannot be made from the partially filled-in pattern?

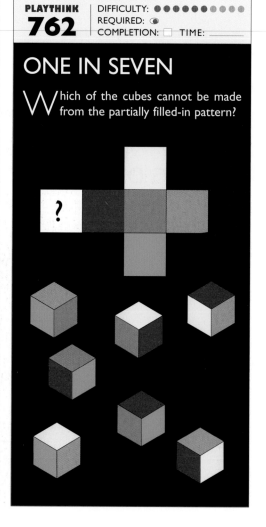

Distortions and Impossibilities

Toward the end of the nineteenth century, biologists noticed that in many cases evolution proceeded in a way that corresponded to a distorted framework—that is, it seemed as if the original plan of the creature had been distorted to form the more modern one. Then, in 1917, D'Arcy Thompson published his classic work, *Growth and Form,* in which he illustrated animal species that differed from one another only by anamorphic distortions—the animals shared a body plan, but certain parts had been stretched or shrunk in a mathematically predictable way.

This was all very intriguing until it was discovered that there are many, many cases in which two creatures that bear a close resemblance in form are not even closely related.

The limits to distortion can be found in mathematics as well. In topology, the way to change a shape is to distort it. Such distortions can be described mathematically: If a grid defines a shape, then a change to the grid will create a new shape. But the logic of the grid can change the shape only so far; push too much and you'll wind up with an impossible shape.

Although the easiest way to change a shape is to superimpose a square grid on the original and then reproduce the shape on a grid of different size, more interesting results can be obtained by redrawing the form on a distorted grid. Deliberate distortions have been found in pictorial representations from the earliest cave paintings to modern art. The sixteenth-century German artist Albrecht Dürer described various geometrical methods of changing the proportions of the human figure by means of altered coordinate systems. That particular method has the effect of producing grotesque but recognizable caricatures.

PLAYTHINK 763

DIFFICULTY: ●●●●●●○○○○
REQUIRED: ◉ ✎
COMPLETION: ☐ TIME: _____

CUBE TO CUBE

1. If a cube can be placed on a table in any of twenty-four different ways, how many different ways can two cubes be placed side by side on a table so that two faces touch each other?

2. When three cubes are placed side by side, what is the total number of different ways the cubes can be turned and still keep the same side by side arrangement?

3. Eight cubes can be stacked four on four to make a larger cube. If the cubes can turn in any way but still maintain their locations within the greater cube, what is the total number of ways the individual cubes can be turned?

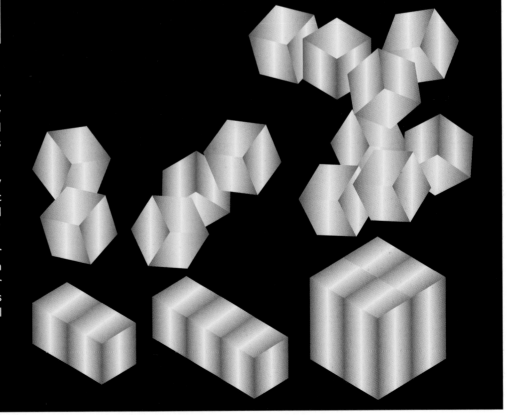

Anamorphic Distortions

When the human visual system is confronted with unusual projections, such as those found reflected in funhouse mirrors, it sometimes has difficulty piecing together the form of the original object. A simple but fascinating way to convey that sense of disorientation in a standard two-dimensional piece of art is through the so-called anamorphic projection.

Viewed from a standard perspective—with the observer's line of sight perpendicular to the picture—a piece of anamorphic art appears as a monstrous distortion. But the original image can be "formed again" (the translation of the Greek *anamorphe*) by viewing the picture on a slant or looking at its reflection in a cylindrical or conical mirror. Those who haven't previously encountered anamorphic art are usually amazed to see the undistorted reflection image seemingly pop out of nowhere.

The first slanted anamorphic image appears in the notebooks of Leonardo da Vinci, but anamorphic pictures were most popular about 300 years ago. Since then people have sometimes found it necessary to create such images for their protection. In England during the reigns of George I and George II, for instance, supporters of the outlawed and exiled pretender to the throne, Charles Edward Stuart, faced imprisonment for treason if they were found with a portrait of their preferred monarch, the "king over the water." Instead, they carried his anamorphic image.

Cognitive researchers have explored the underlying principle of anamorphic art. They asked experimental subjects to wear specially designed glasses that produced extreme topological deformations of the world around them—changing the perspective of things, for instance, or reversing their view of the world upside down or left to right. Their surprising finding was that not only did the subjects eventually adjust to their new "outlook" on the world but when they removed the glasses, their view of the unfiltered world was distorted, at least for a short period. Such experiments suggest that our visual system is more concerned with topologically invariant properties than with Euclidean ones.

PLAYTHINK 764

DIFFICULTY: ●●○○○○○○○○○
REQUIRED: ◉ ✎
COMPLETION: ☐   TIME: ___

DISTORTRIX 2

Can you tell who is the subject of the distorted portrait just by looking at it? If not, redraw the image using the empty grid at the right.

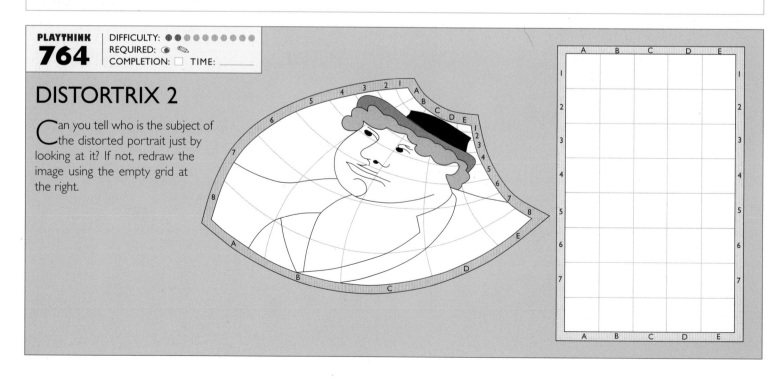

PLAYTHINK 765

DIFFICULTY: ●●○○○○○○○○○
REQUIRED: ◉
COMPLETION: ☐ TIME: _____

DISTORTIONS

This intriguing picture puzzle will test your powers of perception. Can you work out what is hidden in the image?

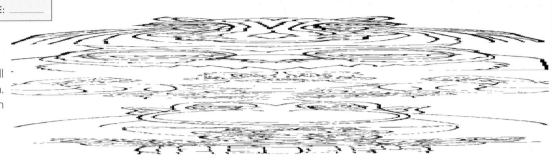

PLAYTHINK 766

DIFFICULTY: ●●●○○○○○○○○
REQUIRED: ◉ ✎
COMPLETION: ☐ TIME: _____

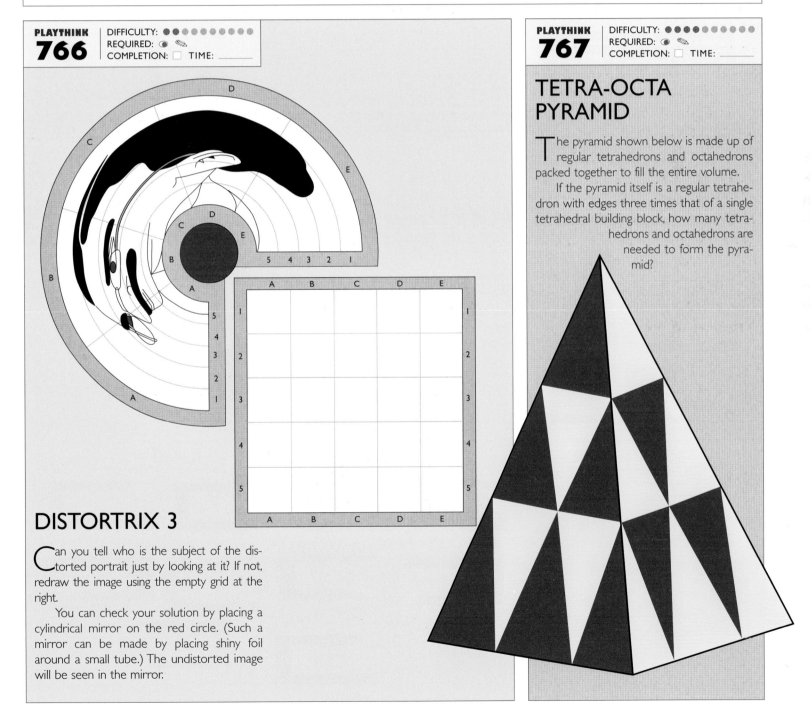

DISTORTRIX 3

Can you tell who is the subject of the distorted portrait just by looking at it? If not, redraw the image using the empty grid at the right.

You can check your solution by placing a cylindrical mirror on the red circle. (Such a mirror can be made by placing shiny foil around a small tube.) The undistorted image will be seen in the mirror.

PLAYTHINK 767

DIFFICULTY: ●●●○○○○○○○○
REQUIRED: ◉ ✎
COMPLETION: ☐ TIME: _____

TETRA-OCTA PYRAMID

The pyramid shown below is made up of regular tetrahedrons and octahedrons packed together to fill the entire volume.

If the pyramid itself is a regular tetrahedron with edges three times that of a single tetrahedral building block, how many tetrahedrons and octahedrons are needed to form the pyramid?

PLAYTHINK 768

DIFFICULTY: ●●●●●●●○○○
REQUIRED: 👁 ✏️ 📄 ✂️
COMPLETION: ☐ TIME: _____

EIGHT-BLOCK SLIDING PUZZLE

The diagram at top shows a group of numbered blocks. Can you rearrange the blocks by sliding them into open spaces so that they form the ordered configuration below? If so, what is the smallest number of moves needed to accomplish this?

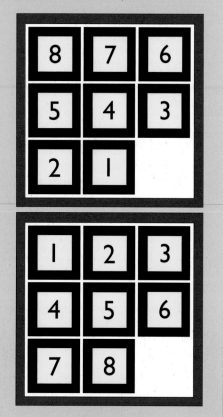

PLAYTHINK 769

DIFFICULTY: ●●●●●●○○○○
REQUIRED: 👁 ✂️
COMPLETION: ☐ TIME: _____

CUTTING WINDOWS 2

Fold a square piece of paper and cut a corner away, as demonstrated in the diagram here.

Can you work out which of the four shapes at right you will see when you unfold the square?

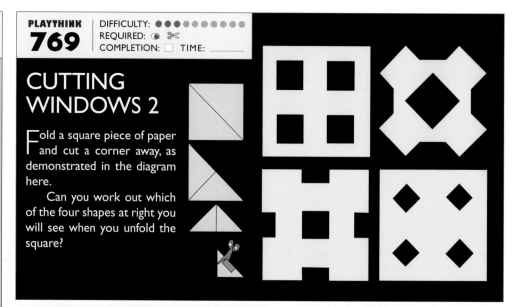

PLAYTHINK 770

DIFFICULTY: ●●●●●●●●●○
REQUIRED: 👁
COMPLETION: ☐ TIME: _____

CUBE RINGS

This cube ring is made up of twenty-two individual cube blocks. Amazingly, it has one face and one edge, like a Möbius strip.

Can you work out the structure of the one-sided block ring made of the fewest cube blocks?

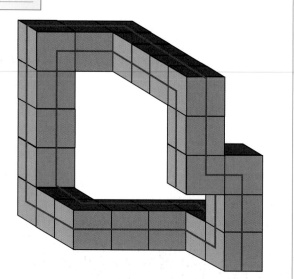

PLAYTHINK 771

DIFFICULTY: ●●●○○○○○○○
REQUIRED: 👁
COMPLETION: ☐ TIME: _____

IMPOSSIBLE RECTANGLES

Of the ten figures shown here, five are identical, counting rotations but not reflections. And another set of three is identical, also counting rotations. Two of the figures are unique. Can you work out which two?

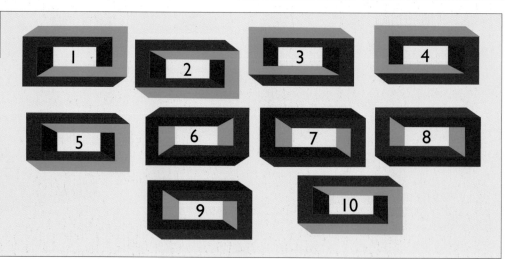

PLAYTHINK 772

DIFFICULTY: ●●●●●●●○○○
REQUIRED: ◉
COMPLETION: ☐ TIME: _____

BIG CUBE THROUGH A SMALLER CUBE

Can you cut a hole through a cube that will enable a bigger cube to pass through it?

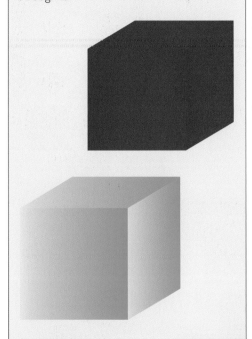

PLAYTHINK 773

DIFFICULTY: ●●●●●●●○○○
REQUIRED: ◉
COMPLETION: ☐ TIME: _____

COUNT THE CUBES

"Putting things into perspective" is such a common phrase that it's easy to forget that perspective does more than bring three-dimensional realism to a two-dimensional representation. It also helps us interpret things we can't see. That's because perspective lets us infer that objects follow certain geometric rules.

In the designs below, various combinations of cubes are stacked together. All the rows of cubes are complete unless you see them end. Most of the stacks are simple heaps, but some require you to understand that one or more rows continue, sight unseen, behind others. Such problems challenge your ability to judge spatial relationships.

Based on the visual evidence given, can you work out how many cubes make up each stack?

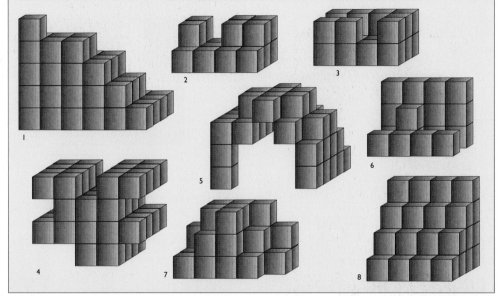

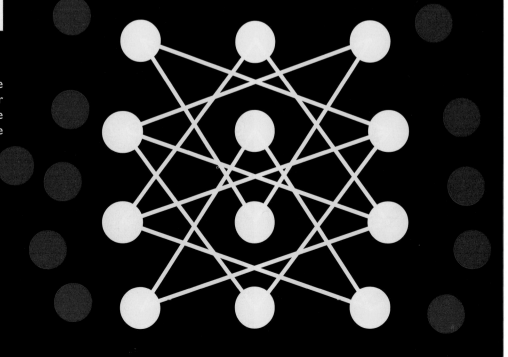

PLAYTHINK 774

DIFFICULTY: ●●●●●●●○○○
REQUIRED: ◉ ✏ 📄 ✂
COMPLETION: ☐ TIME: _____

CROSSROADS 2

Place eleven counters in turn on the twelve circles. You must put each counter on an empty circle and then move the counter immediately to another empty circle connected to the first by a straight line.

PLAYTHINK 775

DIFFICULTY: ●●●●●●○○○○
REQUIRED: 👁 ✎
COMPLETION: ☐ TIME: _____

TWO-COLOR CORNER CUBES

In how many distinct ways can you paint the corners of a cube using only two colors? Rotations do not count as different, but reflections do.

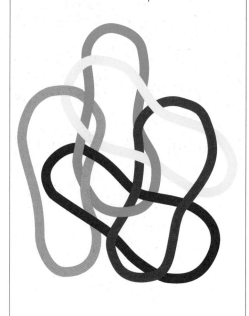

PLAYTHINK 776

DIFFICULTY: ●●●○○○○○○○
REQUIRED: 👁
COMPLETION: ☐ TIME: _____

LINKED OR UNLINKED?

Which of the five loops must be cut so that the other loops will fall free?

PLAYTHINK 777

DIFFICULTY: ●●○○○○○○○○
REQUIRED: 👁
COMPLETION: ☐ TIME: _____

CUBE NETS

A cube has six faces, but does every net made up of six squares fold into a cube? Just by looking at the seven patterns here, can you tell which ones can be folded into a perfect cube box?

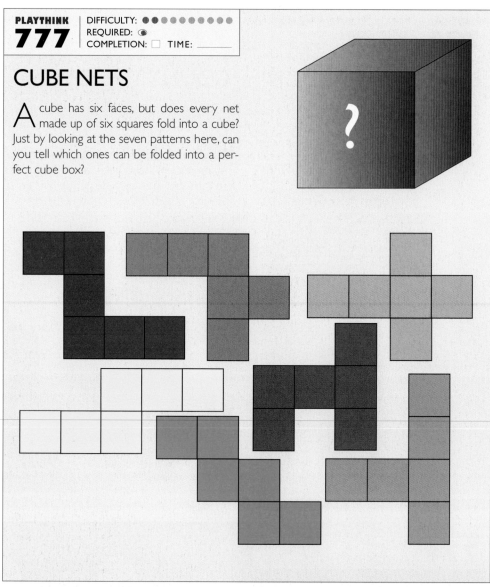

PLAYTHINK 778

DIFFICULTY: ●●○○○○○○○○
REQUIRED: 👁
COMPLETION: ☐ TIME: _____

CUBE FOLD 2

The pattern here can be folded along the creases between the squares to form a cube box. Can you work out which colors will be on opposite faces when the cube is folded?

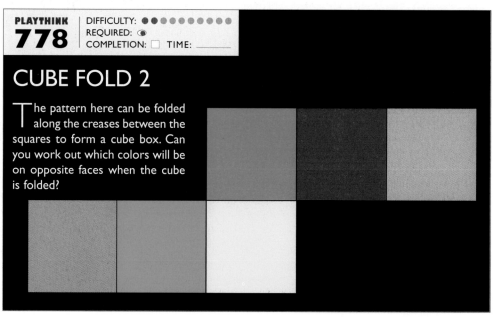

PLAYTHINK
779

DIFFICULTY: ●●●●○○○○○○
REQUIRED: ◉ ✎
COMPLETION: ☐ TIME: _____

FOUR COLOR SQUARES GAME

The object of this two-player game is to fill the entire game board with just four colors and with no two adjacent regions sharing a color.

Players select two of four colors—red, green, blue and yellow—and then take turns filling in one square at a time. Each newly colored section must touch at least one other colored square, but it cannot touch a square of the same color, even at the corner. (See sample game for guidance.) Play continues until no legal moves remain.

Scoring is straightforward: each two-by-two square filled in with one of a player's two colors counts as a point; each three-by-three square counts as two points and so on. One-by-one squares don't count.

PLAYER 1
PLAYER 2

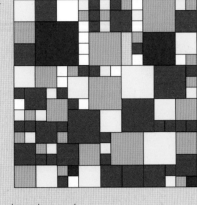

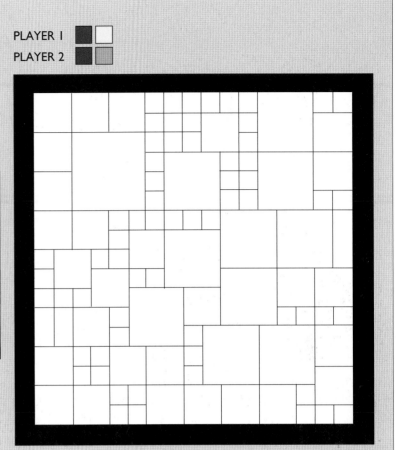

PLAYTHINK
780

DIFFICULTY: ●●●●●○○○○○
REQUIRED: ◉ ✎
COMPLETION: ☐ TIME: _____

DOT WIGGLING 2

The path at left connects all twenty-seven dots with a continuous closed line that possesses twenty-six angles. Can you find another such path that possesses twenty-six angles?

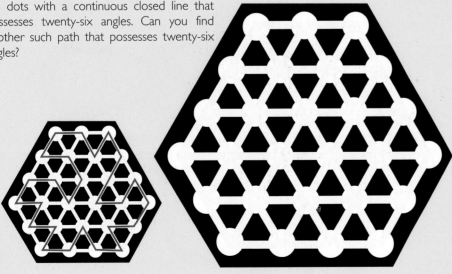

PLAYTHINK
781

DIFFICULTY: ●●●●●●○○○○
REQUIRED: ◉ ✎
COMPLETION: ☐ TIME: _____

TETRA VOLUME

A tetrahedron has been sliced from a cube, as shown. Can you work out how its volume relates to that of the rest of the box?

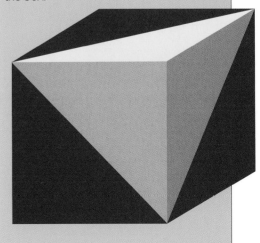

PLAYTHINK
782

DIFFICULTY: ●●●●●●○○○○
REQUIRED: 👁 ✎
COMPLETION: ☐ TIME: _____

HUNGRY MOUSE

Can you find a path so that the mouse eats every vegetable and exits without entering any rooms twice?

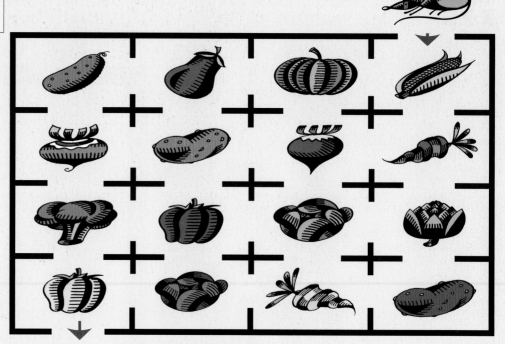

PLAYTHINK
783

DIFFICULTY: ●●●●●●○○○○
REQUIRED: 👁 ✎ 📄 ✂
COMPLETION: ☐ TIME: _____

14-15 PUZZLE OF SAM LOYD

Using only sliding moves, can you rearrange the numbered tiles from the configuration on top to the perfectly ordered one on the bottom? How many moves does it take to exchange 14 and 15?

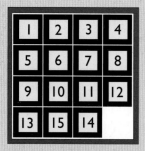

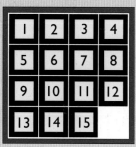

PLAYTHINK
784

DIFFICULTY: ●●●●●●○○○○
REQUIRED: 👁 ✎ 📄 ✂
COMPLETION: ☐ TIME: _____

DAISY GAME

This is a two-person game; if no opponent is available, try figuring out yourself how you can *always* win.

Begin with all thirteen bees in the inward position, toward the center of the daisy. Each player may capture one bee or two adjacent bees each turn, by sliding the bee or bees outward on the petal. The player who captures the last bee wins. Can you work out a strategy so that if your opponent starts first, you will always win?

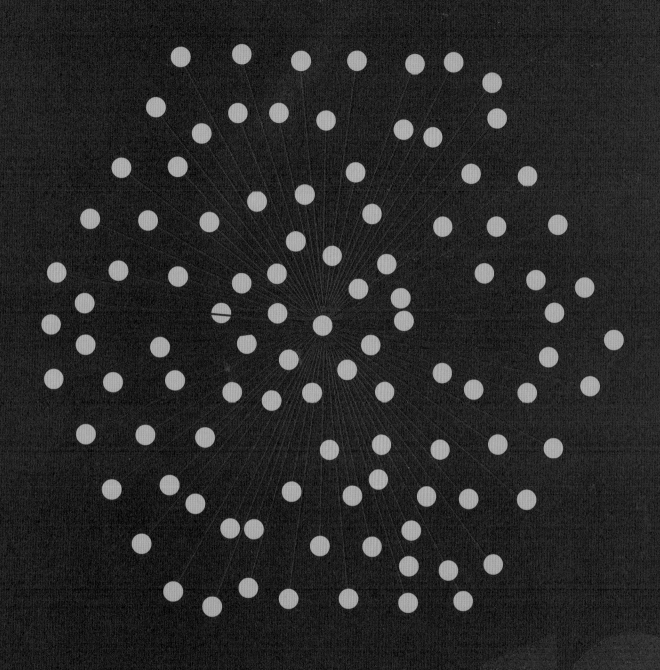

Science

PLAYTHINK 785

DIFFICULTY: ●●●●●●●●●○○
REQUIRED: ◉
COMPLETION: ☐ TIME: _____

GRAVITY TRAIN

It was once suggested that one could build a train that would be powered by gravity alone. Each rail line would be perfectly straight—not only would it not curve left or right, but it would not even curve to follow the surface of the earth. Instead, it would tunnel through the earth from city to city. The middle of each tunnel would, of course, be closer to the center of the earth than either end, so each train would run halfway downhill, giving it enough momentum to run the other half uphill.

Ignoring such factors as friction and air resistance, in theory could such a train work? If so, can you guess how long the fastest and slowest trips would take?

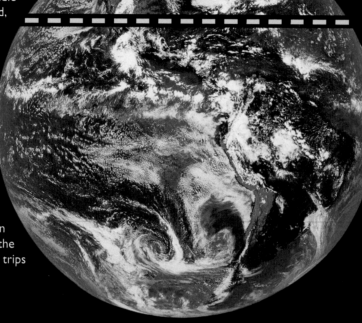

PLAYTHINK 786

DIFFICULTY: ●●●●●●●○○○○
REQUIRED: ◉
COMPLETION: ☐ TIME: _____

INSIDE THE EARTH

If you descend in a shaft to a point far below the earth's surface, what will your weight be?

1. Greater than at the earth's surface
2. Less than at the earth's surface
3. The same as at the earth's surface

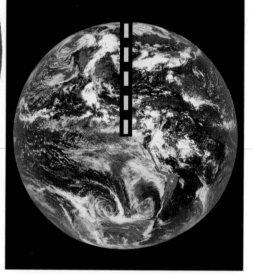

PLAYTHINK 787

DIFFICULTY: ●●●●●○○○○○
REQUIRED: ◉
COMPLETION: ☐ TIME: _____

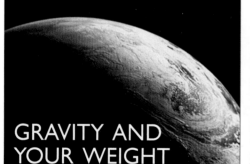

GRAVITY AND YOUR WEIGHT

The earth is not a perfect sphere—it is a bit flat at the top, and it bulges at the equator.

Given that information, can you work out where you weigh more—at the North Pole, at the South Pole or at the equator?

PLAYTHINK 788

DIFFICULTY: ●●●●●●●○○○
REQUIRED: ◉
COMPLETION: ☐ TIME: _____

PLANETARY SCALE

Can you measure your weight anywhere in the universe using a spring scale?

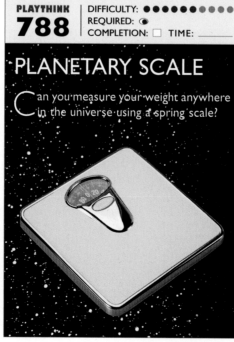

PLAYTHINK 789

DIFFICULTY: ●●●●●●●●●○
REQUIRED: ◉
COMPLETION: ☐ TIME: _____

ASTRONAUT ON THE MOON

Do astronauts on the moon weigh the same as they do on the earth?

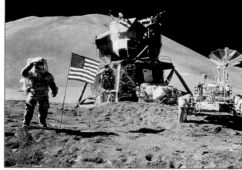

PLAYTHINK 790

DIFFICULTY: ●●●●●●●○○○
REQUIRED: ◉
COMPLETION: ☐ TIME: _____

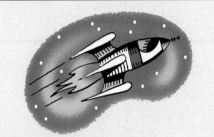

RELATIVITY OF GRAVITY

Imagine you are standing in a small, sealed, windowless room. You drop two objects of different mass, and they fall with the same acceleration and hit the floor at the same time.

Given this information, how can you tell for certain that you are in a room on Earth rather than in a room on a rocket that is undergoing a uniform acceleration equal to 32 feet per second per second (32f/s²)?

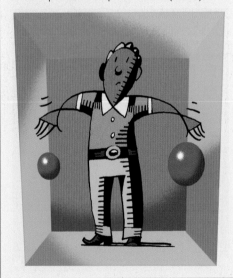

PLAYTHINK 791

DIFFICULTY: ●●●●●●○○○○
REQUIRED: ◉
COMPLETION: ☐ TIME: _____

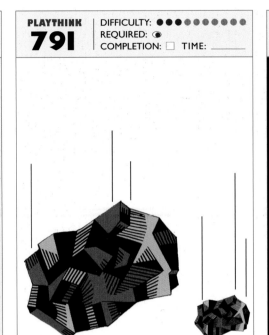

FALLING STONES

A large stone is 100 times heavier than a small rock, but when dropped at the same time, they fall with the same acceleration (ignoring air resistance). Why doesn't the large stone accelerate faster? Is it because of its weight, its energy, its surface area or its inertia?

PLAYTHINK 792

DIFFICULTY: ●●●●●●●●○○
REQUIRED: ◉
COMPLETION: ☐ TIME: _____

FALLING OBJECTS

In 1971 the *Apollo 15* astronaut David Scott performed a famous experiment. He dropped a feather and a hammer at the same time—and they both dropped like the proverbial stone, undergoing the same acceleration. The reason is that he dropped them on the surface of the moon, which has no atmosphere and therefore no air resistance to slow the feather.

The belief that heavy objects fall faster than light ones dates back to Aristotle and dominated thinking until the Middle Ages. Galileo was the first to demonstrate that this belief was false by dropping objects off the tower of Pisa. Since then scientists have tried various ways to counteract the slowing effect of air resistance, though none has gone to as great a length as Scott.

If you drop a coin and a small slip of paper at the same time, the coin will inevitably reach the ground first because of air resistance. Can you find a way to demonstrate that the coin and the paper ought to fall at the same rate in the absence of air resistance, even in a normal room?

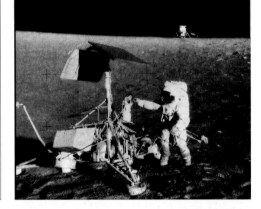

PLAYTHINK 793

DIFFICULTY: ●●●●●●○○○○
REQUIRED: ◉
COMPLETION: ☐ TIME: _____

ANTIGRAVITY

Astronauts in orbit feel weightless as they circle the earth. But the feeling of weightlessness can be achieved in an airplane that performs one of the maneuvers shown here. Can you work out which one?

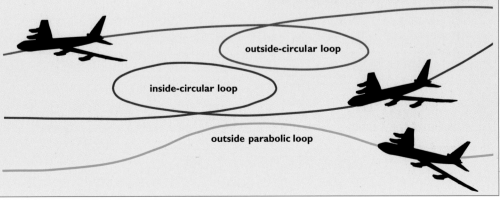

outside-circular loop

inside-circular loop

outside parabolic loop

PLAYTHINK 794 | DIFFICULTY: ●●●●●○○○○○
REQUIRED: ◉
COMPLETION: ☐   TIME: _____

BOOK FRICTION

You are pulling the second book from the top, using the ribbon as shown. Will either the top book or the book underneath stay in place?

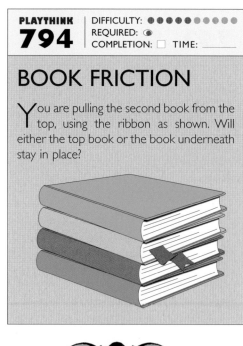

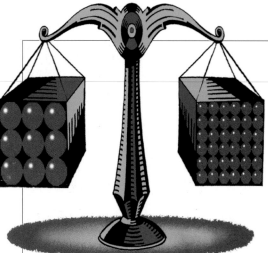

PLAYTHINK 795 | DIFFICULTY: ●●●●●○○○○○
REQUIRED: ◉
COMPLETION: ☐   TIME: _____

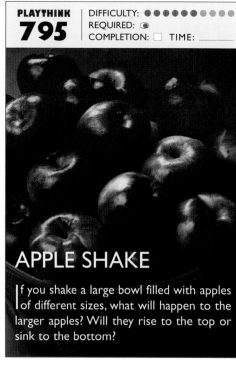

APPLE SHAKE

If you shake a large bowl filled with apples of different sizes, what will happen to the larger apples? Will they rise to the top or sink to the bottom?

PLAYTHINK 797 | DIFFICULTY: ●●●○○○○○○○
REQUIRED: ◉
COMPLETION: ☐   TIME: _____

BALLS BIG AND SMALL

If large steel balls are packed into a one-meter cube and small steel balls are packed into an identical cube, which weighs more?

Do you think it makes a difference that more small balls can be packed into the same space?

PLAYTHINK 796 | DIFFICULTY: ●●●●●●○○○○
REQUIRED: ◉
COMPLETION: ☐   TIME: _____

BREAKING A STRING

I tied some thin thread around a heavy book, as shown in the illustration. As I held both ends of the string, I asked a friend which end would snap when I pulled on the string from the bottom.

If my friend said the upper part, I pulled on the string and the lower part broke. If my friend said the lower part, I pulled on the string and the upper part broke.

Can you figure out how I am able to achieve either feat at will?

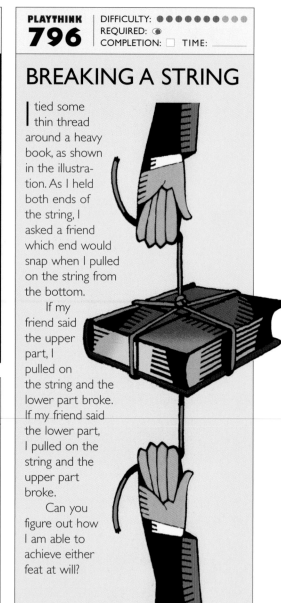

Center of Gravity

The center of gravity of an object isn't always at its center. Most standing lamps have a weighted base so that they won't tip over if you brush against them. Darts are often front-heavy so that they can be thrown with more accuracy.

To find the center of gravity of an irregularly shaped object, simply hang the object by a string from three different points. Because the center of gravity always seeks the lowest position it can reach, it will always be directly below the point from which it is hung—the place where those three vertical lines cross.

Many structures look unstable but are actually in equilibrium, demonstrating the fact that the center of gravity can sometimes exist outside the boundaries of the object itself. For a striking example, think of tightrope walkers, whose long, weighted poles allow them to retain a remarkable amount of stability even when walking upon a wire the diameter of a thumb.

PLAYTHINK 798

DIFFICULTY: ●●●●●●○○○○
REQUIRED: ◉
COMPLETION: ☐ TIME: _____

GOLD SMUGGLERS

Even though every passenger at the customs checkpoint had passed inspection, an observant officer stopped one passenger and reinspected one of his suitcases. The officer found a secret compartment filled with several heavy ingots.

Can you figure out what aroused the officer's suspicion?

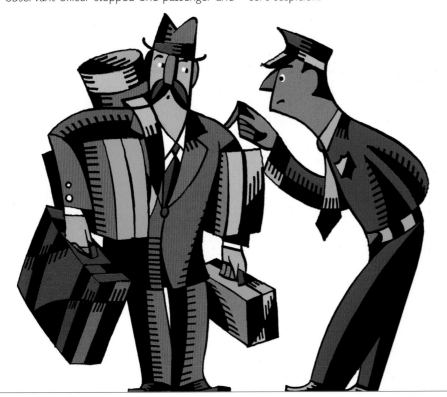

PLAYTHINK 799

DIFFICULTY: ●●●●●●●○○○
REQUIRED: ◉
COMPLETION: ☐ TIME: _____

ODDBALL

The owner of a pool hall is offered five bushels of colored balls, one each of red, blue, green, yellow and orange. All the balls weigh 100 grams, he learns, except for the balls of one color, which all weigh 110 grams.

The owner wants to use a spring scale that is accurate to within 10 grams to find out which color ball is too heavy. Can you work out the minimum number of weighings he must carry out to discover the color of the odd balls?

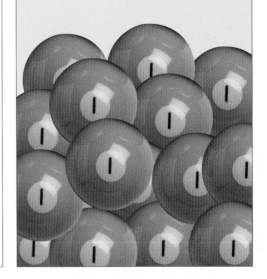

PLAYTHINK 800

DIFFICULTY: ●●●●●●●○○○
REQUIRED: ◉
COMPLETION: ☐ TIME: _____

PULLING STRINGS

In what two different ways can you pull a thread so that the spool rolls either toward you or away from you?

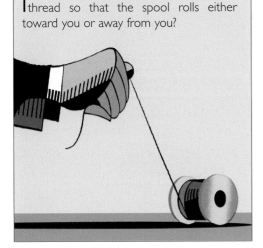

PLAYTHINK 801

DIFFICULTY: ●●●●●●●●○○
REQUIRED: ◉
COMPLETION: ☐ TIME: _____

TOPPLING BOX

A rectangular box is shown in three positions.

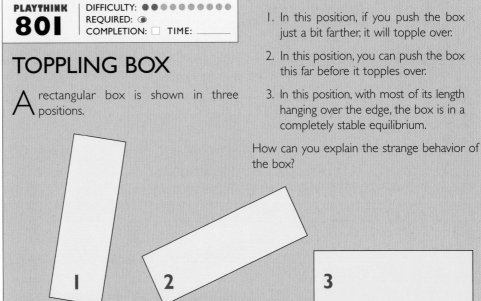

1. In this position, if you push the box just a bit farther, it will topple over.

2. In this position, you can push the box this far before it topples over.

3. In this position, with most of its length hanging over the edge, the box is in a completely stable equilibrium.

How can you explain the strange behavior of the box?

PLAYTHINK 802

DIFFICULTY: ●●●●●●●○○○
REQUIRED: ◉
COMPLETION: ☐ TIME: _____

PRIZE CATCH

You can measure weight—that is, the force of gravity—with a spring balance, the action of which depends directly on gravitational pull. The extension of a helical spring or even a simple rubber band is proportional to the force exerted on it. A twofold or threefold increase in weight leads to a twofold or threefold extension of the spring.

But because spring balances measure force, they don't always read what they mean. Take a look at the illustration here. The scale seems to show that the fisherman's prize marlin weighs 100 kilograms. Can you work out what the marlin really weighs?

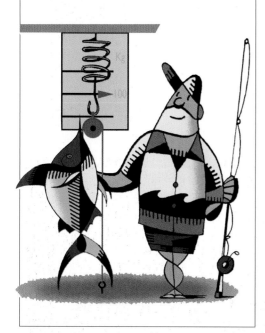

PLAYTHINK 803

DIFFICULTY: ●●●●●●○○○○
REQUIRED: ◉
COMPLETION: ☐ TIME: _____

TOPPLING STABILITY

A very simple device can compare the toppling tendency of various shapes. Each shape is placed in succession on the testing platform; the platform slowly changes angle until the shape topples over. Simple.

Can you figure out which shape stayed on the platform the longest? That is, can you work out which of the shapes below has the greatest toppling stability?

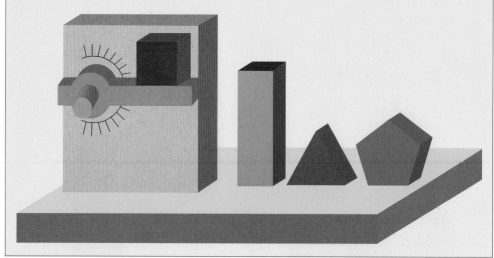

PLAYTHINK 804

DIFFICULTY: ●●●●○○○○○○
REQUIRED: ◉
COMPLETION: ☐ TIME: _____

STICK-BALANCING PARADOX

You and a friend can balance a yardstick on your index fingers, as shown in the illustration. Can you work out what will happen when you both try to slide your fingers toward the middle of the stick? What will happen if you start with both fingers in the middle and slide them toward the ends?

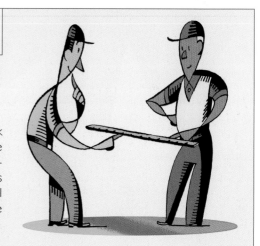

PLAYTHINK 805

DIFFICULTY: ●●●●●●●○○○
REQUIRED: ◉
COMPLETION: ☐ TIME: _____

SPRING BALANCE

A spring balance is hung from the ceiling by a rope. A second rope attached to the floor is tied tightly to the balance, pulling on the spring so that the balance reads 100 kilograms.

With the rope still attached, weights are hung from the hook and measured. Can you work out what the balance will read when weights of 50, 100 and 150 kilograms are hung on the lower hook of the spring balance?

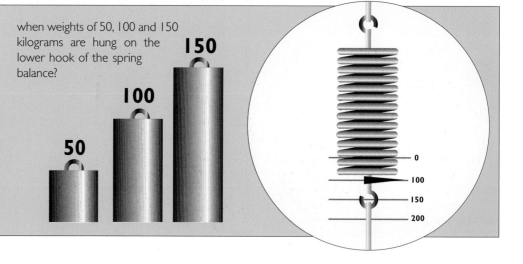

PLAYTHINK 806

DIFFICULTY: ●●●○○○○○○○
REQUIRED: ◉
COMPLETION: ☐ TIME: _____

HALVING MUG

Can you work out how to pour exactly half a mug of coffee from a mug filled to the brim?

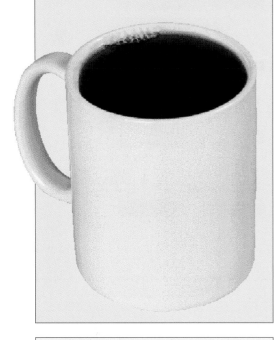

PLAYTHINK 807

DIFFICULTY: ●●●●●○○○○○
REQUIRED: ◉
COMPLETION: ☐ TIME: _____

BOTTLED FLIES

A sealed bottle containing flies is placed on a scale. When does the scale register the heaviest weight: when the flies are resting on the bottom of the bottle, or when all the flies are in flight?

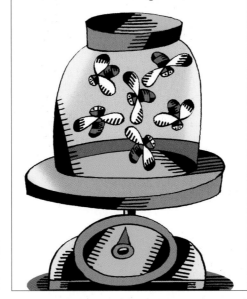

PLAYTHINK 808

DIFFICULTY: ●●●○○○○○○○
REQUIRED: ◉
COMPLETION: ☐ TIME: _____

BOTTLED VOLUME

A tightly sealed cylindrical bottle is partly filled with red wine. (The wine does not rise up past the shoulder level of the bottle.) Using only a standard ruler, can you measure the volume of the entire bottle without opening it or damaging it in any way?

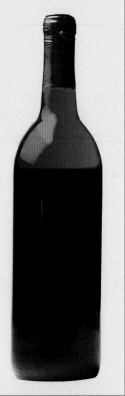

PLAYTHINK 809

DIFFICULTY: ●●●●●●○○○○
REQUIRED: ◉
COMPLETION: ☐ TIME: _____

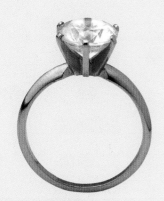

LOST RING

You have sealed the ninth of nine identical parcels of precisely equal weights, only to discover that your diamond ring has accidentally fallen into one of the packages.

You don't want to unwrap every parcel. Can you work out how to find the parcel containing the ring with just two weighings on a balance scale?

PLAYTHINK 810

DIFFICULTY: ●●●●●●○○○○
REQUIRED: ◉
COMPLETION: ☐ TIME: _____

MEASURING GLOBE

Imagine drawing a circle with a giant compass: the point is on the North Pole, and the pencil traces a circle along the equator, as shown. Then, without changing the radius of the compass, imagine drawing another circle on a plane tangent to the North Pole and parallel to the equator.

Can you work out how the surface area of this second circle compares to that of the Northern Hemisphere?

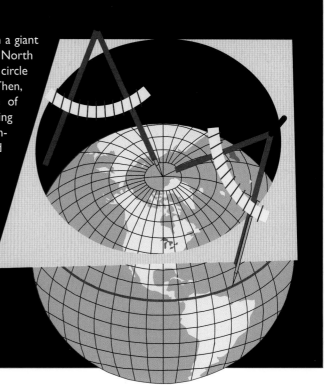

PLAYTHINK 811 | DIFFICULTY: ●●●●●●○○○○
REQUIRED: ◉
COMPLETION: ☐ TIME: _____

MENTAL BALANCE 1

The six identical steel balls are in perfect equilibrium in the balance shown below.

The balls may occupy any of the eleven positions on the balance; those positions are equally spaced and symmetrically arranged from the middle position. Simple equilibrium positions can be achieved through simple symmetrical configurations of the balls, but in these nine puzzles we will avoid such arrangements if at all possible.

In each puzzle some of the balls have already been placed on the balance. Can you place balls on the left side or in the middle position to achieve equilibrium?

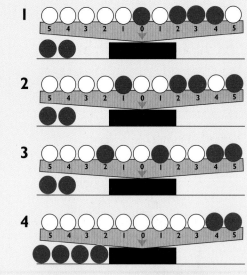

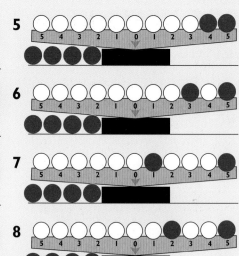

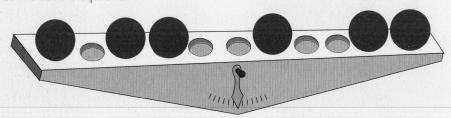

PLAYTHINK 812 | DIFFICULTY: ●●●●●●○○○○
REQUIRED: ◉
COMPLETION: ☐ TIME: _____

MENTAL BALANCE 2

The six steel balls in the balance are in perfect equilibrium. The set of balls comes with the following weights: green is 1 unit, red is 2 units and blue is 4 units.

The balls may occupy any of the eleven positions on the balance; those positions are equally spaced and symmetrically arranged from the middle position. Simple equilibrium positions can be achieved through simple symmetrical configurations of the balls, but in these nine puzzles we will avoid such arrangements if at all possible.

In each puzzle some of the balls have been placed on the right hand side of the balance. Can you place balls on the left side to achieve equilibrium?

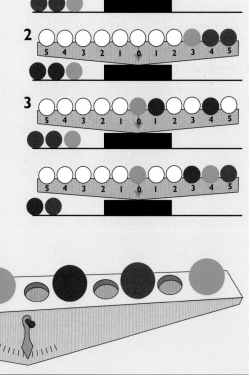

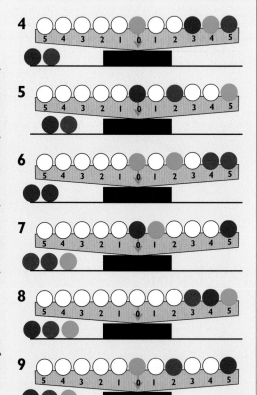

Simple Machines

According to legend, the great Greek mathematician and engineer Archimedes once said, "Give me [a fulcrum and a] place on which to stand, and I will move the Earth," He meant it, too, so impressed was he by the enormous force produced by machines.

Prehistoric humans invented simple devices such as wedges and levers. The ancient Egyptians used roping and ramping to move enormous blocks of stone. The pulley was probably invented along with the first iron tools; Assyrian art from the eighth century B.C. shows the pulley in common use. But it was the ancient Greeks who actually studied simple machines deeply enough to group them into five categories: the lever, the wheel and axle, the pulley, the wedge and the screw.

Simple machines are extensions of the human body, originally invented to augment the muscular efforts of men and animals. Today they are everywhere—and no longer simple!

PLAYTHINK 813

DIFFICULTY: ●●●●●●○○○○
REQUIRED: ◉
COMPLETION: ☐ TIME: _____

BALANCING STICKS

Objects with a low center of gravity are more stable than those with a high center of gravity. Why, then, do acrobats and jugglers—or you—find it easy to balance a long, thin stick on the tip of a finger? Shouldn't pencils and other short objects be easier?

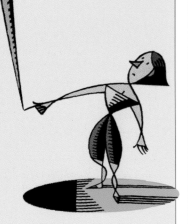

PLAYTHINK 814

DIFFICULTY: ●●●●●○○○○○
REQUIRED: ◉
COMPLETION: ☐ TIME: _____

STRONGER TEAM

Three different types of weights are arranged on the two pulleys at the left so that everything is in equilibrium.

Some of the same weights are used in a different configuration on the pulley at the right. Are these weights in equilibrium, or will one side pull the other?

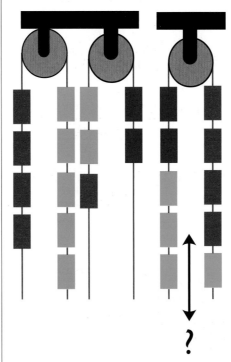

PLAYTHINK 815

DIFFICULTY: ●●●●○○○○○○
REQUIRED: ◉
COMPLETION: ☐ TIME: _____

WATERING CANS

Which watering can holds more water?

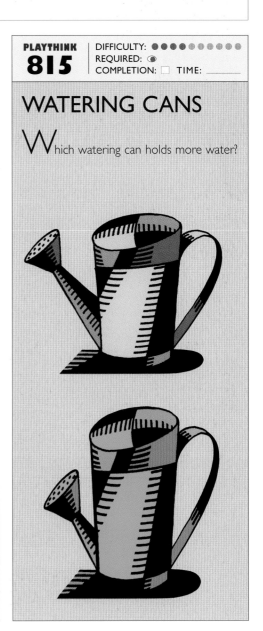

PLAYTHINK
816
DIFFICULTY: ●●●●●●●○○○
REQUIRED: ◉
COMPLETION: ☐   TIME: _____

EGG OF COLUMBUS

Christopher Columbus is said to have stood an egg on its pointy end when he first crossed the equator. I thought of that story several years ago when I saw an ingenious equilibrium toy; The challenge was to re-create Columbus's feat. But as much as I tried, the egg would not balance. Shaking the egg did not reveal any moving parts. In fact, the only way the egg would balance was if one followed the instructions on the box:

1. Hold the egg with the pointed end up for at least thirty seconds.

2. Turn the egg over and wait for another ten seconds, then place it on the pointed end.

The egg would then balance beautifully. It would stay balanced for about fifteen seconds. After that period anyone else who tried to balance the egg would have no luck unless he or she knew the secret of the egg.

From the above description, can you work out the mysterious inner structure of this deeply puzzling egg?

PLAYTHINK
817
DIFFICULTY: ●●●●●●●○○○
REQUIRED: ◉
COMPLETION: ☐   TIME: _____

FIVE-MINUTE EGG

You must boil an egg for exactly five minutes, but all you have is a four-minute timer and a three-minute timer. Can you work out how to use these two timers to measure five minutes?

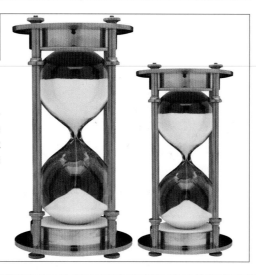

PLAYTHINK
818
DIFFICULTY: ●●●●●●●●○○
REQUIRED: ◉
COMPLETION: ☐   TIME: _____

HOURGLASS PARADOX

A small, enclosed hourglass floats in a sealed, water-filled cylinder, as shown in the diagram. Turn the cylinder over and, surprisingly, the hourglass will not float back to the top. It will sit at the bottom until most of the sand has passed to the lower compartment. Only then will the hourglass float to the top.

Can you work out what delays the floating of the hourglass?

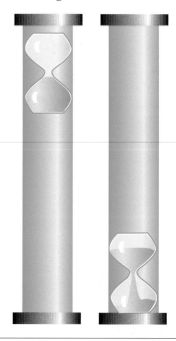

PLAYTHINK
819
DIFFICULTY: ●●●●●●●○○○
REQUIRED: ◉
COMPLETION: ☐   TIME: _____

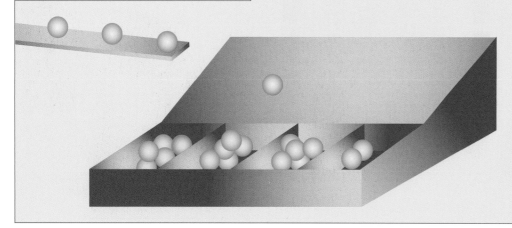

BALL-SORTING DEVICE

A steady supply of balls of the same size but four different weights rolls down a chute. From the chute the balls drop onto the slanted coarse surface of the sorting box. The device easily sorts the balls into four weight groups, eliminating the tedious job of weighing each ball.

From the illustration, can you tell which compartment collects the heaviest balls?

PLAYTHINK
820 | DIFFICULTY: ●●●●●●●●● ●
REQUIRED: ◉
COMPLETION: ☐ TIME: _____

CLOCKWORK

Can you work out what direction the red cogwheel must turn so that the minute hand of the clock will turn clockwise?

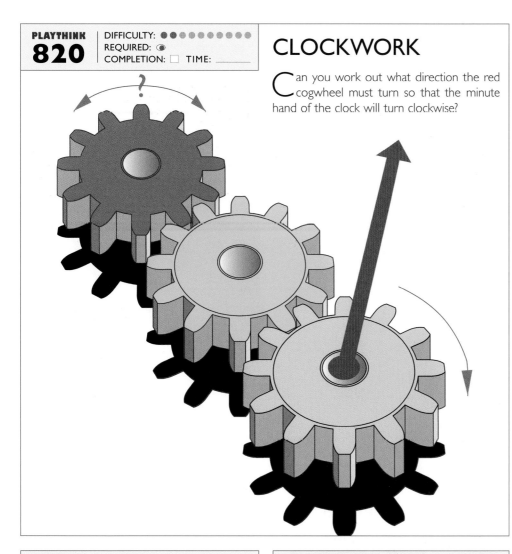

PLAYTHINK
821 | DIFFICULTY: ●●●●●●●● ● ●
REQUIRED: ◉
COMPLETION: ☐ TIME: _____

SCREW ON

Both bolts shown here have right-handed threads and are in constant contact. One hand is turning one of the bolts clockwise, as if screwing it into a nut, while the other hand is turning the other bolt counter-clockwise, as if unscrewing it.

Can you work out whether the two bolts are being drawn together or forced apart?

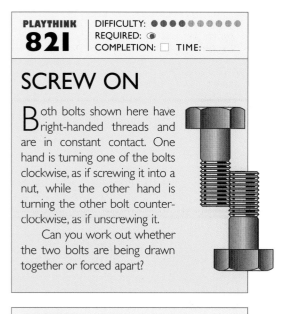

PLAYTHINK
822 | DIFFICULTY: ●●●●●●●●● ●
REQUIRED: ◉
COMPLETION: ☐ TIME: _____

BELT TRANSMISSION

If the green wheel turns clockwise, in what direction must the yellow wheel turn?

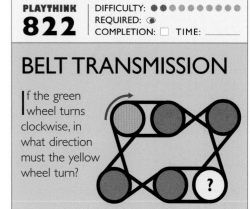

PLAYTHINK
823 | DIFFICULTY: ●●●●●●●●● ●
REQUIRED: ◉
COMPLETION: ☐ TIME: _____

GEAR TRAIN I

The red cogwheel turns in a counter-clockwise direction, as shown. In what direction will the blue cogwheel turn?

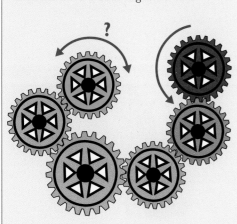

PLAYTHINK
824 | DIFFICULTY: ●●●●●●●●● ●
REQUIRED: ◉
COMPLETION: ☐ TIME: _____

GEAR TRAIN 2

The red cogwheel turns counterclock-wise, as shown. Can you work out which way each of the two racks will move— up or down?

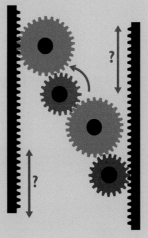

PLAYTHINK
825 | DIFFICULTY: ●●●●●●●●● ●
REQUIRED: ◉
COMPLETION: ☐ TIME: _____

TRAPDOOR

Can you work out which way to push the rack so that the trap-door will open?

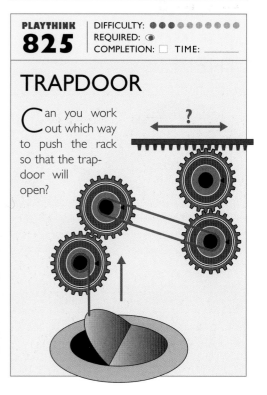

PLAYTHINK 826

DIFFICULTY: ●●●●●○○○○○
REQUIRED: ◉ ✎
COMPLETION: ☐ TIME: _____

GEAR ANAGRAM

Each of the five interlocking gears possesses letters at its contact points. (The number next to the gear specifies how many teeth the gear has.) After a certain number of revolutions, the letters at the four contact points will spell out an eight-letter word, read from left to right.

Can you work out how many revolutions it will take and what the secret word is?

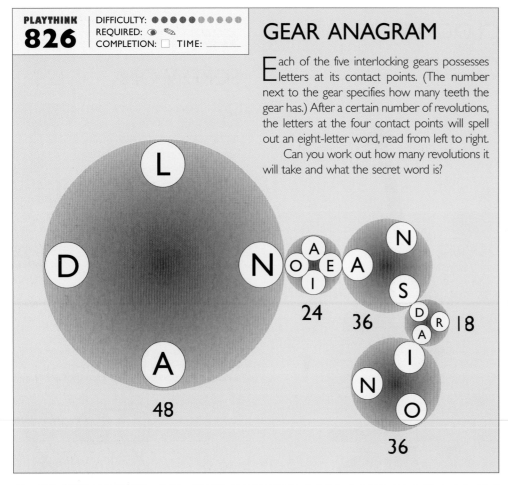

PLAYTHINK 827

DIFFICULTY: ●●●●●●○○○○
REQUIRED: ◉
COMPLETION: ☐ TIME: _____

SATELLITE PRINCIPLE

Imagine you are standing on a 200-mile-high tower, far above the top of the atmosphere. If you throw a Frisbee hard enough, what will happen?

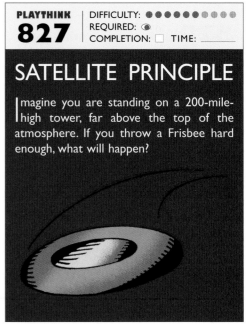

PLAYTHINK 829

DIFFICULTY: ●●●●●●○○○○
REQUIRED: ◉ ✎
COMPLETION: ☐ TIME: _____

JOGGING FLY

Every morning two joggers start out 10 kilometers apart, on either end of a trail. The moment the joggers start running toward the middle of the trail, a fly that sat on the head of one of the joggers flies straight toward the other; once the fly reaches the second jogger, it turns around and heads back toward the first. This back-and-forth flying continues until the two joggers meet.

If each jogger runs at a constant 5 kilometers an hour and the fly travels at 10 kilometers an hour, can you work out how many kilometers the fly covered before the joggers met?

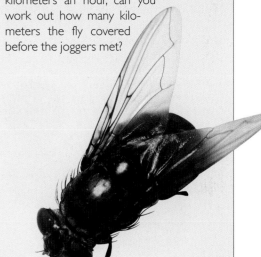

PLAYTHINK 828

DIFFICULTY: ●●●●●●○○○○
REQUIRED: ◉
COMPLETION: ☐ TIME: _____

THE MONKEY AND THE VET

A vet aimed his tranquilizer dart gun directly at a monkey and pulled the trigger. At that exact moment the monkey let go of the branch and began to drop. Ignoring air resistance, can you work out whether the dart will hit the monkey?

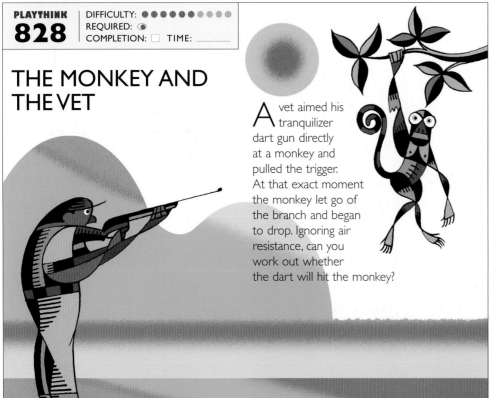

PLAYTHINK 830

DIFFICULTY: ●●●●●●●○○○
REQUIRED: ◉ ✎
COMPLETION: ☐ TIME: _____

ON THE REBOUND 1

You have cleared the pool table of all but your last ball and are on the verge of victory. To celebrate, you plan to sink the last ball in as complex a way as possible, with at least two bounces off the side cushions.

Figuring out where to aim the ball for such a complex trajectory is tricky work. It often helps to have a grid superimposed over the table; the lines can be used as aiming markers at the edge of the table, and the squares can help you measure the angles at which the ball strikes the cushion. (You know, after all, that the angle at which the ball strikes the cushion is identical to the angle at which it rebounds.)

Either of the paths shown below would be too easy—they use only two side cushions. Can you work out a path for the balls that would take it from the bottom left-hand corner, off three cushions, and into either the top left-hand pocket or the bottom right-hand pocket?

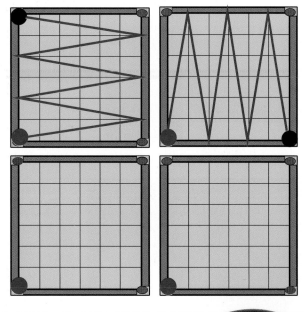

PLAYTHINK 831

DIFFICULTY: ●●●●●●●●○○
REQUIRED: ◉ ✎
COMPLETION: ☐ TIME: _____

ON THE REBOUND 2

Playing pool on an L-shaped table is a challenge, but even then, sinking the ball from the lower left-hand corner to either the upper left or the lower right pocket is easy. The top two diagrams show how it can be done.

But to make things interesting, can you find a way to sink the ball into those pockets by bouncing it off at least four of the six sides? The ball should make five bounces before going into the upper left-hand pocket and seven bounces before going into the lower right-hand pocket.

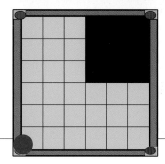

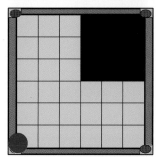

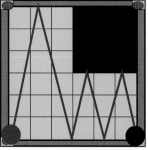

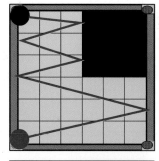

PLAYTHINK 832

DIFFICULTY: ●●●●●●●●●○○
REQUIRED: ◉ ✎
COMPLETION: ☐ TIME: _____

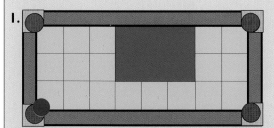

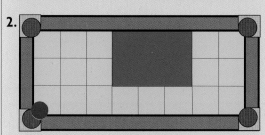

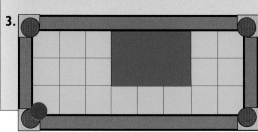

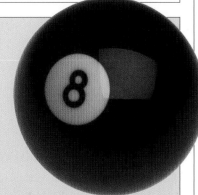

ON THE REBOUND 3

Perhaps you would like to try your luck with even more irregular tables. Starting with the ball in the lower left-hand corner, can you work out how to sink the ball in each instance? You must observe certain restrictions on each shot:

1. Three bounces, each on a different side

2. Seven bounces

3. Thirteen bounces and six different sides

The ball may travel as long as necessary to sink in the pocket.

PLAYTHINK 833

DIFFICULTY: ● ● ● ● ● ● ● ○ ○ ○
REQUIRED: 👁 ✎
COMPLETION: ☐   TIME: _____

REFLECTED BALLS

When a ball hits a side cushion, it rebounds at the same angle at which it struck. With that knowledge, skilled billiard players know the exact path of a cue ball before they hit it.

A number of pool tables of different shapes and sizes are shown here. Can you trace the path of a ball in the lower left-hand corner that has been struck at a 45-degree angle? Can you predict which pocket the ball will land in, based on the dimensions of the individual table?

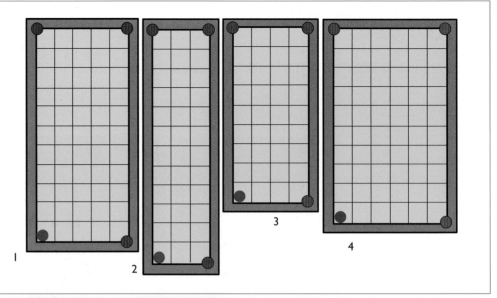

PLAYTHINK 834

DIFFICULTY: ● ● ● ● ● ● ○ ○ ○ ○
REQUIRED: 👁
COMPLETION: ☐   TIME: _____

ROLLING THINGS

Two wooden wheels carry a 10-kilogram weight. One weight is a disk attached to the center; the other is a ring attached near the rim. If the wheels are released simultaneously on an inclined plane, which will reach the bottom first?

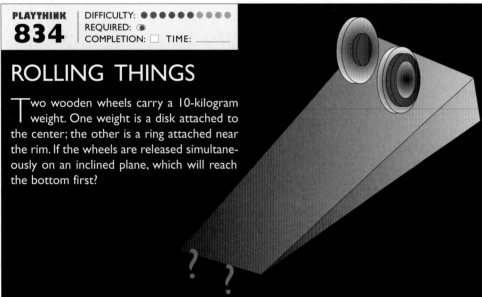

PLAYTHINK 835

DIFFICULTY: ● ● ○ ○ ○ ○ ○ ○ ○ ○
REQUIRED: 👁
COMPLETION: ☐   TIME: _____

BOMBS AWAY

A bomb has just been released from a plane, as shown. Can you work out which path best describes the bomb's trajectory?

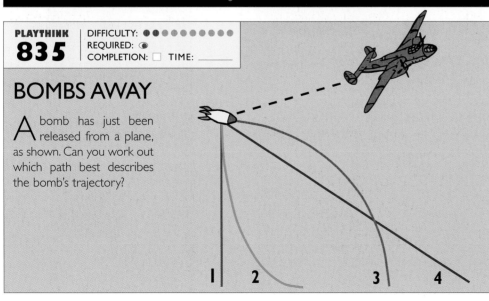

PLAYTHINK 836

DIFFICULTY: ● ● ● ● ○ ○ ○ ○ ○ ○
REQUIRED: 👁
COMPLETION: ☐   TIME: _____

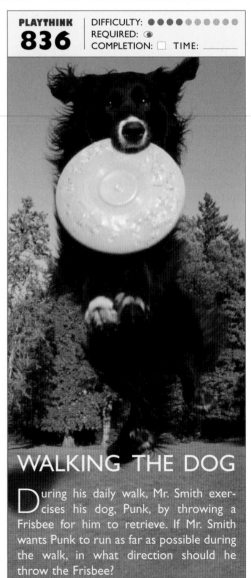

WALKING THE DOG

During his daily walk, Mr. Smith exercises his dog, Punk, by throwing a Frisbee for him to retrieve. If Mr. Smith wants Punk to run as far as possible during the walk, in what direction should he throw the Frisbee?

PLAYTHINK
837 | DIFFICULTY: ●●●●●●●○○○
REQUIRED: ◉
COMPLETION: ☐ TIME: _____

FOLDING LADDER

A folding ladder is placed on the floor with one leg supported by a stick, as shown. A bowling ball rests in the rungs near the end of the leg. A short distance away a bucket is firmly tied to the leg, and near the pivot a heavy weight rests on the leg. The idea behind the setup is a simple one:

You pull the stick away, the ladder collapses, and the ball lands in the bucket.

Can such a trick work? Won't all the objects fall at the same rate?

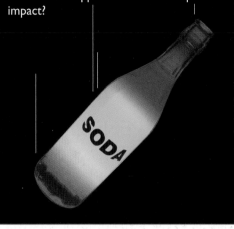

PLAYTHINK
840 | DIFFICULTY: ●●●●●●●●○○
REQUIRED: ◉
COMPLETION: ☐ TIME: _____

DROP

A woman drops a bottle from a second-story window. The bottle hits the ground at a certain speed. Can you work out from what height the bottle should be dropped to double its speed at impact?

PLAYTHINK
841 | DIFFICULTY: ●●●●●○○○○○
REQUIRED: ◉
COMPLETION: ☐ TIME: _____

JUGGLER

A clown who weighs 80 kilograms must carry three 10-kilogram rings across a bridge. Unfortunately, the bridge can support only 100 kilograms. The lion tamer told the clown that he could make it across if he juggled the rings—as long as at least one ring was in the air at all times, he could cross safely.

The clown followed the lion tamer's advice. Did the bridge support his weight?

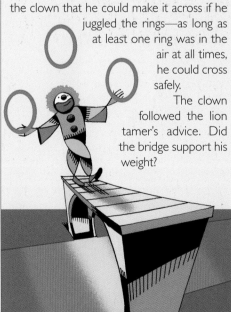

PLAYTHINK
838 | DIFFICULTY: ●●●●●●○○○○
REQUIRED: ◉ ✎
COMPLETION: ☐ TIME: _____

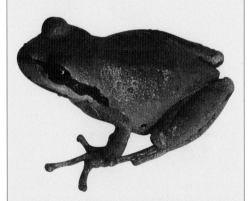

FROG IN THE WELL

A frog falls into the bottom of a 20-meter well. In its struggle to get out, the frog advances 3 meters up the slimy walls of the well; during the night when it rests, the frog slips back 2 meters.

Can you work out how many days it takes for the frog to escape?

PLAYTHINK
839 | DIFFICULTY: ●●●●●●●○○○
REQUIRED: ◉
COMPLETION: ☐ TIME: _____

RADIAL DESCENT

The diagram below shows an experimental device invented by Galileo, in which identical balls are released simultaneously at slanted angles along the chord of a circle. The device can be adjusted to any angle, from horizontal to vertical.

As each ball follows its track, can you work out which will be the first to reach the circumference of the circle?

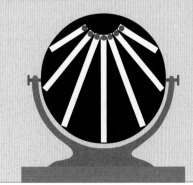

PLAYTHINK 842

DIFFICULTY: ●●●●●●●○○○
REQUIRED: ◉
COMPLETION: ☐ TIME: _____

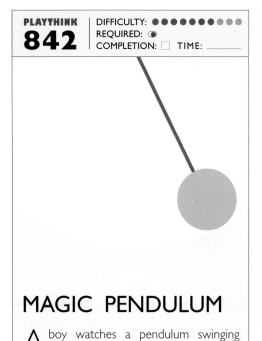

MAGIC PENDULUM

A boy watches a pendulum swinging through a plane. He is wearing a broken pair of sunglasses—the right lens is missing. Can you work out how he will perceive the motion of the pendulum?

PLAYTHINK 843

DIFFICULTY: ●●●●●●●●○○
REQUIRED: ◉
COMPLETION: ☐ TIME: _____

SUPERBALLS

A small superball is temporarily and very loosely affixed to a larger superball, and both are dropped from a height of 1 to 2 meters. What will happen to the smaller ball?

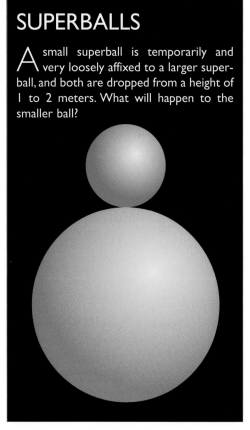

PLAYTHINK 844

DIFFICULTY: ●●●●●●●●○○
REQUIRED: ◉
COMPLETION: ☐ TIME: _____

FOUCAULT'S PENDULUM

Is it possible to watch the earth rotate?

One of the important properties of a pendulum is that once it is set in motion, it will continue to swing through the same plane unless a force acts on it. This is a property of inertia.

That fact became the basis of one of the most beautiful science demonstrations ever performed. The French physicist Jean-Bernard Foucault was invited to arrange a scientific exhibit as part of the Paris Exhibition in 1851. From the dome of the Pantheon, Foucault hung a pendulum consisting of 61 meters of piano wire and a 27-kilogram cannonball. On the floor below the ball, he sprinkled a layer of fine sand. A stylus fixed to the bottom of the ball traced the path in the sand, thus recording the movement of the pendulum.

At the end of an hour, the line in the sand had moved 11 degrees and 18 minutes.

If the pendulum stayed in the same plane, how could it trace different paths in the sand?

Jean-Bernard Foucault

PLAYTHINK 845

DIFFICULTY: ●●●●●●○○○○
REQUIRED: ◉
COMPLETION: ☐ TIME: _____

PENDULUM MAGIC

Pendulums have long fascinated scientists. A well-made pendulum can keep exact time, measure the force of gravity and sense relative motion.

Two pendulums of identical lengths but different masses are released simultaneously, though the heavier pendulum is released from a greater height than the lighter one.

Which pendulum will complete its first full swing first?

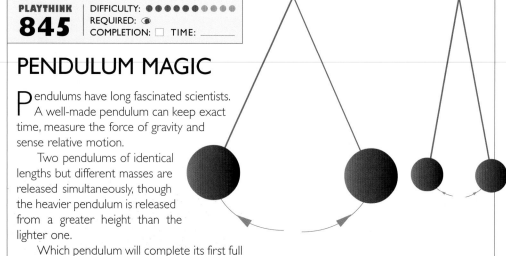

PLAYTHINK 846

DIFFICULTY: ●●●●●●●○○○
REQUIRED: ◉
COMPLETION: ☐ TIME: _____

COUPLED RESONANCE PENDULUMS

Imagine connecting the bobs of two pendulums by a spring, as shown. What happens when one of the pendulums is released? Do the interconnected pendulums eventually have the same amount of energy?

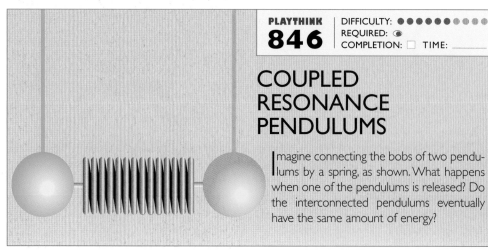

PLAYTHINK 847

DIFFICULTY: ●●●●●●●○○○
REQUIRED: ◉
COMPLETION: ☐ TIME: _____

PECKING WOODPECKER

You may have seen a variation of this toy. Begin with the woodpecker at the top of the rod. If you lift back the woodpecker and release it, the woodpecker will peck the rod and slowly descend to the bottom. Can you explain this behavior?

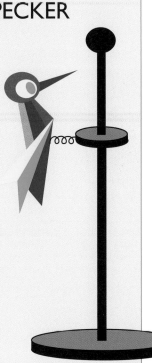

PLAYTHINK 848

DIFFICULTY: ●●●●●●●○○○
REQUIRED: ◉
COMPLETION: ☐ TIME: _____

CIRCLING WEIGHT

A ball on a string is swung in a circle at constant speed. Do the ball's velocity and acceleration stay the same? Can you work out what would happen to the ball if the string suddenly snapped?

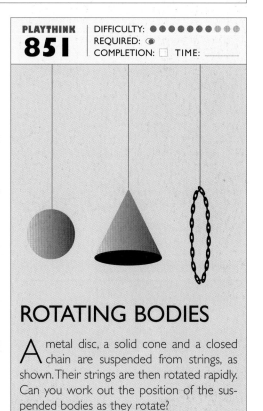

PLAYTHINK 849

DIFFICULTY: ●●●●●●●●○○
REQUIRED: ◉
COMPLETION: ☐ TIME: _____

IMPACT

You must have played with this popular toy, sometimes called Newton's cradle. What happens when you lift up and release one of the balls at the end?

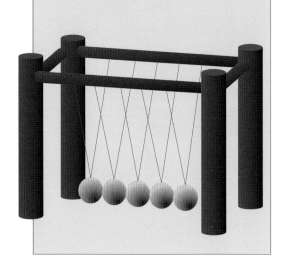

PLAYTHINK 850

DIFFICULTY: ●●●●●●●○○○
REQUIRED: ◉
COMPLETION: ☐ TIME: _____

MARBLE LIFTING MAGIC

Can you lift a marble off a table using only a wineglass?

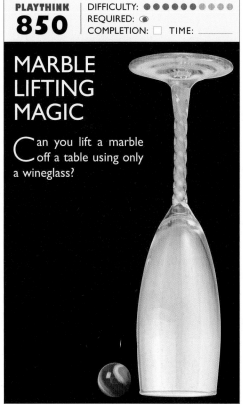

PLAYTHINK 851

DIFFICULTY: ●●●●●●●○○○
REQUIRED: ◉
COMPLETION: ☐ TIME: _____

ROTATING BODIES

A metal disc, a solid cone and a closed chain are suspended from strings, as shown. Their strings are then rotated rapidly. Can you work out the position of the suspended bodies as they rotate?

Gyroscopes

Bicycle wheels, Frisbees, yo-yos, tops—all these spinning objects illustrate the curious properties of the gyroscope, as does any solid object rotating about a fixed point.

A gyroscope has a certain rotational momentum that depends on its mass, on the square of the distance of the individual particles of mass to the axis of rotation, and on the speed of rotation (properties we understand courtesy of Newton's laws of motion). To increase the rotational momentum, a gyroscope can be designed as a disc with a thickened rim; that will concentrate most of its mass as far from the axis of rotation as possible.

The most significant feature of a gyroscope is the way it conserves its momentum and the direction of its rotational axis. As long as no external forces act upon the gyroscope, it will keep the direction of its axis constant in space. It can be used, therefore, to stabilize movement, as well as to measure the change of orientation in three-dimensional space.

PLAYTHINK 852 | DIFFICULTY: ●●●●●●○○○○
REQUIRED: ◉
COMPLETION: ☐ TIME: _____

HUMAN GYRO 1

Can you work out what will happen when a boy who sits on a freely rotating stool holds a spinning bicycle tire as shown?

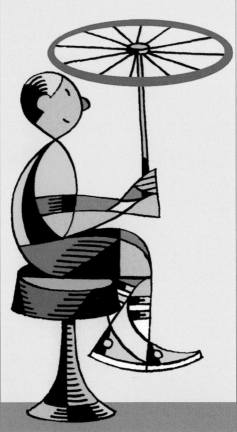

PLAYTHINK 853 | DIFFICULTY: ●●●●●●○○○○
REQUIRED: ◉
COMPLETION: ☐ TIME: _____

HUMAN GYRO 2

Can you work out what will happen when a boy who sits on a freely rotating stool holds a spinning bicycle tire as shown?

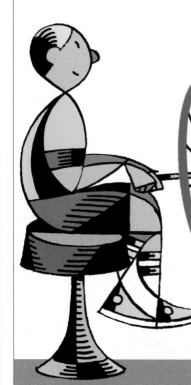

PLAYTHINK 854 | DIFFICULTY: ●●●●●●○○○○
REQUIRED: ◉
COMPLETION: ☐ TIME: _____

HUMAN GYRO 3

A boy sitting on a freely rotating stool holds a spinning bicycle tire vertically with both hands as shown. Can you work out what he should do so that his stool will begin to turn left? Will pushing the handle forward with his right hand and backward with his left accomplish this?

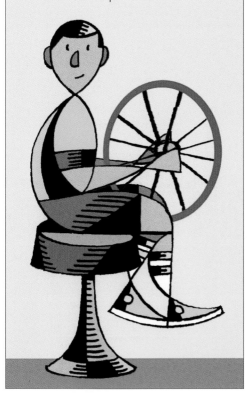

PLAYTHINK 855

DIFFICULTY: ●●●●●●●○○○
REQUIRED: ◉
COMPLETION: ☐ TIME: _____

CENTRIPETAL FORCE

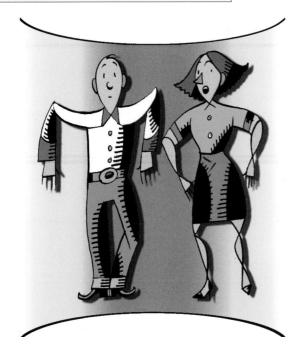

Rotating rides, such as the rotating vertical cylinder shown here, are popular at carnivals. Riders stand with their backs to the wall as the cylinder begins to spin. When the maximum spin rate is reached, the floor drops away. Amazingly, the riders remain stuck to the wall.

Can you work out why this occurs?

PLAYTHINK 856

DIFFICULTY: ●●●●●●●○○○
REQUIRED: ◉
COMPLETION: ☐ TIME: _____

GOLF BALLS

Why does a golf ball have a dimpled surface?

PLAYTHINK 857

DIFFICULTY: ●●●●●●●●○○
REQUIRED: ◉
COMPLETION: ☐ TIME: _____

ICE SKATING

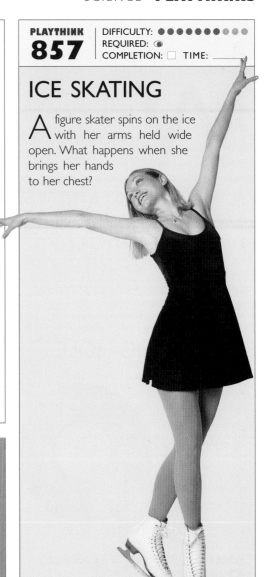

A figure skater spins on the ice with her arms held wide open. What happens when she brings her hands to her chest?

PLAYTHINK 858

DIFFICULTY: ●●●●●○●○○○
REQUIRED: ◉
COMPLETION: ☐ TIME: _____

BALL GAME CAROUSEL

Two jugglers stand on a rapidly rotating carousel, and one throws a ball straight to the other. Can you work out the ball's trajectory and show where it will land?

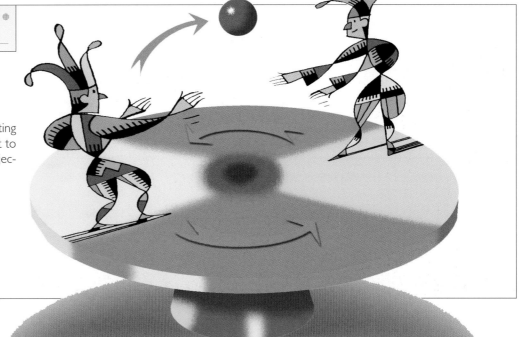

Branched Structures

Whenever one area has an advantage over adjacent areas when it comes to getting more matter, heat, light, or some other requisite for growth, the resultant structure shows signs of the growth of isolated individual sections feeding into a branched form. This is best illustrated by the common tree or a riverbed, but is also found in electric discharges, corrosion and crystal growth.

All such structures start from a point and grow linearly, but they eventually stop as the branches interfere with others already present.

Trees and lungs and river deltas all have the same principle: distribution. And they have all produced the same solution: branching.

PLAYTHINK 859

DIFFICULTY: ●●●●○○○○○○
REQUIRED: ◉
COMPLETION: ☐ TIME: _____

EXPANDING HOLE

A steel washer with a hole in the center is heated until the metal expands by 1 percent. Will the hole get larger or smaller or remain unchanged?

PLAYTHINK 860

DIFFICULTY: ●●●●●●○○○○
REQUIRED: ◉
COMPLETION: ☐ TIME: _____

TREES AND BRANCHES

Can you work out why a tree takes on the form of a branched structure like the one on the right rather than a radial structure such as the one on the left?

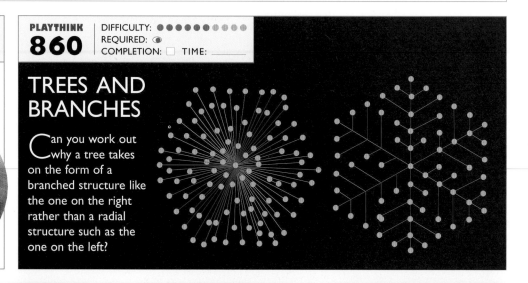

PLAYTHINK 861

DIFFICULTY: ●●●●●●●●○○
REQUIRED: ◉
COMPLETION: ☐ TIME: _____

BALANCING PLATFORM

At many hands-on-science exhibits, you can find balancing platforms that pivot at their centers. The idea is for groups of people to position themselves so that the platforms stay in a balanced position of equilibrium.

Imagine people of uniform weight as red circles distributed in four different configurations on the balancing platform, as shown. Can you work out which arrangements are in equilibrium?

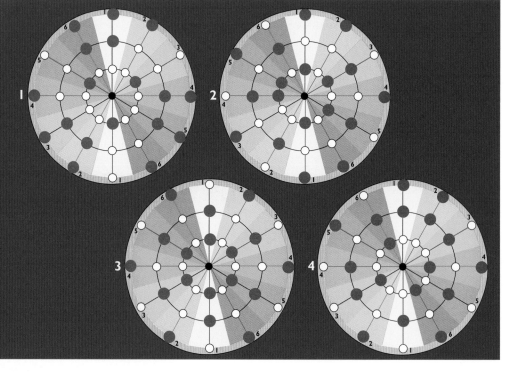

Cracks and Dried Mud

Cracking is inevitably sequential rather than simultaneous. As a result, when a crack is formed, it will typically join an existing crack by forming the ubiquitous three-rayed intersection. The formation of a four-rayed intersection is highly unlikely, though not impossible, since it is improbable that two new cracks would intersect an existing crack from opposite sides at exactly the same point.

It is often possible to determine which of the two lines appeared earlier: the older of the two cracks passes right through the point of junction. Thus, we can follow the splits and eventually find the beginning of the whole system of cracks.

Bubbles and rocks, different as they may seem, break up according to the same principles. Since both are elastic, they divide into segments that meet at 120-degree angles.

When a material is inelastic, like the glaze on a bowl, it cracks first along lines that intersect at right angles. Then, when tension is reduced and elasticity restored, secondary cracks occur, as they do in mud or rock, along lines that run at 120-degree angles.

The patterns of sun-dried mud seem to be quite irregular; nevertheless, they show right angles. This can be explained by assuming that the breaking up of a layer of mud is an effect of contraction: the crack has to follow the line of least work. Because work is proportional to the areas of the sections, the lines must minimize the surfaces laid open by the fissure. The lines will be at right angles if the mud is homogenous. Variations in the thickness of the layer account for the curvature of the lines.

PLAYTHINK 862

DIFFICULTY: ●●●●●●●○○○
REQUIRED: ◉
COMPLETION: ☐ TIME: _____

SOAP BUBBLES

Two soap bubbles of different sizes are blown up in succession. The inlet between the two is closed while they are being blown up. Then the outside inlet is sealed and the passage between the two bubbles is opened.

Can you work out what will happen? Will the smaller bubble grow until the two are of equal size?

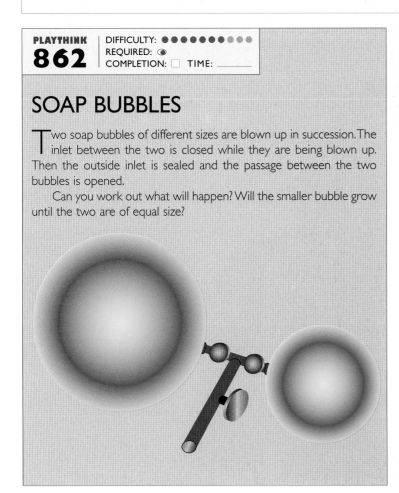

PLAYTHINK 863

DIFFICULTY: ●●●●●●●●●●
REQUIRED: ◉
COMPLETION: ☐ TIME: _____

WHO FIRED THE FIRST SHOT?

Look at the scene as a detective would: The three men each fired a shot. The holes from their shots match the colored dots on their hats. From this information, can you work out who fired the first shot—Joe, John or Jim?

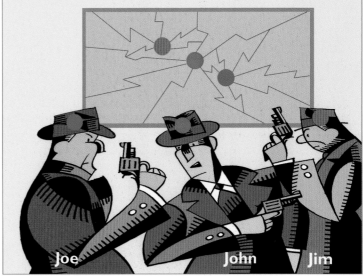

PLAYTHINK 864 | DIFFICULTY: ●●●●○○○○○○○○
REQUIRED: ◉ ✎
COMPLETION: ☐ TIME: _____

CRACKING ROUTE

A collection of twenty-eight blocks can be packed into a seven-by-twenty box, as shown, with each row containing just four boxes.

Can you find the shortest route from the left side of the box to the right, traveling only along the cracks (the heavy black lines)? How long is the shortest route?

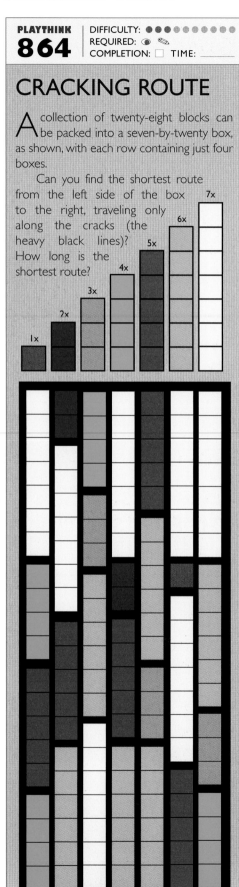

PLAYTHINK 865 | DIFFICULTY: ●●●●●●○○○○○○
REQUIRED: ◉
COMPLETION: ☐ TIME: _____

AIR RESISTANCE

Place a long, thin strip of wood on a table so that about 10 centimeters extend beyond the edge. Lay a few sheets of newspaper over the strip and smooth the paper down to press out all the air from under the newsprint.

Then strike the extended end of the strip. Can you guess what will happen?

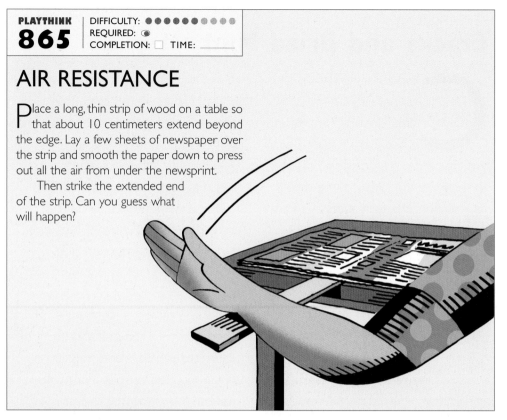

PLAYTHINK 866 | DIFFICULTY: ●●●○○○○○○○○○
REQUIRED: ◉
COMPLETION: ☐ TIME: _____

AIR PRESSURE

Push two sink plungers together as hard as you can. You'll find it is difficult to separate them.

This simple experiment is essentially the same as that of the famous Magdeburg experiment performed in 1654, which first showed that air exerts a lot of pressure. Two hollow half spheres made of bronze were carefully fitted together, and then the air inside was pumped out. Two teams of eight horses each pulling in opposite directions could not separate the hemispheres.

Can you work out why it is so difficult to separate the plungers or the hemispheres?

PLAYTHINK 867 | DIFFICULTY: ●●●●○○○○○○○○
REQUIRED: ◉
COMPLETION: ☐ TIME: _____

NONINFLATABLE BALLOON

Push a balloon into a bottle, stretching its mouth over the opening of the bottle, as shown. If you now try to blow into the balloon, you will find that the balloon can be inflated only partway. It most certainly will not fill the entire volume of the bottle.

Can you work out why this is the case?

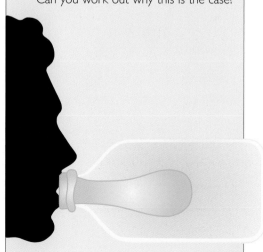

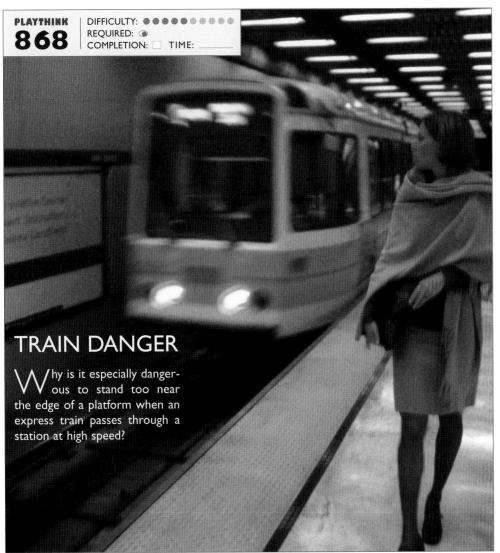

TRAIN DANGER

Why is it especially dangerous to stand too near the edge of a platform when an express train passes through a station at high speed?

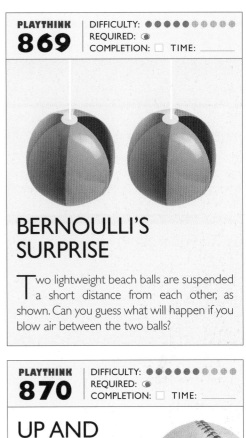

BERNOULLI'S SURPRISE

Two lightweight beach balls are suspended a short distance from each other, as shown. Can you guess what will happen if you blow air between the two balls?

UP AND DOWN

A baseball is tossed in the air. Which takes longer, its flight up or its drop back down?

Fluid Mechanics

Why do most high-speed airplanes have the same general look? It's because they are all subject to the same sorts of intense forces, and the common design is the one that best accommodates them. The designs of aircraft, rockets and ship hulls are based on the principles of fluid mechanics—principles that also help to explain the circulation of blood,

meteorology and oceanography.

The general term *fluid* includes any substance that has no rigidity. Fluids have no definite length or shape—they assume the shape of the vessel that contains them. Thus, both liquids and gases are considered fluids. A distinction can be made between the two: a liquid has a surface and thus a definite volume, while gases have no such volume and expand to fill a container of any size.

The motion of fluids is very complex, which is why engineers need wind tunnels and computer simulations to help them design the most efficient shapes for aircraft and automobiles. The evolution of the scientific understanding of fluid mechanics can be seen in the design of automobiles over the decades: boxy shapes have given way to streamlined silhouettes as ignorance has given way to knowledge.

PLAYTHINK
871
DIFFICULTY: ●●●●●●●○○○
REQUIRED: ◉
COMPLETION: ☐ TIME: _____

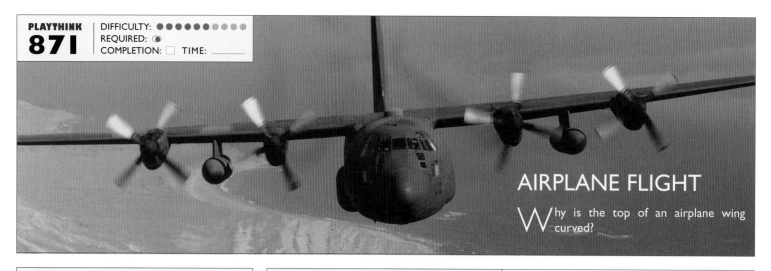

AIRPLANE FLIGHT

Why is the top of an airplane wing curved?

PLAYTHINK
872
DIFFICULTY: ●●●●●●●○○○
REQUIRED: ◉
COMPLETION: ☐ TIME: _____

ASCENDING BALL

Will the time it takes for a Ping-Pong ball to rise to the top of a cylinder of water be different if the water in the cylinder is still or if it is swirling around?

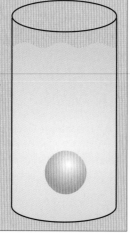

PLAYTHINK
873
DIFFICULTY: ●●●●●○○○○○
REQUIRED: ◉
COMPLETION: ☐ TIME: _____

U-TUBE

Pour water into a transparent U-shaped tube, as shown. Put your thumb on one end of the tube, then carefully tilt the tube back until the water touches your thumb. Press your thumb over the end to make a tight seal.

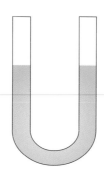

When you return the tube to an upright position, the water will remain touching your thumb. The water level will be unbalanced, as shown in the illustration. Can you explain what causes the water level to be unbalanced?

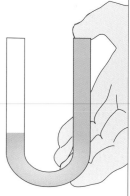

PLAYTHINK
874
DIFFICULTY: ●●●●●●●○○○
REQUIRED: ◉
COMPLETION: ☐ TIME: _____

BATH

Imagine you are in a bathtub checking to see how much weight your toy duck can carry before it sinks. You place a heavy metal ring on the duck, and it doesn't sink. Then the ring slips off and falls to the bottom of the tub.

When the ring falls, does the water level in the tub go up, go down or stay the same?

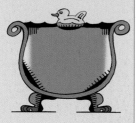

PLAYTHINK
875
DIFFICULTY: ●●●●●●○○○○
REQUIRED: ◉
COMPLETION: ☐ TIME: _____

AIR JET

Put a Ping-Pong ball inside a small funnel. Then tip your head back and blow as hard as you can. Rather than being blown to the ceiling, the ball remains suspended in the air. The harder you blow, the higher it will float above the funnel. Can you work out what causes such strange behavior?

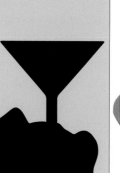

PLAYTHINK
876
DIFFICULTY: ●●●●●●●○○○
REQUIRED: ◉
COMPLETION: ☐ TIME: _____

BLOWING CANDLES

What happens when you blow between two burning candles?

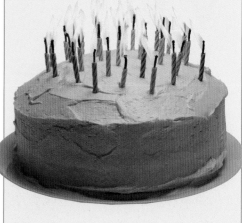

PLAYTHINK 877 | DIFFICULTY: ●●●●○○○○○○ REQUIRED: ◉ COMPLETION: □ TIME: ____

SAILING 1

Suppose you are sailing directly downwind in a 40-kilometer-per-hour wind. If your sail makes a 90-degree angle with the keel of the boat, what is the fastest speed you can achieve?

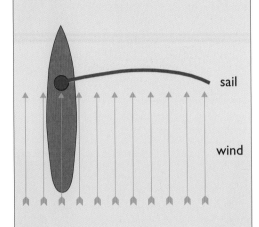

sail

wind

PLAYTHINK 878 | DIFFICULTY: ●●●●○○○○○○ REQUIRED: ◉ COMPLETION: □ TIME: ____

SAILING 2

Suppose you are sailing directly downwind in a 40-kilometer-per-hour wind. If your sail makes less than a 90-degree angle with the keel of the boat, what is the fastest speed you can achieve?

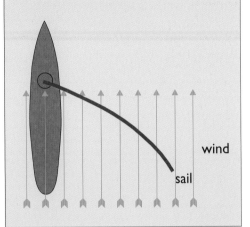

wind

sail

PLAYTHINK 879 | DIFFICULTY: ●●●○○○○○○○ REQUIRED: ◉ COMPLETION: □ TIME: ____

SAILING 3

Suppose you are sailing exactly across a 40-kilometer-per-hour wind. If your sail makes less than a 90-degree angle with the keel of the boat, will you sail faster or slower than you would in a tailwind?

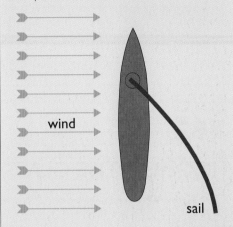

wind

sail

PLAYTHINK 880 | DIFFICULTY: ●●●●○○○○○○ REQUIRED: ◉ COMPLETION: □ TIME: ____

SAILING 4

Which of the four boats moves forward with the greatest speed?

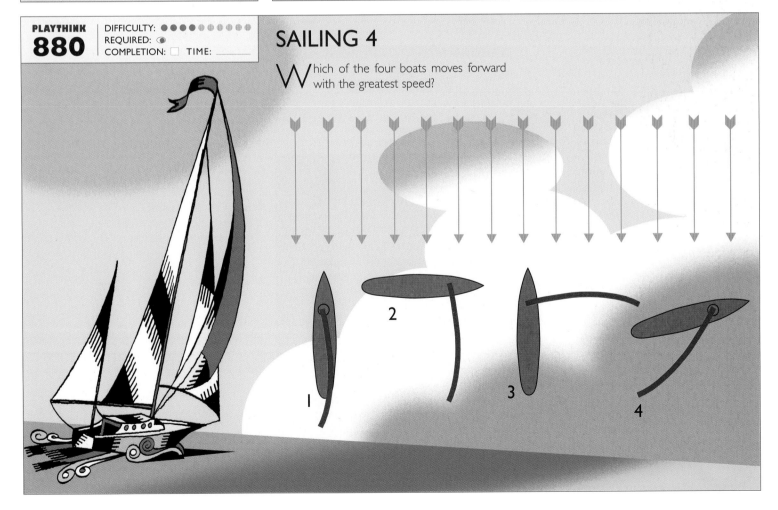

PLAYTHINK 881

DIFFICULTY: ●●●●●●●○○○
REQUIRED: ◉
COMPLETION: ☐ TIME: _____

TEA WITH MILK

You have two glasses, one exactly half full of tea, the other exactly half full of milk. Take a teaspoon of milk from the glass and stir it into the tea. Then take a teaspoon of the tea-milk mixture and stir that into the glass with the milk.

Can you tell whether there is more milk in the tea than there is tea in the milk? Or is there more tea in the milk than milk in the tea?

PLAYTHINK 882

DIFFICULTY: ●●●●●●○○○○
REQUIRED: ◉
COMPLETION: ☐ TIME: _____

FINGER IN THE GLASS

Two glasses filled with water are balanced on a scale, as shown. What happens to the scale when you stick your finger in one of the glasses? Will that side of the balance tip, as if it were heavier?

How would the result change if your finger were made of heavy metal?

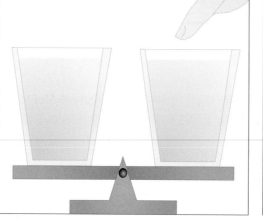

PLAYTHINK 883

DIFFICULTY: ●●●●●●●○○○
REQUIRED: ◉
COMPLETION: ☐ TIME: _____

SHIP IN THE DOCK

A ship in dry dock is left with just a little bit of water around it on all sides. Will the ship touch bottom? What is the maximum amount of water that will support the ship?

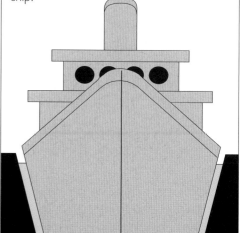

PLAYTHINK 884

DIFFICULTY: ●●●●●○○○○○
REQUIRED: ◉
COMPLETION: ☐ TIME: _____

DIVING BOTTLE

Fill a large plastic bottle up to the brim with water. Then put a small bottle without a top in the big bottle, allowing just enough water in the small bottle so that it will float upside-down. Seal the large bottle tightly.

Can you guess what will happen when you squeeze the big bottle?

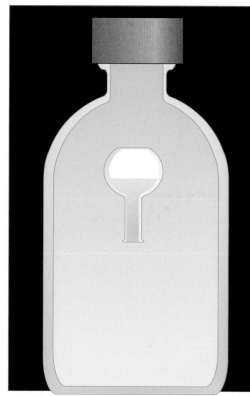

PLAYTHINK 885

DIFFICULTY: ●●●●●●○○○○
REQUIRED: ◉
COMPLETION: ☐ TIME: _____

CORK IN A GLASS

You have no doubt observed that a cork will always drift over to the side of a water glass and stay there. Can you think of a way to make the cork float in the middle of the glass without touching either the cork or the glass?

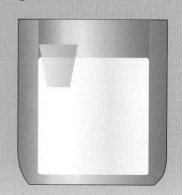

Surface Tension

Why are soap bubbles round? For the same reason that most drops of water are round. Molecules far from the surface of a liquid can be attracted evenly in all directions, but the ones near the surface will be pulled back into the liquid by other molecules. This attraction creates a tendency to minimize the surface area, which becomes as small as possible and behaves like an elastic film. This is surface tension.

Soap has the tendency to reduce the surface tension of water, which is the reason it can pull molecules from a body of water to create soap bubbles and films. When they form, both soap bubbles and drops of liquid contract into the shape that has the least surface area—a sphere, since it is the geometric solid that has the least surface for the same volume.

Surface tension is not the same for all liquids: the force is much stronger in water than in oil. The surface tension of mercury, on the other hand, is about seven times stronger than that of water. That's why spilled mercury forms spherical beads on a tabletop.

PLAYTHINK 886

DIFFICULTY: ●●●●●●○○○○
REQUIRED: ◉
COMPLETION: ☐ TIME: _____

FALLING RAINDROPS

Which raindrops fall faster—the large ones or the small ones?

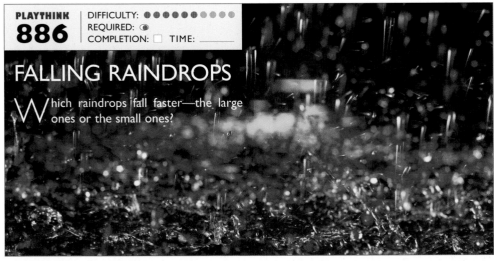

PLAYTHINK 887

DIFFICULTY: ●●●●●●○○○○
REQUIRED: ◉
COMPLETION: ☐ TIME: _____

ICEBERG

A bathtub holding an iceberg is filled to the brim with water. Can you tell what will happen when the iceberg melts?

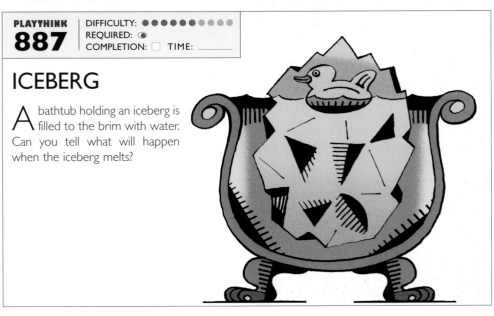

PLAYTHINK 888

DIFFICULTY: ●●●●●●○○○○
REQUIRED: ◉
COMPLETION: ☐ TIME: _____

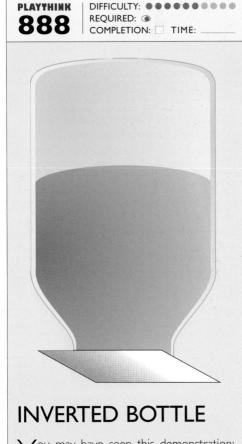

INVERTED BOTTLE

You may have seen this demonstration: The mouth of a jar or bottle full of water is covered with a piece of paper. When the bottle is inverted, the paper remains on the opening and the water does not pour out.

Can you explain why this trick works?

PLAYTHINK 889

DIFFICULTY: ●●●●●○○○○○
REQUIRED: ◉
COMPLETION: ☐ TIME: _____

STORAGE TANK

A tank has two identical holes used to drain water from it. One hole is at the bottom of the tank; the other is a downspout that has a drain hole near the top of the tank but discharges the water at the same level as the other drain.

Ignoring complicating factors such as friction, can you work out which hole discharges water at the faster rate?

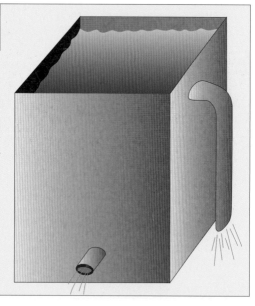

PLAYTHINK 890

DIFFICULTY: ●●●●●●○○○○
REQUIRED: ◉
COMPLETION: ☐ TIME: _____

STORAGE TANKS

Two water tanks are identical in every way except for the size and number of their drains. One tank has one drain that is 6 centimeters across. The other drain has three drains, each 2 centimeters across.

If you open all the drains simultaneously, can you work out which tank will empty first?

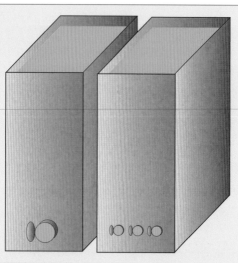

PLAYTHINK 891

DIFFICULTY: ●●●●●●●○○○
REQUIRED: ◉
COMPLETION: ☐ TIME: _____

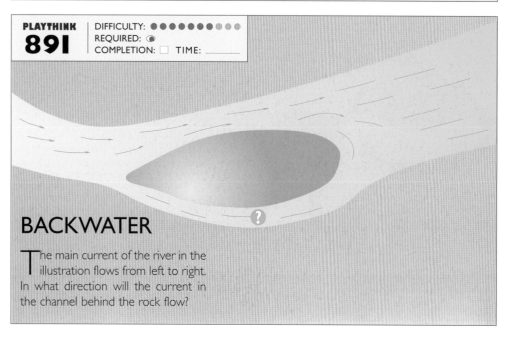

BACKWATER

The main current of the river in the illustration flows from left to right. In what direction will the current in the channel behind the rock flow?

PLAYTHINK 892

DIFFICULTY: ●●●●●○○○○○
REQUIRED: ◉
COMPLETION: ☐ TIME: _____

PENNIES IN A GLASS

Fill a glass with water completely up to the rim. Then slip a penny into the glass—the water will not overflow. Can you guess how many pennies you can slip into the glass before the water spills over the edge?

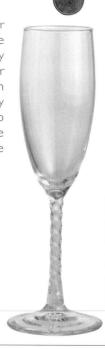

PLAYTHINK 893

DIFFICULTY: ●●●●●●○○○○
REQUIRED: ◉
COMPLETION: ☐ TIME: _____

MARIONETTE'S CONTAINER

A cylinder of water has three holes, spaced as shown in the diagram. A faucet runs into the cylinder to supply enough water to keep the water level constant.

When the holes are unplugged, water will stream continuously from the three holes. Can you work out which stream will shoot out the farthest?

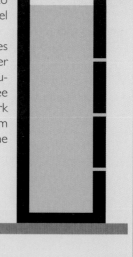

PLAYTHINK 894

DIFFICULTY: ●●●●●●●●○○
REQUIRED: ◉
COMPLETION: ☐ TIME: _____

COANDA EFFECT

What happens when you barely touch the edge of a stream of water with a spoon?

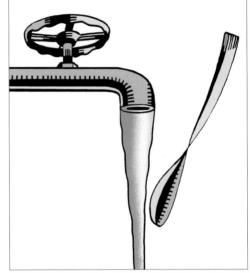

PLAYTHINK 895

DIFFICULTY: ●●●●●●○○○○
REQUIRED: ◉
COMPLETION: ☐ TIME: _____

WATER STREAM

Can you work out why a stream of water becomes narrower as it travels downward from a faucet?

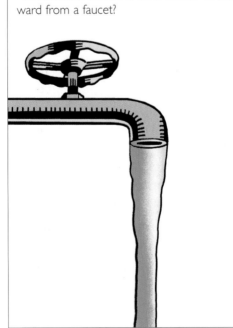

PLAYTHINK 896

DIFFICULTY: ●●●●●●●○○○
REQUIRED: ◉
COMPLETION: ☐ TIME: _____

MUSICAL TUBE

Wave a flexible corrugated tube around in a circle, and it will make a sound. Can you explain why?

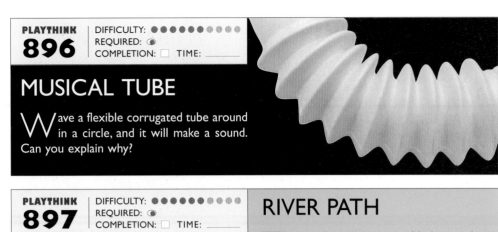

PLAYTHINK 897

DIFFICULTY: ●●●●●●●○○○
REQUIRED: ◉
COMPLETION: ☐ TIME: _____

RIVER PATH

The cowboy must water his horse, then return to his wagon. Can you work out his shortest possible path?

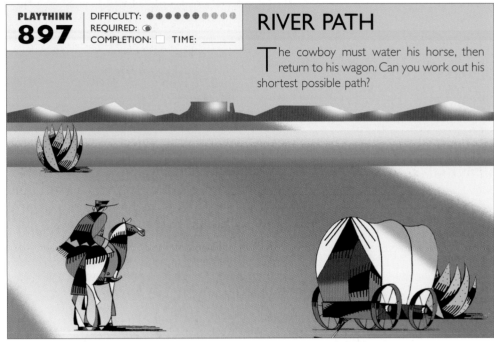

PLAYTHINK 898

DIFFICULTY: ●●●●●●○○○○
REQUIRED: ◉
COMPLETION: ☐ TIME: _____

DISAPPEARING COIN

Put a coin in the bottom of a bucket so that when you peer over the rim, the coin is just out of sight. Without moving the bucket or your vantage point, slowly begin filling the bucket with water. Can you tell what will happen to the coin?

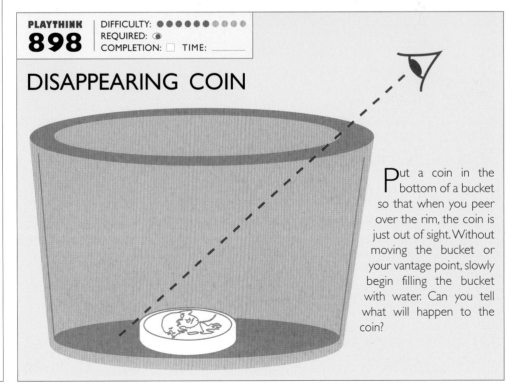

PLAYTHINK 899

DIFFICULTY: ●●●●●●●○○○
REQUIRED: ◉
COMPLETION: ☐ TIME: _____

MAGNIFIER IN WATER

Will a magnifying glass enlarge the image of the knife more if the lens is placed underwater?

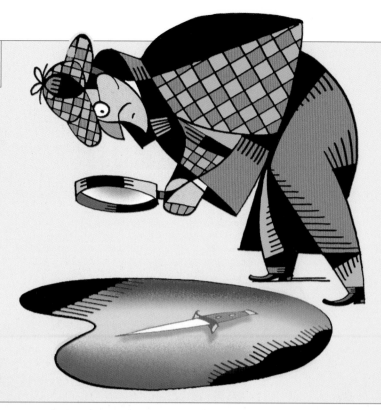

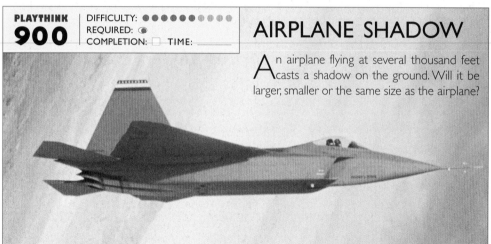

PLAYTHINK 900

DIFFICULTY: ●●●●●●○○○○
REQUIRED: ◉
COMPLETION: ☐ TIME: _____

AIRPLANE SHADOW

An airplane flying at several thousand feet casts a shadow on the ground. Will it be larger, smaller or the same size as the airplane?

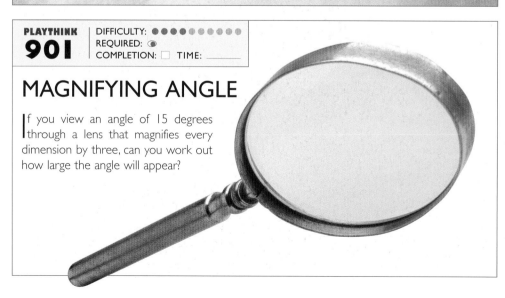

PLAYTHINK 901

DIFFICULTY: ●●●●●○○○○○
REQUIRED: ◉
COMPLETION: ☐ TIME: _____

MAGNIFYING ANGLE

If you view an angle of 15 degrees through a lens that magnifies every dimension by three, can you work out how large the angle will appear?

PLAYTHINK 902

DIFFICULTY: ●●●●●●○○○○
REQUIRED: ◉
COMPLETION: ☐ TIME: _____

FULL-LENGTH MIRROR

Can you work out the minimum height of a mirror that lets you see a full head-to-toe view of yourself?

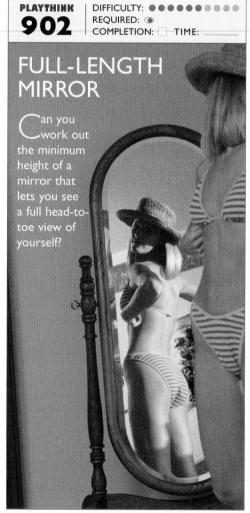

PLAYTHINK
903

DIFFICULTY: ●●●●●●○○○○○
REQUIRED: ◉ ✎
COMPLETION: ☐ TIME: _____

REFLECTION OFF A MIRROR

A ray of light from point A bounces off the surface of a plane mirror and reaches point B.

Can you find the point of reflection on the mirror?

A

B

?

Mirror

PLAYTHINK
904

DIFFICULTY: ●●●●●●●○○○○
REQUIRED: ◉ ✎
COMPLETION: ☐ TIME: _____

MIRROR LABYRINTH

There are six entrances to the labyrinth, each marked with an arrow. All the walls of the labyrinth are covered with mirrors, and if you follow the reflections, you can make your way from each entrance to one of the caged animals.

Can you work out which entrance leads to which animal? (You must enter in the direction of the arrow.)

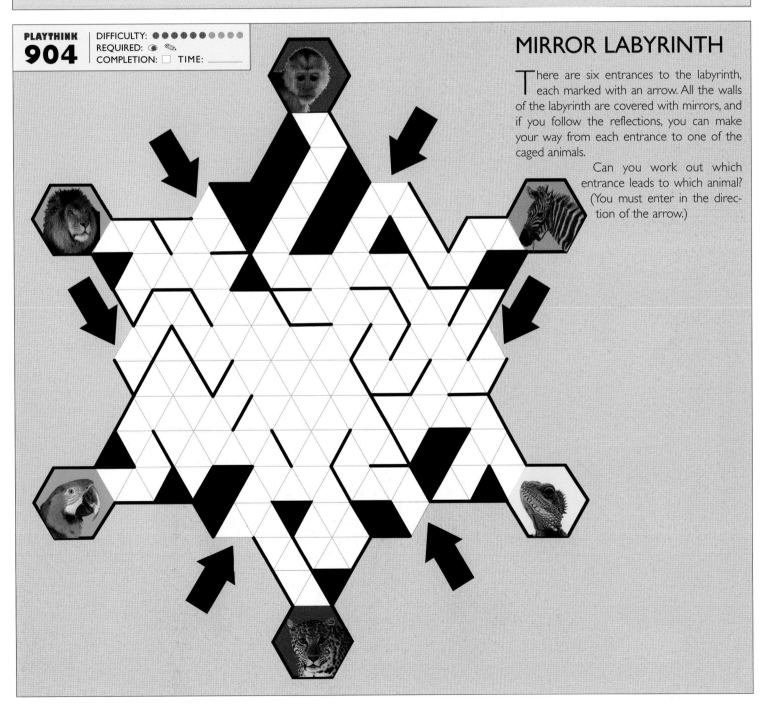

PLAYTHINK 905

DIFFICULTY: ●●●●●●●○○○
REQUIRED: ◉
COMPLETION: ☐ TIME: _____

DESCENT

Identical lead weights are dropped simultaneously into each of five containers that are filled with different substances at the temperatures listed for each.

In which container will the weight take the longest to reach the bottom?

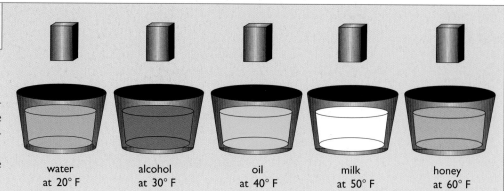

| water at 20° F | alcohol at 30° F | oil at 40° F | milk at 50° F | honey at 60° F |

PLAYTHINK 906

DIFFICULTY: ●●●●●●○○○○
REQUIRED: ◉ ✎
COMPLETION: ☐ TIME: _____

SUPER PERISCOPE

If you rotate ten of the double-sided mirrors by 90 degrees each, you will be able to see the reflection of the lightbulb from the porthole in the top right-hand corner. Can you work out which ten mirrors must be moved?

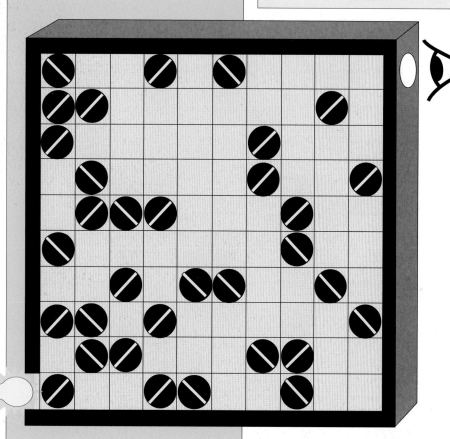

PLAYTHINK 907

DIFFICULTY: ●●●●●●●●○○
REQUIRED: ◉
COMPLETION: ☐ TIME: _____

ARCHIMEDES'S MIRRORS

Mirrors are found in common yet seemingly miraculous objects in science, magic and everyday life. Telescopes, optical scanners and the box in which the magician saws a lady in half all employ mirrors.

One of the most imaginative uses of mirrors is credited to the ancient Greek scientist Archimedes. According to writings from the period, Archimedes used mirrors to repel a fleet of Roman ships that besieged the city of Syracuse in 214 B.C. He is supposed to have used the mirrors to focus the rays of the sun on the ships, setting them on fire.

Is such a feat really possible?

Archimedes

PLAYTHINK 908

DIFFICULTY: ●●●●●○○○○○
REQUIRED: ◉ ✎
COMPLETION: ☐ TIME: _____

FASHION MIRROR

The model stands 2 meters from the dresser mirror and holds a hand mirror half a meter behind her head. How far behind the dresser mirror is the image of the red flower in her hair?

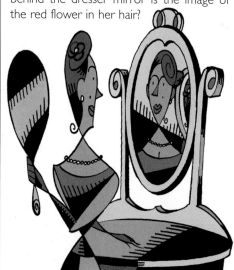

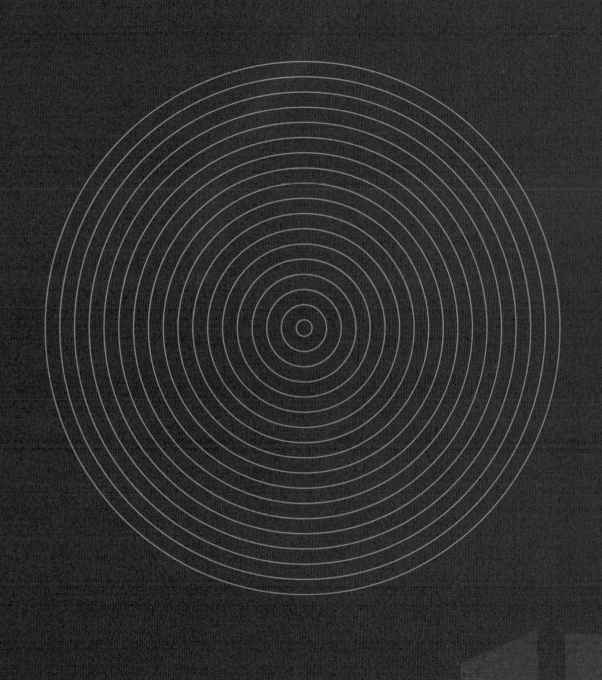

13

Perception

Missing Cubes

You have no doubt seen a room in which a man seems to shrink as he walks from one end to the other. As you quickly realize, the man isn't shrinking—he's walking away from you in a specially constructed room designed to mask the perception of depth.

There are no such tricks included in the following puzzles. These problems depend upon our ability to perceive depth—the three-dimensional effect afforded by perspective—projected into two-dimensional illustrations. Although this ability was either unknown or ignored before the Middle Ages, the effect is so well understood at present that computers can be programmed to recognize three-dimensional objects (such as a particular programmer's facial features) at any angle. And holograms, which don't employ perspective but capture three-dimensional information about an object from the light bouncing off it, are found in demonstrations of science, breathtaking works of art and commercial security systems. Indeed, this last use is now the most common: many a credit card carries a little hologram on its face.

Certainly there are cases when perspective can be misleading. All the same, there is a shortcut to finding the solution to these problems, one that emerges from the vagaries of perspective.

PLAYTHINK
909

DIFFICULTY: ●●●●●●●●○○
REQUIRED: 👁 ✎
COMPLETION: ☐ TIME: _____

MISSING CUBES

The five cubes illustrated here are missing parts. Can you work out how many unit cubes are missing in each case?

Once you have calculated the total number of missing cubes, you should note that some of the missing unit cubes are colored red, blue or green on some of their faces, while others are completely gray. Can you fill in the scorecard below with the number of cubes that fall into each category? Can you work out a visual shortcut for finding that information?

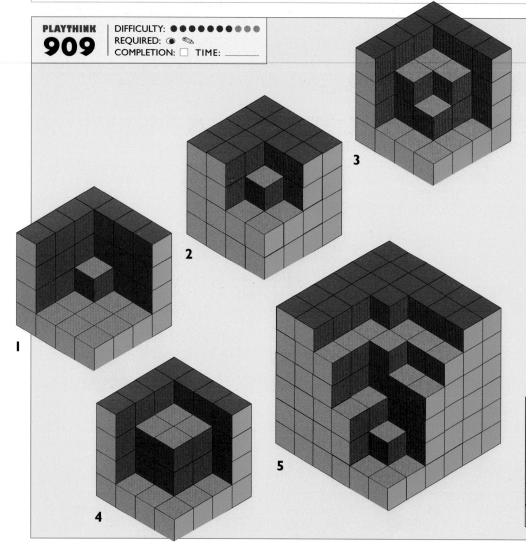

Score Box

Missing Cubes	1	2	3	4	5
Cubes colored on three sides					
Cubes colored on two sides					
Cubes colored on one side					
Cubes not colored					
Totals					

PLAYTHINK
910
DIFFICULTY: ●●●●●○○○○○
REQUIRED: ◉
COMPLETION: ☐ TIME: _____

MISHANDLED SQUARE

In the same way that lines can be distorted by different backgrounds in different ways, so can shapes and polygons. Imagine this perfect square superimposed on the four different background patterns. How will the square be distorted in each case? Will it become convex, concave, bent or skewed?

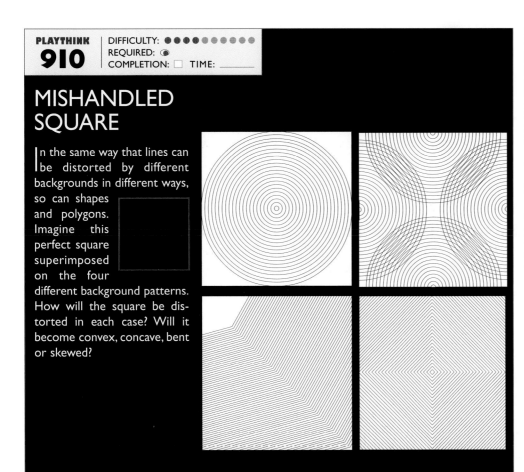

PLAYTHINK
911
DIFFICULTY: ●●●●○○○○○○
REQUIRED: ◉
COMPLETION: ☐ TIME: _____

ILLUSION WHEEL

The twelve lines are identical in length and can be categorized into three groups of four—one group divided by dots, one by arrows and one by semicircles. In each of the three groups, one line is divided exactly in half. Can you find which ones?

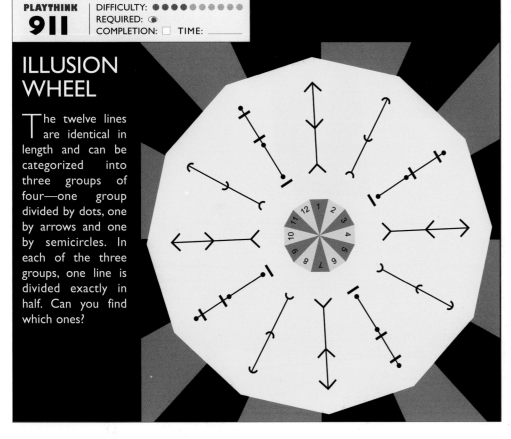

PLAYTHINK
912
DIFFICULTY: ●●●●●○○○○○
REQUIRED: ◉
COMPLETION: ☐ TIME: _____

BLIND SPOT

Is there a way to make the butterfly disappear while keeping it in plain sight?

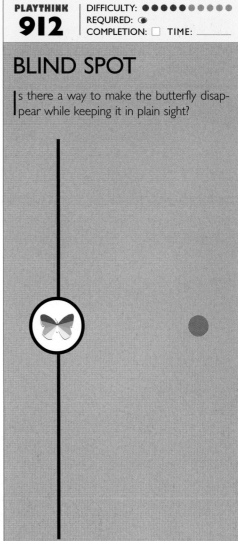

PLAYTHINK
913
DIFFICULTY: ●●●●●●●●●○
REQUIRED: ◉
COMPLETION: ☐ TIME: _____

GREEN BIRD IN THE CAGE

How can you put a green bird in the cage just by looking at this picture?

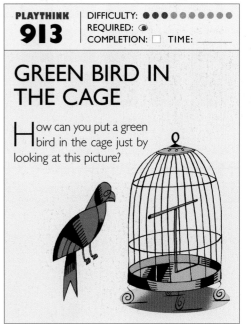

PLAYTHINK 914

DIFFICULTY: ●●●●○○○○○○
REQUIRED: ◉
COMPLETION: ☐ TIME: _____

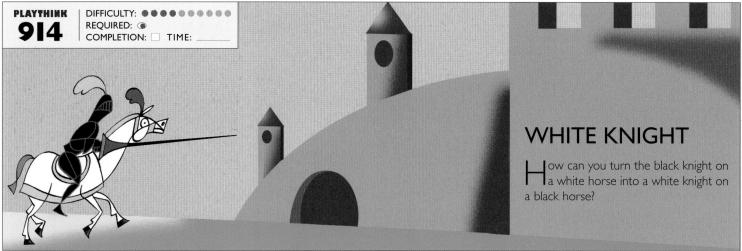

WHITE KNIGHT

How can you turn the black knight on a white horse into a white knight on a black horse?

PLAYTHINK 915

DIFFICULTY: ●●○○○○○○○○
REQUIRED: ◉
COMPLETION: ☐ TIME: _____

ELUSIVE SPOTS

If you look at the grid of black squares, you will see many gray spots at the intersections. But as you look around, you'll find that there is always one intersection that has no gray spot. Can you find which intersection that is?

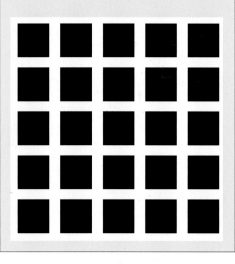

PLAYTHINK 916

DIFFICULTY: ●●●○○○○○○○
REQUIRED: ◉
COMPLETION: ☐ TIME: _____

DRACULA'S COFFIN

Can you work out which lid goes with which coffin?

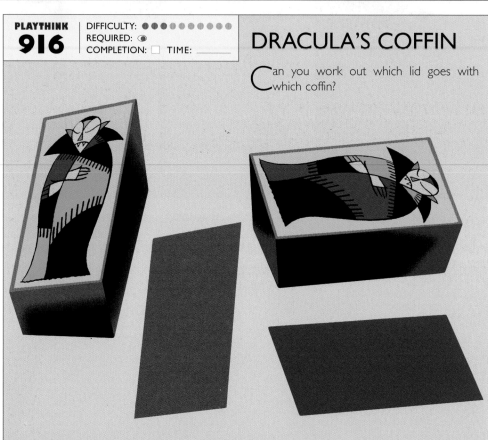

PLAYTHINK 917

DIFFICULTY: ●●●○○○○○○○
REQUIRED: ◉
COMPLETION: ☐ TIME: _____

CROSSING LINES

How can you look at the two intersecting lines to see more than two lines?

PLAYTHINK 918

DIFFICULTY: ●●●○○○○○○○○
REQUIRED: ◉
COMPLETION: ☐ TIME: _____

BROKEN BRIDGE

Can you close the gap in the broken bridge without folding or cutting the page?

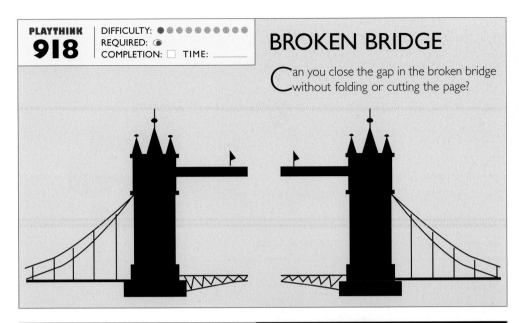

PLAYTHINK 920

DIFFICULTY: ●●●●●●●●○○○
REQUIRED: ◉
COMPLETION: ☐ TIME: _____

POINTILLISTIC SEEING

Can you figure out what's in this picture?

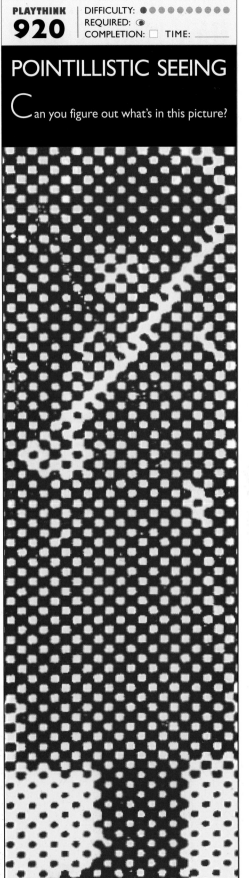

PLAYTHINK 919

DIFFICULTY: ●●●●○○○○○○○
REQUIRED: ◉
COMPLETION: ☐ TIME: _____

SHADOW PROFILES

There are three identical profiles. How quickly can you find them?

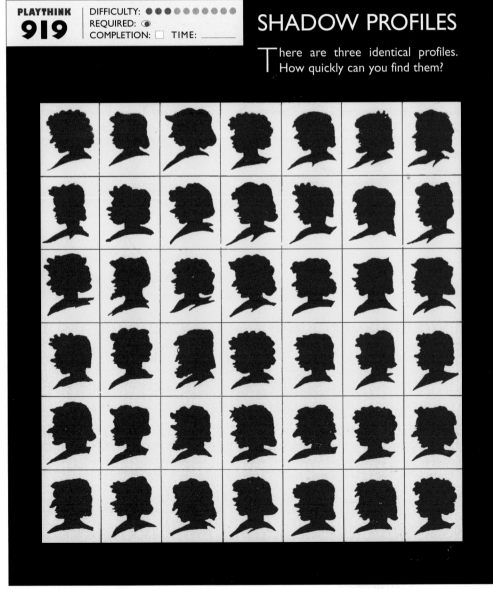

How Many Cubes?

This famous optical illusion is a striking demonstration of the power of the mind to change the orientation of objects. In the same illustration you can see either seven whole cubes or three cubes and several parts of incomplete cubes. If you have a hard time seeing the three-cube orientation, turn the page upside down.

Changing the point of view in this way—or being able to see things the way more literal-minded people can't—is the essence of creative thinking.

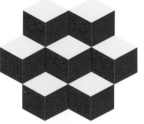

PLAYTHINK
921
DIFFICULTY: ●●●●●○○○○○
REQUIRED: ◉
COMPLETION: ☐ TIME: _____

GUIDED BOMB

In spite of the thick cloud cover, the laser-guided bomb can pinpoint its target. By looking straight at the page, can you tell which numbered position is in direct line with the tank?

1 2 3 4 5 6 7 8 9

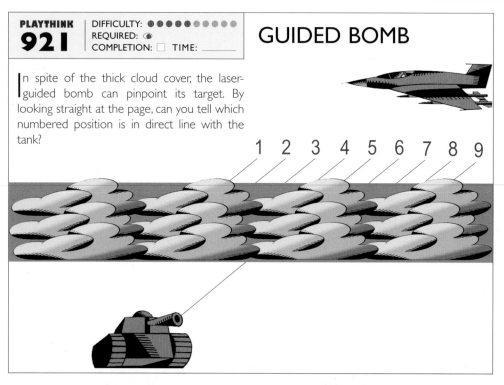

PLAYTHINK
922
DIFFICULTY: ●●●●●●●●●●
REQUIRED: ◉
COMPLETION: ☐ TIME: _____

MISSING SLICE

Can you find the missing slice of cake?

PLAYTHINK
923
DIFFICULTY: ●●●○○○○○○○
REQUIRED: ◉
COMPLETION: ☐ TIME: _____

DIGITS

Can you tell what the pattern of digits represents?

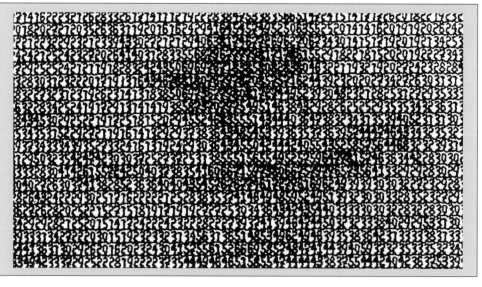

Point of View

Painters often find that the most difficult shape to capture is the familiar one. To see an object as a pure form rather than as a clock or an apple, artists go to great lengths to alter their perception. Many artists will study a still life arrangement through a mirror—or backward, through their legs—to obtain a fresh view of the subject. Such a new perspective can enable them to discover an innovative way to capture a subject's form on canvas.

That artists must struggle to overcome their built-in perception is evidence that our conscious mind stores three-dimensional images, memorizing and categorizing everything we see. Such images are generally available for recall in a way that makes comparison and recognition possible even from unfamiliar angles. This ability is so constant and automatic that it is totally unremarkable—except when that ability is lost. The victims of certain forms of brain damage that impair the normal ability to compare and recognize shapes find, in fact, that everyday life becomes nearly impossible without that aspect of human consciousness.

PLAYTHINK 924

DIFFICULTY: ●●●●●●●○○○
REQUIRED: ◉
COMPLETION: ☐ TIME: _____

CUBES IN SPACE

Isn't it surprising how different something can look from an unexpected angle? Believe it or not, these ten formations of cubes are made up of three identical pairs, one set of three and one unique configuration. It may take you some time to see which ones fall into which category. It sometimes helps to actually turn the book to find the similarities.

Can you identify the three pairs, the set of three identical shapes and the unique configuration?

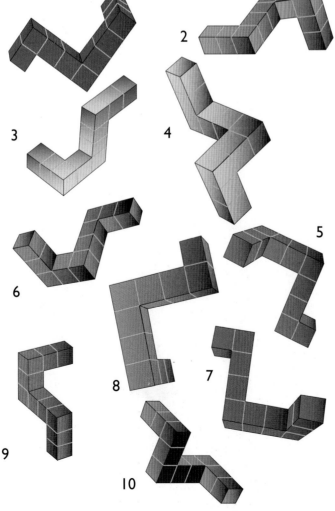

PLAYTHINK 925

DIFFICULTY: ●●●●●○○○○○
REQUIRED: ◉
COMPLETION: ☐ TIME: _____

UPSIDE-DOWN WORDS

Place a mirror along the red line. The words in the top frame will appear reversed right to left, as is normal. But the words in the bottom frame will appear upside-down. Can you explain this?

> **PLACE A MIRROR VERTICALLY ON THE LEFT RED LINE. WORDS IN THE TOP FRAME WILL BE REVERSED RIGHT-LEFT (BUT NOT UPSIDE-DOWN). WORDS AT THE BOTTOM FRAME ARE NOT ONLY REVERSED, BUT ALSO TURNED UPSIDE-DOWN. CAN YOU EXPLAIN WHY ?**
>
> **BOOKIE EXCEEDED HIKED ICEBOX CHOKED COED BOBBED DECK BEECED COD HID BOXED DODO BOB CHOKED COCO EXCEEDED BOOKIE HIKED ICEBOX DID CHOICE BOOKED OBOE HEEDED OX HID COKE EXHOED BOOHOO DOCKED**

The Limits of Seeing

Most people experience seeing as a passive "taking-in" process. But, in fact, perception is an active pattern-seeking process that is closely allied to the act of thinking. The brain is as much a "seeing" organ as the eye. Optical illusions take advantage of the tendency of the human brain to see things as it thinks they should be—based on previous experience—rather than as they are. Although this normalizing property of our perceptional system is widely engaged in science, math, art, design and architecture, the ease with which we can be fooled by a simple optical illusion should be a warning to the general unreliablility of our observations. (Remember that if you should ever have to listen to "eyewitness testimony.") We can be made to perceive things to be larger than they actually are, register depth in a two-dimensional flat surface, see colors in a monochromatic pattern or experience motion in a static image.

There is a limit to the reliability of our senses, and no amount of practice can ever make them good enough for some special tasks. One solution to that problem is to find ways to extend our senses, to invent devices capable of perceiving and recording information without error. Although no one has created a perfect system for doing this, cameras and recorders have proven to be much more reliable and free from bias than even the best human observer.

This human tendency to be tripped up by our perceptions has long been a source of play for the makers of optical illusions (and of inspiration for Op Art painters). For as long as humans have been playing with lines and shapes, colors and patterns, it has been known that we can see disappearing cubes or lines where there are, in fact, none.

PLAYTHINK 926 | DIFFICULTY: ●●○○○○○○○○ REQUIRED: ◉ COMPLETION: ☐ TIME: _____

INSIDE-OUTSIDE FLY

Can you tell where on the box the fly has landed?

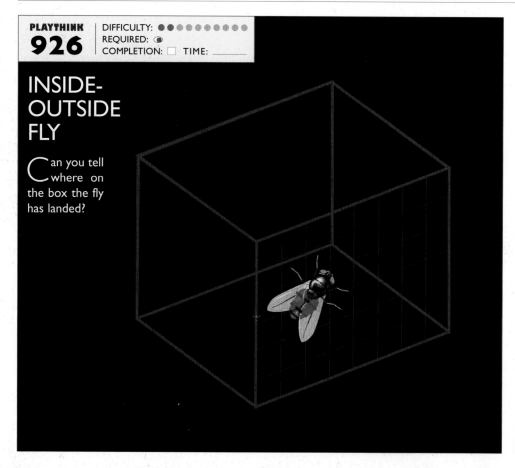

PLAYTHINK 927 | DIFFICULTY: ●●○○○○○○○○ REQUIRED: ◉ COMPLETION: ☐ TIME: _____

BEFORE-AFTER

Below is a portrait of a newlywed couple. Can you find an image that shows how happy they will be in a few years?

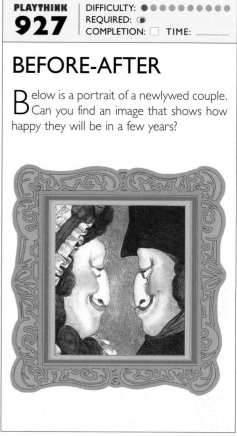

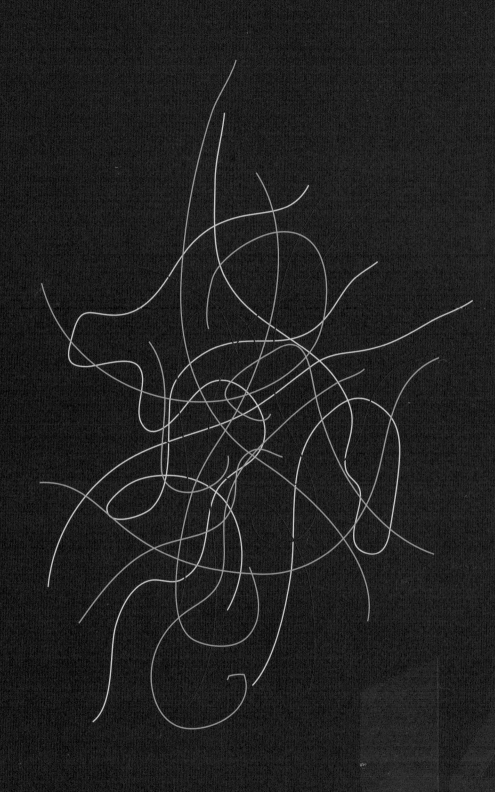

Bonus Round

PLAYTHINK **928** | DIFFICULTY: ●●●●●●○○○○
REQUIRED: ◉
COMPLETION: ☐ TIME: _____

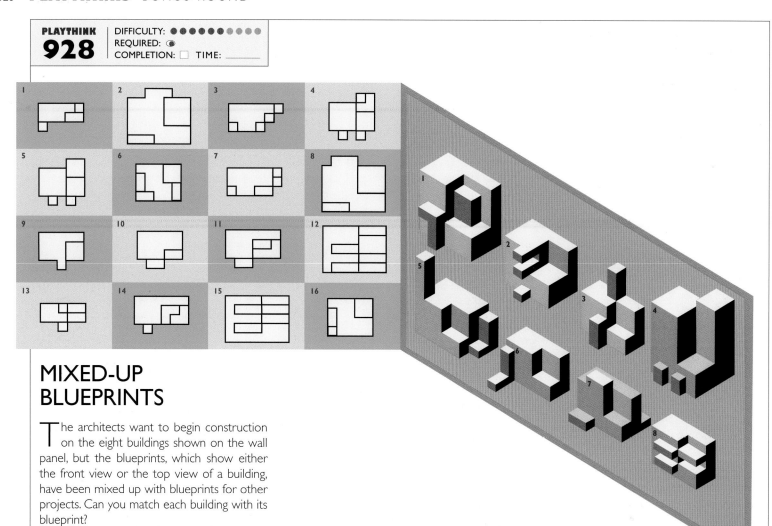

MIXED-UP BLUEPRINTS

The architects want to begin construction on the eight buildings shown on the wall panel, but the blueprints, which show either the front view or the top view of a building, have been mixed up with blueprints for other projects. Can you match each building with its blueprint?

PLAYTHINK **929** | DIFFICULTY: ●●●●●●●○○○
REQUIRED: ◉ ✎
COMPLETION: ☐ TIME: _____

EXHIBITION WIRING

An architect is examining his design for the placement of the electrical outlets in an exhibition hall. The hall is divided into identical unit blocks, and the client needs each intersection to be no more than three blocks from an electrical outlet.

His initial design, shown here, used twenty-five electrical outlets, but the architect is certain that there is a more economical solution. Is he right? Can you find the design that provides the fewest number of outlets yet puts no intersection more than three blocks from an outlet?

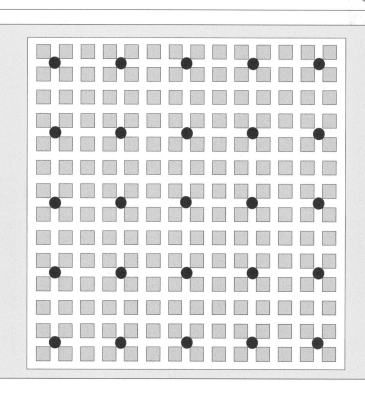

PLAYTHINK 930

DIFFICULTY: ●●●●●●●●○○
REQUIRED: 👁 ✎
COMPLETION: ☐ TIME: _____

FLATLAND RAILWAY

Nine straight parallel railway tracks run between two cities in Flatland. The tracks can connect the two cities without any intersections, which is advantageous for scheduling purposes. The leaders of a third city that is not in line with the existing rail lines have asked for some of the tracks to be re-laid so that their city can be connected to the other two by at least two tracks.

The tracks will be laid out so that one set is parallel in one direction, another is parallel in another direction, and a third set is parallel in a third direction. Can you work out how to design the rail system so that you create the smallest number of intersections?

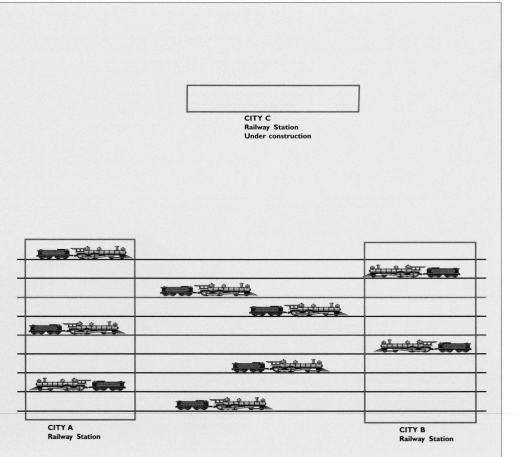

CITY C
Railway Station
Under construction

CITY A
Railway Station

CITY B
Railway Station

PLAYTHINK 931

DIFFICULTY: ●●●●●○○○○○
REQUIRED: 👁 ✎ ✂
COMPLETION: ☐ TIME: _____

MOVING TRIANGLE 2

Two vertices of the triangle are constrained to move along the circumferences of the intersecting circles. As the triangle tips follow their circular paths, the third vertex traces out a complex shape. Can you determine what shape the vertex traces?

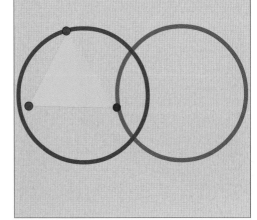

PLAYTHINK 932

DIFFICULTY: ●●●●●●○○○○
REQUIRED: 👁 ✎ ✂
COMPLETION: ☐ TIME: _____

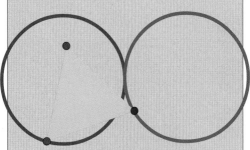

MOVING TRIANGLE 3

Two vertices of the triangle are constrained to move along the circumferences of the two touching circles. As the triangle tips follow their circular paths, the third vertex traces out a complex shape. Can you work out what shape the vertex traces?

PLAYTHINK 933

DIFFICULTY: ●●●●●●●○○○
REQUIRED: 👁 ✎
COMPLETION: ☐ TIME: _____

CRAWLING CENTIPEDE

A centipede sits at the top corner of a three-dimensional solid structure, as shown. Can you find a route along the edges for the bug so that it visits each corner once and only once while not traveling along any edge more than once? (Note that its path will not include every edge.)

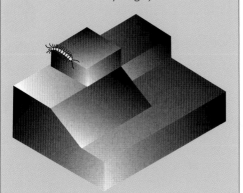

PLAYTHINK 934

DIFFICULTY: ●●●●●●●●○○
REQUIRED: 👁 ✎
COMPLETION: ☐ TIME: _____

CIRCLE DIVISIONS

Using just a compass and a ruler, can you divide this circle into eight regions of equal area?

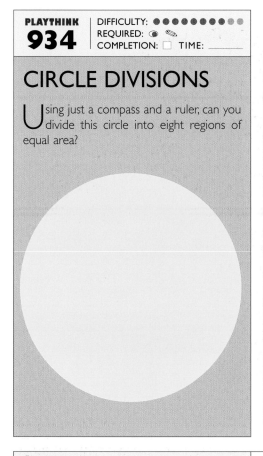

PLAYTHINK 935

DIFFICULTY: ●●●●●●●●○○
REQUIRED: 👁 📄 ✂
COMPLETION: ☐ TIME: _____

FIVE DISKS GAME

Copy (at a 300 percent enlargement) and cut out the five yellow disks. By placing the disks on the red circle one at a time, can you use them to completely cover the area of the circle? Once a disk has been placed, it cannot be moved.

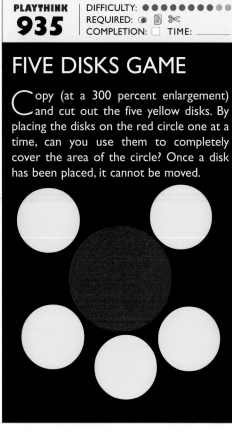

PLAYTHINK 936

DIFFICULTY: ●●●●●●●●○○
REQUIRED: 👁 📄 ✂
COMPLETION: ☐ TIME: _____

THE NINE CIRCLES PUZZLE

Can you fit the nine circles into the red ring in such a way that no circles overlap? Enlarging the puzzle when you copy it may make it easier.

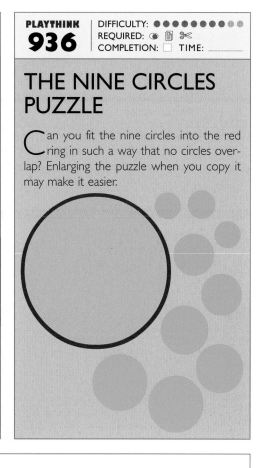

PLAYTHINK 937

DIFFICULTY: ●●●●●●●●○○
REQUIRED: 👁 ✎
COMPLETION: ☐ TIME: _____

ICOSAHEDRON JOURNEY

Imagine holding in your hand the twenty-sided solid known as the icosahedron. Do you think you could find a way to trace a path along its edges so that you visit each of its twelve corners once and only once and end at the point at which you began?

It's difficult to imagine a solution for the three-dimensional solid. But the problem is exactly equivalent—because it is a two-dimensional plane diagram of the three-dimensional icosahedron—and much easier. Can you trace a path along the yellow lines that visits each circle only once and ends on the circle at which you started?

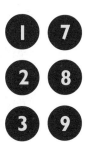

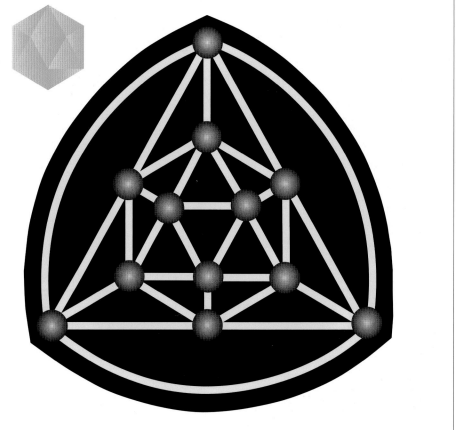

PLAYTHINK 938

DIFFICULTY: ●●●●●●●●○○
REQUIRED: ◉ ✎
COMPLETION: ☐ TIME: _____

TRAVELING IN CIRCLES

Only those who can follow the rules posted in this pentagonal garden are allowed to walk here. First, you may walk only along the paths. Second, you must visit each of the fifteen circles only once and leave a numbered marker to show the order of your visits. Third, as you leave each circle after the first one you decide to visit (which can be any of them), you must change directions so that you are not moving in a straight line. Fourth, you may walk along a path only once.

Can you find a route that will enable you to walk in the garden?

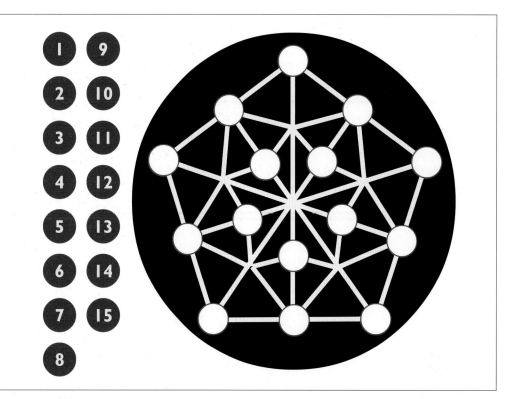

PLAYTHINK 939

DIFFICULTY: ●●●●●●●●○○
REQUIRED: ◉ ✎
COMPLETION: ☐ TIME: _____

OVERLAPPING POLYGONS

For each of the sets of overlapping shapes, can you work out which is larger: the sum of the uncovered red areas or the uncovered blue area in the middle? Refer to the box to figure out the relative sizes of the shapes.

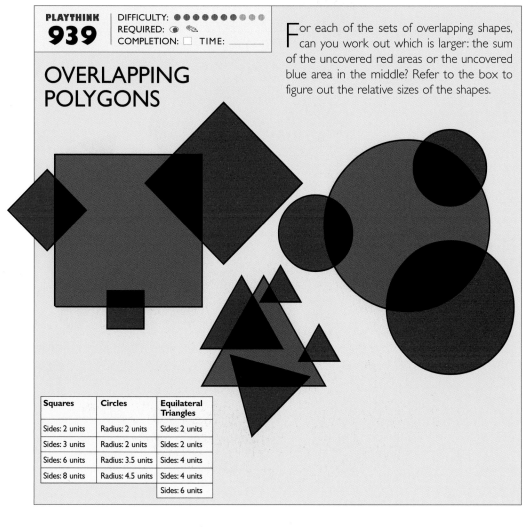

Squares	Circles	Equilateral Triangles
Sides: 2 units	Radius: 2 units	Sides: 2 units
Sides: 3 units	Radius: 2 units	Sides: 2 units
Sides: 6 units	Radius: 3.5 units	Sides: 4 units
Sides: 8 units	Radius: 4.5 units	Sides: 4 units
		Sides: 6 units

PLAYTHINK 940

DIFFICULTY: ●●●●●○○○○○
REQUIRED: ◉
COMPLETION: ☐ TIME: _____

CABLE CONNECTION

A telephone cable has twenty wires—five in each of four different colors. If you are working in total darkness, how many wires must you grab to ensure that you have one of each color?

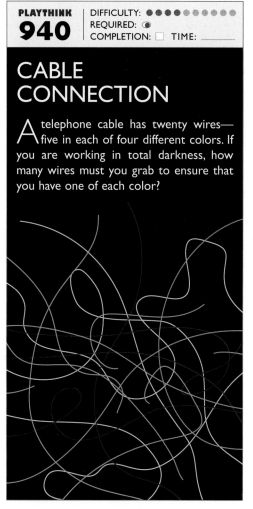

PLAYTHINK 941

DIFFICULTY: ●●●●●●●○○○
REQUIRED: 👁 📄 ✂
COMPLETION: ☐ TIME: _____

TRIANGLES OVERLAP

Three overlapping triangles form eighteen regions, as shown. Can you overlap the same triangles to form even more regions?

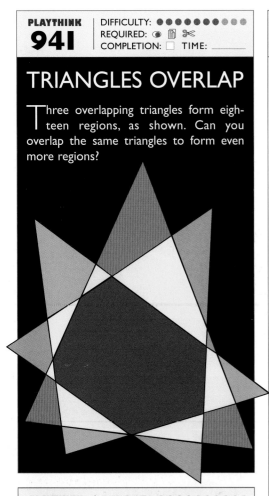

PLAYTHINK 942

DIFFICULTY: ●●●●○○○○○○
REQUIRED: 👁 ✏
COMPLETION: ☐ TIME: _____

WINNING HORSES

If seven horses have entered a race, how many different ways can the first three places be filled?

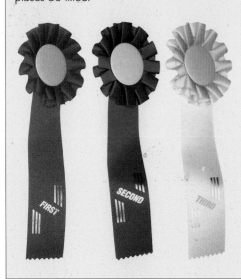

PLAYTHINK 943

DIFFICULTY: ●●●●●●●●●○
REQUIRED: 👁 📄 ✂
COMPLETION: ☐ TIME: _____

POLYGON BRIDGES

Can you connect these polygons to create a bridge connecting the four black triangles at the corners? The polygons can slide around, but they can't be rotated; their sides must make full contact. The black triangles must remain fixed.

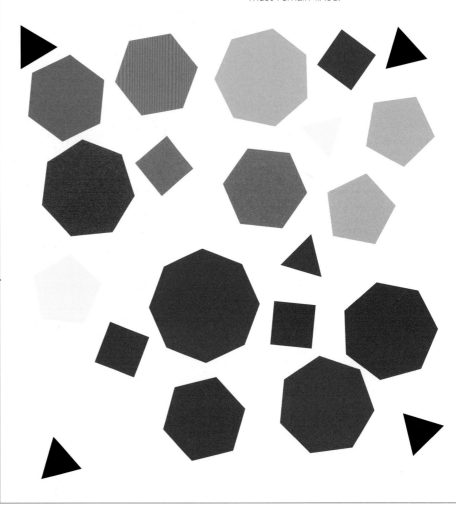

PLAYTHINK 944

DIFFICULTY: ●●●●●●●●○○
REQUIRED: 👁 ✏
COMPLETION: ☐ TIME: _____

COMBINATION LOCK

The lock shown here is opened by selecting the correct nonrepeating three-letter combination. If a bank robber has one guess at opening the lock, what are the chances that he'll guess correctly?

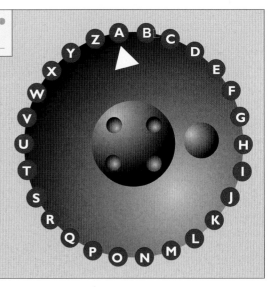

PLAYTHINK 945

DIFFICULTY: ●●●●●●○○○○
REQUIRED: 👁
COMPLETION: ☐ TIME: _____

COVERED TRIANGLE

A right triangle is cut out of paper and folded as shown. Can you work out the relationship of the area visible in red to that of the original triangle?

PLAYTHINK 946

DIFFICULTY: ●●●●●●●○○○
REQUIRED: 👁 ✎
COMPLETION: ☐ TIME: _____

MY CLASS

In a class of fifteen boys, fourteen have blue eyes, twelve have black hair, eleven are overweight and ten are tall. Can you work out how many tall, overweight, black-haired, blue-eyed boys there must be?

PLAYTHINK 947

DIFFICULTY: ●●●●●●●●○○
REQUIRED: 👁 ✎
COMPLETION: ☐ TIME: _____

LICENSE PLATES

In many countries automobile license plates take the form shown here: one letter, followed by three numbers, followed by three letters.

In such a country how many different license plates are possible?

A 234 HIL

PLAYTHINK 948

DIFFICULTY: ●●●●●●●○○○
REQUIRED: 👁 ✎
COMPLETION: ☐ TIME: _____

WALKING DOGS

Beatrice has six dogs to walk. If she walks them two at a time, how many different pairs of dogs can she take out?

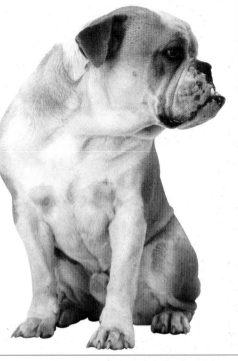

PLAYTHINK 949

DIFFICULTY: ●●●●●●●○○○
REQUIRED: 👁 ✎
COMPLETION: ☐ TIME: _____

MAGIC GRID MATRIX 1

Examine this matrix of numbers. Can you divide it into eight parts in such a way that the digits in each part will add up to the same total?

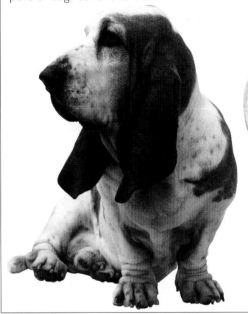

PLAYTHINK 950

DIFFICULTY: ●●●●●●●●○○
REQUIRED: 👁 ✎
COMPLETION: ☐ TIME: _____

MAGIC GRID MATRIX 2

Can you divide this matrix along the grid lines into sixteen identical parts? No two parts may have the same numbers, and the sum of the numbers in each part must total 34.

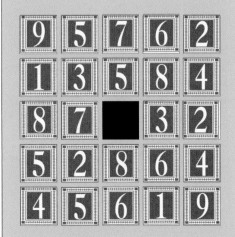

PLAYTHINK 951

DIFFICULTY: ●●●●●●●○○○
REQUIRED: 👁 ✏
COMPLETION: ☐ TIME: _____

EDGE COLORING PATTERN

Imagine you want to color in the lines of this diagram in such a way that no two lines of the same color meet at an endpoint (shown as circles). How many different colors will you need?

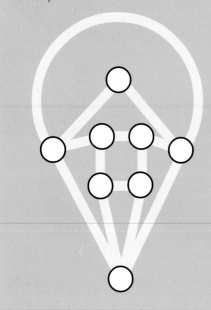

PLAYTHINK 952

DIFFICULTY: ●●●●●●●●○○
REQUIRED: 👁 ✏ 📄 ✂
COMPLETION: ☐ TIME: _____

CUBES IN PERSPECTIVE 2

If you rearrange these twenty-five tiles without rotating them, you can create an image containing a number of cubes. How many cubes does that image contain?

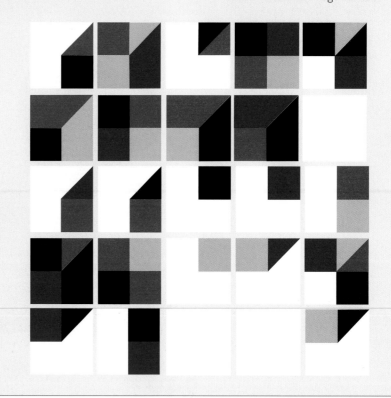

PLAYTHINK 953

DIFFICULTY: ●●●●●●●○○○
REQUIRED: 👁 ✏ 📄 ✂
COMPLETION: ☐ TIME: _____

"THE" PUZZLE

Copy (at a 300 percent enlargement) and cut out the sixteen shapes. Can you work out how to arrange them to form the word "THE"?

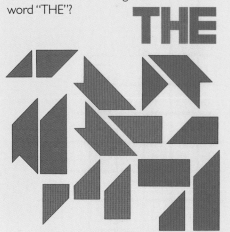

PLAYTHINK 954

DIFFICULTY: ●●●●●●●○○○
REQUIRED: 👁 ✏
COMPLETION: ☐ TIME: _____

CIRCLES COLORING 2

The circles in the inset are filled in according to logical rules. Can you work out those rules and fill in the white circles accordingly?

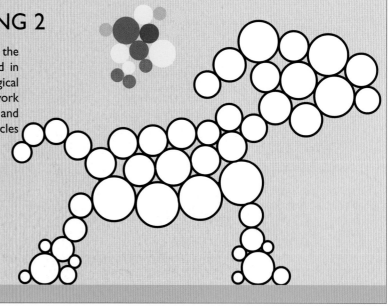

PLAYTHINK 955
DIFFICULTY: ●●●●●●●●○○
REQUIRED: 👁 ✏
COMPLETION: ☐ TIME: _____

DODECAHEDRON EDGE COLORING

How many colors do you need to color each segment of this diagram in such a way that no two segments of the same color meet at a junction?

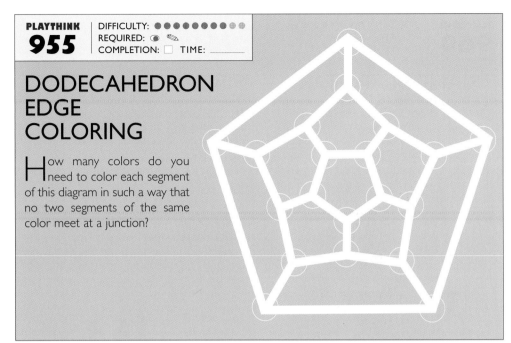

PLAYTHINK 957
DIFFICULTY: ●●●●●●●●●○
REQUIRED: 👁
COMPLETION: ☐ TIME: _____

THREE-DIGIT NUMBER

A toy robot has a three-digit electronic display on its front. The only digits it can display are 1, 2 and 3. Can you work out how many different numbers the robot can display?

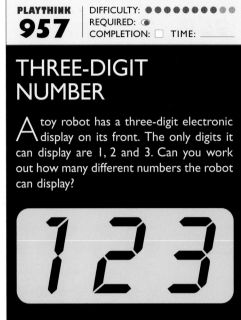

PLAYTHINK 956
DIFFICULTY: ●●●●●●●●○○
REQUIRED: 👁 ✏
COMPLETION: ☐ TIME: _____

PARQUET

The floor plan of an odd room is shown at right; the black squares and rectangles indicate where columns and fixtures fit into the floor. Can you find a way to completely cover the floor with uncut wooden planks that are 1 unit by 4 units?

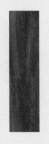

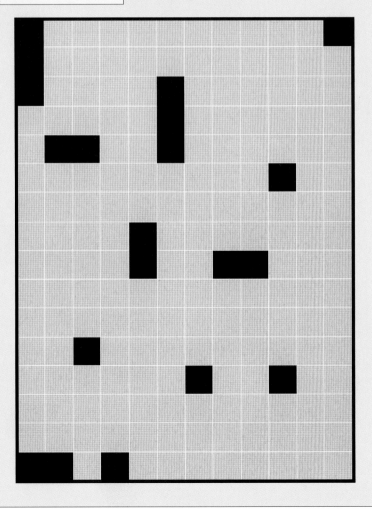

PLAYTHINK 958
DIFFICULTY: ●●●●●●●○○○
REQUIRED: 👁
COMPLETION: ☐ TIME: _____

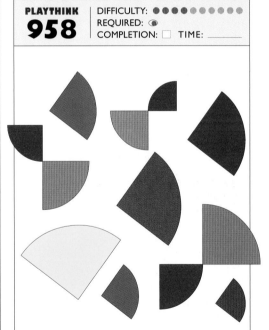

EQUAL AREAS 2

This diagram shows three pairs of quarter circles in contact with each other, as well as a number of isolated quarter circles of various sizes. It turns out that the sum of the area of each pair of quarter circles is equal to the area of one of the single quarter circles shown. Can you work out which quarter circle goes with which pair? Can you guess which geometric property ensures that the areas are exactly equal?

PLAYTHINK 959

DIFFICULTY: ●●●●●●●○○○
REQUIRED: 👁 ✏
COMPLETION: ☐ TIME: _____

FRUITS ON FOUR PLATES

A hostess has four pieces of fruit and four identical unlabeled plates. Can you find all the different ways she can serve those four pieces of fruit? You can use the blank diagram below and four colors of pencil to help you find them all.

Fruit 1 - Yellow ○
Fruit 2 - Red ●
Fruit 3 - Blue ●
Fruit 4 - Green ●

PLAYTHINK 960

DIFFICULTY: ●●●●●●●●○○
REQUIRED: 👁 ✏ 📄 ✂
COMPLETION: ☐ TIME: _____

TRIANGULAR STAR

Polyamonds are triangular counterparts to polyominoes. They are created by joining identical equilateral triangles side by side.

Can you fill the outline of this six-pointed star with the five polyamonds shown here?

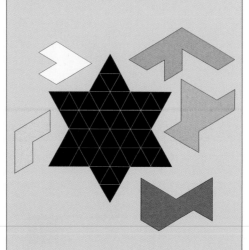

PLAYTHINK 961

DIFFICULTY: ●●●●●●●○○○
REQUIRED: 👁 ✏
COMPLETION: ☐ TIME: _____

FIBONACCI RABBITS

In 1202 Leonardo Fibonacci, a twenty-seven-year-old Italian mathematician, published a book called *Liber Abaci*. In that groundbreaking work, he wrote the following puzzle:

Every month a breeding pair of rabbits (one male, one female) produces one new pair of rabbits—also one male, one female. That new pair begins breeding two months later. How many pairs of rabbits can be produced from a single pair of rabbits in one year, assuming no rabbits die and every pair has one male and one female?

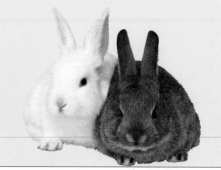

PLAYTHINK 962

DIFFICULTY: ●●●●●●●●●○
REQUIRED: 👁 ✏ 📄 ✂
COMPLETION: ☐ TIME: _____

HEXIAMONDS

Hexiamonds are created by joining six identical equilateral triangles side by side. There are exactly twelve different hexiamonds, shown at right.

In each of the black outlines here, three hexiamonds have been placed. Can you fit in the nine remaining hexiamonds?

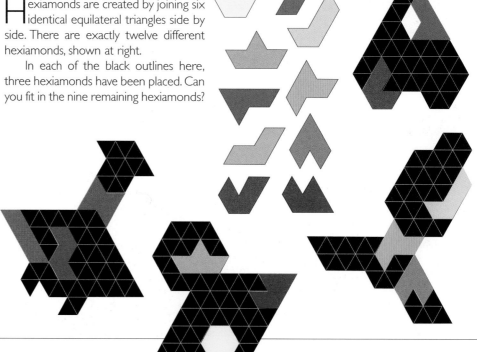

PENTAHEX HONEYCOMB

All 22 different ways to join five regular hexagons edge to edge are shown here. Such combinations are called pentahexes.

If you're by yourself, try to cover the entire 110-hex board below with the 22 possible pentahexes.

If you're with a friend, take turns placing pentahexes along the grid lines of the board. The last player able to place a shape successfully wins the game.

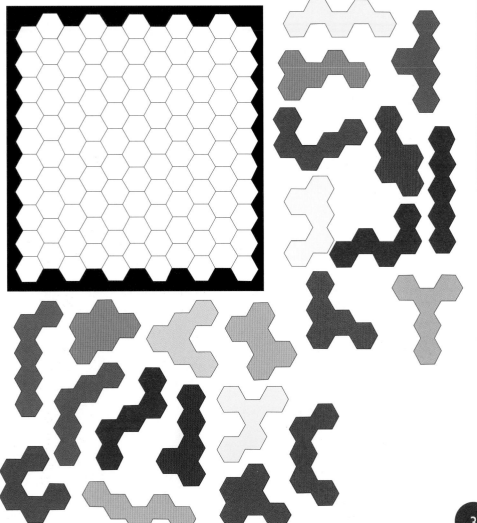

SUM-FREE GAME

In this two-person game, which I heard described in a lecture by American graph theorist Frank Harary, players alternate placing consecutive numbers (starting with 1) in either of the two columns. A player can place a number in a column only if it does not already possess two numbers that add up to that number. For example, in this sample game, the player whose turn it is must play an 8 but is blocked from doing so because the first column contains 1 and 7 and the second column contains 3 and 5. The last player to place a number wins.

Can you work out the moves for player 2 so she or he will win every time no matter what player 1 does?

Can you work out the longest possible game?

Sample	
COLUMN 1	**COLUMN 2**
1	3
2	5
4	6
7	

MATHEMAGIC HONEYCOMB

Can you place the numbers 1 through 9 in this honeycomb so that, for any given hexagon, the sum of the numbers in the adjacent hexagons will be a multiple of that hexagon's number? For example, if a hexagon contains a 5, the adjacent hexes must total 5, 10, 15, 25 and so on.

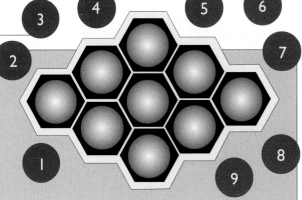

PLAYTHINK 966 | DIFFICULTY: ●●●●●●●○○○
REQUIRED: 👁 ✎
COMPLETION: ☐ TIME: _____

AN ARRAY OF SOLDIERS

Each of eleven army units (represented here by the green squares) has an identical number of soldiers. If you add the general to the total number, the soldiers can be rearranged to form a single perfect array of fighting personnel.

What's the minimum number of soldiers that must be in each army unit? How many soldiers—including the general—are in the array?

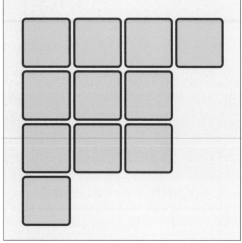

PLAYTHINK 967 | DIFFICULTY: ●●●●●●●●○○
REQUIRED: 👁 ✎
COMPLETION: ☐ TIME: _____

HAILSTONE NUMBERS

Think of a number. If it is odd, triple it and add 1; if it is even, divide it by 2. Apply this rule to each new number you obtain. Can you see what eventually happens?

Starting with 1, you get: 1, 4, 2, 1, 4, 2, 1, 4, 2 and so on.

Starting with 2 gives you: 2, 1, 4, 2, 1, 4, 2, 1, 4 and so on.

Starting with 3: 3, 10, 5, 16, 8, 4, 2, 1, 4, 2, 1 and so on.

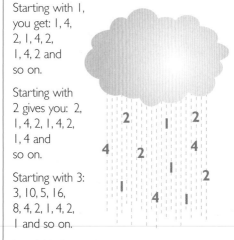

It quickly becomes apparent that the above sequences get stuck in a loop of 1-4-2-1-4-2. But will every sequence run into that inescapable routine? Test your idea by starting with 7.

PLAYTHINK 968 | DIFFICULTY: ●●●●●●●●●○
REQUIRED: 👁 ✎
COMPLETION: ☐ TIME: _____

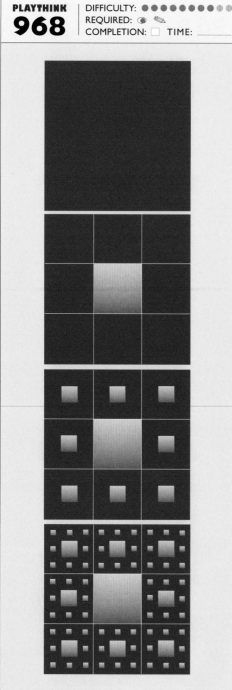

SQUARES IN SQUARES

A blue square is divided into nine smaller squares, and the middle one is painted gold. The eight remaining blue squares are divided into nine, and the middle square of those is painted gold. If this process continues indefinitely, can you work out the eventual area of the gold squares in relation to the original blue square?

PLAYTHINK 969 | DIFFICULTY: ●●●●●●●●○○
REQUIRED: 👁 ✎
COMPLETION: ☐ TIME: _____

MAXIMUM OVERHANG

Nine identical planks, each 1 meter in length, are stacked with the bottom plank nailed to the floor, as shown. Can you move the eight other planks to achieve the maximum overhang for the top plank? Will that overhang be sufficient for the mouse to cross over the planks to reach the cheese on a platform 1.4 meters away?

1 meter

1.4 meters

PLAYTHINK
970
DIFFICULTY: ● ● ● ● ● ● ● ● ○ ○
REQUIRED: ◉
COMPLETION: ☐ TIME: _____

TRUTH AND MARRIAGE

The king has two daughters—the virtuous Amelia, who always tells the truth, and the wicked Leila, who always lies. One of them is married, and one of them is not—but the king has kept the details of the marriage a secret, even down to which of the daughters is wedded.

To find a suitable mate for the other daughter, the king has organized a joust. The winner gets to name which of the daughters he wants to marry; if she is available, they will wed the next day. The man who wins asks the king if he may talk to the daughters. The king says he may ask one of the daughters one question, but it can be no more than three words long.

What question should he ask?

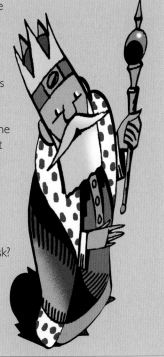

PLAYTHINK
971
DIFFICULTY: ● ● ● ● ● ● ● ● ○ ○
REQUIRED: ◉
COMPLETION: ☐ TIME: _____

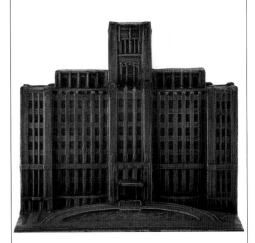

HOTEL INFINITY

This problem is a favorite introduction to the weirdness of infinite numbers:

You are the manager of the Hotel Infinity, an inn that has an infinite number of rooms. No matter how crowded the hotel is, you know that you can always make room for one more guest: you simply move the person in room 1 to room 2, the person in room 2 to room 3, the person in room 3 to room 4 and so on. After all the guests have been moved, you check the new guest into room 1.

Unfortunately, just as you are about to go off-duty, a group of people arrive for a convention. The topic must be very popular, because there are an infinite number of new guests. If you already *have* an infinite number of guests, how can you accommodate the newcomers?

PLAYTHINK
972
DIFFICULTY: ● ● ● ● ● ● ● ● ○ ○
REQUIRED: ◉
COMPLETION: ☐ TIME: _____

TRUTH CITY

You are on your way to Truth City, where the inhabitants always tell the truth. At one point you reach a fork in the road, with one branch leading to Truth City and the other leading to Lies City, where the citizens are all liars. The road signs at the junction are, as you can imagine, confusing, but there is a man standing there from whom you can ask directions. The only problem is, you don't know where he is from—the city where everyone always gives the right answer or the city where everyone lies.

If you have time to ask him only one question, what question will ensure that you will be headed in the right direction?

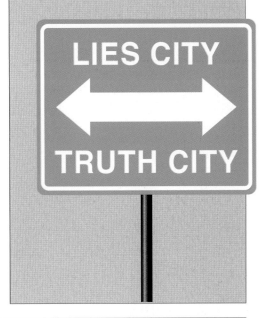

PLAYTHINK
973
DIFFICULTY: ● ● ● ● ● ● ● ● ● ●
REQUIRED: ◉ ✎
COMPLETION: ☐ TIME: _____

MAGIC PRIMES SQUARE

Can a magic square be made up of only prime numbers and 1? Henry Ernest Dudeney, the greatest English puzzle inventor, was the first to construct such a square, using the numbers 1, 7, 13, 31, 37, 43, 61, 67 and 73. Can you fit those numbers into a three-by-three grid to form a magic square?

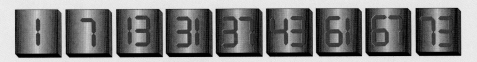

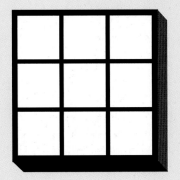

PLAYTHINK 974

DIFFICULTY: ●●●●●●●●●●○○
REQUIRED: ◉
COMPLETION: ☐ TIME: _____

GUESS CHESS

Five chess pieces—a king, a queen, a bishop, a knight and a rook—are to be placed on a chessboard. The pieces must each occupy a square marked with a red circle, and they must be placed in such a way that two of the pieces can attack the squares marked with a red 2.

Can you work out where each of the pieces must be placed?

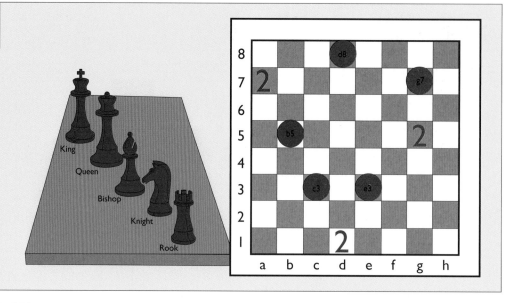

PLAYTHINK 975

DIFFICULTY: ●●●●●●●●●○○○
REQUIRED: ◉
COMPLETION: ☐ TIME: _____

TRUTH, LIES AND IN BETWEEN

There are three types of people in the city of Las Wages: those who always tell the truth, those who always lie and those who alternate between lying and truth telling. If you meet an inhabitant on the streets of Las Wages and can ask only two questions, what two questions will enable you to determine what sort of person he or she is?

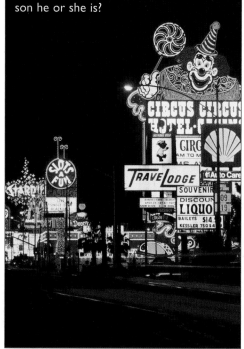

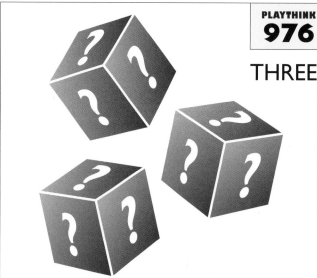

PLAYTHINK 976

DIFFICULTY: ●●●●●●●●●○○○
REQUIRED: ◉
COMPLETION: ☐ TIME: _____

THREE DICE

You see three faces on each of three dice, for a total of nine faces. If the sum of the dots on each die is different, and you see a total of forty dots altogether, then can you work out which faces must be visible on each die?

PLAYTHINK 977

DIFFICULTY: ●●●●●○○○○○○○
REQUIRED: ◉
COMPLETION: ☐ TIME: _____

COUNTING LETTERS

Read the following sentence:

FINISHED FILES ARE THE RESULT OF YEARS OF SCIENTIFIC STUDY COMBINED WITH THE EXPERIENCE OF YEARS.

Now read it again, this time counting every *F* you see. How many did you find?

FLIPPING COIN GAME

Two boys play a simple game: They take turns flipping a coin, and the first to throw "heads" wins. Can you work out whether one player can gain an advantage even if the coin is fair?

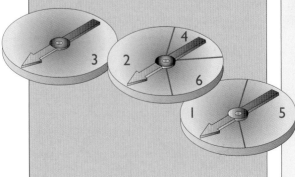

SPINNERS GAME

The object of this game is simple: spin the higher number. You and your opponent may each choose one of three spinners. The first spinner has only one number, 3. The second spinner is divided 56 percent for number 2, 22 percent for number 4 and 22 percent for number 6. The third spinner is divided 51 percent for number 1 and 49 percent for number 5.

Can you work out which spinner is the best to choose?

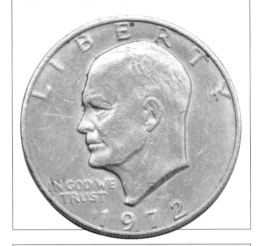

BALLS IN BOXES

When a girl throws four balls randomly into any or all of four boxes, what are the chances that each box will contain a single ball?

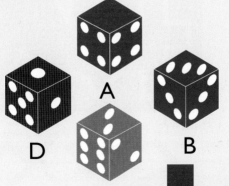

NONTRANSITIVE DICE

The mathematical property of transitivity states that if A is greater than B, and B is greater than C, then A is greater than C. But certain games appear to flout this logic. One common nontransitive game is "Rock, Paper, Scissors," the children's game that displays circular logic: Scissors cut paper, paper wraps rock, rock breaks scissors.

A special set of dice, shown here, also displays this nontransitive logic. If you play a two-person betting game with these dice, always allow your opponent to select his or her die first. No matter which die your opponent chooses, you can select a die that will give you an advantage. Can you work out how?

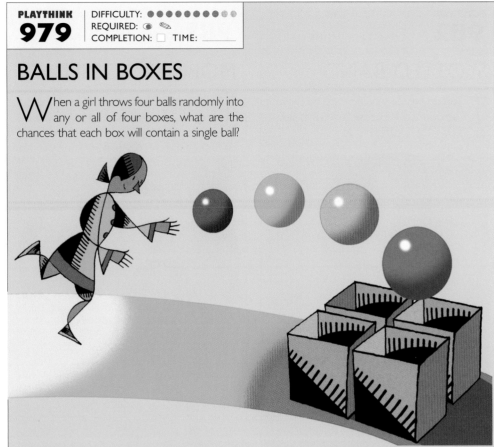

PLAYTHINK 982

DIFFICULTY: ●●●●●●○○○○
REQUIRED: 👁 ✂
COMPLETION: ☐ TIME: _____

SLOTTED BAND

This strip passes through itself, as shown. Can you work out what will happen if you divide it along the red line?

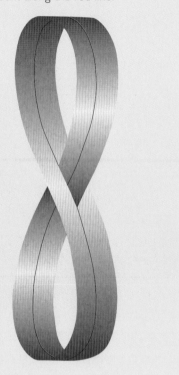

PLAYTHINK 983

DIFFICULTY: ●●●●●●○○○○
REQUIRED: 👁 ✂
COMPLETION: ☐ TIME: _____

MÖBIUS CROSSED

This figure is made up of two closed loops: a Möbius strip and a cylindrical band. Can you work out what structure will be formed if you cut the figure along the red line?

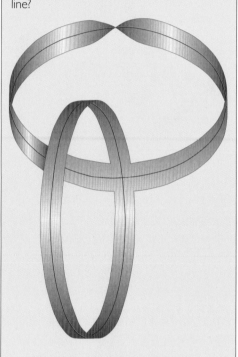

PLAYTHINK 984

DIFFICULTY: ●●●●●●○○○○
REQUIRED: 👁
COMPLETION: ☐ TIME: _____

LINKED OR NOT?

Could the elements of the structure below be separated without making a cut?

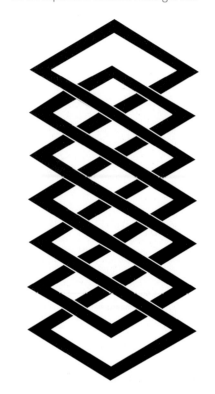

PLAYTHINK 985

DIFFICULTY: ●●●●●●○○○○
REQUIRED: 👁 ✏
COMPLETION: ☐ TIME: _____

LINKS

The closed white line is made up of sixteen links, each of which is shown separately and in color. The separate links may be in a different orientation than they appear in the line, but none of the links overlap. Can you color in the line according to the colors of the sixteen links?

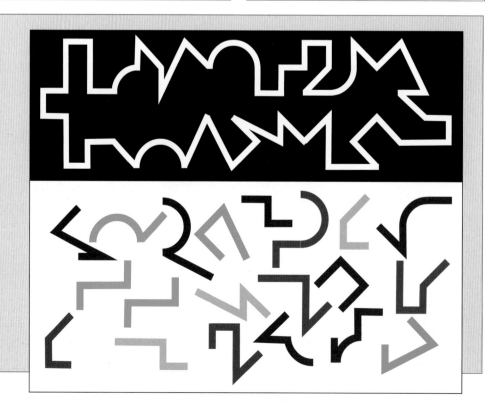

PLAYTHINK
986
DIFFICULTY: ●●●●●●○○○○
REQUIRED: 👁 ✎ 📄 ✂
COMPLETION: ☐ TIME: _____

WAR OF THE PLANETS

You are the leader of an alien society fighting hostile invaders. The many planets in your star system are linked by gravity currents. You need to keep your spaceships moving from one planet to another and avoid falling into a gravity well from which there is no hope of escape.

That's the scenario for this two-person game. Each player gets six spaceships and places them, in turn, on any planet—though a planet can hold just one spaceship at a time. After all the spaceships have been placed, players take turns moving their ships along a gravity current. The ships must follow

the direction of the arrows; if all the currents point toward the planet, the ship cannot leave. The last player who can make a move is the winner.

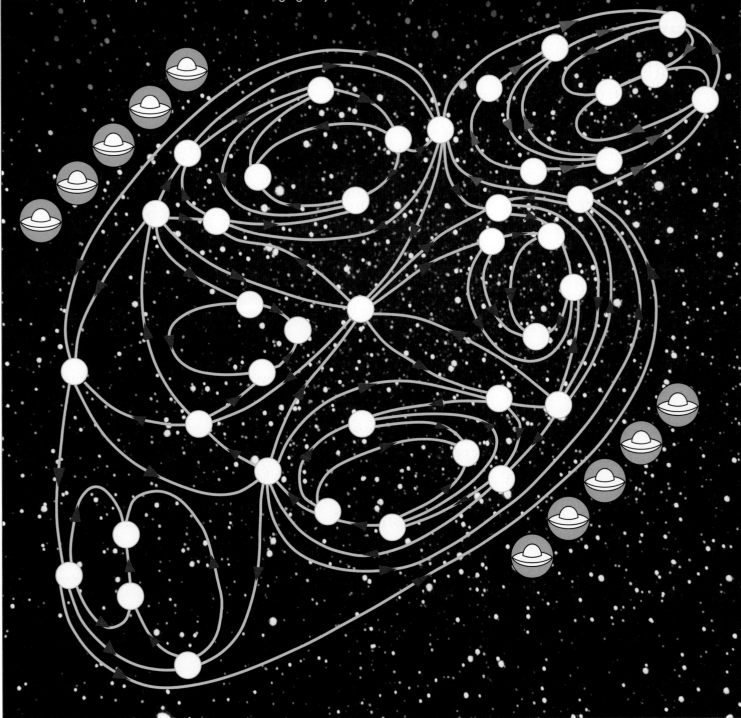

PLAYTHINK 987

DIFFICULTY: ●●●●●●●●○○○
REQUIRED: ◉ ✎
COMPLETION: ☐ TIME: _____

TRIANGLES IN A CUBE

Choose any three corners of a cube at random. Can you work out the chances that those points will form a right triangle?

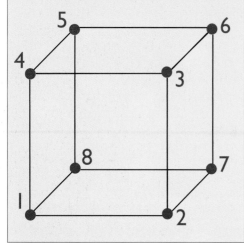

PLAYTHINK 988

DIFFICULTY: ●●●●●●●●○○
REQUIRED: ◉ ✎
COMPLETION: ☐ TIME: _____

MINIMAL ROUTES

Three, four and five towns are represented by red points on the three maps shown here. For each map, can you draw the shortest possible road system that links all the towns?

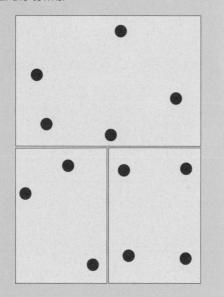

PLAYTHINK 989

DIFFICULTY: ●●●●●●●○○○○
REQUIRED: ◉
COMPLETION: ☐ TIME: _____

ANTIGRAVITY CONES

Galileo devised many ingenious inventions, but none so magical as the simple device shown in this illustration. When you place the double cone on the inclined tracks at their lowest point, the cone will start rolling uphill to the high ends. Can you work out how this double cone can seem to defy gravity?

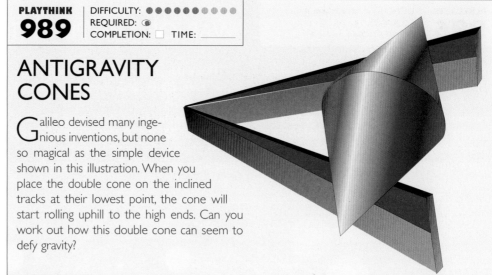

PLAYTHINK 990

DIFFICULTY: ●●●●●●●●○○○
REQUIRED: ◉ ✎
COMPLETION: ☐ TIME: _____

MINIMAL WEIGHTS

Suppose you need to have the ability to weigh any integral weight from 1 to 40 grams on a scale like the one shown here. Can you work out the minimum number of weights you must have?

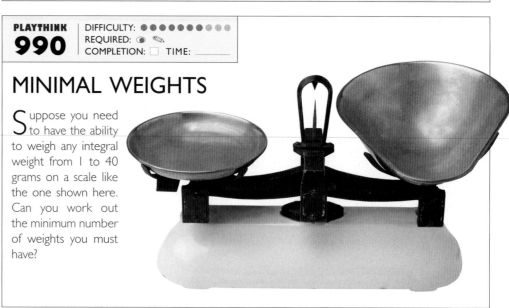

PLAYTHINK 991

DIFFICULTY: ●●●●●●●○○○○
REQUIRED: ◉
COMPLETION: ☐ TIME: _____

BOTTLENECK

The red valve will open in a second to allow the water in the reservoir to flow through the tubes at the right. Can you predict the water levels in the three thin vertical tubes?

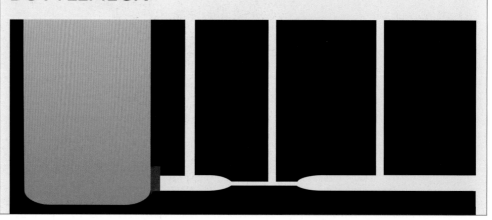

PLAYTHINK
992

DIFFICULTY: ●●●●●●●○○○
REQUIRED: 👁 ✎
COMPLETION: ☐ TIME: _____

PYTHAGOREAN HEXAGONS

A set of regular hexagons with sides 3, 4 and 5 is extended on the sides of a right triangle. This seems to suggest that the Pythagorean theorem can be extended beyond squares and is valid for hexagons as well. Is that really the case?

A related problem was posed by American mathematician James Schmerl. He noted that a hexagon of side 5 can be dissected so that the pieces can form two smaller hexagons, one of side 3 and one of side 4. What is the smallest number of pieces that will accomplish this?

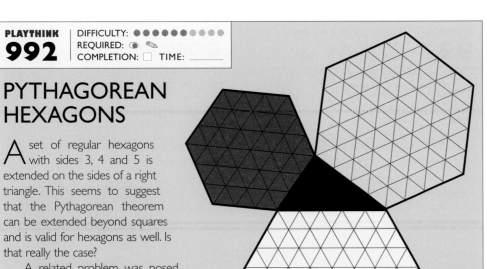

PLAYTHINK
993

DIFFICULTY: ●●●●●●●●○○
REQUIRED: 👁 📄 ✂
COMPLETION: ☐ TIME: _____

SILHOUETTE 2

If you move the four yellow shapes over the black grid, you can create the silhouette of a familiar figure. Can you work out what it is?

PLAYTHINK
994

DIFFICULTY: ●●●●●●●●○○
REQUIRED: 👁 ✎
COMPLETION: ☐ TIME: _____

SEPARATING GHOSTS

Can you separate the fifteen ghosts into fifteen private compartments just by moving the five straight lines?

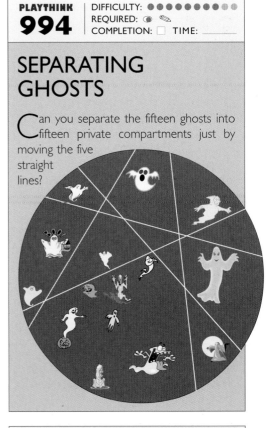

PLAYTHINK
995

DIFFICULTY: ●●●●●●●●○○
REQUIRED: 👁 ✎
COMPLETION: ☐ TIME: _____

BIRD NEST

Seven birds live in a nest. They are very organized and send three birds out each day in search of food. After seven days every pair of birds will have been in exactly one of the daily foraging missions. For example, on the first day birds 1, 2 and 3 go out; that means the pairs 1-2, 1-3 and 2-3.

Can you work out how every pair can be so matched over the course of a week?

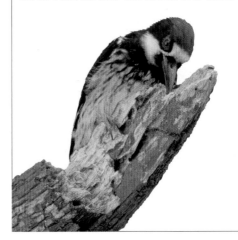

PLAYTHINK 996

DIFFICULTY: ●●●●●●○○○○
REQUIRED: 👁
COMPLETION: ☐ TIME: _____

LINKED TUBES

Several tubes of various shapes are linked in such a way that liquid can pass from one to another. The network of tubes is connected to a reservoir of water, at left. If the reservoir is opened and the water flows into the tubes, can you work out what the water level will be in each tube?

PLAYTHINK 997

DIFFICULTY: ●●●●●●○○○○
REQUIRED: 👁
COMPLETION: ☐ TIME: _____

PROGRESSING SQUARES

Start with a small square of side 1. Employ the diagonal of that square as the side of a second square. Employ the diagonal of the second square as the side of a third square. Continue in this manner to create an infinite progression of squares.

Without measuring, can you work out what the length of the sides of the eleventh square in the series will be?

PLAYTHINK 998

DIFFICULTY: ●●●●●●●●○○
REQUIRED: 👁 ✎
COMPLETION: ☐ TIME: _____

THE TOSS OF THE DIE

If you toss a die six times, what are the chances that all six faces will turn up?

PLAYTHINK 999

DIFFICULTY: ●●●●●●●○○○
REQUIRED: 👁 ✎ 📄 ✂
COMPLETION: ☐ TIME: _____

MOVING TRAINS

Two trains meet at a switch, each needing to pass the other. No locomotive or carriage may stop on the diagonal section of tracks, and only two carriages or a locomotive and a carriage may park on either side of the switch. Employing only the locomotives to move the carriages, how many moves will it take you to get the red train to exchange places with the green train? Locomotives can back up and push, and be positioned anywhere on the train. A locomotive and the car or cars it's pulling can, as one move, separate; however, cars cannot separate while the train is moving.

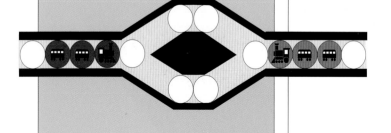

PLAYTHINK 1000

DIFFICULTY: ●●●●●●●○○○
REQUIRED: 👁
COMPLETION: ☐ TIME: _____

THE LAST PUZZLE

This last challenge was very carefully selected. The puzzle is a classic that contains the best elements of recreational mathematics. The solution requires thinking, concentration, creativity, logic, insight and attention to the smallest detail. Enjoy!

Two Russian mathematicians meet on a plane.

"If I remember correctly, you have three sons," says Ivan. "What are their ages today?"

"The product of their ages is thirty-six," says Igor, "and the sum of their ages is exactly today's date."

"I'm sorry, Igor," Ivan says after a minute, "but that doesn't tell me the ages of your boys."

"Oh, I forgot to tell you, my youngest son has red hair."

"Ah, now it's clear," Ivan says. "I now know exactly how old your three sons are."

How did Ivan figure out the ages?

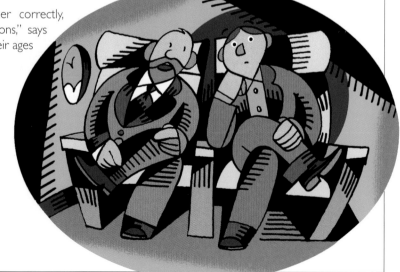

SOLUTIONS

CHAPTER 1 SOLUTIONS

1 The Roman numeral for seven (VII) can be made by cutting the Roman numeral for twelve (XII) in half horizontally.

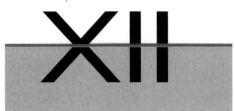

2 The solution given in the *sangaku* tablet is as follows: Imagine that the perpendicular line is drawn separately from the line specified in the puzzle. If they are in fact different lines, then they would start at the center of the blue circle and run to different points on the diameter. As is the case with most of the surviving *sangaku* puzzles, the proof of the theorem is not given, making them difficult (if not impossible!) for us to understand. Take heart. I have included this example only as a means of explaining the inspiration behind my book; all other PlayThinks have answers. I promise.

3 16,807 measures of flour. That's 7 × 7 × 7 × 7 × 7. This puzzle, which comes from the ancient Egyptian "Rhind Papyrus," was written by the scribe Ahmes in 1850 B.C. Perhaps the world's oldest puzzle, it has inspired a great many variations over the thousands of years since its creation.

4 The frames are exactly identical. Because the frames are three-dimensional, they can be arranged in a nontransitive way so that A is inside B, B is inside C, and C is inside A.

5 Door number 5 is the right answer. In many instances people choose a door that is more square than the original. That is because the background figure often influences one's perception of the door's shape.

6 The egg. The riddle does not specify that the eggs in question are chicken eggs and, according to paleontologists, reptiles and dinosaurs existed long before birds and chickens. Fossilized eggs dating back one hundred million years have been uncovered. Thus it can be said that eggs came before chickens.

7

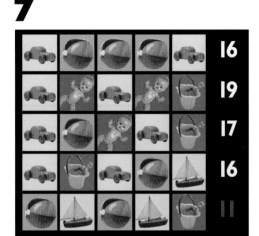

8 The answer is four. The outlines of the four sets of rectangles are shown next to their corresponding squares.

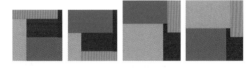

9 The frowning clown is the thirteenth clown from the right in the second row.

The human perceptual system is designed to detect an item that stands out as different without a systematic search. This principle is used in the design of instrument panels: under normal conditions, in which all indicators point in the same direction, any change is easily spotted.

10 The winning sequence is yellow, orange, red, pink, violet, light green, dark green, light blue and dark blue.

This puzzle was created in much the same way that animated cartoons are drawn. Many elements of the scene were painted on transparent cells, then stacked on top of one another in the correct order to create the illusion of one seamless drawing.

11

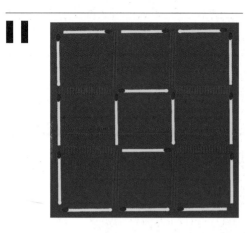

12 One of the many possible solutions for each puzzle.

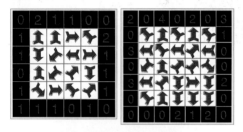

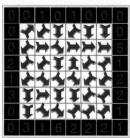

13 The choices offer identical odds. But in a psychological experiment, about four in ten people preferred the single draw and held to this view even when the other choice was altered to provide fifty draws from the box of 100.

14

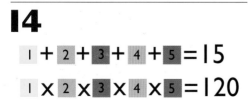

15 The number 2,520 is obviously divisible by 5 and 10. But since all five of the numbers are single-digit, 10 is excluded. So the third number must be 5.

Adding the known numbers (8 + 1 + 5) gives us 14. Since 30 − 14 = 16, the total of the remaining two numbers must be 16.

Multiplying the known numbers (8 × 1 × 5) gives us 40. Since 2,520 / 40 = 63, the product of the two remaining numbers must be 63.

Only 9 and 7 can be added to make 16 and multiplied together to make 63.

So the answer is 5, 7 and 9.

16 This puzzle is another that often creates a conceptual block. But, as you can see, the solution is quite simple.

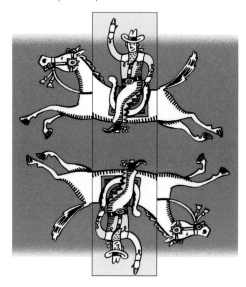

17 The key to constructing the bridge is to set up two dominoes as temporary supports, as shown in the illustration below. When enough dominoes have been placed to give the structure its overall stability, the supports can be removed and placed on top.

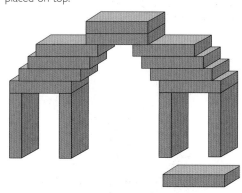

18 If the drawer contained socks, then you would need to select only four to get a matching pair. But gloves have an attribute that socks don't: handedness. It is not enough to have two gloves that are the same color—they must be of complementary handedness. So to ensure that you have one pair of gloves, you must select one more than the number of gloves of one-handedness, or twelve. Assuming that you can distinguish in the dark between right- and left-handed gloves, you may need to select only eleven.

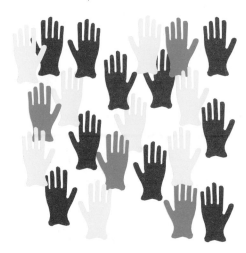

19 The outlines of the six overlapping squares for one six-by-six square, six three-by-three squares, three two-by-two squares and eight one-by-one squares—eighteen squares altogether.

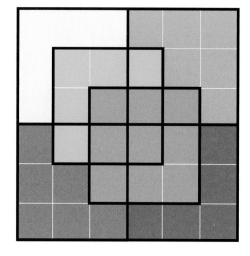

20 Sam Loyd, widely acclaimed as the greatest American puzzle inventor, created the classic T-Puzzle. In terms of elegance and simplicity, the T-Puzzle has never been surpassed. It is deceptively simple because it has few pieces. But it is a good example of a problem that looks easy at first but possesses elements that often lead to a conceptual block. Once the block is in place, it is often impossible to find the solution even if the pieces are cut out and handled.

The solution may come eventually, in a flash of inspiration. Such a moment of insight—the "Aha!" experience—is usually accompanied by a feeling of achievement for one's own act of creative thinking.

21 A three-move solution (with thanks to Joe DeVicentis). All the moves are clockwise.

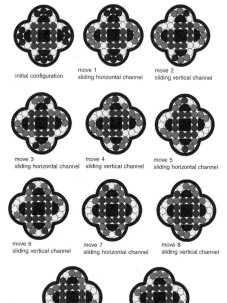

22 There are sixteen possible combinations of choices for the firing of the four lasers. Four combinations will form a closed energy field around the man:

left, left, left and left
left, right, left and right
right, left, right and left
right, right, right and right

The probability of success, then, is one in four.

23 The best way to work out the solution is with a diagram such as the one at the right.

As you can see, both statement 1 (Gerry's) and statement 3 (Anitta's) can be true, *so the number cannot be more than 100.*

Statement 3 and statement 2 (George's) can be true if the total is between 100 and 1.

But only statement 2 is correct if the total is 0.

Ivan is hiding in an anamorphic picture. To find him, look at the page from the bottom at a highly slanted angle.

24 If the treasure were buried on the orange island, then all the statements would be false. And if the treasure were buried on the purple island, then all the statements would be true. But if the treasure were buried on the yellow island, then only the statement for the purple island would be false. Therefore, the treasure is on the yellow island.

25 If the horses were not circling, there would be seven factorial (7!, or 5,040) possible arrangements. But because they form a circle, each arrangement is identical to six others that could be formed by declaring one horse or another is the "first" horse in the circle. That means the answer is 7!/7 or 6! (6× 5 × 4 × 3 × 2 × 1). Six factorial is still a large number: 720.

26 The trick here is looking at the way the books are lined up. The bookworm eats through only the front cover of volume 1, all of volumes 2, 3 and 4, and only the back cover of volume 5. The total distance is 19 centimeters.

27 The first step you must take to solve the problem is to find the number of combinations of three colors you can make from five colors. Plugging the values into a general formula for the number of combinations gives you:

$$5!/(3! \times (5-3)!) = (5 \times 4 \times 3 \times 2 \times 1) / (3 \times 2 \times 1 \times (2 \times 1)) = 120/12 = 10$$

That result tells us there are ten possible combinations of three colors out of five. But the number of combinations tells us nothing about the order in which the colors are placed on the mask. The different orders in which the three colors can be painted on the mask is 3!(3 × 2 × 1), or six for each color combination. That means there is a total of sixty possible ways the mask could be painted using three colors out of five.

28

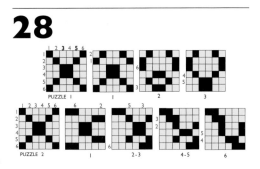

29

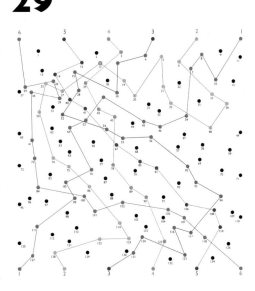

30 Your friend is wrong. Because the odds for each coin is independent of the others, there are in fact two possible outcomes for a single coin, four possible outcomes for two coins and eight possible outcomes for three coins:

1	2	3
H	H	H
H	H	T
H	T	H
H	T	T
T	H	H
T	H	T
T	T	H
T	T	T

In only two tosses out of eight will the coins land all heads or all tails.

31

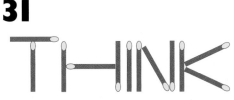

32 The message is hidden as an anamorphic image. If you hold the page at a very slanted angle, you will be able to read it: HELLO.

33

$$2 + 2 = 4$$
$$2 + 3 = 5$$
$$5 - 2 = 3$$
$$6 - 3 = 3$$

34 The message is a statement that mathematical concepts are understood, as well as an attempt to convey logic.

$$1 + 2 = 3 \rightarrow \text{true}$$
$$2 + 2 = 4 \rightarrow \text{true}$$
$$3 + 2 = 4 \rightarrow \text{false}$$

The triangle stands for "plus"; the diamond stands for "equals"; the pentagon stands for "true"; and the hexagon stands for "false."

35

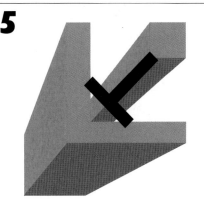

36 The hostages can easily separate themselves. One of the hostages grabs his rope with both hands so that a loose, untwisted loop is made in his rope on the other side of his partner's rope. Then he tucks the loop through the circle of rope around his partner's wrist; as you'll soon discover, it's only possible to keep the rope untwisted by moving toward one wrist, not the other. Next, he moves the loop up toward his partner's fingers. When the first hostage then passes the loop over his partner's hand and tucks the loop back through the rope, they are free.

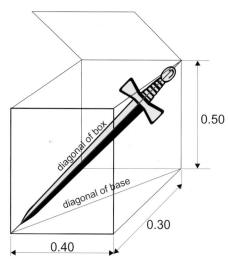

37 $6 + \frac{6}{6} = 7$

38 The solution uses the Pythagorean theorem (the square of the length of the hypotenuse of a right triangle equals the sum of the squares of the lengths of the other two sides) to calculate the length from the lower front left-hand corner of the chest to the upper back right-hand corner. First the diagonal of the base is determined to be 50 centimeters; then that length and the height of the chest can be used to calculate the maximum length through the box. That turns out to be 70.7 centimeters—just long enough for the sword to fit!

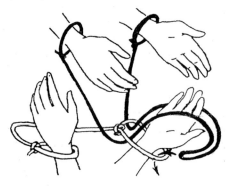

diagonal of box
diagonal of base
0.50
0.30
0.40

39 The solution is so obvious that many people overlook it.

40

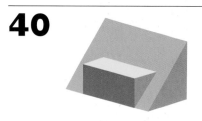

41 The answer is a man. A man crawls on all fours in the morning of his life (when he is a baby), walks upright in middle age, and uses a cane in old age.

42

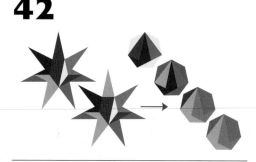

43 "With two statements there are four possible combinations of truth or falsehood:

true/true
true/false
false/true
false/false

The first combination can't be right because at least one of the statements is false. The second and third can't be right either because if one of the statements is false, it's impossible for the other to be true. The only logically consistent possibility is that they both lied. That means Mister Ladybug has the yellow dots and Miss Ladybug has the red dots.

44

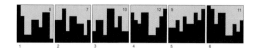

45 It can't be done. If you start drawing a line outside the black closed line and cross it an odd number of times, you will end up inside the black line. To close the new line, you must intersect the black line, making an even number of intersections. Not only are nine intersections impossible; all odd numbers of intersections are impossible.

46 The larger rug covers exactly 25 percent of the smaller one. The proof of this is shown in the diagram at right.

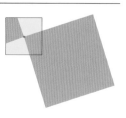

47

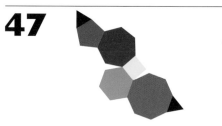

48 The best-case scenario—that the two missing socks make a pair, leaving you with four matched pairs—can happen in only five different ways. If the socks can be labeled A1, A2, B1, B2, C1, C2, D1, D2, E1 and E2, then the best-case scenario occurs only when the missing socks are A1-A2, B1-B2, C1-C2, D1-D2 or E1-E2.

The worst-case scenario—that the two missing socks do not make a pair, leaving you with only three matched pairs and two orphan socks—occurs when the missing socks are A1-B1, A1-B2, A2-B1, A2-B2, A1-C1, A1-C2, A2-C1, A2-C2, A1-D1, A1-D2, A2-D1, A2-D2, A1-E1, A1-E2, A2-E1, A2-E2, B1-C1, B1-C2, B2-C1, B2-C2, B1-D1, B1-D2, B2-D1, B2-D2, B1-E1, B1-E2, B2-E1, B2-E2, C1-D1, C1-D2, C2-D1, C2-D2, C1-E1, C1-E2, C2-E1, C2-E2, D1-E1, D1-E2, D2-E1, D2-E2.

That's forty different ways to get the worst-case scenario. As you can see, the worst-case scenario is eight times more likely to occur than the best-case scenario.

49 Mark the card as shown, fold in half along the horizontal line and cut along the red lines. The result will be a long, thin loop of paper.

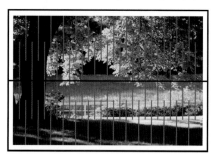

50 The total number of possible permutations in a seven-digit phone number is seven factorial (7!, or $7 \times 6 \times 5 \times 4 \times 3 \times 2 \times 1$), which equals 5,040. So the probability of any given combination being the right phone number is 1 in 5,040, or about .02 percent. For a complete discussion of factorials, see "Combinations and Permutations," p. 140.

51
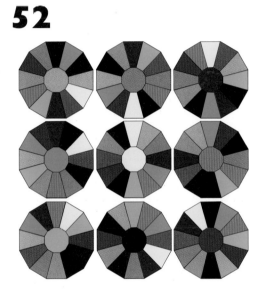

52

53
There were six people at the meeting. Each person shook hands five times, but that makes for fifteen handshakes, not thirty, since each shake was shared by two people.

54
Five, as illustrated below.

55
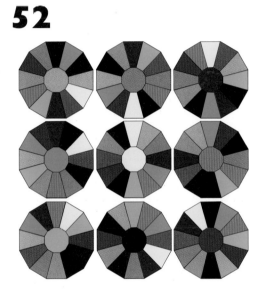
triangle   quadrilaterals   pentagons

hexagons

56
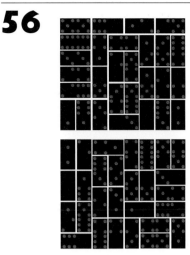

57
Change the word *man* to *person*. Otherwise, it is possible that the man has a wife and many daughters and that one of them knocked on the door.

58
The maximum number of attempts can be found by adding:

$8 + 7 + 6 + 5 + 4 + 3 + 2 + 1 = 36$ attempts

59
In each row the yellow wedges add up to make a complete square.
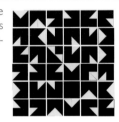

60
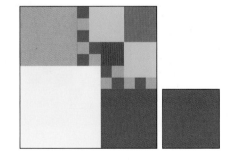

61
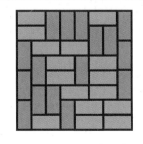

62
Pentahex 2 is not part of the honeycomb.

63
Since the nine bananas, nine oranges and nine apples in the three fruit baskets together cost $4.05, the cost of one of each fruit should cost just one-ninth of that, or $0.45. (There's no need to know that apples are 10 cents each, bananas are 20 cents each and oranges are 15 cents each.)

64
There were seven people at the reunion: a man and his wife, their three children (two girls and a boy) and the man's mother and father.

Without the stipulation that both halves of the relationships were present, there could be as few as four people; after all, one man can simultaneously be a father, a grandfather, a son, a brother and a father-in-law.

65
Based on her remark, we know that Miss Blue's dress is either pink or green. Since the woman who replied to her was wearing a green dress, that means Miss Blue must be wearing pink. That leaves the blue dress for Miss Green and the green dress for Miss Pink.

66
You can write four numbers:

a. $2^{2^2} = 2^4 = 16$, the smallest number
b. 222
c. $22^2 = 484$
d. $2^{22} = 4,194,304$, the largest number

Using powers is an efficient way to write very large or very small numbers. Raising a number to a power simply means multiplying it by itself as many times as is indicated by the power. So:

$2^{22} = 2 \times 2 = 4,194,304$

67
If you shake one of the coins out of the bank labeled "15¢," you can figure out how to correctly label all the banks. Since you know that the bank is mislabeled, it cannot hold 15 cents—instead, the bank contains either two dimes or two nickels. The coin that drops out will tell you what the other coin is. Say the answer is two dimes; that leaves you with three nickels and a dime between the two remaining banks, one labeled "20¢" and one labeled "10¢." Since the bank labeled "10¢" cannot have two nickels in it—because it is mislabeled—it must contain a nickel and a dime, and the other bank must have the two nickels.

68

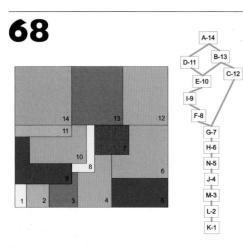

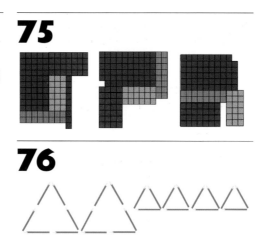

The relative layering of D-11 and B-13 cannot be determined. Similarly, the position of C-12 can actually be anywhere from 8 to 12. See chart.

69

View 5 is inconsistent with the other views.

70

Fold 3 is impossible. In general, it is not possible to fold the strip so that stamps that touch only at the corners will appear next to each other in the stack.

71

Card number 3 is not found in the colored pattern.

72

Each letter has been shifted one place down alphabetically. A becomes B, B becomes C and so on. The secret message is ONE THOUSAND PLAYTHINKS.

73

74

When overlapped, the strips can create a six-pointed star.

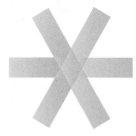

75

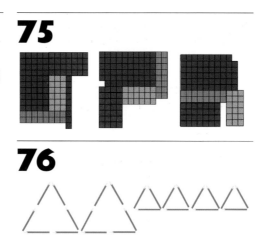

76

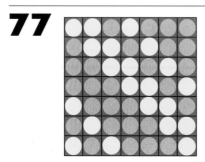

77

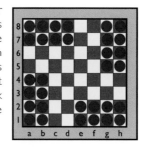

78

The missing animal is the donkey. The pattern is made of six animals running across the five-by-four grid. Each time the pattern is repeated, the first animal in the series is omitted. If each animal were a number, the series would read: 12345623456345645656.

79

The odd one out is the third in the first row.

80

The answer is yes. As pictured, it is possible to place a maximum of thirty-two knights on the board so that each piece can attack one and only one other piece.

81

One in six. Three hats can be distributed among three people in six different ways: ABC, ACB, BAC, BCA, CAB, CBA.

82

In every second row some of the letters differ from those in the row above it. Those letters spell out the message:

"There is only one good—knowledge—and one evil—ignorance."

—SOCRATES

83

The probability of the coin landing on a corner is about 50 percent. You can verify this by tossing the coin onto the board many times. In general, the probability that a coin will cover a corner can be calculated by dividing the area of the coin by the area of a single square of the game board.

84

The five numbers between 1 and 100 that have twelve factors:

60: 1, 2, 3, 4, 5, 6, 10, 12, 15, 20, 30, 60
72: 1, 2, 3, 4, 6, 8, 9, 12, 18, 24, 36, 72
84: 1, 2, 3, 4, 6, 7, 12, 14, 21, 28, 42, 84
90: 1, 2, 3, 5, 6, 9, 10, 15, 18, 30, 45, 90
96: 1, 2, 3, 4, 6, 8, 12, 16, 24, 32, 48, 96

85

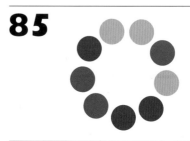

86

Four cuts, as shown, will be sufficient. Notice that the lengths are equal to the place numbers in the base 2, or binary, number system.

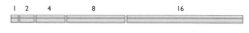

87

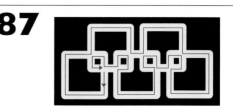

88

The sequence of colors the guide shouted was:

red, blue, blue, blue, blue, red.

The tourists all met in the central cave. Note that even a tourist who started in the central cave would wind up back there at the end of the sequence.

The two roads emanating from each point of the pentagonal labyrinth represent a type of mathematical problem—a strictly bifurcated directed graph. This particular PlayThink, which is based on the "road coloring problem" of graph theory that mathematicians such as R. L. Adler, L. W. Goodwin, B. Weiss, J. L. O'Brien and J. Friedman have tackled so intensively is like other problems of this sort, still unsolved in general. When mathematicians say "in general," they mean they don't have a ready formula for solving every problem of that sort; instead, the answers are found through trial and error.

CHAPTER 2 SOLUTIONS

89

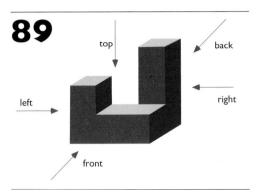

90

The sixteen views are combined correctly in the table:

A/15	E/10	I/14	M/13
B/11	F/12	J/7	N/1
C/8	G/16	K/9	O/4
D/6	H/3	L/2	P/5

The multiview problems combine spatial awareness with logic—the ability to visualize in three-dimensional views.

In fact, the overhead views and front views given correspond fairly well to what architects call a plan and front elevation. The plan represents the shape as laid out horizontally on the ground; the elevation is a front view that is derived exactly and immediately from the dimensions of the plan.

Other elevations derived by architects in the same way are those of the remaining sides of the building, each seen as a direct face-on-view, with no perspective.

91

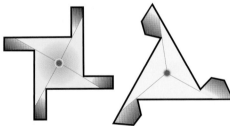

92

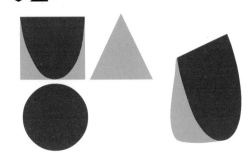

93

The large central figure was also traced along the lines of the center grid.

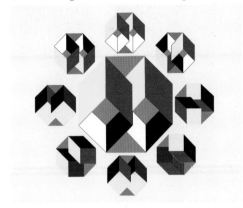

94

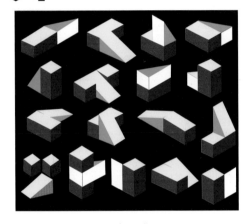

95

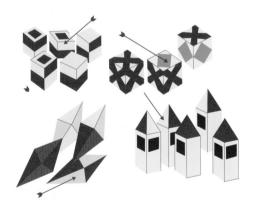

96

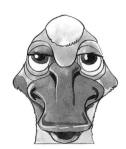

97

As seen from the point marked in red, the sculpture resolves into a perfect square divided into seven colored pieces that fit together seamlessly.

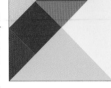

The sculpture was designed using the laws of perspective and the rules for perspective design, all to demonstrate the importance of point of view when observing a three-dimensional object.

98

Each number is the sum of the two numbers immediately above it. This mathematical tree is called Pascal's triangle.

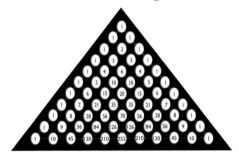

99

There can be many shapes of squares in taxicab geometry. Shown below are several squares that are six blocks on a side.

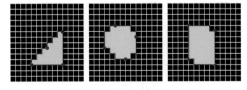

100

In the geometry of Gridlock City, the shortest route that links all four points is twenty blocks long. And there are 10,000 different routes that you could take that are that short.

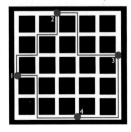

101 There is generally more than one shortest path between two points in a place like Gridlock City. For example, to go to a point halfway around the block, you can move clockwise or counterclockwise—both paths are equally short.

To work out the number of paths of minimum length to each intersection in the grid, you begin by marking the starting point with a 1, which represents the fact that standing still is the shortest path to where you started. The shortest path to the corner is a straight line, so mark each of the nearest corners with a 1 as well. But as was mentioned above, there are two equally short paths to the corner opposite the starting point, so mark that point with a 2. If you carefully fill in the grid and then tilt the grid a bit as shown, you should see part of the famous Pascal's triangle (PlayThink 98).

As seen in the image below, when the plan of Gridlock City is superimposed on Pascal's triangle, point B is located at the point marked 210. Thus, there are 210 equally short paths between point A and point B.

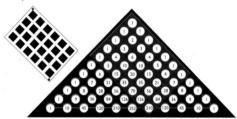

102 In taxicab geometry circles are squares. The circle of 1 kilometer radius is shown in red, with an intersecting circle with radius ⅔ kilometer (but a center that is two blocks to the east) shown in green. The two circles intersect at nine different points.

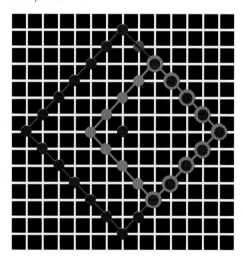

Although Euclidean geometry states that any two intersecting circles can have at most two points in common, taxicab geometry allows circles to intersect at any number of points. The larger the squares, the more points they can have in common.

103 A configuration with nine frowning faces and four smiling faces.

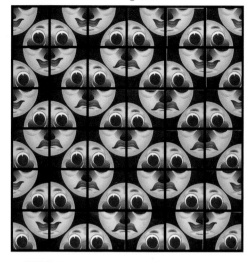

105 In Flatland a law was passed requiring women to constantly twist and turn. In that way they would always be visible.

106 The Flatlanders would not be able to sense the approach of the ball until it intersected with the plane of their world. Those at a distance would see a point appear from nowhere, and that point would grow into a circle that would eventually reach the size of the ball itself. Then the circle would begin to diminish, shrinking to a point and eventually disappearing.

For some Flatlanders the event would be a catastrophe: if they were at the point where the ball intersected their world, they would be lifted off their world into the mysterious "third" dimension. Indeed, if someone from our dimension wanted to take objects from Flatland, they would encounter few problems. Even the most secure vault in Flatland is simply a two-dimensional box with heavy walls. Someone from our dimension could reach into that vault and take anything without disturbing the walls or picking the lock.

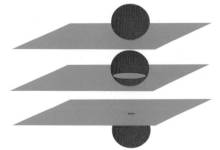

107 The answer sounds trivial—you can bring them together by closing the book—but some physicists speculate that if our three-dimensional space could be made as malleable as the pages of a book, folding space itself may be the means by which humans can travel from star to star.

108 A cube sitting on one side can face in four different directions. A cube has six sides. So four directions per side multiplied by six sides gives a total of twenty-four possible orientations.

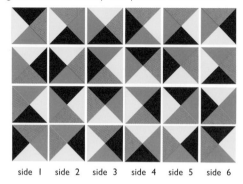

side 1   side 2   side 3   side 4   side 5   side 6

109 There are sixty different ways a dodecahedron can be placed on a table.

110

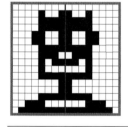
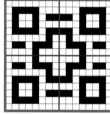

111 The square can undergo eight transformations; the star can undergo ten.

The operations involved are called symmetries. When speaking of symmetry, a mathematician is talking about the way of transforming an object so that it preserves its shape. The object can be rotated or flipped about an axis; the set of transformations of that sort for a specific object is called the symmetry group.

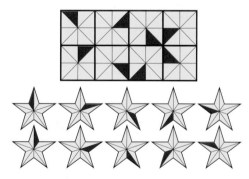

112 The player making the first move can always win by following these instructions: Place the first coin on the exact center of the table. After that move, always respond to the opponent's move with a symmetric move, which will always be possible.

Since the first player's moves are always safe, he or she can't lose. The second player will eventually run out of safe moves.

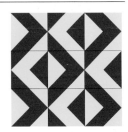

113

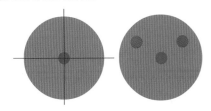

114 The last two tiles don't follow the rule.

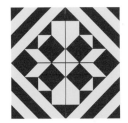

115

isosceles triangle	▲	▲	2
scalene triangle	◣	◿	1
equilateral triangle	▲	▲	6
square	■	▢	8
greek cross	✚	✚	8
rhombus	◆	◇	4
parallelogram	▰	▱	2

116 The red letters are the capital letters in the alphabet that have only vertical symmetry. The blue letters are the capitals that have only horizontal symmetry.

117 The parallelogram has no symmetry axes. The circle has an infinite number of symmetry axes.

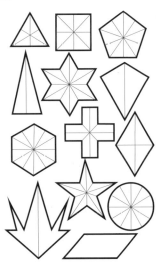

118

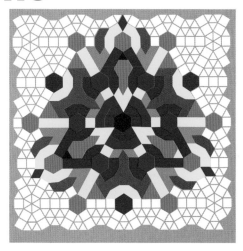

119 The symmetries of the capital letters can be categorized as follows:

1. Letters that are symmetrical only in the vertical plane: A, M, T, U, V, W, Y

2. Letters that are symmetrical only in the horizontal plane: B, C, D, E, K

3. Letters symmetrical in both the vertical and horizontal planes: H, I, O, X

4. Letters that possess only rotational symmetry: N, S, Z

5. Asymmetric letters: F, G, J, L, P, Q, R

120

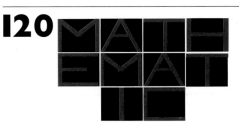

121 The blue letters are the capital letters that have both horizontal and vertical symmetry. The red letters are asymmetrical.

122 The red letters are asymmetrical. The blue letters have a twofold rotational symmetry. Although some shapes—and letters— have no bilateral symmetry, they still possess rotational symmetry.

123 The first face in the first row, the second face in the seond row and the third face in the third row are impossible to re-create.

124 The ancient Greeks proved that the pentagram comprised two golden triangles with sides equal to the golden ratio —approximately 1.618—often symbolized by the Greek letter ø.

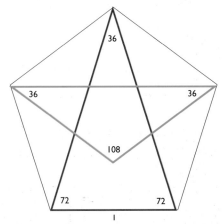

125 The cube has three fourfold axes of rotational symmetry, four threefold axes and six twofold axes. In general, having a certain number-fold of rotational axes means that if you rotate the object through part of a full rotation equal to the inverse of that number (for example, one-third rotation for a three-fold axis), you get a figure identical to the original.

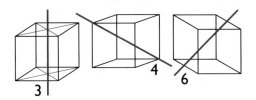

126
At the end of the game, only one green square remains on top of the board.

I hope that you anticipated from the outset that the triangles, circles and semicircles would fall through the square holes. I also hope you noticed that in some cases differences in orientation would prevent triangular and semicircular shapes from falling through similarly shaped holes.

Number of shapes initially on top	16	16	16	16
SHAPES	▦	◣	●	◖
Number of shapes initially falling through	6	4	8	12
Number of shapes falling through after ¼ turn clockwise	5	6	7	0
Number of shapes falling through after ½ turn clockwise	3	1	1	3
Number of shapes falling through after ¾ turn clockwise	1	5	0	1
Number of shapes falling through after one full turn clockwise	1	0	0	0
Number of shapes staying on top	1	0	0	0

CHAPTER 3 SOLUTIONS

128
One of many possible solutions.

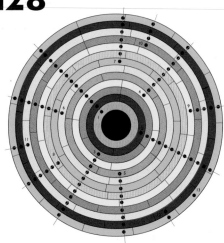

129

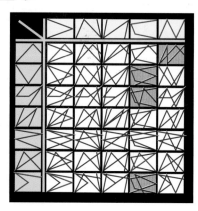

130

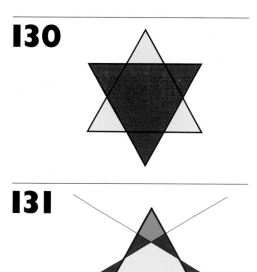

131

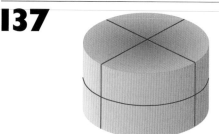

132
The sets of straight lines will blur into concentric circles of different sizes. That baffling result is due to an optical illusion. You no doubt have seen such an illusion before, but you may not know why it works. Don't feel bad: even scientists who study human perception are not sure why straight lines can be perceived as circles.

The most important element of the illusion is something you don't really see—the center point around which the rest of the disc revolves. The distance from that center point to the middle of the line will give you the approximate radius of the circle you see when the turntable begins its motion.

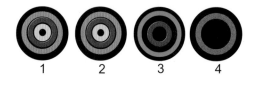

133
A solution with seven triangles is illustrated.

In general, what is the largest number of nonoverlapping triangles that can be enclosed by *n* straight line segments? Trial and error will quickly lead you to the discovery that for *n* = 3, 4, 5 and 6, the maximum number of triangles enclosed is one, two, five and seven, respectively. When the problem reaches *n* = 7, trial and error no longer provides the easy answer. And the general problem for *n* of any number has yet to be solved.

134
A simple closed curve is one that does not cross itself. A loop of string that follows that rule can always be stretched into a circle; likewise, a circle of string can be pulled to form a loop. But with a loop or a circle, there is always an inside and an outside.

One way to determine whether a point is on the inside or the outside is to carefully shade in all the interior spaces of the loop. But that is time-consuming. A short and elegant solution is to draw a line connecting the point to an area clearly outside the loop and count the number of times the line crosses a curve. If it crosses an odd number of times, the point is inside the loop; if it crosses an even number of times, it is outside the loop.

This rule is known as the Jordan curve theorem.

135
You can check with your own randomly drawn lines, but the intersections will always align. That surprising result is known as Pappus's theorem.

136
There is only one convex polygon: the hexagon in the lower right-hand corner.

The figure-eight-shaped polygon is different from all the other objects because its lines intersect.

137

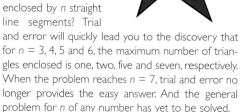

138
An eleven-triangle solution is illustrated.

139
A fifteen-triangle solution is shown.

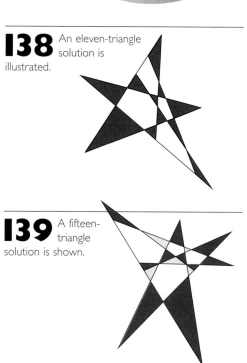

140

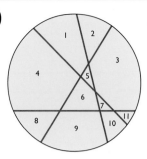

The illustration above shows four cuts dividing a cake into eleven pieces. As a general rule, try to place each new cut across all the previous cuts. In that way every *n*th cut creates *n* new pieces.

Lines	Pieces	Total
0	1	1
1	1 + 1	2
2	2 + 2	4
3	4 + 3	7
4	7 + 4	11
5	11 + 5	16
and so on		

The general principle can be written as a general formula for *n* number of cuts: $(n(n+1))/2 + 1$.

141

If you understand the general rule (see PlayThink 140), this should be easy: if four cuts can make eleven pieces, then a fifth cut across the previous four will make five new pieces, for a total of sixteen.

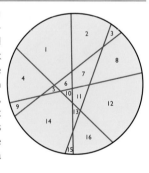

142

In spite of the answers for the smaller numbers of points, the answer for six points is thirty-one, not thirty-two.

This is a beautiful example of why guessing at an answer is not the best way to solve a problem. The sequence of the partitions created for the series from zero points to nine points is 1, 2, 4, 8, 16, 31, 57, 99, 163, 256.

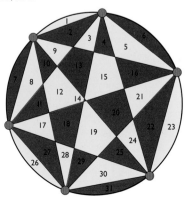

143

In general, the number of compartments crossed by the laser equals the sum of the two sides of the box minus the greatest common divisor of those two numbers. In this instance:

$$10 + 14 - 2 = 22.$$

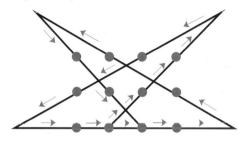

144

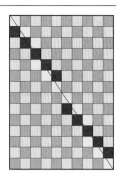

145

Minimizing the number of intersections is easy: make all the lines parallel. Maximizing the number of intersections is much more difficult. Two lines can meet at only one point; three lines at exactly three points; four lines at six and so on. A little trial and error with drinking straws, pencil and paper or computer graphics will lead you to the maximum solution. All you need to do is avoid making any line parallel to another—eventually every line will intersect with every other line.

So for five lines there is a maximum of ten intersections.

146

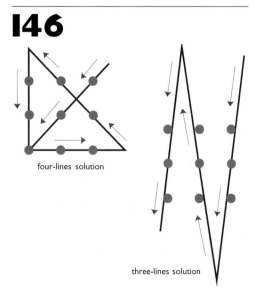

four-lines solution

three-lines solution

147

Once gained, a valuable insight can be generalized. If you have solved the problem of the nine points, the answer to problems involving greater numbers of points should come easily. For this problem five lines are needed.

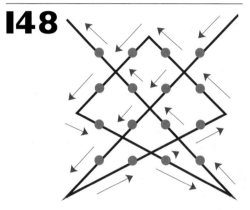

148

149

150

Most people think that three is the best answer. But if the three trees surround a steep hill or valley, then a fourth tree can be planted at the top of the hill or at the bottom of the valley, forming a tetrahedron. A tetrahedron is a three-dimensional shape made of four equilateral triangles, and therefore all four of its points are equidistant.

151

Since Fido is tied to a tree, he can reach anywhere within a ten-foot radius of the tree. His bowl is five feet from the tree, on the opposite side from where Fido started.

152 Begin by creating a triangle that connects points B and C to point D. You will find as you move points B and C around—careful to make sure that line BC always runs through point A—that the angles BDC, DBC and BCD remain the same. That means that the way to make line BAC the longest is by making lines BD and CD the longest they can be. Lines BD and CD are at their longest when they are the diameters of their respective circles. It is then that line BAC is at its longest.

It just so happens that when BD and CD run through the diameters of the circles, line BAC is perpendicular to line AD.

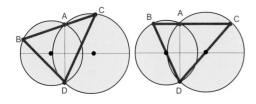

153 Sample game in which green wins.

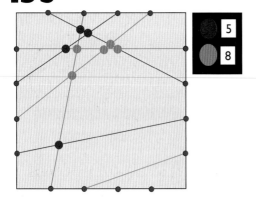

154 Two solutions are possible. The hidden snake is either green or blue.

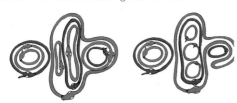

155

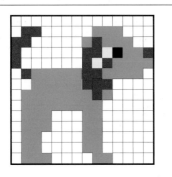

156

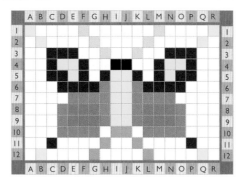

157 This is another example of a problem concerning lines, intersections and restrictions on possible configurations. With n lines, a maximum of (n (n − 1))/2 intersections is possible. Fewer intersections are also possible, down to (n − 1) intersections, a case in which all but one of the lines run parallel.

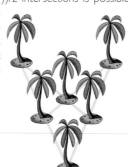

158 There are exactly eight two-distance sets; all eight are illustrated here. In each figure the red lines have one length, and the blue lines have another.

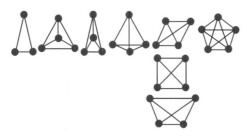

159

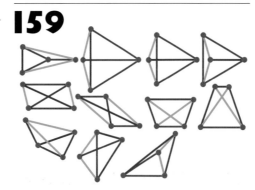

160

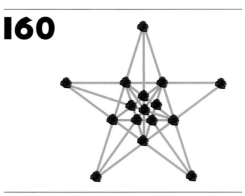

161 The Hungarian mathematician Ilona Palásti discovered the eight-point multidistance graph in 1989. It is the largest set known: an eight-point, seven-distance set.

Distance 1 is black; 2, red; 3, cyan; 4, green; 5, magenta; 6, yellow; 7, blue.

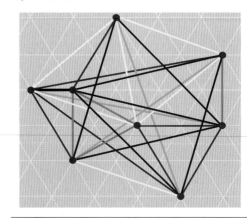

162 The key to solving this sort of puzzle is to visualize the answer before you pick up the first match. Some answers involve squares of different sizes; some overlap; many have common sides. But if you have trouble imagining the answer, the trial-and-error approach will help you work toward a solution and better understand the principles behind the puzzle. Once you have mastered these games, you can devise more complex versions on your own.

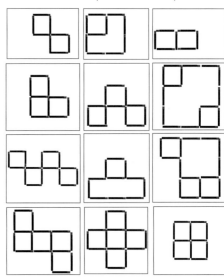

163

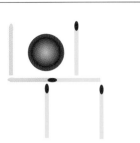

164

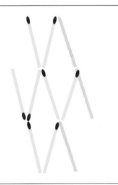

165

The solution shown here requires twelve matches meeting at eight points in the plane. A triangular pyramid with six matches meeting at four points would do it in space.

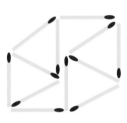

166

With four matchsticks five configurations are possible. With five matchsticks there are twelve possible configurations.

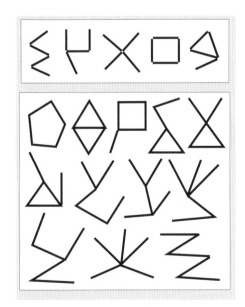

167

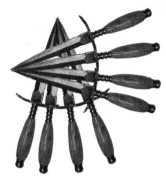

168

As you can see, area and perimeter have little bearing on each other. The way the area and angles vary as other elements of the shape change introduces the concept of function, which you will see more of later.

	CONSTANT	CHANGE
AREA	NO	YES
PERIMETER	YES	NO
SIDES	YES	NO
ANGLES	NO	YES

169

The linkage illustrated below is a schematic representation of the famous Watt's linkage, which draws a figure-eight-shaped curve. Part of that curve—called Bernoulli's lemniscate—is a nearly straight line.

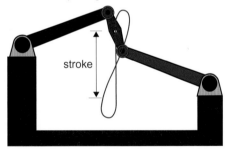

stroke

170

The path is approximately a straight line.

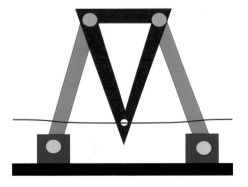

171

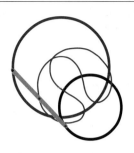

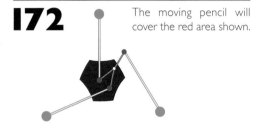

172

The moving pencil will cover the red area shown.

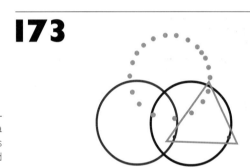

173

CHAPTER 4 SOLUTIONS

174

The only way to get to the ladybug's friend is through the red flower at the top of the diagram, so red must represent up.

Purple cannot be up, and if it were down, the ladybug's first move would be off the diagram. If purple meant left, then the ladybug would move to a yellow flower and the only allowable direction for pink would be right—a never-ending loop! So purple must represent right.

After figuring out that, it is easy to tell that blue represents left and yellow represents down.

175

A pirate with one peg leg pushed a two-wheeled cart. The pirate's dog walked beside him.

176

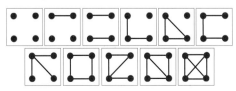

177 There are twenty allowable paths between the pillars, but no matter how many different ways I ran, I could never get past seventeen legs. If the courtyard had had seven pillars or nine pillars, I would have been able to reach the mathematical maximum. As it was, I later discovered through my study of topology, the full complement of paths is impossible to achieve in a courtyard with eight pillars.

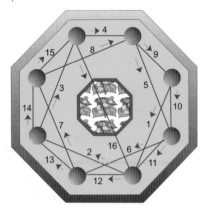

178 If you have trouble solving this problem, it may be because it is often difficult to visualize the hidden edges and corners of a solid figure. It may be useful to draw a topologically equivalent two-dimensional diagram of the three-dimensional solid. Such a diagram makes each edge and corner visible and enables you to see the relationships between them.

Our solution is drawn on that sort of diagram.

179 When he solved the problem of the Seven Bridges of Königsberg (see page 71), Leonhard Euler discovered the general rule for tackling this class of puzzle. The secret is to count the number of paths leading from each point of intersection, or junction. If more than two junctions possess an odd number of paths, the pattern is impossible to trace.

In this instance, paths 4 and 5 are impossible.

If there are exactly two junctions that have an odd number of paths, the problem may be solved, but only if you begin and end at those two junctions. Path 7 has this property; to fully trace it, you must start at one of the lower corners and finish at the other.

180 There are ten allowable routes.

181

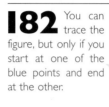

The Hamiltonian Circuit: 1-5-6-2-8-4-10-11-9-3-7-1

182 You can trace the figure, but only if you start at one of the blue points and end at the other.

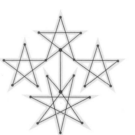

183

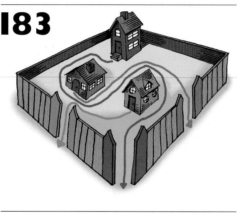

184

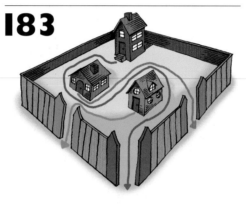

185

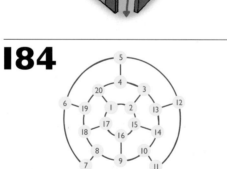

186 It is, in fact, impossible to connect each house to each utility without at least one pair of lines intersecting. Or, as one ingenious solution has it, tunneling under some of the houses.

187

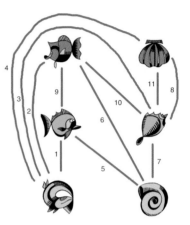

188

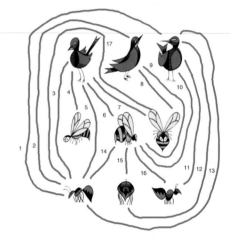

189

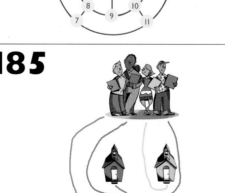

190 The worm can crawl 22 centimeters, as shown below.

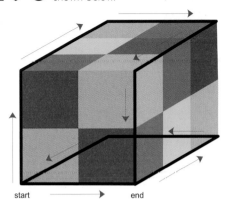

start → end

191

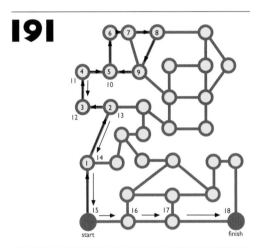

192 To travel from A to B will take thirteen minutes; from C to D also thirteen minutes; from E to F nine minutes; and from G to H fifteen minutes, as shown.

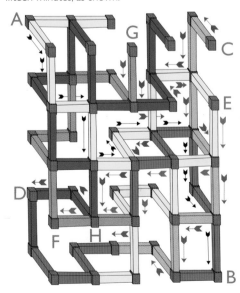

193 The two guideways that, when missing, make the puzzle impossible are numbers 10 and 13.

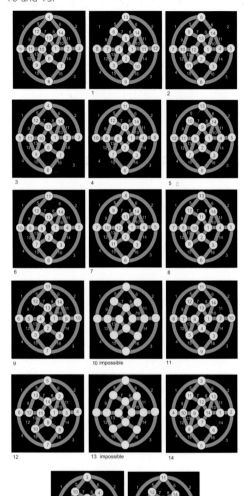

194 Puzzle master Sam Loyd first published his Mars puzzle in *Our Puzzle Magazine* in 1907; ten thousand readers wrote in saying they had tried to solve the problem and found "there is no possible way." Those ten thousand readers had solved the puzzle—THERE IS NO POSSIBLE WAY.

195 The four arrows in each row and column point in a different direction.

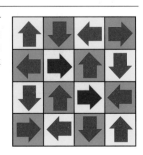

196

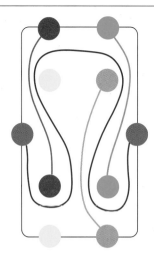

197

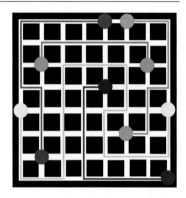

198

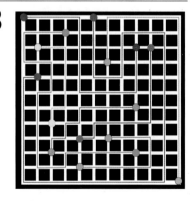

199 Circuit board #3 is the right one.

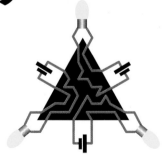

200 Before taking into account the symmetries of the cube, you can place the arrows in 4,096 (4⁶) different ways. But eliminating configurations that are symmetrical duplicates leaves you with just 192 different ways to label the cube with arrows.

201 Line number 5 can be moved so that it crosses only one other line. That makes for nine intersections, which is the fewest possible when interconnecting seven different points. Mathematicians have their own way of saying that: The minimal crossing number for seven points is nine.

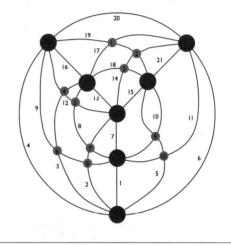

202

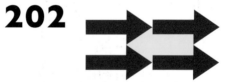

203 The sixteen tree graphs that connect the four points are illustrated below.

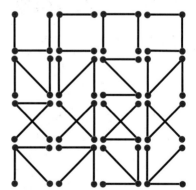

204 The topologically distinct trees for six and seven points are illustrated below.

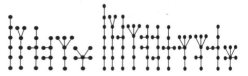

206 TREE GAME CARD SETS:
1-20-35-61
2-5-32-56
3-29-47-75
4-17-24-25
6-8-21-59
7-11-30-31
9-36-41-45
10-22-38-49
12-19-26-63
13-27-50-55
14-39-43-48
16-42-46-62
18-23-53-64
28-34-40-58
33-44-51-60
15-37-52-54

207 One solution is shown. There are many others, but all will have eighteen branches.

In the case of strings and beads, the correct answer can be suspended in the manner shown, and each bead will hang from exactly one piece of string. Therefore, the number of strings or lines or branches is equal to the number of beads or points, minus one.

No matter how you draw your tree, that is both the maximum and the minimum number of lines.

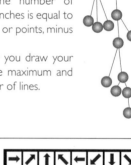

208 Each row and column contains arrows that point in the eight main directions.

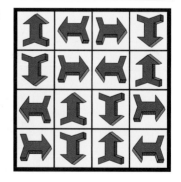

209

210 One of many possible solutions.

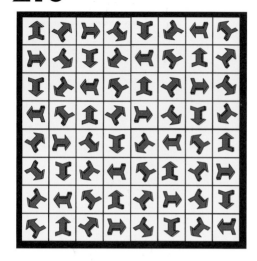

211 The route is 5, 1, 2, 4, 3.

212 One route is 6, 1, 5, 3, 2, 4; another one is 6, 1, 4, 5, 3, 2.

213 There are many solutions, including the one shown here.

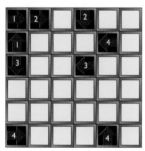

214 No matter how the arrows are placed, there will always be a path that interconnects the six cities. This is because this is a complete digraph puzzle.

215

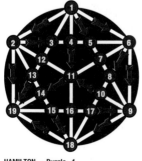

HAMILTON - Puzzle 1

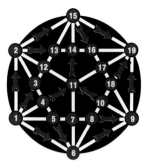

HAMILTON - Puzzle 2

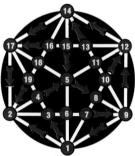

HAMILTON - Puzzle 3

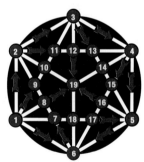

HAMILTON - Puzzle 4

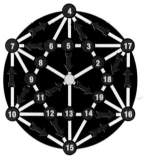

HAMILTON - Puzzle 5

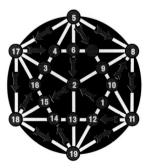

HAMILTON - Puzzle 6

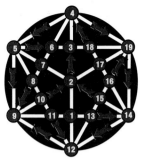

HAMILTON - Puzzle 7

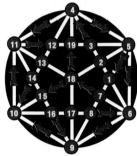

HAMILTON - Puzzle 8

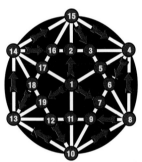

HAMILTON - Puzzle 9

216 You can avoid love or hate triangles in groups of four or five, as shown at right. For any three points there are always two different types of relationships represented.

For the group of six, however, there is no way to avoid having a love triangle or a hate triangle. As you can see, no matter which color you choose for the uncolored line, you will be forced to create either a blue triangle or a red one.

This is one of the applications of Ramsey theory. There are quite a few others.

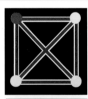

218

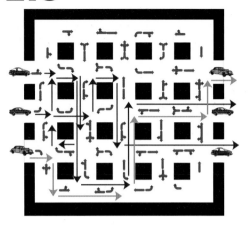

CHAPTER 5 SOLUTIONS

219 The secret of the puzzle is in the color sequence: yellow, orange, red, pink, blue, violet, light green, dark green, purple. The sequence moves in a clockwise direction. The pieces are put together so that the next piece continues the sequence where the last piece left off.

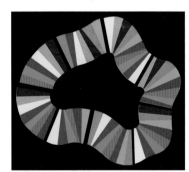

220 The pattern that emerges is a 1:2 web, though it is also known by a grander name: cardioid, or heart curve.

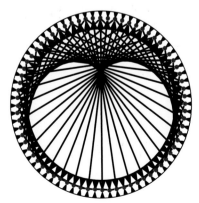

221 This pattern is the 1:3 web, also known as the nephroid, or kidney curve.

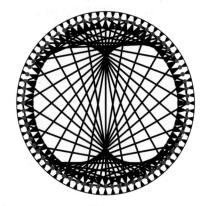

222 The pattern will be a cardioid.

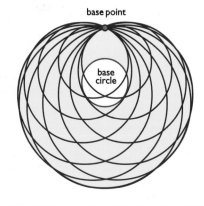

223 The pattern that emerges is a nephroid.

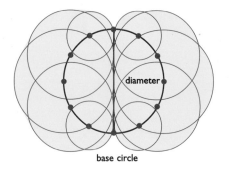

224
Center
Circumference
Radius
Diameter
Tangent
Arc
Chord
Segment
Semicircle
Sector
Quadrant

225 The path formed when one object chases another object that moves in a predetermined way has a special name: the pursuit curve, or tractrix.

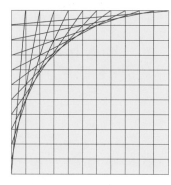

226 The red fluid completely fills the circle of radius a/2, but it only partly fills the square. By observation we can see that the fluid fills an area equal to $3 + \frac{1}{7}(\frac{1}{2})^2$, from which it follows that π equals $3 + \frac{1}{7}$.

The area of the triangle is $(a^2)/2$.

227

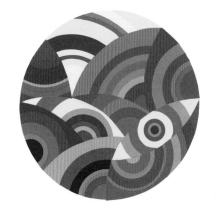

228 1. Round manhole covers cannot fall through their round holes accidentally. Square or other polygonal covers can.

2. Heavy round covers can be rolled into position, while other shapes would have to be carried.

3. Round covers can cover holes no matter how they are oriented vis-à-vis the hole. Square covers fit only when they are positioned in one of four orientations.

229 As the rollers are moved forward, their point of contact with the weight moves backward at a rate of 1 meter a turn. But the rollers are also in contact with the ground and moving forward in comparison with it at a rate of 1 meter a turn. Together, that means that the weight moves forward in relation to the ground at a rate of 2 meters per full turn.

230 The circumference of every circle is approximately $3 + \frac{1}{7}$ times the diameter. That number is famously known as π and is the best known of the irrational numbers—numbers that continue an infinite number of decimal places without repeating.

$$\pi = 3.14159265358 \ldots$$

Most students learn about the number π when a teacher simply gives its definition. Here you discovered it yourself, much as the ancient Greeks did thousands of years ago.

231 The combined areas of the two red crescents—which are the areas of the two small semicircles not covered by the large black semicircle—equal the area of the right triangle itself.

Although the circle itself cannot be squared, other figures bounded by circular arcs can be. That fact arouses false hope in those who would still like to square the circle.

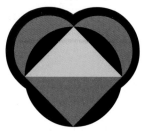

232 The area of the red parts is slightly more than 1.3 times greater than that of the black areas. The black areas seem larger because of an optical illusion.

233

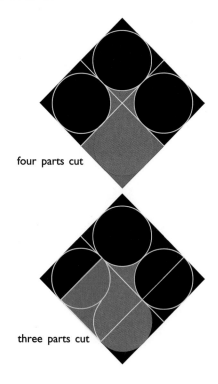

four parts cut

three parts cut

234 The area of the sickle is equal to the area of a circle that has a diameter of *L*. The famous Greek scientist Archimedes first solved this problem, which now bears his name.

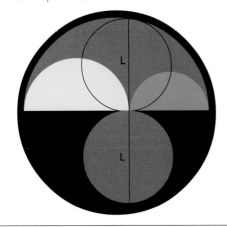

235 Rather than count all the lines, you can calculate the total. Fourteen lines emanate from each point, and $14 \times 15 = 210$. But since each line is shared by two points, the actual number of lines is half that, or 105.

According to Euler's Problem (PlayThink 179), it is possible to trace the design in one continuous line.

Mystic roses may be considered to be all the diagonals and sides of a regular polygon of a given number of sides.

236 The area of the circle is πr^2.

237 Triangle 1 provides the largest total area of circles.

This puzzle is a special case of the famous Malfatti's problem. In 1803, Gian Francesco Malfatti, an Italian mathematician, asked for the three largest cylinders (in volume) that could be placed in a prism.

238

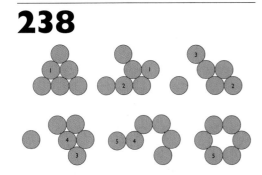

239

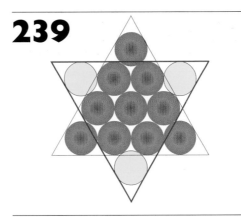

240 There are basically five ways to arrange two circles on a plane.

There are ten common tangents, as illustrated at right.

Yes. If the circles were identical, cases 4 and 5 would not be possible.

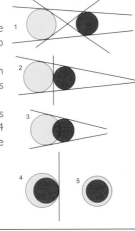

241 The three yellow circles will grow so large that they become, in the limit, the sides of a triangle. The red circle will become an inscribed circle in that triangle.

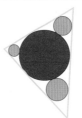

242 Surprisingly enough, there are only eight different ways that three circles may touch a fourth on a plane. All eight are illustrated below.

For the general case, take three circles and move them together so that they are mutually tangent; then, in the space between the three, draw a circle that touches all of them. In that way four circles can be mutually tangent. You may also draw a circle around all three that is mutually tangent.

Four is also the maximum number of circles that may be mutually tangent on a plane.

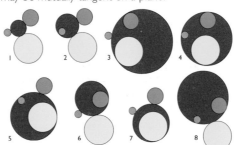
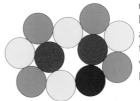

243 The color of the circle depends upon the number of circles it touches.

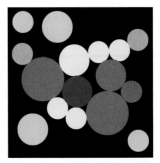

244 Five intersecting circles will divide a plane into twenty-two regions, as shown.

Euler's formula for polyhedra (see below) is also valid for this sort of connected graph; simply imagine the polyhedra distorted and flattened on a plane.

A circle can intersect another

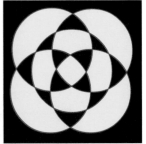

circle at two points. For each circle, that makes for $2(n-1)$ points of intersection. Counting all the circles and dividing by 2 (since each point was counted twice) gives $n(n-1)$ points of intersection, or vertices. Each circle is also divided into $2(n-1)$ segments, giving a total of $2n(n-1)$ edges.

Euler's formula gives:

$$\text{Regions} = \text{Edges} - \text{Vertices} + 2, \text{ so}$$
$$= 2n(n-1) - n(n-1) + 2$$
$$= n^2 - (n-2) \text{ regions}$$

245 There are twelve polygons possible with these five points. Only two of the polygons are regular; the rest can be divided into two groups—essentially, two shapes in five different orientations each.

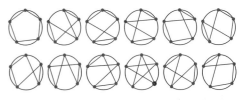

246 It takes only eleven circles, as illustrated, to form a configuration that requires four colors. No matter how you arrange the colors, a fourth will be needed where the blue chip is located.

247

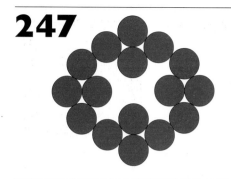

248

The bigger circle has twice the area of the smaller one. Simply put, a diagonal running from the center of the square is equal to the square root of two times the distance from the center of the square to the middle of one side. That diagonal is the radius for the large square; the distance to the middle of a side is the radius of the other. Since the area of a circle is proportional to the square of the radius, the larger circle has twice the area of the smaller one.

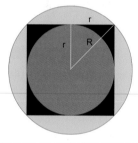

249

You will see a perfect circle.

250

One of many solutions.

251

The top roller will always remain exactly above the other, regardless of their size.

252

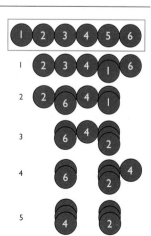

253

Six identical circles, as shown.

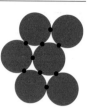

254

Red circle's diameter = ½
Yellow circle's diameter = ¼
Green circle's diameter = ¼ (2 − √2), or about ⅛

255

One of many solutions.

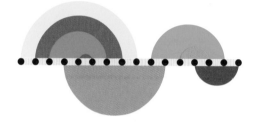

256

The perimeter of the rosette is exactly equal to the circumference of the larger circle. This is true no matter how the circles in the rosette are arranged (as long as they all pass through the same point) or how many circles there are in the rosette.

257

Every triangle has this property. The nine-point circle is half the size of the circumcircle (the circle that passes through all three vertices of the triangle), and its center is halfway between the center of the circumcenter and the orthocenter.

Charles-Julien Brianchon and Jean-Victor Poncelet first published this theorem in 1821, though the Englishman Benjamin Bevan proposed an equivalent problem in 1804.

258

Because of the great size of the sphere, there is quite a bit of safe space where the wall of the tunnel meets the floor. If he squeezes himself into that space, he can let the stone roll past him and escape.

259

No matter how you triangulate the polygon, the sum of the diameters of the circles will always be the same. To verify this, simply measure the circles and add the diameters together.

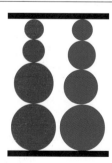

260

The common chords of three intersecting circles will always pass through a single point.

261

The three intersections of the tangent lines will always lie on a straight line. Imagine that the circles are three spheres of unequal size upon a flat plane. The lines between the circles are lines of perspective, which converge on the horizon.

262

The optimal solution is
Turn 1: 1, 2, 3, 4, 5
Turn 2: 2, 3, 4, 5, 6
Turn 3: 2, 3, 4, 5, 7

263

As a circle rolls a distance equal to its circumference, it makes one complete revolution. The perimeter of the rectangle is 12 circumferences. That means that the outside circle will make 12 revolutions as it rolls along the rectangle's sides; it will also make a quarter turn at each corner. So the outside circle will make a total of 13 revolutions.

The inside circle travels a distance equal to 12 circumferences minus 8 radii. Each radius is the circumference divided by 2π. That makes the total travel $12 - (4/\pi)$, or about 10.7 revolutions.

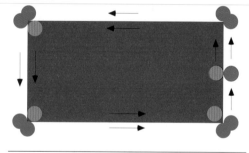

264

This is the best solution, proven by Michael Mallard and Charles Payton in 1990. In cases of packing circles into squares, mathematicians have found that as the size of the circles decreases, the density of circle to square approaches .9069. That is the limit obtained for the familiar tight packing of circles so that their centers form a lattice of equilateral triangles.

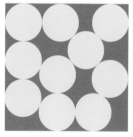

265

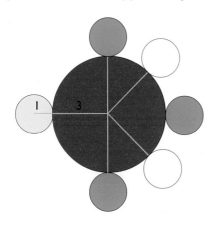

266

In an earlier puzzle we saw that one coin rolling over another rotates twice as much as one might have anticipated. In this instance the coin rolls through two full circumferences (a third of a circumference for each coin), so it makes four revolutions.

And it will once again face left.

267

The small circle travels on a path that is three times longer than its circumference; if it were a straight line, it would make three revolutions. But because it is rolling over the surface of a circle, the smaller circle "gains" an extra revolution. This would be true even if the smaller circle did not roll but simply kept the same point of contact as it slid along the circumference of the larger circle—the circle would make one complete revolution without rolling at all. The circle makes a total of four revolutions.

The concept of the revolution is a mind trap in this puzzle; a revolution is simply a 360-degree turn.

268

The intuitive answer is that the coin will be upside down because the coin has rolled along an edge equal to half its circumference. But if you try the puzzle experimentally, you will find that the coin rotates twice as much. It winds up facing left in the orientation it started with.

269

The density of the rectangular packing is π/4, or about 78 percent. The density for the hexagonal packing is π/(2 × √3), or about 90.7 percent. The hexagonal packing is the most efficient of all possible packings.

270

It is possible for one sphere to simultaneously touch twelve other spheres of the same size: six spheres around the equator and three around each pole. This is the maximum number of spheres that can "kiss" at one time. Therefore, the number of spheres that may be packed into a sphere three times as large is thirteen.

The number of identical spheres that can touch a single sphere of the same size is called the kissing number. Problems involving kissing numbers are related to many important fields, including error-correcting codes—codes employed to send messages over noisy electric channels.

271

Curiously enough, the point will trace a straight line—the diameter of the larger circle.

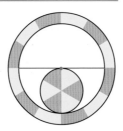

272

The plane is 50 kilometers from the North Pole. During its eastbound leg, the plane remained a constant distance from the pole.

273

Just take the first or last coin from the vertical row and place it on top of the coin in the middle.

274

The three points trace examples of a family of curves called orthocycloids. The point on the circumference traces a cycloid. The point on the inside traces a curtate cycloid. And the point on the flange traces a prolate cycloid.

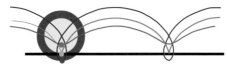

275

Imagine that the four cuts have created a tetrahedron in the interior of the sphere. Based on that tetrahedron, the sphere has been divided into the following regions: four at the vertices, six at the edges, four at the faces of the tetrahedron, and the tetrahedron itself. The total is fifteen regions.

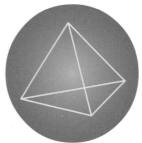

276

The point will trace a near-perfect square. This property was exploited in the invention of a tool that drills square holes.

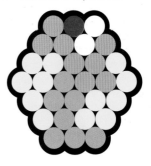

277

The final board layout for one solution reached in fifty moves.

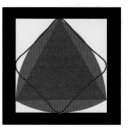

278

Imagine that you can split the cylinder and lay it flat, as shown. According to the Pythagorean theorem:

$$c^2 = a^2 + b^2 = 9 + 16 = 25 \text{ meters}$$

$$c = 5 \text{ meters}$$

Thus, length of the rope is 4 × 5 meters, or 20 meters.

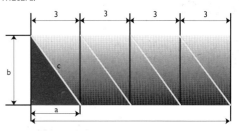

279

The intuitive answer is that since 2 meters is inconsequential compared to the circumference of the earth, the belt would hardly budge. But in this case intuition is wrong.

A little analysis shows why. The circumference of the earth is 2π times its radius, and the length of the belt is 2π times both the radius of the earth and the height that the belt is pulled off the surface. If the difference between those two lengths is 2 meters, then:

$$2\pi(r + x) - 2\pi r = 2 \text{ meters}$$

$$2\pi r + 2\pi x - 2\pi r = 2\pi x = 2 \text{ meters}$$

$$x = 1/\pi \text{ meters, or about .33 meters}$$

The same answer would hold for an "earth" of any size, even one the size of a tennis ball.

280

The sphere and the cylinder have the same surface area: $4\pi r^2$.

281 The volume of the cylinder is exactly equal to the volume of the sphere plus the volume of the cone. This is a fundamental theorem on which the determination of the volume of the sphere depended. Archimedes considered it one of his greatest triumphs.

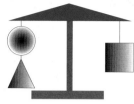

The ratio of a cone, sphere and cylinder of the same height and radius is quite elegant:

1:2:3

282 The area of the cycloid is three times that of the generating circle. That answer shocked mathematicians when it was first discovered.

The length of the cycloid arch, from cusp to cusp, is four times the diameter of the circle, which was also an unexpected result. Mathematicians were certain that it would be an irrational number, much like the circumference of the circle. As a curve, the cycloid is much more complex than the circle, so it is little wonder that the discovery that its length is so simple would be surprising.

In 1664, Evangelista Torricelli, a student of Galileo, wrote the first treatise on the cycloid.

283 Six spheres can be removed, as shown.

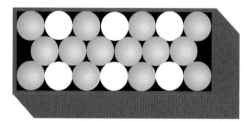

284 The shortest path—the straight line—is not the quickest. Instead, the ball that rolls on the cycloidal track will be the first to arrive. Amazingly, the cycloidal path is the longest of the four.

The cycloid is called the curve of quickest descent, or brachitochrone. The ball descending the cycloid reaches a high speed early in its descent and uses that speed to race ahead of the others.

285 All except the last curve will turn like a circle.

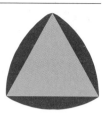

286

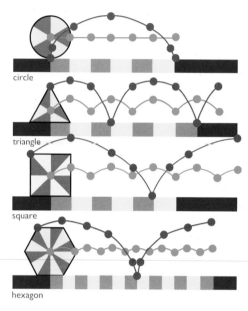

circle

triangle

square

hexagon

Reuleux triangle

287 The problem lies in drawing the swords from the scabbards. It is impossible for the warrior with the wavy sword to pull it out of its scabbard. The other swords will go in and out of their scabbards, although the helical sword must be "unscrewed," a time-consuming act that would leave its owner at a bit of a disadvantage.

288 1. A cut parallel to the base makes a circle.

2. A cut parallel to a line generating the cone makes a parabola.

3. A cut inclined to the axis at an angle greater than the semivertical of the cone makes an ellipse.

4. A cut inclined to the axis at an angle less than the semivertical of the cone makes a hyperbola.

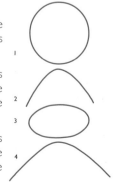

289 An ellipse is formed by slanted cuts through cones or cylinders. The man can make such a cut by picking up his water glass and tilting it. The surface of the water will form a perfect ellipse.

290 The resultant curve will be a nephroid, or kidney curve.

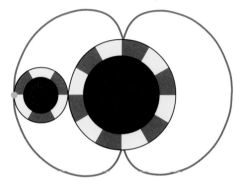

291 Mark a point on the circle, then fold the circle along any line so that the edge of the circle just touches the point. Make a crease in that fold line. Repeat the process of folding and creasing. Before too many folds, you will begin to see an ellipse surrounded by all the fold lines.

The fold lines are tangents to the ellipse and form an envelope around it. With other circles of paper, investigate what happens to the ellipse as you move the mark nearer the center of the circle.

In the illustration below, the points marked A and C are the foci of the ellipse.

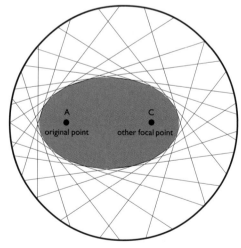

A
original point

C
other focal point

292 No matter where you hit a ball placed at one focus of the ellipse, it will always travel to the other focus, which is where the pocket is (as long as you don't strike the obstacle). On the other hand, if the ball sits between the two focal points, striking the ball off the ellipse will send it on a path that never gets closer to a focus.

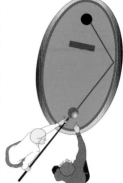

The reflection property of the ellipse is employed in the architecture of so-called whispering galleries—elliptical rooms in which even faint sounds made at one focus can be heard clearly at the other.

CHAPTER 6 SOLUTIONS

293 The pink shape is the only polygon shown that is not regular; not all of its sides and angles are identical.

294

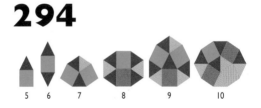

295

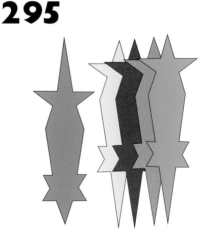

296 The missing number is 5. The sum of the numbers on the convex angles of each polygon is five times greater than the sum of the numbers on the concave angles.

297 The mechanism cannot make the pentagonal profile.

298 The result will always be 1. The operation you worked out,

$$points - sides + regions = 1$$

is Euler's formula. It is an important mathematical relationship and a beautiful example of simplicity amid complexity.

299 The only square with a perimeter equal to its area has four sides of 4 units. The only rectangle with that property measures 3 by 6 units.

300 One might imagine that the shrinking circles would eventually approach a size of 0. But, surprisingly, the limit is somewhat farther out. It takes very advanced mathematics to produce the result, but the ultimate solution is that the radii of the shrinking circles approach a limit approximately 1/8.7 that of the radius of the first circle, or about .115 units.

301 Both areas are identical. The total area of the small triangles is equal to that of the big triangle. And the overlapping parts in white decrease both equally.

302 The key to understanding this problem is realizing that for a rectangle divided by a diagonal, the area on one side of the diagonal is equal to that of the other side. For a one-by-two rectangle, that means each side has an area of 1 square unit. There are nine squares divided in this way; that means 4.5 square units are enclosed by the band and 4.5 are outside the band. Add the 4.5 to the three squares completely enclosed by the band to get the total area, which is 7.5 units squared.

303 The first step to solving the puzzle is turning the inner hexagon so that its corners touch the outer hexagon. Then divide the inner hexagon into six equilateral triangles, and each of those equilateral triangles into three identical isosceles triangles. It is clear that the six 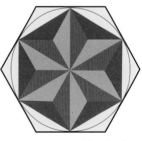 areas of the outer hexagon uncovered by the inner hexagon are equal in size to those isosceles triangles. From that, it is easy to see that the outer hexagon has an area of 4 square units.

304 There are exactly fifteen identical overlapping equilateral triangles. If you counted the triangles formed by the overlap, there would be a total of twenty-eight.

305

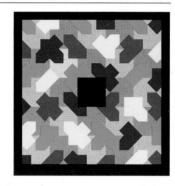

306 If you inscribe a number of different regular polygons on a circle, each shape will envelop a circle bearing a definite ratio to the original circle. For example, a triangle will envelop a circle 50 percent the size of the original; a square, 71 percent; a pentagon, 82 percent, and a hexagon, 87.5 percent.

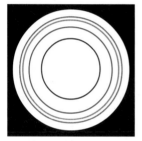

The astronomer Johannes Kepler was fascinated with the idea of inscribing regular polygons and three-dimensional polyhedrons in circles and spheres. Kepler believed the results might somehow lead to a better understanding of the arrangement of the planets in our solar system; utimately, no relationship could be found.

307 Yes. This mysterious and completely unexpected fact was discovered by English mathematician Frank Morley in 1899—which is why it's called Morley's triangle.

308 Four points are not enough—imagine a triangle with an interior point. It takes five points to guarantee a convex quadrilateral. This fact was demonstrated by the Erdös-Szekeres theorem in 1935. If you surround the five points with a rubber band, there are three possible outcomes:

1. The band forms a convex quadrilateral with the fifth point tucked inside.

2. The band forms a pentagon; connecting two of the vertices will result in a convex quadrilateral.

3. The band forms a triangle with two points inside. Connect the two interior points with a line—on one side of the line, there will be one vertex of the triangle; on the other side, two vertices. Connect those two vertices to the interior points to make a convex quadrilateral.

309 A total of 213 goats can graze in the orchard.

Mathematics provides a quick and elegant way to solve this kind of problem, which involves lattice polygons. In 1898 the Czech mathematician Georg Pick discovered a simple method for finding the area of a polygon whose vertices lie upon the points of a square grid plane: simply count the number of lattice points inside the polygon, then count the number of lattice points on the boundary, including the vertices. The area is then equal to the number of enclosed points, plus half the boundary points, minus 1. This is called Pick's theorem.

In this problem there are 115 enclosed lattice points and 198 boundary points, so 115 + (198/2) − 1 = 213.

310 The area of the triangle to the area of the hexagon is 2:3.

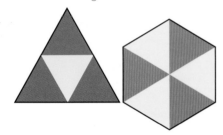

311
1. 36 triangles
2. 52 triangles
3. 36 triangles and 13 squares
4. 22 squares
5. 76 triangles
6. 9 triangles and 6 squares
7. 15 regular hexagons
8. 29 squares
9. 31 squares

312
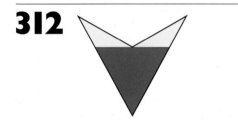

313 There are twenty-seven triangles.
In general, the number of triangles of different sizes in a triangular grid follows the sequence 1, 5, 13, 27, 48, 78, 118, etc., for triangles of increasing size. For triangles with an even number of levels, the general formula is

$$\frac{n(n + 2)(2n + 1)}{8}$$

For odd numbers of levels, the general formula is

$$\frac{n(n + 2)(2n + 1) - 1}{8}$$

314 To enclose the most area, the panels should be opened at 135 degrees. The area is one-quarter of a regular octagon.

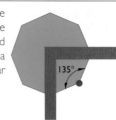

315
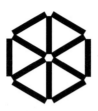

316 The midpoints and the reconstructed squares are shown here.

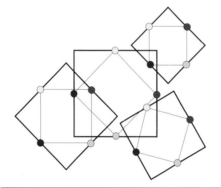

317
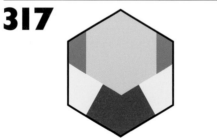

318
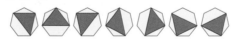

319
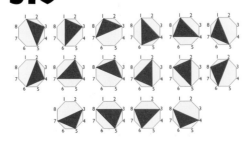

320 The order is circle, pentagon, square and triangle. The circle is the polygon that encloses the most area per unit of perimeter. It is the most economical shape for a fence or enclosure.

321 The answer is triangle, square, pentagon and circle. The circle, of course, has the shortest perimeter to enclose a given area.

322
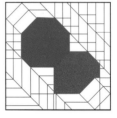
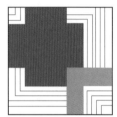
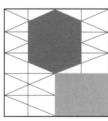
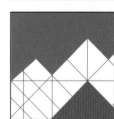
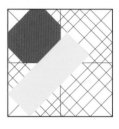
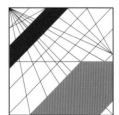

One common form of camouflage found in nature blurs the outlines of an object so it simply fades into the background. But another kind, featured in this problem, involves the deliberate creation of a pattern that distracts the eye; in that way the shape of the object is somewhat less obvious. Redundant lines attract the attention of the eye with their regularity and angularity. Also, a number of shapes within the pattern are misleading: they are close to but not identical to those that are sought.

323 It takes just one cut, as shown. Join the triangle created by the cut to the other end of the parallelogram to form the rectangle.

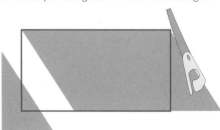

324

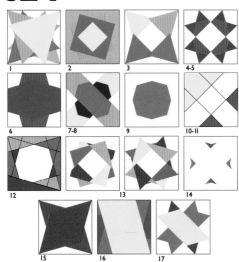

325

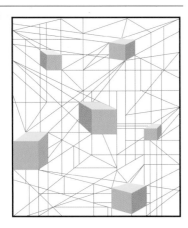

326

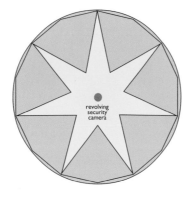

327

In general, a convex polygon of *n* sides needs n – 3 diagonals to triangulate it, and those diagonals create n – 2 triangles. Thus, for the heptagon, four diagonals make five triangles; the nonagon needs six diagonals to make seven triangles; the undecagon employs eight diagonals to make nine triangles.

328

A five-by-five square can be so inscribed on the seven-by-seven square, as shown.

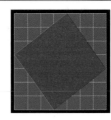

329

To create a triangle from three strips, it is necessary that the sum of the lengths of any two sides be greater than the length of the third side. The green and blue sets of strips do not follow this rule and thus cannot form triangles.

330

A simple solution would be walls that form a polygon of fourteen sides. Another solution, one requiring the least amount of floor area, would be to make the walls form a seven-pointed star.

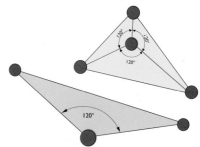

331

The minimum solution, discovered by the late Andrei Khodulyov, uses fifteen additional linkages, to be added as shown.

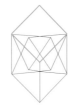

332

Each trisecting line divides the triangle into ⅓ or ⁷⁄₂₁, which is again divided into three parts, which simple observation tells us can be only ¹⁄₂₁, ⁵⁄₂₁ and ¹⁄₂₁. It follows that the central triangle is ³⁄₂₁.

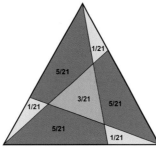

333

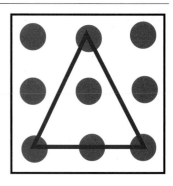

334

The two problems are related, since the three villages—no matter how they are arranged—can be said to be the vertices of a triangle. For the triangles and the villages, the most economical path will have three arms that meet at a point that is at the minimum total distance from the villages, or vertices.

In the case of a triangle in which all three angles are less than 120 degrees, the paths will be straight lines that meet at a point where they form angles of exactly 120 degrees, as illustrated above. For a triangle in which one angle is 120 degrees or more, the minimum path will pass through that vertex.

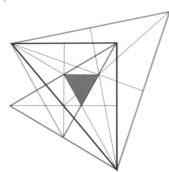

335

This will work with every triangle. In the example shown, the triangles are constructed inward; as you can see, the centers still form an equilateral triangle that has the same center as the original triangle. Interestingly, the difference in the area of the three constructed triangles is equal to the area of the original triangle.

336

Curiously enough, the line from the vertex that bisects the median will divide the opposite side in a 2:1 ratio.

337 Four cameras are sufficient (see the red dots in the diagram). There are many ways to arrange them.

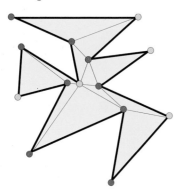

338 The three blue points are the solution.

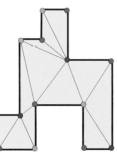

The question of how many cameras are needed to always cover every point on the floor was first posed by Victor Klee in 1973. Within a few days Rutgers University mathematician Vasek Chvátal had proved that if the shape of the floor has *n* vertices, then there are n/3 positions from which it is possible to view the whole gallery. The question became known as the "Chvátal Art Gallery Problem" until Bowdoin College mathematician Steve Frisk used his ingenious triangulation proof to figure out the exact placement of the cameras.

Here's what you do: Triangulate the layout and color the vertices of each triangle in three colors. The same three colors should be used for each triangle, and the same color should be used for every vertex that occupies a given point. The cameras should be placed at the points that have the color that appears the fewest times.

339

area (T) = area (JLNM) − area (JKM) − area (KLN)
= (a + b)(2a + 2b)/2 − ab − ab
= a² + b² = EB² = area (S)

$$\text{area (T)} = \text{area (JLNM)} - \text{area (JKM)} - \text{area (KLN)}$$
$$= (a + b)(2a + 2b)/2 - ab - ab$$
$$= a^2 + b^2 = EB^2 = \text{area (S)}$$

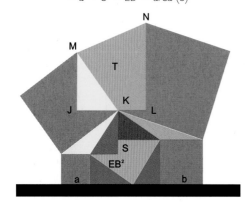

340

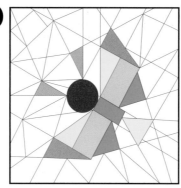

341

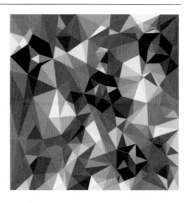

342 No. The divisions of Cake 1 and Cake 3 are equal, but the red group gets bigger slices from Cake 2.

If the number of chords (or cuts through the cake) is even and equal to four or more, the areas (or pieces of cake) are always equal.

If the number of chords is odd or less than four, the areas will not be equal—unless the chords go through the center of the circle, as they do in Cake 1.

This puzzle was inspired by the "Pizza Problem," which was discovered by L. J. Upton in 1968, and proved by Larry Carter and Stan Wagon in 1994.

343 The order is yellow, orange, red, pink, violet, light green, dark green, light blue, dark blue and lime. The order is also that of an increasing number of sides, from the triangle with three to the dodecagon with twelve.

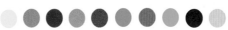

345 Miraculously, yes!
This gem of geometry is known as von Auble's theorem, and it will work with nonconvex quadrilaterals and even quadrilaterals in which three or four corners are colinear.

346 In a quadrilateral the length of each side is always less than the sum of the other three sides. Thus, the blue set of strips, of lengths 2, 3, 3 and 8, cannot form a quadrilateral.

347 The solution begins with drawing a line between two points, such as the one between points 1 and 2. Then draw a line from point 3 that is both equal in length and perpendicular to the line between 1 and 2. The endpoint of that line, marked as 5, is obviously on the line of the square.

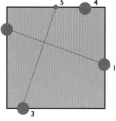

Draw a line through points 4 and 5, and draw a parallel line through point 3. To complete the square, draw lines perpendicular to these lines through points 1 and 2. The four lines will intersect to form a square.

348

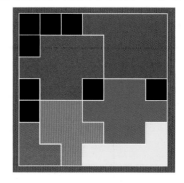

349 Given a pentagon with sides of 1 unit, the square shown in the problem has a side larger than 1.0605. But the square shown here, which is a solution published by Fitch Cheney in the *Journal of Recreational Mathematics* in 1970, has a side greater than 1.0673.

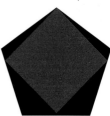

350 Twenty-one squares are possible.

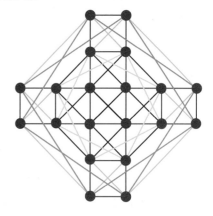

351

1. 1½ square units
2. 2½ square units
3. 1 square unit
4. 2 square units
5. 3 square units
6. 2½ square units
7. 4½ square units
8. 6½ square units
9. 5½ square units
10. 2 square units
11. 5 square units
12. 18 square units
13. 5½ square units
14. 7 square units
15. 7 square units
16. 7½ square units

352

There is a total of 204 squares of various sizes:

1 square unit—64
4 square units—49
9 square units—36
16 square units—25
25 square units—16
36 square units—9
49 square units—4
64 square units—1

The total number of different squares on a square matrix with n units on a side is simply the sum of the squares of the first n integers.

353

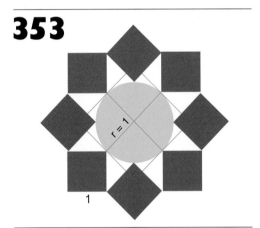

354

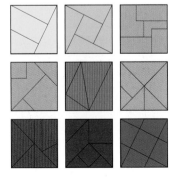

355

To find the incenter, bisect the three angles of the triangle, as shown.

To find the circumcenter, bisect each side with a perpendicular line.

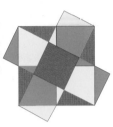

356

The figure can be rearranged into five identical squares, as shown. Therefore, the red square has one-fifth the area of the original figure.

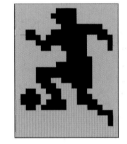

CHAPTER 7 SOLUTIONS

357

You can make three actual words. The first letter can be any one of the three; the second can be either of the two remaining letters; the third is the letter left over: $3 \times 2 \times 1 = 6$ possible words. The possibilities are

OWN, ONW, NOW, NWO, WON, WNO.

For n different letters, numbers or objects, the number of possible arrangements can be calculated:

$$n \times (n - 1) \times (n - 2) \times \ldots 3 \times 2 \times 1$$

This number is called n factorial and is abbreviated as $n!$.

358

If rotationally similar configurations had been allowed, the answer would have been 7!, or 5,040. But because any of those 5,040 arrangements is the same as 6 others through rotation, the total number of different diadems is $7!/7$, which equals 6!, or 720.

Had we outlawed similar configurations available by flipping the diadem, the answer would have been half of 720, or 360.

359

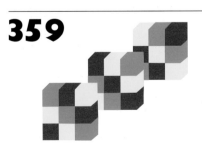

360

With four children per group, there are six different permutations in which every girl sits next to another girl, as shown. There is also the possible arrangement of four boys and no girls.

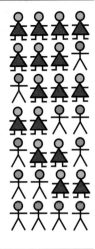

361

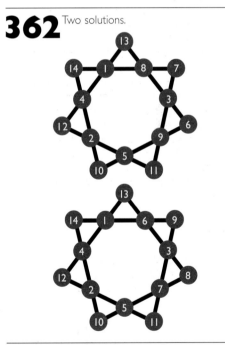

362

Two solutions.

363

There are eight symbols. Horizontally row by row, the sequence is 1; 1-2; 1-2-3; 1-2-3-4; 1-2-3-4-5; and on so up to 1-2-3-4-5-6-7-8. At that point the pattern repeats.

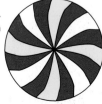

364

There are sixteen possible pairs.

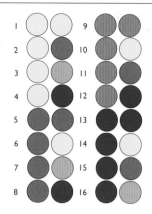

365

There are just six different arrangements for the three objects. There are three different possibilities for the leftmost fruit. For each fruit, there are two different possibilities for what goes in the middle; and for each left and middle, there is just one possibility for what goes on the right.

$$3 \times 2 \times 1 = 6$$

The operation from one arrangement to another is called a permutation.

366

In 5,040 different ways.

367

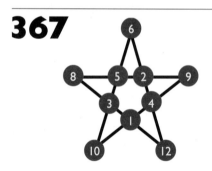

368

Once you cut out the strips, you will find that there are only twelve unique patterns.

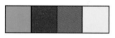

369

Mathematicians call this a universal cycle for 2-sequences. It exists for any number of colors or objects; the cycle is the square of the number of colors.

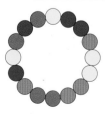

370

Note that the four strips in the square outlined in red and the square below it can be placed horizontally or vertically.

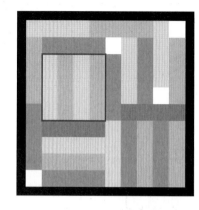

371

One of many ways.

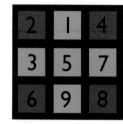

372

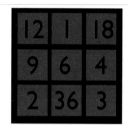

373

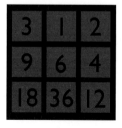

374

One of many solutions is shown. This one was obtained by taking the "Magic Square of Dürer" (PlayThink 377) and subtracting 17 from every value greater than 8.

-1	3	2	-4
5	-7	-6	8
-8	6	7	-5
4	-2	-3	1

375

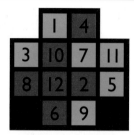

376

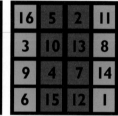 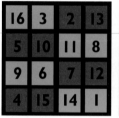

377

There are two solutions, shown below. In Dürer's "diabolic" magic squares, there are many sets of numbers that add up to the magic constant. Look, for instance, at the two-by-two square in the top left-hand corner: 16, 3, 5 and 10 add up to 34.

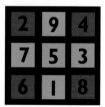

378

The sum of all nine digits is 45; distributed across three rows or columns, that means the "magic constant" is 15.

In general, the constant for magic squares with any number of rows and columns

2	9	4
7	5	3
6	1	8

can be found without adding the digits. For any number of rows n, the magic constant is

$$(n^3 + n)/2$$

To solve the Lo-Shu, you should first realize that there are eight possible triads of digits that add up to 15:

9-5-1; 9-4-2; 8-6-1; 8-5-2; 8-4-3; 7-6-2;
7-5-3; 6-5-4

The digit in the center of the square appears in four lines (a column, a row and both horizontals). Since 5 is the only digit that appears in four triads, it must be the center digit. Since 9 appears in only two triads, it must go into the middle of a row or column, which is completed with 1 to make the 9-5-1 triad. Similarly, 3 and 7 are in only two triads, so they must be in the middle of a row or column. The remaining four numbers can fit in only one way—an elegant proof of the uniqueness of the Lo-Shu solution.

379

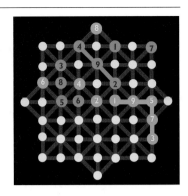

380 Only the flipped hinges are shown.

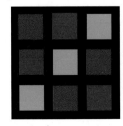

381

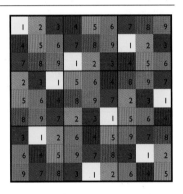

382 There are fifteen different combinations. For each monkey you could choose any of the three donkeys, so there are three possible pairs. Since this is true with each of the five monkeys, that leads to fifteen possible pairs.

383 It is not always possible to complete magic color squares or diagonal color squares. In many cases one can find only the best solution—the one that fits the most tiles onto the grid.

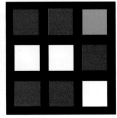

384 A magic color square extended to the two main diagonals is shown here. It is impossible, however, to extend it to all diagonals.

385 Diagonal magic color squares of order 6 are impossible

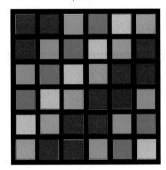

386

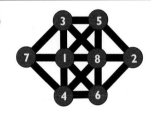

387 A full diagonal magic color square, with the rule extended across all the smaller diagonals as well as the two main ones, is shown here. In general, complete magic color squares are possible only when the order is not divisible by 2 or 3.

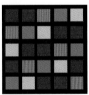

388

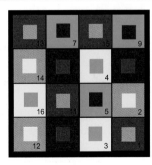

389

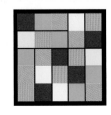

391 There are twelve different clowns, as identified below.
The clowns numbered 1, 2, 3, 6, 7, 8, 9 and 11 each appear three times; the rest show up only twice.
There are thirty-two complete clowns, but only twenty-four can be put together at any given time.

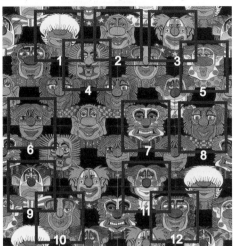

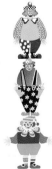

392

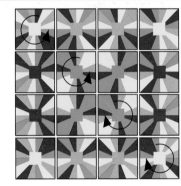

393 It is the only combination they haven't tried.

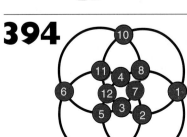

394

395

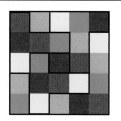

396

Here are two of an infinite number of solutions.

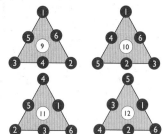

397

Excluding rotations and reflections, four unique solutions exist.

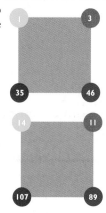

398

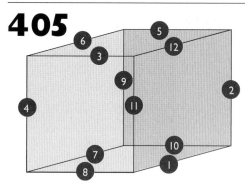

399

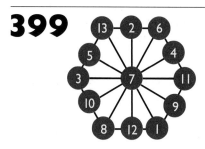

400

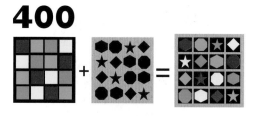

401

$n = 5; k = 11; p = 12$

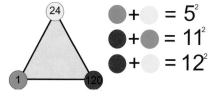

$$+ = 5^2$$
$$+ = 11^2$$
$$+ = 12^2$$

402

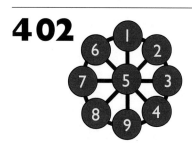

403

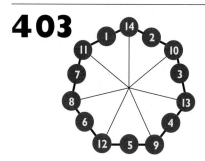

404

No square and no alien appears more than once in any row, column or diagonal. The middle alien with the red background will complete the pattern.

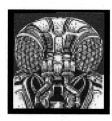

405

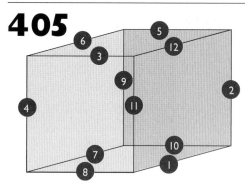

406

407

Two solutions are shown; many are possible.

9	8	4
7	5	3
6	2	1

16	12	8	4
15	11	7	3
14	10	6	2
13	9	5	1

408

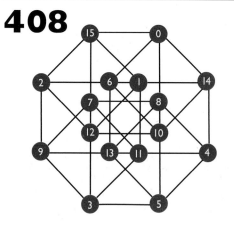

409

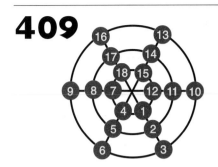

410

The sum of all nineteen numbers is 190, which is divisible by 5, and there are five parallel rows in each direction. Thus, the magic constant is 190 divided by 5, or 38.

In general, it is possible to arrange a set of positive integers from 1 to *n* in a hexagonal honeycomb array of *n* cells so that every straight row has a constant sum—that is, a magic constant.

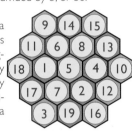

As we see illustrated above, an order 3 magic hexagon is possible. But an order 2 hexagon, one that has seven cells, is impossible. The sum of the numbers from one to seven is 28, and 28 divided by three (the number of rows in each direction) is not an integer. Likewise, magic hexagons of order 4 and order 5 are also impossible. In fact, an extremely complicated proof has shown that no magic hexagon of a size greater than order 3 is possible. What is even more astonishing is that the magic hexagon shown above, which was discovered in 1910, is the only possible solution.

411

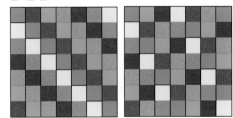

412

Two solutions.

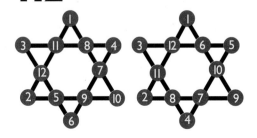

413

Top right octagon: one quarter turn counterclockwise

Bottom left octagon: one half turn

Bottom right octagon: one quarter turn clockwise

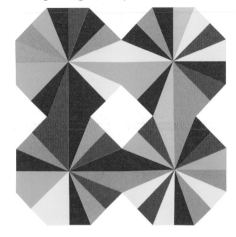

414

The octagons in the lower left and right can each be positioned in two ways, making for four solutions.

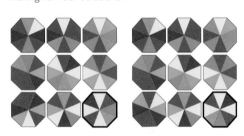

415

The arrows show the motion of the squares in each pattern. The missing pattern from each sequence is shown in red.

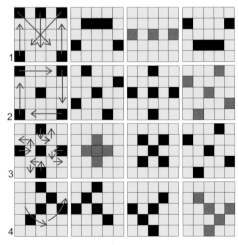

416

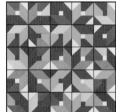

417

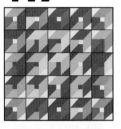

418

419

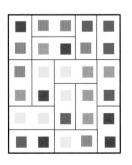

420 A simple proof shows why it is impossible: Each domino has a red square and a yellow square, so the number of squares of each color must be equal. But the chessboard was truncated in such a way that there are thirty-two red squares and only thirty yellow ones.

421 There are four different ways to distribute two desserts on two plates, as illustrated below.

422 The yellow dot stands for the pineapple; the red dot, for the apple. There are nine different ways to distribute them among the three bowls, as shown.

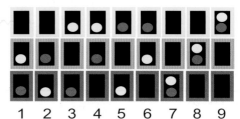

423 Two slightly different solutions are shown.

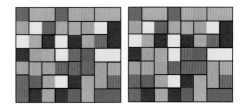

424

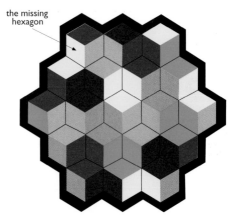
the missing hexagon

425 The missing triangle is yellow in all three segments.

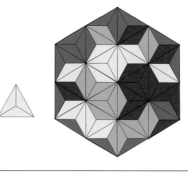

426 It is possible, but only if the monomino covers one of the squares, shown in black.

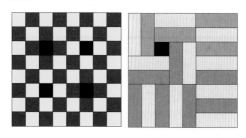

427

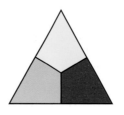

428 The missing square is all yellow.
There are many possible arrangements of the squares. One is shown here.

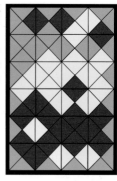

429 The zigzag runs through the greens.

430

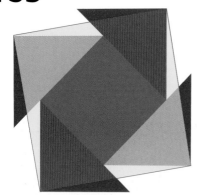

432

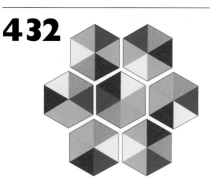

433

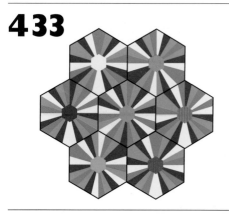

434 Card 3 is not found in the pattern.

CHAPTER 8 SOLUTIONS

435

436 THE

437 One of many solutions.

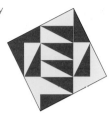

438 The result is the solution to the classic "T-Puzzle" (PlayThink 20).

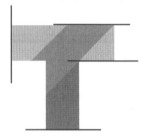

439 Although the minimum answer for the three squares problem involves making just five pieces, no one has yet found it. This solution, using six pieces, is the current record.

440

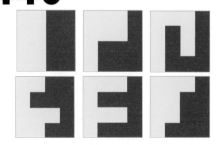

441

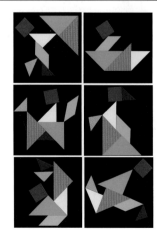

442

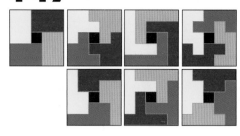

443 One of many possible solutions.

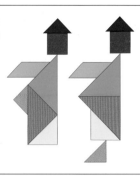

444

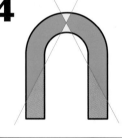

445

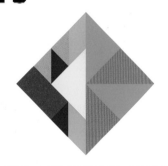

446

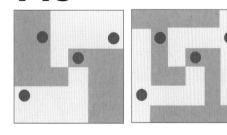

447

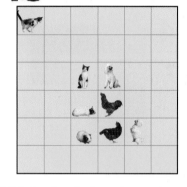

448

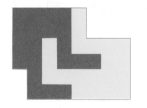

449

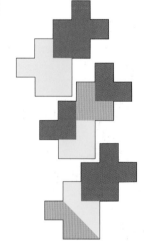

450

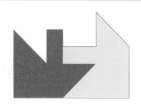

451

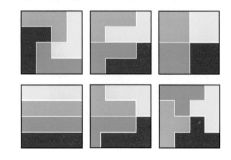

452

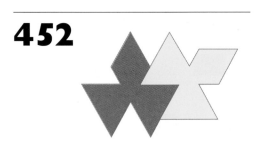

453 It turns out that every line drawn through the yellow dot divides the perimeter in half.

454

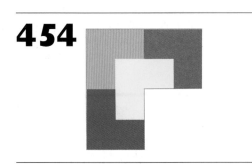

455

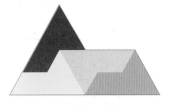

456

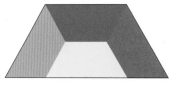

457

458

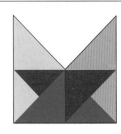

459

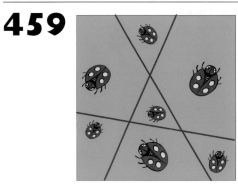

460

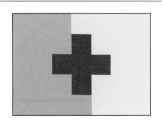

461

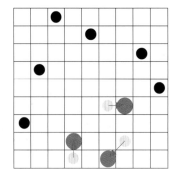

462

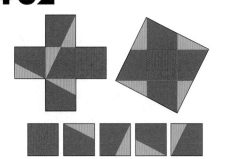

463

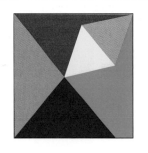

464 You can make the two squares from four pieces: one for the smaller square and three for the larger one.

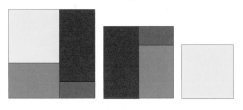

465 The pieces form a chain—when they are swung in one direction, they form an equilateral triangle; when swung in the opposite direction, they form a square.

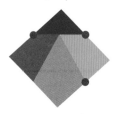

The inventor of this gem of recreational mathematics was Henry Ernest Dudeney, England's most accomplished puzzle maker. Born in 1857, Dudeney was extremely successful with dissections and set many records. This dissection, however, is his most famous discovery.

466 The task requires only seven cuts.

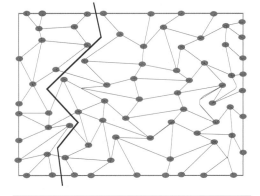

467

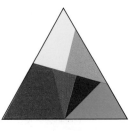

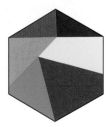

468 You can make the three squares from just five pieces.

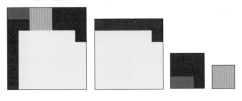

469 Congratulations! You have demonstrated the truth behind the Pythagorean theorem.

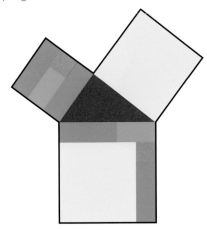

470 This puzzle is derived from one of the most beautiful proofs of the Pythagorean theorem, discovered by Henry Perigal (1801–1898). His proof involved dropping a perpendicular from the center of square B to the line c, and constructing a line parallel to line c through the center of B.

The four pieces of that dissection, plus square A can be rearranged to make square C, as shown. This construction works for every set of squares about a right triangle.

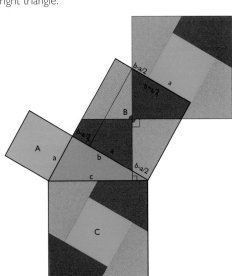

472

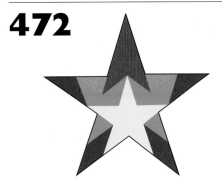

473

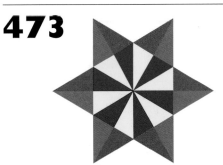

474

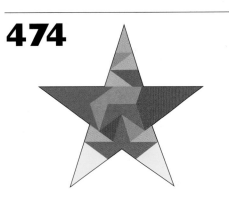

475

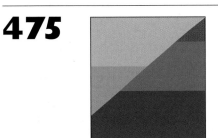

476

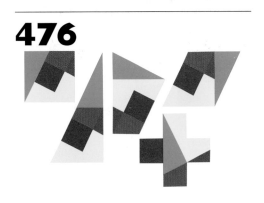

477 The solution involves six pieces.

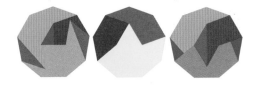

478

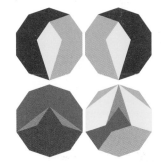

479

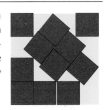

480 The German mathematician Walter Trump found the solution shown here. Some of the red squares are inclined by 40.18 degrees.

481 When you swap the lower parts of the drawing, you have six red pencils and seven blue pencils. A close examination will reveal which pencil changed color.

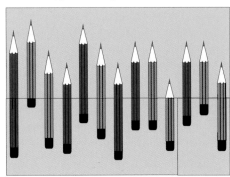

482 Each star contains the same arrangement of pieces.

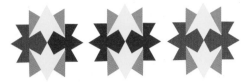

483 Each star contains the same arrangement of pieces.

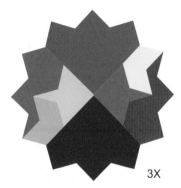

3X

484
Area 1—1.5 units
Area 2—4.5 units
Area 3—1.5 units
Area 4—2.5 units
Area 5—2.5 units
Area 6—3 units
Area 7—4 units
Area 8—15.5 units

Since the area not taken up by the red triangle totals 19.5 units, it is larger.

485 The thirty-two-by-thirty-three perfect rectangle is the smallest known.

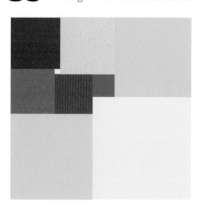

486 Surprisingly, in spite of the coincidence that the sum of the squares and the area of the big square are both 4,900, there is no known solution in which all twenty-four squares can be placed on the larger square without overlap. The best solutions known to date can fit only twenty-three of the twenty-four squares; in each instance it is the seven-by-seven square that must be left out. One such solution is illustrated here.

Although there are other sets of consecutive squares that add up to a square number; none is less than the sequence from one to twenty-four.

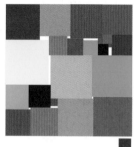

487 The minimal solution for an eleven-by-eleven square consists of eleven smaller squares, shown at right.

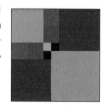

The minimal solution for a twelve-by-twelve square consists of four smaller squares, each six-by-six.

The minimal solution for a thirteen-by-thirteen square consists of fourteen smaller squares.

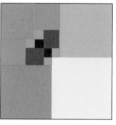

The minimal solution for a fourteen-by-fourteen square consists of four smaller squares, each seven-by-seven. I hope you've caught on to the pattern for even-sided squares.

488 The covered square can be anywhere on the board. Three sample arrangements are shown below; through reflection and rotation, one of the arrangements will uncover any given square.

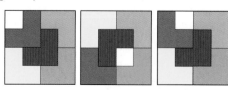

489

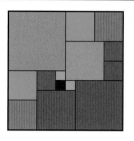

490 It takes eleven smaller triangles to completely cover the eleven-by-eleven triangle. One solution is shown.

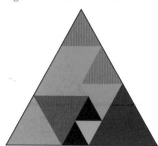

491

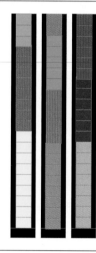

492 The maximum number of holes that can be made on a board cannot exceed the number of dominoes. In fact, if the length of one side of the board is evenly divisible by three, then the maximum number of holes is the product of the two sides, divided by three.

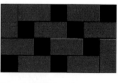

493

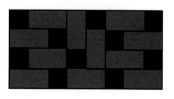

494

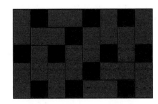

495

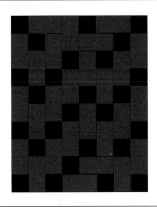

496

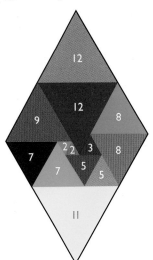

497 In the first and third examples, about three-quarters of the triangle is covered. In the other two, much less is covered.

498 This solution has the fewest number of triangles, with thirteen.

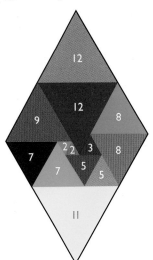

499

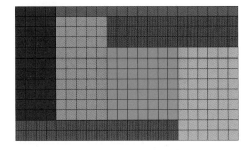

500 The twelve different ways of joining five identical squares are shown above. Such shapes are called pentominoes.

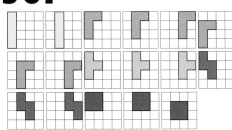

501

502

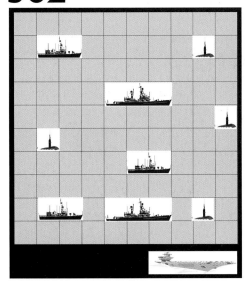

503 The two squares seem to be identical, but since 2 minus 1 does *not* equal 2, it's obvious that the second square must be smaller, though not by much. The missing area, equal to that of the small square that was removed, is spread so thinly around the remaining pieces that it is almost impossible to notice its absence.

By the way, the secret to putting together the smaller square is to swap the two triangles along every edge of the square. After you do that, the arrangement of the rest of the pieces is fairly obvious.

One thing to learn from such vanishing puzzles is that, in order to fool the eye and the mind, you have to be very subtle. Although humans are adept at spotting differences, they can easily overlook very small changes that are deftly hidden.

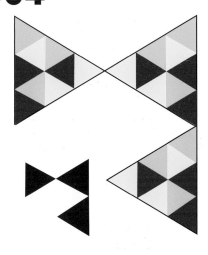

504 Nine small figures, as shown.

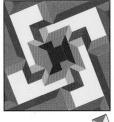

505
There are many ways to fit the twelve pentominoes on the board.

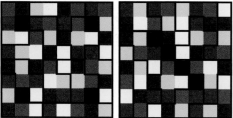
Puzzle 1- Solution   Puzzle 2-Solution

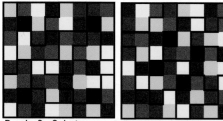
Puzzle 3 - Solution   Puzzle 4 - Solution

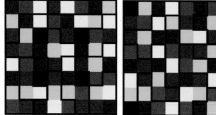
Puzzle 5 - Solution   Puzzle 6 - Solution

506

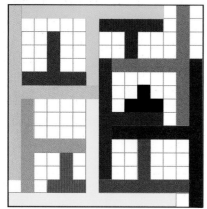

507
The large replica holds sixteen smaller T-tiles.

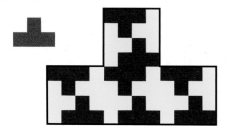

508
In this, one of many solutions, a yellow pentomino has been formed at the top.

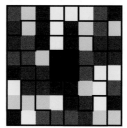

509
One of the most counterintuitive facts in geometry is that only three regular polygons—the equilateral triangle, the square and the regular hexagon—are capable of tessellating a plane.

There is a beautiful logic behind the rarity of regular tessellations. At every point in which the vertices of the tessellating polygons meet, the sum of the angles of those vertices must equal 360 degrees. The only regular polygons that can tessellate, then, are the ones whose angles are factors of 360.

Six equilateral triangles, each with angles of 60 degrees, can meet at a point—and so they can tessellate.

 Four squares, each with angles of 90 degrees, can meet at a point—and so squares can tessellate.

Pentagons have internal angles of 108 degrees—not a factor of 360—and so pentagons cannot tessellate.

Three hexagons, each with angles of 120 degrees, can meet at a point, and so hexagons can tessellate.

As you can see, the next whole number that can meet at a point is 2—making for 180 degrees on each side. That's not a tessellation—it is a bisection. Therefore, only an equilateral triangle, a square and a regular hexagon are capable of tessellating a plane.

510
The medium-sized fish can hold nine smaller ones, and the large fish can hold nine medium-sized fish. That means all eighty-one small fish can fit inside the large fish. But even that fish should not rest easy, because there is always an even bigger fish somewhere!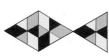

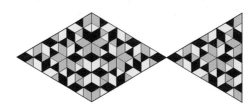

CHAPTER 9 SOLUTIONS

511
The numbered objects of the tetraktys can be arranged in (10!)/(2 × 3), or 604,800, different ways.

512
Triangular numbers are the sum of any number of consecutive positive integers, beginning with 1. The fourth triangular number, 10, equals 1 + 2 + 3 + 4.

Babylonian cuneiform tablets show that the formula for deriving triangular numbers has been known since antiquity. For any number n, its triangular number can be calculated as $n(n + 1)/2$.

To find the eighteenth natural number, then, simply find $18(18 + 1)/2$, which is 171.

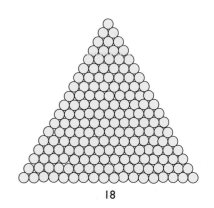
18

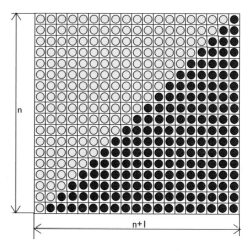

513 $99 + \frac{99}{99} = 100$

514 Each successive ring has $6(n - 1)$ elements. That means the next hexagonal number is $37 + 6(5 - 1) = 61$.

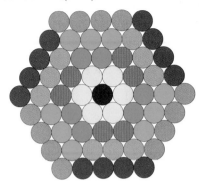

515 Squares are formed by the sum of the series of odd numbers, beginning with 1.

$1^2 = 1$
$2^2 = 1 + 3 = 4$
$3^2 = 1 + 3 + 5 = 9$
$4^2 = 1 + 3 + 5 + 7 = 16$ and so on

The seventh square would be $7^2 = 1 + 3 + 5 + 7 + 9 + 11 + 13 = 49$.

516 The sixth and seventh triangular numbers, 21 and 28, add together to make 49.

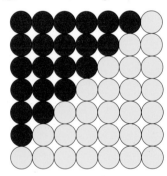

517 It is the fifth triangular number: 15. $(15 \times 8) + 1 = 121$

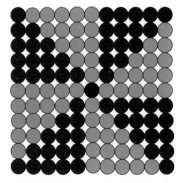

518 The tetrahedral series can be expressed by the formula $n(n + 1)(n + 2)/6$. That gives a series 1, 4, 10, 20, 35, 56, 84 . . .

The square pyramidal series can be expressed in the formula $n(n+1)(2n+1)/6$. That gives a sequence of 1, 5, 14, 30, 55, 91, 140 . . .

519 You can use the principle of one-to-one correspondence to find the answer without counting. Simply mark off pairs of sheep—one right-facing, one left-facing—until no more of one type remain.

520 The numbers are 1, 3, 9 and 27. This problem is a good exercise in getting the maximum work from a minimal number of elements.

1	=	1	9+3-1	=	11
3-1	=	2	9+3	=	12
3	=	3	9+3+1	=	13
3+1	=	4	27-9-3-1	=	14
9-3-1	=	5	27-9-3	=	15
9-3	=	6	27-9-3+1	=	16
9-3+1	=	7	27-9-1	=	17
9-1	=	8	27-9	=	18
9	=	9	27-9+1	=	19
9+1	=	10	27-9-3-1	=	20

27-9+3	=	21	27+3+1	=	31
27-9+3+1	=	22	27+9-3-1	=	32
27-3-1	=	23	27+9-3	=	33
27-3	=	24	27+9-3+1	=	34
27-3+1	=	25	27+9-1	=	35
27-1	=	26	27+9	=	36
27	=	27	27+9+1	=	37
27+1	=	28	27+9-3-1	=	38
27+3-1	=	29	27+9+3	=	39
27+3	=	30	27+9+3+1	=	40

521 Gauss realized that the series $1 + 2 + 3 + 4 \ldots 97 + 98 + 99 + 100$ could be written as:

$1 + 100 + 2 + 99 + 3 + 98 + 4 + 97 \ldots$

or 101 times 50, to get the total, 5,050.

This trick works for any sum of sequential integers. Indeed, the general formula is simply $n(n + 1)/2$, which is the equation for triangular numbers.

This problem is a beautiful illustration of the importance of understanding the patterns underlying ordinary routines. If you grasp what a question is really asking, you can avoid a lot of drudgery in answering it.

522 The concept of mathematical equivalence, or isomorphism, is the key to winning this game. Think back to the famous Lo-Shu magic square (PlayThink 377): the square is filled with the numbers from 1 through 9, and each row, column and main diagonal adds up to 15. As you can see, then, maneuvering to mark off three numbers that total 15 is the equivalent to playing tic-tac-toe.

The best strategy, then, is to keep that fact in mind—perhaps even to memorize the Lo-Shu magic square—and attack and defend as if you were playing tic-tac-toe. The best first move, for instance, is to color in 5.

523

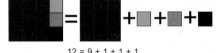

$12 = 9 + 1 + 1 + 1$

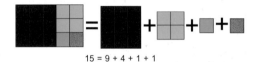

$15 = 9 + 4 + 1 + 1$

524 With the Pythagorean theorem, it is quite simple to calculate the length of the hypotenuse: $1^2 + 1^2 = c^2 = 2$; so $c = \sqrt{2}$.

But finding a rational number that equals $\sqrt{2}$ is impossible. The Pythagorean disciple Hippasus first showed that the diagonal of a square with rational sides does not have a rational length. Numbers like $\sqrt{2}$, $\sqrt{3}$ and so on, which cannot be expressed by the fraction of two whole numbers, are now known as irrational numbers. Although this discovery shook the foundations of Greek mathematics, the study of length later became a bridge between geometry and algebra. Attempts to measure the properties of curves eventually gave rise to calculus.

525 $4 - 1 + 2 \times 3 + 5 = 20$

526 Two odd numbers added together result in an even number. But that means that the sum of an odd number of odd numbers will always be odd. So five odd numbers cannot add up to 100. But six odd numbers can; the numbers 1, 3, 45, 27, 13 and 11 are just one set of odd numbers that total 100.

527 Just five. The same pickers who can pick five apples in five seconds can pick sixty apples in sixty seconds; they average an apple a second.

528
The second perfect number is 28, the sum of 1, 2, 4, 7 and 14.

Students of the Bible have noted that the first two perfect numbers are embedded in the structure of the universe. After all, God created the universe in six days, and the moon circles the earth every twenty-eight days.

The third perfect number is 496.

No one knows whether the supply of perfect numbers is inexhaustible, nor do we know whether there are any odd perfect numbers. That question has been vexing mathematicians since the time of Pythagoras.

529
The unique solution for four pairs of blocks is shown here.

The Scottish mathematician C. Dudley Langford first laid out the general form of this problem in the 1950s after watching his son play with colored blocks. It turns out that the problem has a solution only if the number of pairs of blocks is a multiple of 4, or is 1 less than a multiple of 4.

531

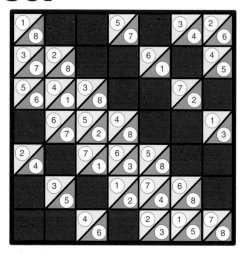

532
Regardless of how steeply the plane is inclined, a ball rolling for two seconds will always travel four times as far as it does after one second, and after three seconds, it will go nine times as far. The pattern becomes quite obvious: if the ball goes one unit after one second, then for every n number of seconds, the ball will travel n^2 units.

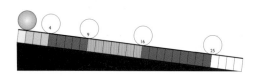

533

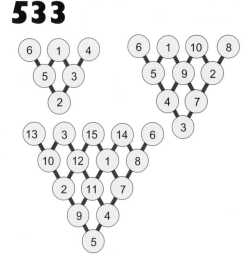

534
Twenty ladybugs.

535
Swap the 8 and the 9, then turn the 9 upside-down so it reads as a 6. Both columns will then total 18.

536
Since there are seven pages before page 8, there must be seven pages after page 21. The newspaper has twenty-eight pages.

537
One of many possible solutions.

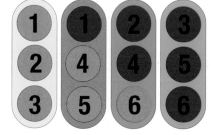

538

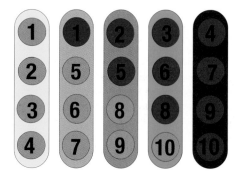

539

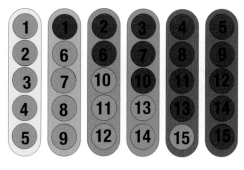

540
There are many examples: 243 + 675 = 918; 341 + 586 = 927; 154 + 782 = 936; 317 + 628 = 945; 216 + 738 = 954 . . . and so on.

541
The ten digits can be permutated in 10!, or 3,628,800, ways. But since all the ways that start with 0 must be dropped, the actual number is 362,880 lower, for a total of 3,265,920.

542
Four neighboring cells form a diamond in which $A \times D - B \times C = 1$.

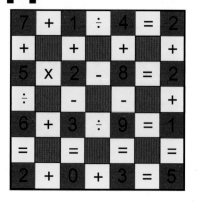

543
One, of course, is the smallest number of persistence. Twenty-five is the smallest number that has a persistence of 2; 39 is the smallest that has a persistence of 3; and 77 is the smallest that has a persistence of 4.

544

545 Each number is the sum of its neighbors immediately above, to the left and to the upper left diagonal. Following this rule, the missing number is 63.

546
$$0 = 4 - 4$$
$$0 = 4 - 4$$
$$1 = 4 \div 4$$
$$2 = (4 + 4)/4$$
$$3 = 4 - (4/4)$$
$$4 = 4$$
$$5 = 4 + (4/4)$$
$$6 = ((4 + 4)/4) + 4$$
$$7 = (44/4) - 4$$
$$8 = 4 + 4$$
$$9 = 4 + 4 + (4/4)$$
$$10 = (44 - 4)/4$$

547
$$20 = 1 + 1 + 1 + 1 + 1 + 1 + 1 + 13$$
$$20 = 1 + 1 + 1 + 1 + 1 + 1 + 3 + 11$$
$$20 = 1 + 1 + 1 + 1 + 1 + 1 + 5 + 9$$
$$20 = 1 + 1 + 1 + 1 + 1 + 3 + 3 + 9$$
$$20 = 1 + 1 + 1 + 1 + 1 + 1 + 7 + 7$$
$$20 = 1 + 1 + 1 + 1 + 1 + 3 + 5 + 7$$
$$20 = 1 + 1 + 1 + 1 + 3 + 3 + 3 + 7$$
$$20 = 1 + 1 + 1 + 1 + 1 + 5 + 5 + 5$$
$$20 = 1 + 1 + 1 + 3 + 3 + 3 + 5 + 5$$
$$20 = 1 + 1 + 1 + 3 + 3 + 3 + 3 + 5$$
$$20 = 1 + 1 + 3 + 3 + 3 + 3 + 3 + 3$$

548 Six darts:
$$17 + 17 + 17 + 17 + 16 + 16 = 100$$

549

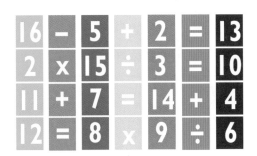

550 Surprisingly, both sums are 1,083,676,269.

551 The next four numbers are 21, 34, 55 and 89.
Each number is the sum of the two numbers preceding it. As the sequence continues, the ratio of successive terms approaches the famous golden ratio, 1:1.6180037.

552 The first digit can be any digit from 1 to 9; the second can be any of those digits except the consecutive one. That makes for eighty-one nonconsecutive two-digit numbers.

553 This problem has been around for a long time, and mathematicians have found several answers. Our solution is just one of them.

$$1 \cdot 2 + 3 - 4 + 5 + 6 + 78 + 9 = 100$$

554 $2,520 = 5 \times 7 \times 8 \times 9$

555 Most people who approach this problem see each number as the difference between the two numbers feeding into it. But that can't account for the 7, since $21 - 13 = 8$.
Instead, examine the individual digits of the numbers feeding into each circle. You will find that 9, 9, 7 and 2 add up to 27, and that 4, 5, 2 and 7 total 18. Thus, the missing number can be found by adding 3, 6, 2 and 1. The missing number is 12.

556 | 312211 |

Each term is a description of the number preceding it: "11" means there's one 1; "21" means there are two 1s; "1211" means there is one 2 and one 1; "111221" means there is one 1, one 2 and two 1s.

557 The numbers make up the cake-cutting sequence—the maximum number of pieces that can be made from a given number of straight cuts through a plane. As a general rule, each nth cut will make n number of new pieces. Thus, for the sixth cut, the number of pieces will be $16 + 6$, or 22.

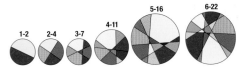

558 The sequence is based on the principle of persistence, in which the digits of a number are multiplied together to get another number; the function is carried out until only a one-digit number remains.
Thus, the last number in the sequence is 8.

559 The answer is 20 years old because 210 is the twentieth triangular number, equal to the sum of all the numbers from 1 to 20.

560 The numbers double as they run from left to right horizontally; the numbers go up by 2 as they run from top to bottom diagonally.

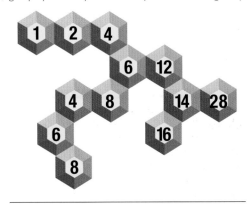

561 The possible answers are 52 and 25, 63 and 36, 74 and 47, 85 and 58, or 96 and 69. But the ages that match up with how long my friend has been practicing magic are 74 and 47.

562

IOTOIO

563 $17 \times 4 = 68 + 25 = 93$

$$\begin{array}{r} 1\boxed{7} \\ \times \boxed{4} \\ \hline = 6\boxed{8} + \boxed{2}5 = \boxed{9}\boxed{3} \end{array}$$

564 Add 40 to both.

170		30
+40		+40
210		70

$$\frac{Y}{Z} = \frac{210}{70} \quad \boxed{X = 40}$$

565
$$2^6 - 63 = 1$$

566 The puzzle begins with one hundred separate pieces and ends with one complete cluster. Since each move reduces the number of pieces or clusters by one, only ninety-nine moves are needed.

567

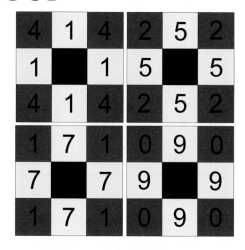

568

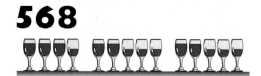

569 In a single-elimination tournament, one team is knocked out in each match. So if there are fifty-eight teams and one champion, then fifty-seven teams must be eliminated over the course of the tournament. Therefore, fifty-seven matches must be played.

The principle of identifying a one-to-one correspondence between two sets crops up in probability theory, enumeration and everyday problem solving.

570 Yes, there is enough information to work this out. If there are even two red flowers, then it will be possible to pick a pair without one being purple. So there is only one red flower, and the rest are purple.

571 There can't be even two red flowers, or else it will be possible to pick two reds and a yellow and not have any purple flowers out of three. Similar logic dictates that there can't be more than one purple or one yellow flower. Therefore, there are only three flowers in the entire garden.

572

Top Floor

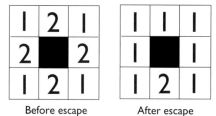

Ground Floor

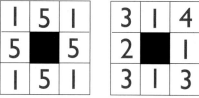

Before escape   After escape

573 There were twenty-three emus and twelve camels.

574 I saw twenty-two two-legged birds and fourteen four-legged beasts.

575 Yes. There is a unique solution; you simply have to remember that every leg is counted—stool legs, chair legs and people legs!

Thus, for every occupied stool, there are five legs (three stool legs and two people legs). And every occupied chair counts for six legs. So 5 × (number of stools) + 6 × (number of chairs) = 39.

From that it is easy to work out that there are three stools, four chairs and seven people.

576 Yes.

577 To solve this problem, you have to work out the number of possible pairs for the nine friends. In mathematical language the problem involves a "Steiner triple system of order nine." But in more simple terms, for any given friend, four separate dinners are necessary to see all eight cohorts.

Day 1—Kate, David, Lucy
Day 2—Emily, Jane, Theo
Day 3—Mary, James, John
Day 4—Kate, Emily, Mary
Day 5—David, Jane, James
Day 6—Lucy, Theo, John
Day 7—Kate, Jane, John
Day 8—Lucy, Jane, Mary
Day 9—David, Theo, Mary
Day 10—Lucy, Emily, James
Day 11—Kate, Theo, James
Day 12—David, Emily, John

578 Since the mother cat has two lives left, the kittens must divide up the remaining twenty-three. That means there are two possible answers: seven kittens (one has five lives left and six have three lives) or five kittens (one with three lives and four with five lives).

579 There are 9 one-digit numbers, 90 two-digit numbers and 900 three-digit numbers, for a total of 2,889 digits. That leaves 40 more digits, or 10 four-digit numbers: 1,000 to 1,009. The book must have 1,009 pages.

580

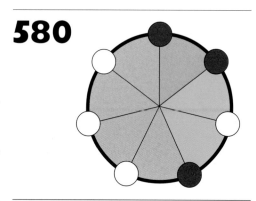

581 The four points on the circle must be distributed in one of two ways: 1-2-6-4 or 1-3-2-7.

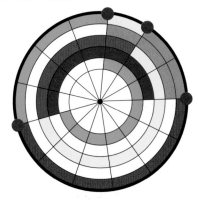

582 For five points on a circle to represent twenty-one different units of length, they must be distributed with the spacings 1-3-10-2-5.

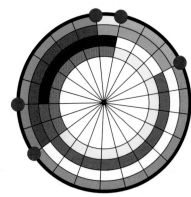

584
Day 1—4-5-2 7-1-9 6-8-3
Day 2—7-8-5 4-3-1 6-9-2
Day 3—8-1-2 4-7-6 9-3-5
Day 4—1-5-7 3-2-8 9-4-6
Day 5—8-4-1 5-6-2 3-7-9
Day 6—7-2-4 8-9-5 1-6-3

585 The secret is to look at the eight coins in the shaded areas. With any given move, either two or none of those coins will turn over. That means if the number of Jekylls is even, the configuration can be solved; if the number of Jekylls is odd, it cannot.

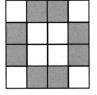

586 Minimal length rulers, invented by Solomon W. Golomb, can only be "perfect" up to length 6. All higher length rulers are "imperfect," since some distances occur more than once or don't occur at all. Using an 11-unit ruler, it is impossible to place the markers so that a 6-unit distance is measured.

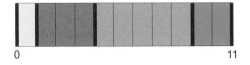

0   11

587 There were fifteen ladybugs:
3 + 5 + 6 + 1 = 15

588

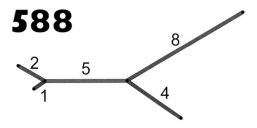

589

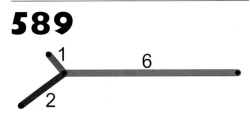

590 When you double the linear measurements of a two-dimensional object, its area increases by a factor of 4 (2^2). Similarly, doubling the linear measurements of a three-dimensional object increases the volume by a factor of 8 (2^3). Assuming that the density of that volume remained constant, your weight would also increase by a factor of 8. Or, to find your new weight, simply multiply your present weight by 8.

591 The red triangles occupy an area that is roughly one-third that of the square.

592 The red arm occupies exactly one-fourth of the square. You can divide the entire square into four such spiral arms.

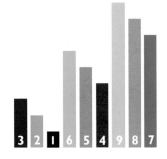

593 There are some eighty-four different solutions. The one illustrated below involves lengths of 3, 2, 1, 6, 5, 4, 9, 8, 7.

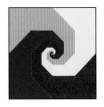

594 Any arbitrary sequence of ten numbers or lengths will always have an increasing or decreasing sequence of at least four members. Although nine lengths can be arranged in such a manner, the tenth member will complete either an ascending or descending run, no matter where it is placed.

595 The beaker was half full after 39 minutes.

596 You might want to experiment with other initial configurations to try to find out if the outcome will always be a checkerboard pattern. But a word of warning: The answer has never been proved.

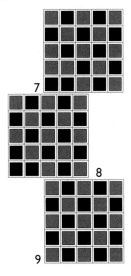

597 The initial configuration of five red, or live, cells transforms over five generations to four identical copies, as shown below.

This system, called a cellular automaton, has a fascinating property: virtually any starting configuration will, after a few generations, replicate into four, sixteen and sixty-four copies of itself. It is remarkable that a system so simple can possess a property as "lifelike" as self-replication.

Edward Fredkin of MIT created this self-replicating system in 1960. The Game of Life, invented by Princeton mathematician John Horton Conway, is a subtler cellular automaton that works on similar principles. In it, whether a given square "lives" or "dies" depends upon the number of "live" squares around it. Finding configurations that will live, grow and even replicate is an interesting mathematical problem.

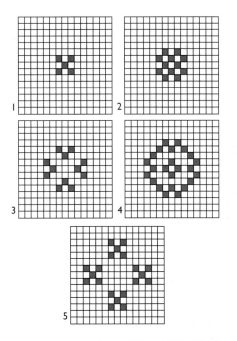

598

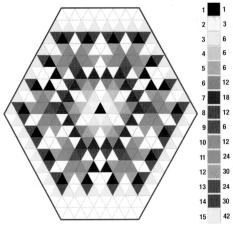

599

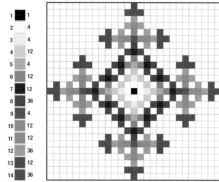

1	1
2	4
3	4
4	12
5	4
6	12
7	12
8	36
9	4
10	12
11	12
12	36
13	12
14	36

600

The ladybugs return in games 1, 2, 3 and 5 but not in game 4.

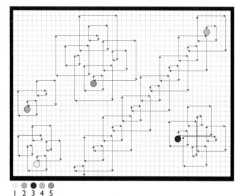

1 2 3 4 5

601

Sallows found this eight-sided golygon to be the simplest possible; it has the interesting ability to tessellate in the plane. The next simplest golygon has sixteen sides; there are twenty-eight variations of it. Martin Gardner proved that the number of sides in a golygon must be a multiple of 8.

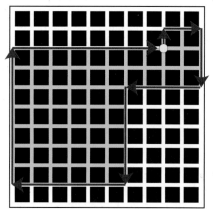

602

Although many properties of primes remain unproven, one famous proof has demonstrated that there is always a prime between every integer greater than 1 and that integer's double.

603

None of the 362,880 numbers will be prime.

In each case the sum of their digits is 45, which is divisible by 9. And any number that has digits adding up to a multiple of 9 is itself a multiple of 9. This simple divisibility check shows why none of the numbers can be prime.

604

The limit on the area approaches about 1.6 times that of the original triangle. Amazingly, the curve will not extend beyond a circle that circumscribes that triangle.

As for the perimeter, say each side of the initial triangle is 1 unit in length, for a total of 3 units of perimeter. The polygon that replaces the triangle after one generation consists of twelve sides, each one-third the length of the original sides, for a total of 4 units. Every successive step sees the perimeter increasing by the same factor of $\frac{1}{3}$. Thus, there is no ultimate boundary on the perimeter—if you take infinite steps, you will have an infinite perimeter.

The yellow in the problem shows the opposite process; it will form the "antisnowflake" curve.

605

The stack of images would approach a height twice that of the original picture, but it would never actually reach that point. The sum of $1 + \frac{1}{2} + \frac{1}{4} + \frac{1}{8} + \frac{1}{16} \ldots$ is less than 2.

606

Examine the sum of the divisors of 220:

$$1 + 2 + 4 + 5 + 10 + 11 + 20 + 22 + 44 + 55 + 110 = 284$$

Now look at the divisors for 284:

$$1 + 2 + 4 + 71 + 142 = 220$$

If the sum of the divisors of a number is equal to a number whose divisors are equal to the first, the pair is said to be amicable. The smallest known pair is 220 and 284.

Pythagoras knew about amicable numbers, and Arab mathematicians investigated such pairs during the Middle Ages. Euler himself published 60 pairs, and some 5,000 pairs are known today.

Although amicable numbers have been the subject of intense study over the millennia, Nicolo Paganini, an Italian schoolboy, discovered the second smallest pair—1,184 and 1,210— in 1866. This goes to show that there are sometimes great rewards awaiting even amateur mathematicians.

607

The complete decomposition of 420 is $42 \times 10 = 6 \times 7 \times 2 \times 5 = 2 \times 3 \times 7 \times 2 \times 5$.

608

Anne's neighbors can be either two boys or two girls. If they are girls, then each of them must be neighbored by another girl, since they are both next to Anne. So in the instance where Anne's neighbors are girls, the entire circle must be girls.

Since there are boys in the circle, the circle is obviously not all girls. That means Anne's neighbors must both be boys, each of whom is neighbored by Anne and another girl. This alternating pattern continues around the circle, so that the circle contains twelve boys and twelve girls.

609

The best way to avoid false moves in this game is to move the smallest disk from one column to the next and then any disk other than the smallest. Although such a recipe seems arbitrary, it ensures that there will always be one legal move. And repeating the pattern over and over will miraculously bring you to the solution. There is some deep connection between the cyclical movement of the disks and the mathematical underpinnings of this game.

For Puzzles 1 through 4, the minimum number of moves is, respectively, three, seven, fifteen and thirty-one.

For Puzzle 5, which has the restriction against placing disk 1 on disk 4, nineteen moves are required.

For Puzzle 6, which has restrictions against placing disk 1 on disk 3, and disk 2 on disk 4, the minimum number of moves required is only fifteen—the same as if there were no restrictions.

610

The answer is 24, composed of 1, 2, 3, 4, 6, 8, 12 and 24.

611

$$1 + 2 + 3 = 1 \times 2 \times 3 = 6$$

612

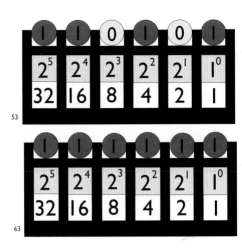

613

Before you turn your back, you check to see how many coins are showing heads. You know that the number of heads will increase by two, decrease by two or stay the same for every pair of coins that is turned over. Therefore, if the initial number of heads is odd, the number will remain odd, no matter how many pairs of coins are turned.

When you turn back around, you count the number of heads that are now showing. If the number is odd, as at the start (or even, as at the start), the covered coin must be a tail. If the number of heads is even for an odd start (or odd for an even start), the covered coin must be a head.

This simple trick helps demonstrate the importance of parity: the odd-even parity of this system is preserved as long as pairs of coins (not individual coins) are turned over.

614

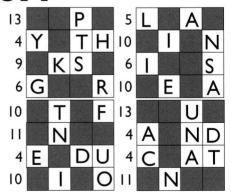

"*PlayThinks* is great fun and education."

615

The filled-in two-by-two matrices are a visual representation of the numbers from 0 to 15 in the binary number system: 0000, 0001, 0010, 0011, 0100, 0101, 0110, 0111, 1000, 1001, 1010, 1011, 1100, 1101, 1110 and 1111.

But are the sixteen tiles really different? On close inspection you may notice that there are only six different tiles, three of which are present in four different orientations.

616

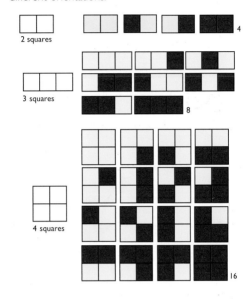

Shown above are fifty solutions to the Q-Bits color-matching game. Rotations, reflections and color reversals are not considered different.

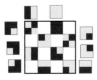

The shortest possible two-person game can end in eight moves, and there can be a great number of solutions, one shown. It can be seen that none of the remaining eight tiles can be fitted in the board.

617

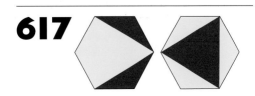

618

1	100	26	89
2	72	27	95
3	90	28	69
4	59	29	93
5	94	30	63
6	77	31	96
7	86	32	91
8	85	33	73
9	80	34	81
10	51	35	78
11	58	36	76
12	68	37	99
13	92	38	74
14	53	39	79
15	84	40	83
16	62	41	82
17	98	42	87
18	67	43	64
19	97	44	55
20	52	45	57
21	71	46	54
22	61	47	88
23	75	48	70
24	56	49	60
25	66	50	65

619

620

Try as they might, they will fail. That is because turning over two glasses at a time changes the number of upright glasses by two or by zero. And although the number of upright glasses in the first setup was one, so that adding two gave you a total of three, the number of upright glasses in the second setup is zero. Changing two at a time will allow your friends to fluctuate between zero glasses and two glasses, but they will never get to three glasses. In other words, the first setup has an odd parity, while the second setup has an even parity. In both instances, turning over two glasses at a time will not change that parity.

621

The parity of the initial setup is odd, and an even number of moves will not change that. Therefore, both all-upright and all-inverted conclusions are impossible.

622

The thief will always stay one step ahead unless the policeman moves first and changes the parity of the game. He can do that by going around the triangular block just once, catching the thief in seven or fewer moves.

623

Hexagon 19 is the odd one out.

624

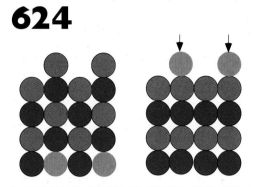

625

Since a loop of gears turns alternately clockwise and counterclockwise, an even number of gears is required for the setup to work. An odd number of gears, as in this puzzle, can't rotate at all.

626

Many people claim that there is not enough information provided to solve this problem. But that is because they have taken too narrow a view.

The key is understanding what a lightbulb does: it produces not only light but heat, and it remains warm many minutes after it has been switched off.

With that in mind, you can find the solution fairly easily. First, turn on switch 1 and leave it on for several minutes so that the bulb will get good and hot. Next, turn off switch 1 and turn on switch 2, and then go quickly to the attic. If the light is on, then switch 2 works the lamp; if the bulb is dark but warm, switch 1 works the lamp. If the bulb is both dark and cold, switch 3—the one that has not been used—works the lamp.

627

Such a bet is a losing proposition. Only three out of six possible random settings allow for the light to be turned on with the flip of just one switch.

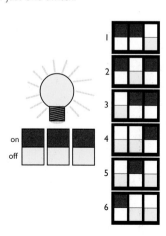

628

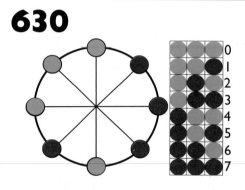

629

Just five moves: 1-2-3, 4-5-6, 7-8-9, 8-9-10 and 8-9-11.

630

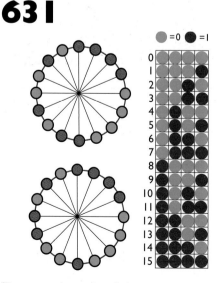

This solution is the only one possible.

Longer binary wheels are used to code messages in telephone transmission and radar mapping. University of California—Davis mathematician Sherman K. Stein called such binary structures memory wheels; they have also been called Ouroborean rings, a name derived from the mythological snake that ate its tail.

631

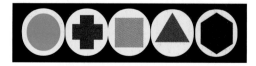

There are at least two solutions:
1-1-1-1-0-0-0-0-1-1-0-1-0-0-1-0 and
1-1-1-1-0-0-0-0-1-0-0-1-1-0-1-0.

632

The missing necklace.

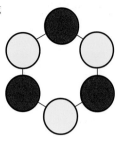

633

There are three different necklaces possible. The different necklaces can be described by the number of red beads between the green ones: either none, one, or two.

CHAPTER 10 SOLUTIONS

634

You have to attack problems like this one in a systematic fashion, or the complexities will boggle your mind. The best way to visualize the variables is to draw a cell chart with, say, the positions across the top and the names down the side. Put an X in a cell that has been logically ruled out, and put a * in a cell you believe is correct.

	CHAIRMAN	DIRECTOR	SECRETARY
Gerry	X	•	X
Anita	X	X	*
Rose	*	X	X

Then work your way through the premises:

Gerry has a brother, and the secretary is an only child, so Gerry can't be the secretary.

Rose earns more than the director, and the secretary earns less than anyone, so Rose can be neither the director nor the secretary.

The conclusions, then, are that Anita is the secretary, Gerry is the director and Rose is the chairman.

635

The clerk forgot to mention that the parrot was deaf.

636

The first three rules eliminate 118 of the 120 possible permutations of the five disks. The last rule selects one of the remaining two possibilities.

637 The reflexive answer is that if boys and girls are equally likely, the probability that the other child is a girl is ½.

But the reflex is wrong. There are four possible combinations for the Smiths' two children: boy-boy, boy-girl, girl-boy and girl-girl. One possibility (boy-boy) can be ruled out, but the other three are equally likely. Of the possibilities that remain, only one involves a second girl, so the likelihood that the Smiths have a second girl is only ⅓.

This problem is an example of conditional probability—that is, the probability of one event given the fact that another event has occurred. The results are counterintuitive and generally misunderstood.

638 The question is, rather, *where* can you build it? Only on the North Pole.

639 Fish.

640 Green.

641 He married the sister first.

642 The note meant: "I ought to owe nothing for I ate nothing."

643 Fifty percent of the birds will be watched by one other bird, and another 25 percent will be watched by two other birds. That leaves 25 percent unwatched.

644 The first child says he is a truth teller. The statement is true if he's telling the truth and false if he is lying.

What the second child says is true no matter whether the first child is telling the truth. She is therefore a truth teller.

The truth of the third child's statement depends on the truthfulness of the first child. If the first child is lying, the third is telling the truth; if the first is telling the truth, the third is lying.

The possibilities are either (from left to right): liar–truth teller–truth teller or truth teller–truth teller–liar. Either way, two are telling the truth and one is lying.

645 The two heirs swapped horses.

647 The chances of drawing a red ball are ²⁰⁄₅₀, or 40 percent. The chances of drawing a blue ball are ³⁰⁄₅₀, or 60 percent.

648 "Solve PlayThinks."

649 You should take the bet. The probability of at least one man getting his own hat back is almost .632.

650 86.

651 The fifth row of Pascal's triangle provides the answer. The average number of balls that reaches each juncture corresponds to a Pascal's triangle for which each successive row from the bottom is multiplied by an additional factor of 2, so that each row has the same sum.

In a full-sized probability machine, which possesses a large number of balls and branches, the distribution pattern approaches the famous Gaussian curve, also known as the bell curve.

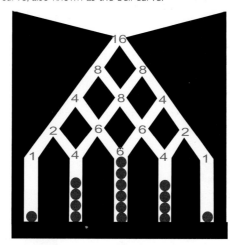

652 You are better off fighting the brontosaurus. Although your chances of beating any stegosaur is ½, beating three in series brings the probability to ½ × ½ × ½, or ⅛.

653 His reasoning was wrong. Sure, the chance of an unlikely event happening twice is fairly low, but the sailor's safety can't be calculated just by looking at the random nature of another shell landing in that hole. For one thing, the destination of a shell is not entirely random—the guns are being aimed, and gunners who have success with one shot may try sending another round in the same direction. For another, each time a random phenomenon occurs, the probability of the specified event happening again is exactly the same. So even if the guns were not being aimed, the spot where the shell hit is just as likely to be hit with the next round as any other spot.

654 The ladybug should start at the fifth aphid from the bumblebee—either clockwise or counterclockwise, depending on which direction she travels.

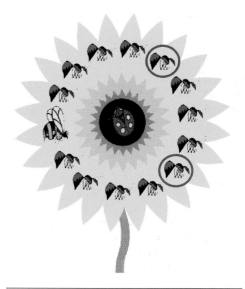

655 It took only seven trips, four to the ship and three back.

1. I took the Denebian to the spaceliner airlock and left it there.

2. I returned alone.

3. I took the Rigellian up to the spaceliner airlock.

4. I returned with the Denebian.

5. I took the Terrestrial up to the spaceliner airlock.

6. I returned alone.

7. I took the Denebian back up to the spaceliner airlock. Then all three could enter together.

656

Number 1 is Jerry, who likes chicken.
Number 2 is Ivan, who likes cakes.
Number 3 is Jill, who likes salad.
Number 4 is Anita, who likes fish.

657

The probability that the underside matches the top is ⅔. If you see heads, there are three, not two, equally possible scenarios:

1. You see the head half of a head-tail coin.

2. You see one side of a double-headed coin.

3. You see the other side of a double-headed coin.

In two of the three cases, the underside matches the top.

This result is so counterintuitive that many people refuse to believe it. If you are skeptical, try experimenting with "coins" cut out of cardboard. Keep track of your results and see if your probabilities match what I've outlined above.

658

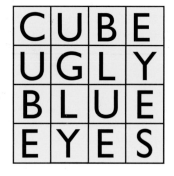

659

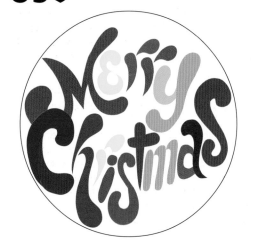

660

Puzzles like this depend as much on logic as they do on observation. Logic is required to sort out the visual evidence and make sure there is enough information to draw a conclusion. In this instance, even though all the information is not there, logic can help you deduce a symmetrical answer.

I want to emphasize logic here, because many particularly observant or logical people are perplexed if they are asked to solve a puzzle without all the pieces. They are often hesitant to use deduction or even intuition to come up with an answer.

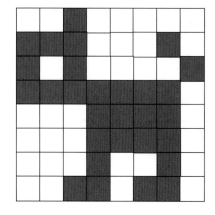

661

Own the casino!
The math of roulette and other casino games guarantees that, over time, the casino owners make far more money than they pay out. For every person who leaves the casino richer, there are many others who have lost considerable sums.

662

"Just between you and me" and "Split second timing."

663

A possible solution:

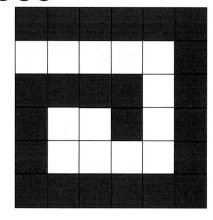

664

There are six possible outcomes for rolling three marbles, and in four of those instances Peter wins. So his chances of winning are ⅔.

665

1. The word *three* is misspelled.

2. The word *mistake* should be plural.

3. There are only two mistakes in the sentence, which is the third mistake.

666

RANGE and ANGER.

667

If you count the letters, you will find there is 1 D, 2 I's, 3 S's, 4 C's, 5 O's, 6 V's, 7 E's and 8 R's. The secret word is DISCOVER.

668

This puzzle is somewhat related to the birthday paradox. The usual answer people give is that it should take about 100 links. But research conducted at Harvard University in Massachusetts demonstrates that any two strangers in the United States can be linked by a chain of intermediate acquaintances only five to six people long.

This problem, known as the "Small World" problem, is the basis of the popular trivia game in which one tries to link any actor to Kevin Bacon in just six steps. Both Hollywood and the world at large are examples of networks, a system with many interconnections. Chains of acquaintances have always been important, but with the revolution in travel and communication that has taken over the world in the last fifty years, people are connected through a very few steps to almost every other person on earth.

669

B\A	2	4	5
1	L	L	L
3	W	L	L
6	W	W	W

The player with die A will, over the long run, win 55 percent of the time, as demonstrated in the chart above.

670
In the last composition the rectangle and the oval do not overlap.

671
"Take us to your leaders."

	HAIR	EYES	NOSE	MOUTH
T				
A				
K				
E				
U				
S				
T				
O				
Y				
O				
U				
R				
L				
E				
A				
D				
E				
R				
S				

672
There were fourteen squares on the sheet, six on one side and eight on the other.

673
Only the second statement is true. Statement number 3 rules out both number 1 and number 3.

674
The passenger realized that if his face were clean, one of the other passengers would have realized that his own face was blackened by soot. Since neither of them stopped laughing, he realized his face must be sooty as well.

675

$$
\begin{array}{ccccc}
6 & + & 6 & + & 8 & + & 8 & = 28 \\
+ & & + & & + & & + & \\
6 & + & 6 & + & 6 & + & 6 & = 24 \\
+ & & + & & + & & + & \\
12 & + & 12 & + & 10 & + & 8 & = 42 \\
+ & & + & & + & & + & \\
\underline{8} & + & \underline{10} & + & \underline{12} & + & \underline{6} & = 36 \\
32 & & 34 & & 36 & & 28 &
\end{array}
$$

676

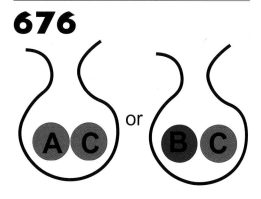

At first glance it seems the chances of a red ball remaining in the bag are 50 percent. But there are actually three—not two—equally possible states:

1. The initial red ball (A) was drawn, leaving the added red ball (C).

2. The added red ball (C) was taken, leaving the initial red ball (A).

3. The added red ball (C) was taken, leaving the blue ball (B).

As you can see, in two out of the three cases, a red ball remains in the bag.

In the initial draw, the chances of pulling out a red ball are 75 percent. But once the first ball is drawn, the odds change.

677
The chances are not ⅔ but ⅓. The reasoning is simple. Choose any card. Of the three remaining cards, only one is the same color, so the chances of picking it are just one in three.

Your friend's reasoning is incorrect because the three possibilities he or she considered are not equally likely.

678
Although Amos and Butch are sure shots, Cody's chances of survival are twice as good as the other cowboys'.

The reason is straightforward. If Amos or Butch gets the first shot, the one who gets it will eliminate the other (since they represent the greatest threat) and take his chances with Cody. Cody then has a 50 percent chance of shooting the survivor and a 50 percent chance of missing and getting shot. If Cody draws the first shot, he'd be well advised to miss, because if he actually shouts either Amos or Butch, the other could gun him down.

So Cody's chances of surviving are 50 percent.

Amos and Butch both have the same chances: If they lose the draw, they are shot in the first round; if they win the draw, one shoots the other and take his chances with Cody. Since both outcomes are equally likely, the chances for either Amos or Butch turn out to be 0 percent plus 50 percent, divided by two—or 25 percent.

679
The formula for solving such problems has eluded mathematicians for centuries. Practical solutions are best found through simple trial and error. In the circle of thirty-six prisoners, the proper positions to plant your enemies are numbers 4, 10, 15, 20, 26 and 30.

680
In the case of our coin-flipping experiment, a surprising probability is found in Benford's law. The odds are overwhelming that at some point in a series of 200 tosses, either heads or tails will come up six or more times in a row. Most fakers don't know this and will not put such nonrandom occurrences in their fake results.

681
In calculating probability, mathematicians generally limit themselves to four possible outcomes: heads-heads, tails-tails, heads-tails and tails-head. But there is can be a fifth possible result—uncountable. For example, one coin could land on edge. Or it could be lost down a grate. Or be carried off by a bird in midflight. Perhaps mathematicians should account for such occurrences when they calculate probabilities in the future.

682

The answer is ONE WORD.

683

There are six possible even numbers that can come up—2, 4, 6, 8, 10 and 12—and only five possible odd numbers—3, 5, 7, 9 and 11. In spite of that, as the diagram shows, there are eighteen ways to throw an even number and eighteen ways to throw an odd number. So the odds of an even number are even.

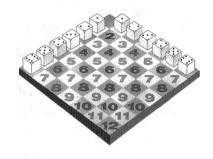

684

In any given roll of a die, the odds that a 6 will *not* come up are ⅚. Since each roll of a die is independent of the others, the chances of not rolling a 6 in a given series can be calculated as:

Two rolls: ⅚ × ⅚ = .69

Three rolls: ⅚ × ⅚ × ⅚ = .57

Four rolls: ⅚ × ⅚ × ⅚ × ⅚ = .48

which means that more often than not, you will roll at least one 6 after four rolls.

685

Remarkably, the probability of two people sharing a birthday is about .5 in a group of just twenty-three people.

To calculate this, you have to look at the probability that everyone has a *different* birthday. For a group of two people, the probability is extremely high—about ³⁶⁴/₃₆₅—that they will have different birthdays. With a group of three, the probability is not as high—³⁶³/₃₆₅—and since the group of three still contains the group of two, the two probabilities are multiplied. Continue along this track until the probability of everybody in the group having different birthdays drops below .5, which means the probability of two people sharing a birthday is now more than .5.

The probability approaches near certainty with ninety people or more.

687

In the seventeenth century Antoine Gombaud Chevalier de Méré, a French nobleman with an interest in gambling, suspected that the odds were not in his favor, so he checked his suspicions with the famous mathematicians Blaise Pascal and Pierre de Fermat, who found that the probability of rolling double 6 after twenty-four throws was ³⁵/₃₆ to the twenty-fourth power, or about .49, which meant losing in the long run.

Gombaud's small request marked the birth of the science of probability.

688

Martin Gardner has presented several versions of this paradox, but the *Parade* magazine columnist Marilyn vos Savant is most famously associated with it. Her 1990 column on the subject provided the right answer but provoked thousands of letters of disbelief and accusation.

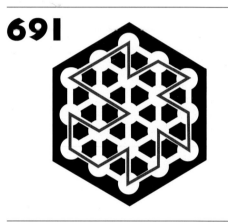

Why? Because the answer seems so wrong!

If you stick with your initial choice, your chances of winning are one in three. That is easy to understand: one car, three doors.

That means the chance of the car being behind one of the doors you did not initially choose is two in three. Of course, if you were to switch to one of the two other doors without any additional information, that ⅔ would be divided between two doors, for a ⅔ chance with each door—no better than if you stuck with your initial choice.

But when the host reveals the monkey behind one of the two doors, that additional information suddenly changes the odds. The host, of course, will not open a door to reveal a car. And the host's choice of doors depends greatly on your initial choice: if your door hides the car, the host can pick either remaining door; but if your door hides a monkey, the host must pick one and only one door to open. As you can see from the chart above, the possibilities for the doors you did not pick—monkey-monkey, car-monkey and monkey-car—have now been constrained to just monkey–open door, car–open door and open door—car. Therefore, if you switch, you have a ⅔ chance of selecting a door with a car behind it.

Again, if you are not convinced, try playing a number of games with and without swapping to check the validity of this proof. Remember, this is a case of conditional probabilities—the probability of something happening given that something else already has.

689

When the letters are arranged so that the arrows follow a clockwise order, they spell out TONY BLAIR.

690

It isn't a fair bet, even with 3-to-2 odds.

I can ensure that my chances of winning are at least ⅔ and are sometimes as high as ⅞. All I have to do is let you pick your triplet. Then I pick my triplet so that it starts with the opposite of your second coin, then copies your first two. If you select HTH, I'll pick HHT and have a ⅔ advantage. If you choose TTT, I'll pick HTT and will have a ⅞ advantage—you can win only if the first three tosses are all tails.

CHAPTER 11 SOLUTIONS

691

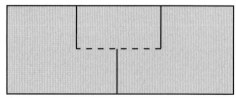

692

a-5, b-1, c-9

693

There are two different lengths—ten long and ten short. Each color comes in two lengths. The sequence that removes them all is short yellow, short orange, short red, short pink, short purple, short light green, short dark green, long light blue, short dark blue, long yellow, long orange, long red, long pink, long purple, long light green, long dark green, short light blue, long dark blue, short violet and long violet.

694

695 A sample game in which the map could not be fully colored is shown below. Six regions had to be left blank.

If you started with a blank map, could you do better?

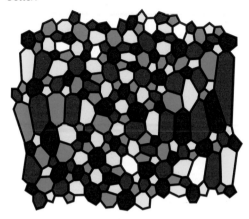

696 Only 2 and 9 are topologically identical.

698 You will need at least three colors. One of the many possibilities is shown here.

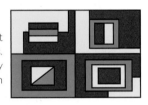

699 The solution illustrates the two-color theorem.

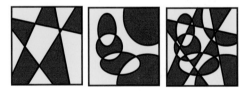

700 Clockwise: yellow triangle, orange pentagon, red heptagon, pink nonagon, violet square, light green hexagon, blue octagon and purple decagon.

701

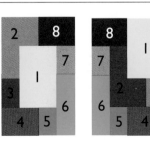

703 The minimum number of colors is eight, as shown.

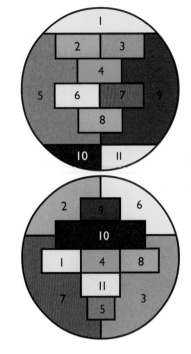

704

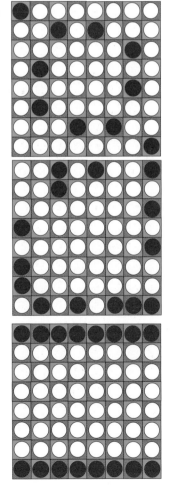

705 First the yellow horizontal strip is laid down. On top of that go the orange, red, light green, dark green, light blue, dark blue and pink strips, respectively. See the diagram here for the location of the strips on the grid.

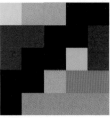

706

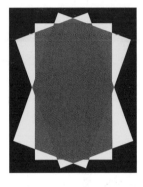

707 It takes at least six moves for the eye to swap ends.

708 The strip will stay in one piece. It will be twice as long and have two complete twists.

709 The strip will break into two linked bands, one a Möbius strip of the same length and the other a band that is twice as long and has two complete twists.

710
1. Four colors
2. Three colors
3. Two colors
4. Two colors
5. Four colors
6. Two colors
7. Two colors
8. Three colors

711 To make the model, make three sets of hypercard cuts, as shown, on a strip of paper and then twist the strip to create the three flaps. Glue the ends of the strip together to make the ring.

Once the glue dries, you can change the number of outside benches from one to two by turning the entire ring inside out.

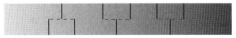

712

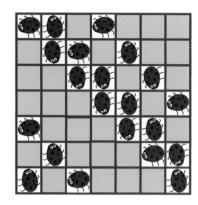

713

The quartets are 1-9-11-14; 2-3-7-13; 4-5-6-8. That leaves the pair: 10-12.

714

Each 2-pire touches each of the other eleven; therefore, twelve is the minimum number of colors needed to complete this puzzle.

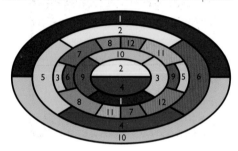

715

The capital E is topologically equivalent to F, G, J, T and Y.

ABCDE
FGHIJ
KLMNO
PQRST
UVWXYZ

716

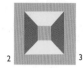

717

There are two different solutions, one of which is shown below.

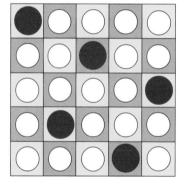

718

There is just one solution.

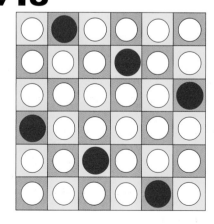

719

The unique solution is shown below.

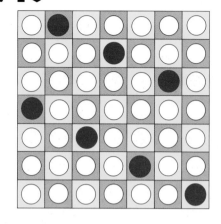

720

The diagram below shows one of the twelve different solutions, not counting rotations and reflections.

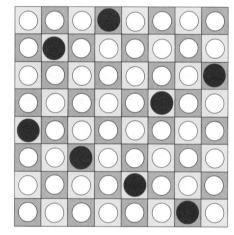

721

The illustration below shows one of four possible solutions.

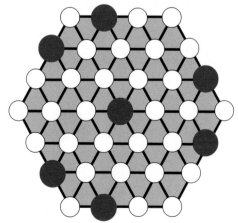

722

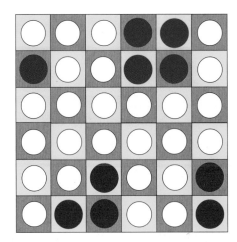

723

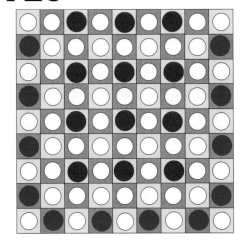

724
Every shape but the pentagon can be made by slicing a cube.

725
Two disconnections, as shown, will form five lengths of one, one, three, six and twelve beads. Combining these lengths in various ways can form necklaces of one to twenty-three beads.

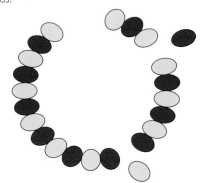

726
With three points of intersection for the rope to overlap, there are eight different configurations for the loop. Only two of those will form a knot, as shown below. Therefore the probability is 1/4.

727
Only two of the loops will be knotted if the hose is pulled tight: the one at the bottom right and the one on the middle left.

728

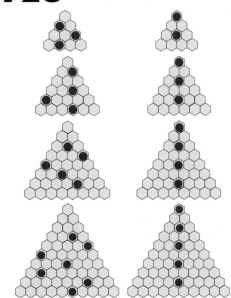

729
The twenty-four connected cubes represent an ordinary overhand knot.

730
Just one cut is needed. If she cuts the fourth ring from the left, the chain will fall into four pieces—of lengths one, one, three and six links, respectively. Those pieces, alone or in combination, can cover the amounts owed for each day. For example, on day three, she can trade the two loose links for the three-link piece.

732
The keys spell out P-L-A-Y-T-H-I-N-K-S.

733
If you reshape all the marked keys the same way, you will need to mark three key handles. Two of the marked keys should be grouped together, and the third should be separated by one key with an unmarked handle. In that way, you can identify both the starting point—the single marked key—and the direction—toward the two marked keys—in which the memorized sequence progresses.

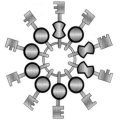

734
The solution for the ten-by-ten board is unique.

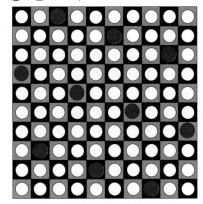

735
It will take nineteen moves to remove the piston.

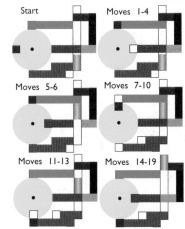

736 It takes thirteen moves.

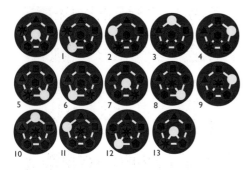

737 It takes twenty moves to get all the animals to their proper cages. In general, the moves should create a cyclic order to solve the puzzle in the fewest possible moves.

738

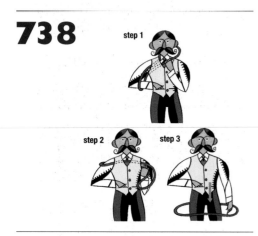

step 1

step 2   step 3

739 A winning strategy for the maximizer is to always play on the face of the distorted dodecahedron opposite the position last played by the minimizer—and to copy the color the minimizer used.

The game illustrated below began with the maximizer filling in the center pentagon and then following the outlined strategy. As you can see, this player won the game, as the last two regions cannot be filled in with any of the five colors.

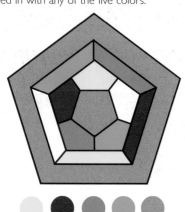

740

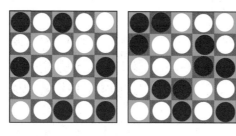

741

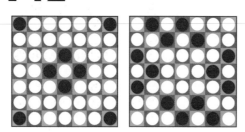

742

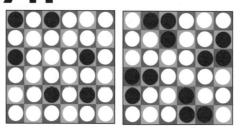

743

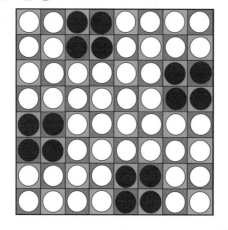

744 The three possible folds are shown.

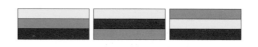

745 The four possible folds are shown.

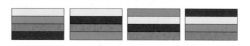

746 It turns out that it is nearly impossible to fold a sheet of newsprint in half more than eight or nine times, no matter how large or thin the sheet.

Every time you fold the sheet, you double the number of pages in the stack. One fold makes two pages, two folds make four pages; Nine folds will produce a stack of newsprint 512 pages thick—the size of a small phone book. A stack that thick prevents any additional folding.

747 The eight possible folds are shown above.

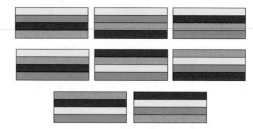

748 The message is CREATIVE PLAY IS PURE FUN.

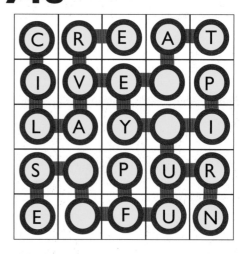

749
One of sixteen possible solutions is shown.

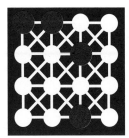

750
One of twenty-eight possible solutions is shown.

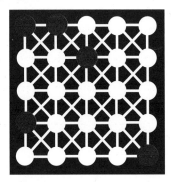

751
There are only two possible answers, both of which are shown below.

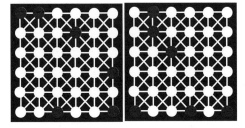

752
There is only one possible solution, shown below. No solution has been found for a matrix larger than this.

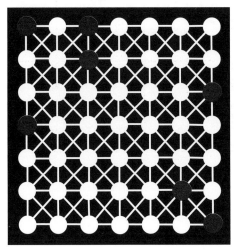

753
The key is to place each coin on a circle that is connected to the starting position of the previous coin. There will always be one pathway free, according to this strategy.

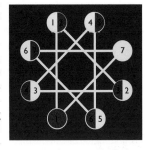

A more trial-and-error approach involves filling the star with seven coins and playing the puzzle in reverse, noting the moves. You could also imagine untangling the star to form a circle, which would enable you to visualize the solution easily.

This puzzle offers an introduction to "clock arithmetic" and finite number systems. Its star track can be described as a modulus 8 with a linking operation of +3 (or −5). That is, there are eight points spaced around a circle, and every third point is joined to form a single continuous track.

754
There are ten distinct ways.

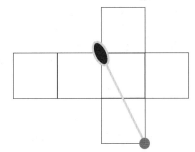

755
The shortest route will not follow the edge of the cube. To envision the shortest route, imagine flattening out the faces of the cube, as shown below. If you draw a straight line from the ladybug to the aphid, you will see that the shortest path does not run down the edge.

756
One of the small chains was separated into its three separate links, and then that was used to link together the other four chains.

757
The cars can be transferred in as few as thirty moves.

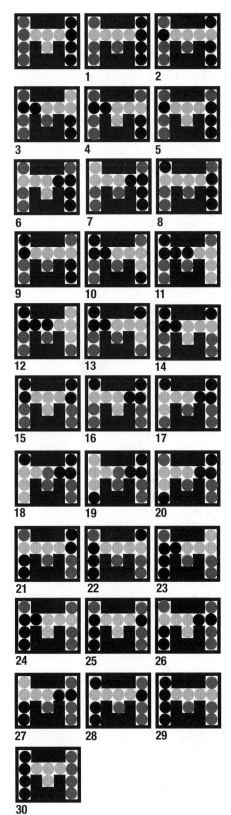

758 Did you notice that the numbers below each set of disks add up to 15 and 24, respectively? The sequence shows the number moves that must be made in succession by each color group (for instance, one red, two blues, three reds, three blues, three reds, two blues, one red). If you follow the sequences, you will come to the solution—which otherwise may remain elusive—in the fewest possible moves.

For example, the first puzzle can be solved by first moving the red disk into the center space, followed by two moves of the blue disks, then three moves of the red disks, and so on. Because of the restrictions on the movements of the disks, the moves will be obvious.

759

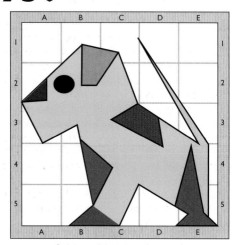

760

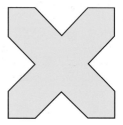

761 Yellow and orange, red and green, pink and blue.

762 Only the bottom left cube.

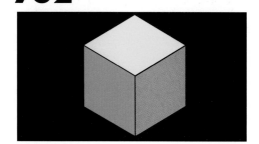

763 1. There are twenty-four ways to place the first cube. In any of those twenty-four ways, the second cube can be in one of four locations. And at any given location, the second cube can turn in one of twenty-four different ways. So $24 \times 4 \times 24 = 2,304$ different ways.

2. As long as the cubes stay in the same order, the variations possible with three cubes are simply $24 \times 24 \times 24$, or 13,824, different ways.

3. As long as the eight cubes maintain their relative position—and counting each individual turn of one face of a cube as a variation on the entire pattern—the number of variations is 24^8, or 110,075,314,176.

It is little wonder, then, that there are so many cube games on the market, or that Rubik's Cube, involving twenty-six joined cubes, has proved so difficult.

764 Harpo Marx.

765 To reveal the true form of the distorted images, simply hold the outer edge of the page about 15 centimeters from your nose and look at the page from a very slanted angle. Close one eye and everything will be clear.

766 Groucho Marx.

767 Regular tetrahedrons will not fill the space. When four pyramids are grouped together to define a larger tetrahedron, the central space is a regular octahedron.

Therefore, the pyramid is made up of eleven tetrahedrons and four octahedrons.

768 As you learned from the previous puzzles, a simple parity check can determine whether one configuration can be obtained from another. Simply switch pairs of blocks until the desired pattern is achieved. If the number of swaps is even, the puzzle can be solved; if the number of swaps is odd, it is impossible.

For this puzzle, the solution is possible in thirty moves.

769

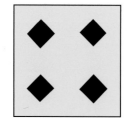

770 The minimal prismatic one-sided ring is made up of ten unit cubes.

771 Numbers 2, 3, 4, 5 and 10 are identical. And numbers 7, 8 and 9 are identical. But number 1 and number 6 are unique.

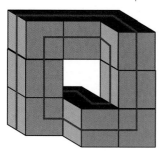

772 If you hold a cube so that one corner points directly toward you, its edges outline a hexagon. It then becomes obvious that the cube has ample space for a square hole slightly larger than one of its faces.

If a cube has sides of 1 unit, a square hole can be drilled through it with sides of almost 1.06 units.

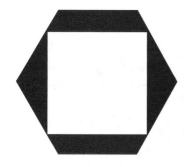

773 1. Fifty-eight cubes
2. Eighteen cubes
3. Twenty cubes
4. Fifty-six cubes
5. Thirty-three cubes
6. Eighteen cubes
7. Thirty cubes
8. Forty cubes

774

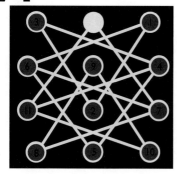

775 To solve this difficult problem in a systematic fashion, you can create a table that shows the number of different cubes possible for each combination of colors.

Number of red corners: 8 7 6 5 4 3 2 1 0

Number of yellow corners: 0 1 2 3 4 5 6 7 8

Number of different cubes: 1 1 3 3 7 3 3 1 1

Therefore, twenty-three different cubes are possible.

776 The green loop.

777 Only the yellow, green and orange nets can be folded into a perfect cube.

778 Orange and green, yellow and pink, blue and red.

780

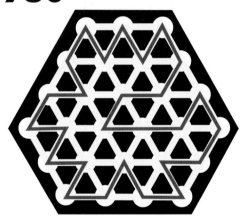

781 The sliced-off tetrahedron has one-sixth the volume of the whole box.

782 No path exists. The next best answer is a path that leaves one room unvisited.

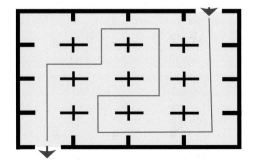

783 The famous sliding-block puzzle and the story behind it.

If you put in some effort to solving the 14-15 puzzle, you may be disappointed that you didn't find an answer. Don't be. This famous puzzle, designed by Sam Loyd, is impossible to solve. Loyd knew this when he introduced the puzzle some 120 years ago—but he offered a $1,000 reward to anyone who could devise a solution and thereby touched off an international craze. Indeed, the only other instance of such a worldwide involvement in recreational mathematics was the Rubik's cube fad in the 1980s.

Loyd's 14-15 configuration is just one of 600 billion possible arrangements of the numbered tiles, and like Loyd's, half are impossible to bring into sequential order. A simple parity check can determine whether a given configuration has a solution. Simply swap the misplaced tiles, then count the number of swaps—if the number is even, it's possible; if it's odd (as in this case), it's not.

In the language of computer science, the 15 puzzle, as it is generally known, is a model of a sequential machine. Each movement of a block is an input; each configuration of the blocks, a state.

784 By playing correctly, the second person will always win. If the first player takes one bee, the second player takes two bees on the exact opposite side of the daisy. If the first player takes two bees, the second player takes one bee, again on the opposite side of the daisy. Either way, this leaves two equal sets of bees placed symmetrically around the daisy. All the second player has to do now is keep the two patterns symmetrical for the rest of the game, and he or she will never lose.

CHAPTER 12 SOLUTIONS

785 In theory, the gravity train would work as planned. And interestingly enough, every trip would take the same amount of time—about forty-two minutes. In fact, if the earth were hollow, an object dropped through the earth would arrive on the other side in just forty-two minutes as well.

Of course, the earth isn't hollow. Friction and air resistance cannot be ignored.

786 Less than at the earth's surface. Even though you are closer to the center of the earth's mass, there is enough mass above you to cancel out the effects of some of the mass below you.

787 Your weight is a measure of the gravitational pull of the earth's mass upon your body. The closer you are to the earth's center of mass, the more strongly you will feel its pull.

Because of the earth's bulge, then, you weigh about .5 percent less at the equator than you do at the poles.

788 Yes. Weight is a relative magnitude, and your weight may change from planet to planet, but a spring scale will always be able to measure that weight—even though your weight will often be 0.

789 No. At the surface the moon's gravitational pull is only one-sixth that of the earth's, so astronauts on the moon will weigh only ⅙ of what they did on the earth.

790 This thought experiment was devised by the great Albert Einstein and demonstrates his equivalence principle: The effect of being at rest in a gravitational field is the same as the effect of being at rest in an accelerated system.

If you are in an accelerating rocket as described, you will feel yourself pulled toward the floor with the same force—and watch objects fall at the same speed—as if you were in a room on the earth, though it is the floor that is actually rising up to meet the objects.

In the absence of other information, then, it is impossible to tell whether you are on the earth or in an accelerating rocket.

791 Common sense tells us that heavy objects should accelerate faster than lighter ones, but experimental science has proven this is not the case.

Newton's second law of motion shows that acceleration is directly proportional to force (weight, in this case) and inversely proportional to mass. The equation can be written as:

$$a = f/m$$

where a is acceleration, f is force and m is mass.

The resistance to motion due to mass is called inertia. Therefore, even though a large stone may weigh 100 times more than a small rock, it has 100 times more mass (and inertia), and so the two factors cancel out.

In general, and ignoring air resistance, the acceleration of every falling body near sea level is 32 feet per second per second.

792 To eliminate the difference in air resistance, place the slip of paper on top of the coin. Then drop the coin, giving it a slight spin to keep it horizontal as it falls. The coin and the paper should fall together.

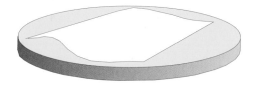

793 Weightlessness can be achieved for up to a minute in an airplane flying a controlled parabolic course. The pilot steers the plane so it follows the path of a free fall. Because every object in the plane—including the plane—is falling at the same rate, the effect is simulated weightlessness.

794 The book underneath will probably stay in place, but the book on top will move along with the book you are pulling.

The reason is friction. The frictional force is proportional to the normal (or perpendicular) force, and the normal force is equal to the amount that an object presses down on a surface. The normal force on the book underneath the one you are pulling is equal to the weight not only of that book but of the two books on top of it as well. The friction between that book and the book on the bottom is then greater than the friction between that book and the one sliding across its top (that is, the one you are pulling), so the book will tend to stay put.

795 The biggest and heaviest apples will rise to the top.

The arrangement that is most stable is one in which the most densely packed apples are at the bottom. The smaller an object is, the more likely it is to find a space to drop into at a lower position. Therefore, in a group of mixed apples, the smaller apples can be more densely packed than the large ones and will eventually sink to the bottom.

796 When I pull on the string from the bottom slowly and steadily, the top part of the string must bear both the weight of the book and the strength of the pull. The tension on it is greater than the tension on the lower half, so the top thread will break first.

If I pull with a sharp jerk, inertia comes into play. The book is little affected by the jerk at first, so the force of the jerk is not transmitted to the top string. The tension is therefore greater on the bottom thread and it breaks first.

797 Whether large or small, packed spheres will occupy about .5235 cubic meters for every cubic meter of space they are packed in. This is independent of the size of the ball, as long as the radius is small in relation to the size of the box.

Even though each void is smaller for tightly packed small spheres, there are more voids altogether. Each box will weigh the same.

798 A false bottom filled with heavy items will noticeably affect the center of mass of a suitcase. This will cause the suitcase to hang at an odd angle, as shown.

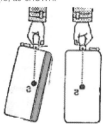

799 One weighing will do. He simply needs to place one red, two blue, three green, four yellow and five orange balls on the scale. If red is the color of the odd balls, the scale will read 1510 grams; if it's blue, 1520 grams and so on.

800 If you pull up at a sharp angle, a torque is created that turns the spool away from you. If you pull instead at a more shallow angle, the opposite torque is created, and the spool will roll toward you.

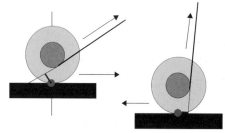

801 A very heavy weight is fixed to the red end of the box. As you can see in the diagram, such a weight greatly affects the behavior of the box.

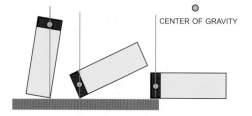

CENTER OF GRAVITY

802 The fish actually weighs 50 kilograms. Each end of the rope pulls down on the spring with the same force, so two "marlins" are being weighed in the setup shown in the illustration: the real marlin tied to one end of the rope and the restraint on the dock attached to the other end. The restraint on the dock may be an imaginary fish, but the force it exerts on the balance is real. To get an accurate weight, the fisherman should have tied the fish directly to the scale.

803 The triangular shape is the one where the angle (as measured from the center of gravity) is the greatest between the force of gravity and the point around which the shape will topple. That also means it is the most stable.

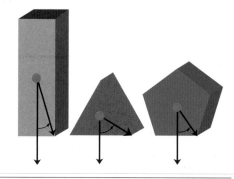

804 Friction will always keep the stick from falling. The finger that is farther from the stick's center of gravity carries a lighter load and therefore experiences less friction, so that finger moves first. As it is brought closer to the center, more and more weight is borne by that finger until the kinetic friction between the stick and the finger is greater than the static friction between the stick and the other finger. At that point the first finger stops and the second finger begins to slide. The stick will first slide over one finger, then on the other, switching back and forth until both fingers meet at the stick's center of gravity.

Starting from the middle, the finger that moves first immediately bears less weight and continues to bear less weight as it moves. There will be no alternating motion in this case.

805 If you hang weights of 50 or 100 kilograms on the hook, nothing will change and the balance will continue to read 100 kilograms. The tension in the rope lessens as more weight is placed on the hook and becomes 0 when the 100-kilogram weight is added.

When more than 100 kilograms are placed on the hook, the rope becomes slack, and the readings on the scale will equal the suspended weights. So for a 150-kilogram weight, the scale will read 150 kilograms.

806

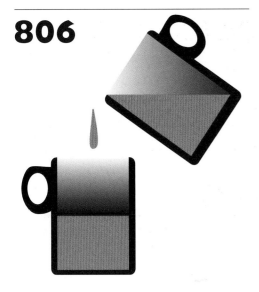

807
The weight is the same in both instances. The weight depends on the mass of the bottle and its contents, and that does not change. When flies are in flight, their weight is transmitted to the bottle by air currents, especially the downdraft generated by moving wings.

808
First, measure the diameter of the bottom of the bottle. Halve that, square the answer and multiply that number by 3.14159 to get the area of the base.

Then measure the height of the liquid, turn the bottle upside-down and measure the height of the air. Add those numbers together and multiply the sum by the base to get the volume of the entire bottle.

809
Weigh three parcels against three parcels. If one side is heavier than the other side, one of those three must contain the ring. If both sides are equal, the ring must be in one of the three that were not weighed. From the group of three with the ring, weigh one against another. The heavier of the two has the ring; if both are equal, the ring will be found in the unweighed parcel.

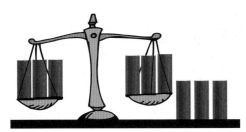

810
Both areas are identical.

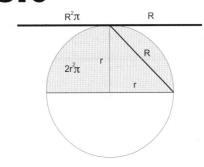

811

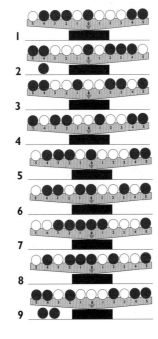

812

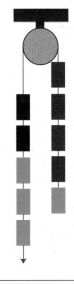

813
The rule that objects with a low center of gravity are the most stable relates to static equilibrium. Balancing a stick is a more dynamic situation, one in which the finger is constantly moving to stay under the stick's center of gravity. A long stick has a large "moment of inertia" (the property of an object to resist turning). Because of this resistance to turning, the stick's center of gravity will shift slowly, giving you time to move your finger back under the center. Short objects have smaller moments of inertia and can turn more quickly than you can respond.

814
The left side of the pulley is heavier by the difference between one red and one green weight.

815
The spout of the yellow can reaches to its rim and so may be filled completely. The green can, while taller, has a low spout and thus may be only partially filled. The yellow can will hold more.

816
The ingenious inner structure, shown below, is quite simple. A small cylinder filled with a very viscous liquid is embedded in the egg at a slanted angle. The cylinder also contains a small but heavy piston that will move very slowly through the liquid—it takes about seventy seconds for it to travel from one end of the cylinder to the other. The piston is heavy enough to throw the egg off balance except during the middle of its transit. Then, for about ten seconds, the egg can be placed in equilibrium on its pointed end.

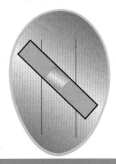

817 Start both timers simultaneously. When the three-minute timer ends, turn it over quickly. When the four-minute timer ends, turn the three-minute timer over once again—there will be one minute's worth of sand to add to the four minutes to make a full five minutes.

818 When this paradox was first discovered, complex explanations were advanced to account for the hourglass's behavior. But its workings are quite simple.

When the cylinder is turned over, the hourglass's high center of gravity makes it topple over, and its buoyancy helps wedge the glass against the sides of the cylinder. Friction between glass and glass holds the hourglass in place until enough sand has passed to the lower compartment to drop the center of gravity. Only then will the hourglass free up and rise to the top.

819 The heaviest balls will not be slowed as rapidly by the coarse surface. Therefore the heaviest balls will collect in the compartment farthest from the chute, and the lightest will collect nearest the chute.

820 Clockwise.

821 The two bolts will not move in relation to each other.

822 Clockwise.

823 Clockwise.

824 Both racks will move up.

825 To the left.

826 After 1¼ clockwise turns of the leftmost gear, the letters will spell out LEONARDO.

827 If you throw your Frisbee with real gusto, it will travel all the way around the earth without falling. Since there is no friction from the air, it will continue to orbit without any need of additional propulsion. It will become a satellite.

The moon and communication satellites circle the earth in much the same way as the planets circle the sun.

Sir Isaac Newton studied the paths taken by objects in ballistic flight and theorized that a cannonball fired parallel to the horizon with a great enough force from a great enough height could achieve a path that would match the curvature of the earth. Such a path would take objects completely around the earth, ignoring factors such as air resistance.

Newton, then, was the first to describe how an artificial satellite could be launched. It was an idea that would take centuries to finally realize.

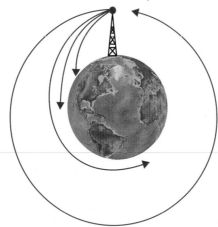

828 The vertical fall of the dart (from a straight-line trajectory) and the vertical fall of the monkey will be exactly the same. No matter what the velocity of the dart is, it will strike the monkey.

829 Many people are boggled by this puzzle and try to sum up an infinite series straight out of advanced math. But the answer is simple: it takes the joggers an hour to meet, and the fly travels 10 kilometers in an hour.

In his fascinating book, *Time Travel and Other Math Bewilderments*, Martin Gardner tells a story about the Hungarian mathematician John von Neumann, who was asked this puzzle at a party. Neumann gave the correct answer in an instant. The person who posed the question was disappointed; he usually could count on mathematicians to overlook the obvious answer and try instead to solve the problem through the time-consuming process of summing up an infinite series.

Von Neumann was startled. "But that's how I solved it," he said.

830

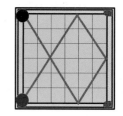 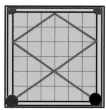

831

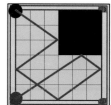 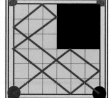

832

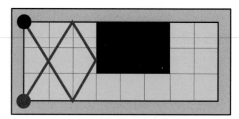

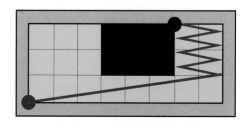

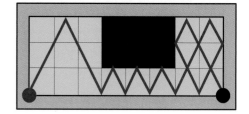

833 If we strike a ball in the corner at a 45-degree angle, it will land in one of the three other corners after a finite number of rebounds. To find out which corners, color in the starting point and every other intersection point of the unit grid. In the first three tables, only one of the other corners will be filled in—a sign that that is the corner in which the ball will eventually land. If all the pockets are filled in, double the size of the unit squares and repeat the process.

In general, if the dimensions of the table are odd-odd, the ball will end up in the opposite pocket; if the dimensions are even-odd, it will end up on the side the ball started from. If the dimensions are even-even, divide by 2 until at least one of the dimensions is odd.

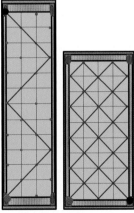

odd-odd

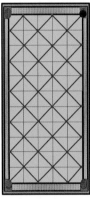

even-odd

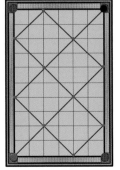

even-even

834 The wheel with the weight at the center will arrive first. Because the weight is at the center, it will not resist turning as much as the weight placed near the rim. That means the wheel will speed up much more quickly. But the wheel that has the weight near the outside, though it doesn't speed up as quickly, will not slow down as quickly either: it will roll longer than the other wheel.

835 The bomb will follow a parabola (trajectory 3). The vertical component is the same as a free fall (trajectory 1), but the bomb also carries a horizontal motion imparted by the airplane. Since the vertical motion is accelerating, the curve will become steeper, as in trajectory 3, rather than shallower, as in trajectory 2.

836 Mr. Smith should throw the Frisbee backward so that the dog will have to run the additional distance Mr. Smith walks while he retrieves the Frisbee.

837 The trick works. There's more than gravity working on the bucket: the falling arm of the ladder has its center of mass near the pivot point because of the heavy weight. The resultant torque causes the end of the arm to descend faster than a free fall. As long as the bucket lands in the line of the falling bowling ball, the ball will land in the bucket.

838 The frog advances 1 meter a day. After seventeen full days the frog is 3 meters from the exit. The frog escapes on the eighteenth day.

839 The balls will reach the circumference simultaneously.

Gravity is acting on any given ball in a direction in which it is free to move. The force may be resolved into two components: one parallel to the chord and one perpendicular to the chord. The force that is pulling the ball along the chord turns out to be proportional to the length of that chord. Therefore, the time of travel down one chord will be the same as that down any other.

This experiment prompted one of Galileo's most important discoveries: If balls are released simultaneously from the highest point in a vertical circle along its radial chords, all the balls will arrive at the circumference of the circle at the same time.

Galileo's demonstration proved that the time of descent along any chord from the top to the circumference is independent from its slope.

840 The bottle must be dropped from a height four times as great.

Doubling the height seems intuitively sufficient. But to double the speed, one must double the time of the fall, which means that four times the potential energy must be put into the system.

841 The bridge did not support the clown. Newton's third law of motion states that every action has an equal and opposite reaction; the clown applied a force to the rings to lift them into the air—a force that was greater than the weight of the rings. That force, plus the weight of the clown and the other ring, broke the bridge.

842 The pendulum will appear to swing in a counterclockwise three-dimensional elliptical path. If the lenses are reversed, the pendulum will appear to swing clockwise.

The illusion shows how the intensity of light influences the judgment of distance and depth. Darkened retinal images are transmitted to the brain more slowly than are bright images. This has nothing to do with the speed of light, which is constant. The image seen through the dark lens is recognized a fraction of a second later than the bright image.

When the brain gets two pictures of the pendulum in slightly different positions at the same time, it perceives them stereoscopically, creating an illusion of depth where none exists. The effect is the greatest in the middle of the swing, when the pendulum is at its fastest, because at that point the difference between the two pictures is the greatest.

843 The small ball will rebound nearly nine times the original height.

This works because momentum and energy are conserved. When the balls hit the floor, the bottom ball reverses its velocity an instant before the top one. The small ball is moving downward with speed V and strikes a large ball moving upward with speed V after the rebound, making the two balls' relative speed 2V.

If their relative speed is 2V before the top and bottom balls collide, then their relative speed must be 2V after impact. Since the bottom ball is already moving at V, that means the top ball must be moving now at 3V. Because the top ball's velocity has tripled as a result of the impact, its maximum height after the rebound is nine times its original height.

The alignment of the ball at release is very important to achieve this full height. Releasing the balls through a tube or similar arrangement will enable you to get the maximum effect.

844 The apparent rotation of a pendulum varies with the latitude at which it is installed. Its rate at points between the poles and the equator is equal to 15 degrees per hour multiplied by the sine of the latitude. This can be explained only by the fact that the earth turns beneath the pendulum.

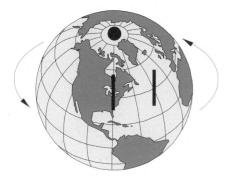

845 Surprisingly, the two pendulums will swing back and forth in the same period of time. This may seem counterintuitive, but the time of a pendulum's swing depends only on the length of the pendulum's arm. Whether it makes a long swing or a short one, the period will be the same.

The strange motion of the pendulum obeys certain laws:

1. The period of oscillation does not depend on the weight of the bobs.

2. The period does not depend upon the distance traveled.

3. The period of oscillation is proportional to the square root of the length of the pendulum.

The time for a pendulum to go through one cycle is $2\pi\sqrt{(L/g)}$, the length and g is the rate of acceleration due to gravity.

Since the acceleration due to gravity is the only variable besides the length, a pendulum is a simple way to measure the gravity of a planet. A 1-meter-long pendulum will complete a swing in about 1 second on earth and 2.5 seconds on the moon.

846 Surprisingly, the pendulums will not end up with the same amount of energy. Instead, energy will be periodically exchanged between them in such a way that sometimes one and sometimes the other of them stops.

As one of the pendulums is set in motion, after some time its energy will pass over to the other pendulum, which will gradually overtake the first swing. Eventually the first pendulum will be stationary. Then the whole procedure starts over again.

847 The woodpecker is a simple mechanical oscillator. The hole in the ring around the vertical rod is slightly larger than the diameter of the stick. When the woodpecker is at rest, friction keeps the ring in place on the rod. But when it moves, the ring becomes vertical at the midpoint of each oscillation. Because the ring is now not wedged in place, it slips down a bit along the rod. This slight drop gives enough of a jolt to the bird to keep it vibrating. So at each drop, potential energy is converted into movement—kinetic energy.

The oscillating woodpecker also demonstrates the basic principle of a grandfather clock: the simple escape mechanism.

848 Velocity is speed in a particular direction, so the velocity of the ball is constantly changing because its direction is constantly changing.

A change in velocity means acceleration. And the ball is accelerating toward the center of the circle. In fact, anything that moves in a circle accelerates toward the center of the circle. The acceleration changes the velocity just enough to make the ball follow the path of a circle.

If the string broke, the ball would move off in a straight line tangent to the circle at that point.

849 Pull out a ball on one end and release it, and another will pop off at the opposite end. If you pull two to the side and release them, two will pop out at the other end.

Can the balls count?

The collision between two bodies where relatively large forces act during a very short interval of time is called an impact. When the highly elastic steel balls collide, they exchange velocities. Faster than the eye can follow, the energy of the impact is passed along to each neighboring ball, and the ball on the end receives that energy and swings into the air.

The effect is the same regardless of the number of balls that are released. The toy demonstrates Newton's third law of motion: To every action there is always an equal and opposite reaction.

850 Place the glass over the marble and move it around so that the marble starts to spin around the inside of the glass. Once the marble starts rotating, it will begin to rise off the table. When the marble is spinning fast enough, you can lift the glass off the table. The marble will not drop immediately; it will continue to spin around under its own momentum.

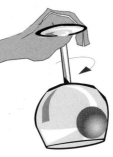

851 Suspended bodies tend to rotate around the axes of the greatest moment of inertia (see answer to PlayThink 813). This property will make the three objects rotate as shown below.

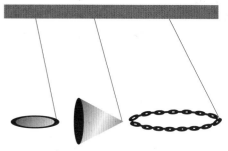

852 The stool—and the boy—will start rotating in the opposite direction. The angular momentum is conserved by having the two opposite rotations cancel out.

853 Nothing will happen! The response to the tire's angular momentum will try to drive the stool into the ground.

854 Pushing the handle forward with his right hand and backward with his left one will cause the wheel to tilt to the left.

As paradoxical as it may sound, to turn the stool, the boy must push upward on the right side of the handle and down on the left side. He will then feel the gyroscopic precession: the property of the axis of a spinning body to resist a tilting force by moving in a direction at right angle to that force. The bicycle wheel, which is no different from a gyroscope, resists the tilting force, and its axis begins to rotate at a right angle to what one might expect. The turn of the wheel to the left is transferred to the revolving stool with the boy.

A turning wheel resists any change in speed and direction. Unless you push it in some specific way, the wheel will keep spinning in the same direction. If you turn it, it tilts. If you tilt it, it turns.

Indeed, any fast-spinning object will act like a gyroscope—bicycle and motorcycle riders often experience gyroscopic effects.

855 The centripetal force caused by the rotating cylinder is perpendicular to the wall, creating friction. When the circular acceleration is high enough, the friction force can overcome the force of gravity and prevent the carnival riders from falling when the floor is removed.

856 Golf balls always fly with backspin. The dimples trap a layer of air that spins the ball. The top layer of trapped air moves faster than the bottom layer, giving the ball greater lift. This is called Bernoulli's principle, which is also the basis of airplane flight.

A smooth golf ball would travel about half the distance that a dimpled golf ball can cover.

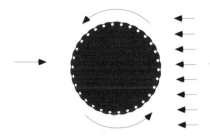

857 The skater will spin much faster. By bringing her arms to her chest, she decreases the moment of inertia of her body because more of her weight is now concentrated near the center. To compensate for this, there is an increase in her angular velocity. If the spin becomes too fast for her, she can stretch her arms back out to slow down.

All moving objects have energy of movement, or kinetic energy. The kinetic energy stored by something spinning depends on two things: the way its weight is distributed and how fast it spins.

Flywheels utilize this idea, though in the opposite way. They are designed to store as much energy as possible when they spin. Most of their weight, therefore, is concentrated near the rim.

858 The ball will miss the juggler and land to the right of him.

The trajectory will appear to be curved because the jugglers are in motion themselves. The ball will not even start toward the other juggler because it carries the thrower's velocity, which further deflects the ball to the right. This deflection, called the Coriolis effect, is associated with things in a turning frame of reference. There is even a slight Coriolis effect on everything that moves around us because the earth itself is turning.

Although the two jugglers see the ball curve, an outside observer will report that it went straight.

859 Every dimension of the washer will expand, so the hole will get larger too.

860 The branching pattern is more economical than the radial pattern. The branching pattern has a much shorter total length than the radial pattern, at the expense of only a slightly longer average path length. Thus, trees, blood vessels, rivers and even subway networks are all examples of branching patterns.

861 Arrangements 1 and 3 are in equilibrium.

862 The pressure inside a bubble decreases with increasing size. It is inversely proportional to the radius. Thus, the smaller bubble has more internal pressure than the larger one; it will send air through the passageway and into the larger bubble and will shrink as the larger bubble expands. Thus, paradoxically, the smaller bubble will blow up the larger one, collapsing in the process.

This is quite unexpected and different from a similar experiment that involves blowing up two balloons.

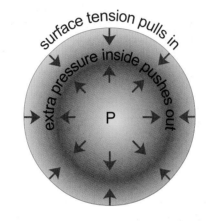

surface tension pulls in
extra pressure inside pushes out
P

863 Since the lines radiating from John's shot are the source for the others that branch off from them, John was first.

864 The shortest route along the cracks is 13 units long.

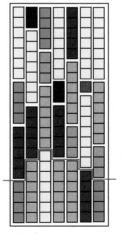

865 The end of the strip under the paper will not move. In fact, if you strike the wood hard enough, it may snap, but the newspaper won't budge.

The weight of the atmosphere presses on the newspaper and resists being squeezed up suddenly. This holds the stick firmly to the table.

The pressure of air is 1 kilogram on every square centimeter. The force of air pressure on the newspaper—about 2.25 metric tons over its entire surface—is strong enough to hold the newspaper and stick firmly in place for the split second it takes you to break the stick.

866 When you push the plungers together, you remove most of the air between their cups. The air on the outside presses in on the plungers and forces them together.

867 The pressure of the air in the balloon increases as you blow into it—but so does the counterpressure of the air enclosed in the bottle.

The air around the balloon inside the bottle takes up a certain amount of space and has nowhere to escape. As you try to inflate the balloon, the balloon compresses the air inside the bottle until the inside air pressure becomes so great that you cannot inflate the balloon any further.

868 Bernoulli's principle shows that the train carries low-pressure air around it, and atmospheric pressure may force you toward the train.

869 The balls will actually move toward each other. The air moving between the balls has a lower pressure than the surrounding air, which pushes the two balls together.

This is a simple demonstration of the Bernoulli's principle, which links air speed and air pressure. This is also the basis of airplane flight.

870 It takes longer to drop than to fly up.

The ball has to work against air resistance on its way up and so continuously loses energy. Thus, the total energy of a ball at a point on its way up is greater than its energy at the same height on its way down. Since the potential energy (its energy due to its height) is the same at both instances, the difference in energy must be due to a reduced kinetic energy. That means the falling ball is moving more slowly and will take more time to cover the same distance.

871 The wings of an airplane are designed so that air will rush across their upper surface faster than it rushes past the lower surface. For this reason the top surface of the wings is made longer than the bottom.

As described in Bernoulli's principle, that extra speed lowers the pressure above the wings, producing a net force from below called lift. That force keeps the airplane in the air as it moves forward. When an airplane is in midflight, the combined weight of the plane, fuel, passengers and cargo exerts a heavy pull downward. However, that total weight is overcome by the lift, allowing the airplane to remain airborne.

872 The lightweight Ping-Pong ball will rise very quickly in still water.

But when the water is agitated, the buoyancy of the ball is drastically reduced. The movement of the liquid produces higher pressures that make the displacement of the water by the ball more difficult.

873 Your thumb prevents the surrounding air from entering one end of the tube. The open end of the tube allows air to enter and press down on the water on that side. The weight of the air pressing down on the water prevents the level from returning to its initial balanced position.

This is a simple proof that air has weight.

874 According to Archimedes's principle, an object floats because it displaces an amount of water equal to the weight of the object. So to float when the ring was placed on it, the duck must displace a volume of water that equals the weight of the ring.

Since the metal ring is denser than water, the volume of the displaced water is greater than the volume of the ring. When the ring falls in the water and sinks, it displaces only its own volume of water.

The water level, then, drops when the ring slips off the duck and into the tub.

875 Rapidly moving air has low pressure, and a column of upward-rushing air can actually imprison a lightweight object like a Ping-Pong ball. As soon as the ball wobbles a bit to one side, the greater pressure outside of the airstream forces the ball back to the middle.

876 The stream of air creates a low-pressure area, drawing the flames together.

877 You can attain a speed of nearly 40 kilometers per hour. If the forces of water friction on the boat were 0, you could attain the speed of the wind, but no higher.

If the boat were traveling as fast as the wind, there would be no impact of air against the sail. The sail would sag, as on a windless day, because there would be no wind relative to the sail.

878 This configuration will decrease the speed of the boat for two reasons. First, the impact of the wind against the sail is lessened because the sail catches less wind at such angles. Second, the direction of the wind impact force is not in the direction of the boat's motion, as shown in the parallelogram of forces.

Whenever any fluid—gas or liquid—interacts with a smooth surface, the force of interaction is perpendicular to the surface. Not only is this magnitude of force smaller than what it would be if the wind were hitting the sail face on, but only a fraction of the force is directed along the direction of the boat's motion. That's the component that drives the boat forward. The other component simply tips the boat.

As the sail is pulled farther in, this force vector decreases until it reaches 0, when the sail is pulled in so that it is parallel to the keel.

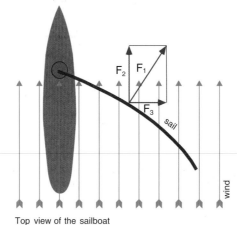

Top view of the sailboat

879 You can go faster. The force vector is greater because the sail doesn't catch up with the wind speed, so it will not eventually sag.

Even when the boat is traveling as fast as the wind, there is still an impact of wind against the sail, so it can sail even faster than the wind. The boat will reach its maximum speed when the relative wind—the vector made by the natural wind and the "artificial wind" caused by the boat's motion through the air—is directed parallel to the sail.

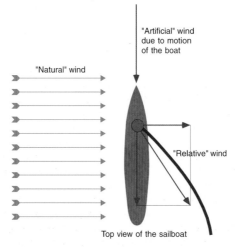

"Artificial" wind due to motion of the boat

"Natural" wind

"Relative" wind

Top view of the sailboat

880 Surprisingly, only boat 4 will move in a forward direction, even though it is sailing into the wind.

The force vector has a small component that will propel the boat. In fact, the faster the boat travels, the greater the force of the wind's impact. As counterintuitive as it may seem, a sailboat's maximum speed comes at an angle upwind. The boat cannot sail directly into the wind, so to reach a straight upwind destination, it has to zigzag back and forth. That strategy is called tacking.

881 As tricky as the problem sounds, there is exactly the same amount of milk in the tea as there is tea in the milk. As you can see in the diagram above, the total volume in each glass is unchanged by the transfer; the net volume transferred from glass A to glass B exactly cancels that which went from glass B to glass A.

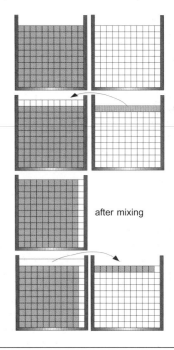

after mixing

882 When you stick your finger in the water, your finger takes the place of some of the water, and so the water level goes up.

Your finger not only takes the place of some of the water but also stands in for the weight of that water. The glass weighs more, by the weight of that displaced water. The weight of the object displacing the water is not a factor; it could be a balloon or a lead cylinder.

883 The ship will float as long as there is enough water to surround it completely. The amount of water does not matter. The ship's hull cannot tell whether it is surrounded by an ocean or by just a thin layer of water. The water pressure on the hull is the same in both cases.

To float, the ship must displace its weight in water. The displacement refers to the water that would fill the ship's hull if the inside of the ship's hull were filled to the waterline.

This principle is exploited at the Mount Palomar Observatory, where the 550-metric-ton telescope actually floats on a thin cushion of oil.

884 The small bottle will drop. The pressure exerted on a confined liquid is transmitted in all directions. When you squeeze the big bottle, you increase the pressure on the water. The air bubble in the small bottle is compressed and gets smaller. As more water rises into the small bottle, it sinks to a depth where water pressure is greater. When you loosen your grip on the large bottle, the pressure is released and the small bottle rises to its original position.

885 Fill the glass with water until it forms a convex lip above the rim. Then place the cork in the glass. The cork will seek the highest point, which is now in the middle, and stay there.

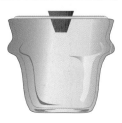

886 Large raindrops fall faster. A falling drop is subject to two opposing forces—gravity and air resistance. Air resistance is proportional to the drop's cross section, and it increases with velocity. At first, the slowing effect of air resistance is very small, and the drop keeps falling faster because of the constant force of gravity. As the speed increases, so does air resistance—until the speed is so great that the force of air resistance equally opposes the force of gravity. From that point the drop starts falling at a uniform speed, the so-called terminal velocity.

The force of gravity grows in proportion to the drop's volume, which is the cube of the radius. On the other hand, air resistance builds up at the cross-section area of the drop, which is the square of the radius. As the drop's radius increases, the force of gravity increases faster than the opposing force of air resistance. The drop can reach a greater terminal velocity before the air resistance catches up with it.

887 The water level will stay exactly as before.

The weight of the water displaced by the iceberg exactly equals the weight of the iceberg. When the iceberg melts, it turns back into water and fills the volume of water it displaced.

The volume of the iceberg above the water must exactly equal the increased volume of the water that froze and expanded to become ice.

888 When the bottle is inverted, the paper will bulge a bit. That bulge causes a change in the volume of the air inside the bottle. According to Boyle's law, any change of volume is accompanied by a change in pressure. What is really surprising is that such a small change in volume as that caused by the bulge in the card is sufficient to drop the pressure enough to prevent water from pouring out.

It should be noted that the necessary change in volume is easier to achieve when the bottle is nearly full.

889 The speed of the flow depends on how far below the surface the outlet is located. The depth is the same for both outlets, so water will leave both holes at the same speed.

890 The 6-centimeter drain has a cross section that is three times that of the total for the three smaller drains, so it will drain three times as fast.

891 The current will flow backward. The flow actually speeds up through the narrow passage but slows down where the channel widens. Where does that excess speed go? The water sheds the speed by flowing uphill. The water flows back around behind the rock from a section of lower elevation to one of slightly higher elevation.

Such backwaters create dangerous turbulence behind boulders in fast rivers.

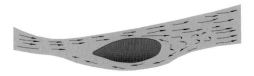

892 The last time I tried this, I was able to add fifty-two pennies to a supposedly full cup of water before it overflowed.

Water has a high surface tension. It behaves as though it had a flexible skin on its surface; that skin pulls inward and resists breaking. Not only can a glass of water develop a great bulge before it flows over the edge of the container, but the surface tension can support the weight of light objects. If you place a clean razor blade flat against the surface of a glass of water, the blade can actually "float"—not because of buoyancy but because of the support of surface tension.

893 The distance the water will squirt depends on the exit speed of the water out of the hole multiplied by the time it takes the water to reach the table. The middle hole has the greatest range because speed increases with the square root of the water depth (because of water pressure), while time increases with the square root of the distance to the surface. This product is highest at the halfway point.

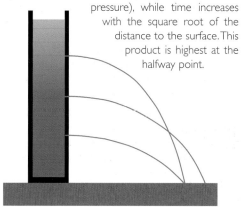

894 The stream will follow the curve of the spoon; that's called the Coanda effect.

On a microscopic scale, a minuscule electrostatic force is generated when two molecules come close, a force that tends to draw the molecules together. This attraction, called the van der Waals force, is the reason why poured liquids often dribble down the side of a glass rather than exit cleanly over the side.

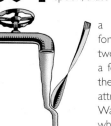

895 If the flow of water is continuous, the volume of water that is discharged is constant along the entire stream. The same volume of water per second must pass through any given cross section of the stream, including the top and the bottom. But as the velocity of the falling water increases (because of the acceleration due to gravity) the cross section of the stream becomes thinner.

896 The air pressure at the moving end of the tube is lower than the pressure at the end being held. That pressure difference causes the air to flow through the tube, and the air vibrates as it passes over the corrugated walls of the tube.

897 The path is shortest when angles A and B are equal, as shown below. (This is the same as the reflection of light off a mirror.) In fact, if the cowboy imagined that the wagon was on the other side of the riverbank but the same distance from it, he could ride toward that point to reach the proper spot to water his horse.

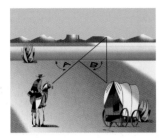

898 As the container fills with water, the coin will come into view.

Light travels at different speeds through different substances. It travels more slowly through water or glass than it does through air. When light passes across the border between two different "speed zones," it changes direction. This change in direction is called refraction; it makes light rays look like they "bend" at the point where two substances meet.

When the light from the coin reaches the surface of the water, it is bent back toward your eyes. But since your brain does not sense what is happening, you perceive the light as coming from a place that is higher and farther back than the coin actually is.

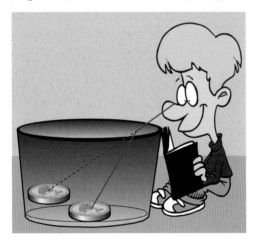

899 The magnification will actually decrease. The amount by which a lens can bend rays of light depends on both the curvature of the glass and the difference in the speed of light between air and glass. The difference in speed from water to glass is less than that between air and glass, so the lens will not bend the light as powerfully and therefore will not magnify the image as much.

900 Because the sun is so large, the shadow will be smaller, but the difference in size is imperceptible. But if the sun is at an angle to the shadow surface, such as an hour or less before sunset, the shadow can be much larger.

Light rays from a distant object may appear parallel, but this is not necessarily the case. If the light source is larger than the object, the shadow (on a flat surface perpendicular to the light source) will be smaller. If the light source is smaller than the object, then the shadow will be larger. The difference in size, however, is scarcely perceptible if the distance between the two objects is great.

901 The angle will remain 15 degrees. Some measurements do not change when dimensions are magnified.

902 It doesn't matter how far you are from the mirror, as long as it is hung at the correct height—with the lower edge at half the height of the eyes of the person looking in the mirror.

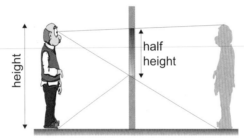

half height

height

903 The ancient Greek geometer Euclid also studied optics. Euclid found that light travels through space along straight lines, and he laid down the fundamental laws of reflection:

- The plane of incidence of the ray coincides with its plane of reflection.

- The angle of incidence of the ray equals its angle of reflection (in the diagram, angle a = angle b).

- Light always travels via the shortest path.

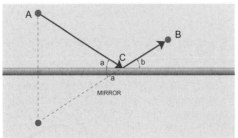

904

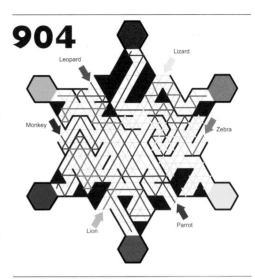

Leopard   Lizard

Monkey   Zebra

Lion   Parrot

905 In the water container—because at 20° F, water is frozen solid.

906 One way to route the light rays is shown; ten mirrors have been rotated.

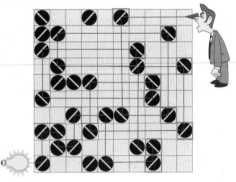

907 Scientists and historians have long dismissed the story as an impossible feat. But over the centuries a few enthusiasts have tried to prove otherwise. Rather than using one giant mirror, these people say, Archimedes created the effect of a large mirror by using a great number of small reflectors that were aligned in the proper way. The highly polished shields of the Syracuse army may have done the job, they say.

But even if Archimedes lined up his men and had them focus the sun's rays on the Roman ships, was it physically possible for the ships to catch fire?

In 1747 the French naturalist Georges-Louis Leclerc de Buffon conducted an experiment using 168 ordinary rectangular flat mirrors. Aligning them in just the right way, he was able to ignite a piece of wood at a distance of about 100 meters. The port of Syracuse was not nearly that large; the Roman ships were probably less than 20 meters from land.

A Greek engineer conducted a similar experiment in 1973, employing 70 mirrors to focus sunlight on a rowboat some 80 meters from shore. Within a few seconds after the mirrors were properly aligned, the boat burst into flames. Those mirrors were slightly concave, but it is likely that Archimedes could have built such mirrors.

908 Three meters.
The image of the flower in the hand mirror is as far behind that mirror as the flower is in front of it: .5 meter. That puts the image of the flower .5 + .5 + 2, or 3 meters, in front of the large mirror, so that is the distance behind the large mirror that its reflected image forms.

CHAPTER 13 SOLUTIONS

909 Your scorecard should look like the chart below. The visual shortcut requires turning the page upside down. That makes the missing cubes appear solid.

SCORE BOX

Missing Cubes	1	2	3	4	5
Cubes colored on three sides	1	1	1	1	1
Cubes colored on two sides	6	3	6	6	10
Cubes colored on one side	12	3	12	12	19
Cubes not colored	7	0	1	0	6
TOTALS	26	7	20	19	36

910 1, concave; 2, convex; 3, skewed; 4, bent

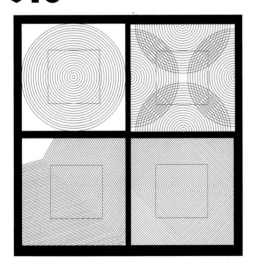

911 Dots, number 9; arrows, number 7; semicircles, number 5.
The Illusion Wheel was inspired by one of the simplest and most striking optical illusions, the so-called Müller-Lyer illusion and its variants.

912 To make the butterfly disappear, close your right eye and stare at the red dot with your left eye. From a certain distance, the circle containing the butterfly should disappear, and the line should appear to be continuous. The disappearance of the butterfly is sudden and striking.
This illusion is due to a phenomenon called the blind spot. Researchers have shown that one eye cannot cover the entire visual field. There are no visual receptors over an area of about 1.5 millimeters in diameter at the place where the optic nerve enters the retina.
When the incomplete signal from the eye reaches the brain, the brain uses simple rules to calculate what the blind spot of the retina ought to be seeing. In this case the brain extrapolates between the two black lines and deduces that it is one straight line and fills the gap. Although the brain behaves in this way to enable us to make sense of the world, sometimes this property can be exploited to make nonsense, such as illusions.

913 Stare at the red bird for a minute and then look at the center of the birdcage. You will see an illusory afterimage—a green bird—in the cage.
There are three types of color receptors in the eye—one each for red, green and blue. The red of the bird in the picture causes the red receptors to adapt, temporarily decreasing their sensibility to red. Since the figure does not reflect much green or blue light, receptors for those colors become considerably more sensitive. When you shift your gaze to the gray area, the effect of adaptation makes your green and blue receptors overly sensitive—and the red receptors dulled—and therefore you see the gray area temporarily as green.
In short, afterimages are a signal that our visual receptors have become fatigued from seeing too much of the same color.

914 Stare at the black knight for a while, then look at the gray area at right. You'll see the afterimage reversal—a white knight on a black horse.

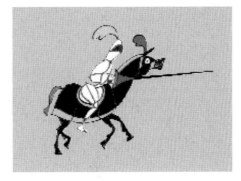

915 It's always the one you are looking at. Look steadily at the pattern, and you'll see a positive afterimage effect that results in an illusion of small gray spots at the intersections. But if you try to look directly at a spot, the new visual information from the center of your field of vision erases the afterimage effect—and the spot.

916 The blue lid fits the red coffin, and the red lid fits the blue coffin.

917 When you look at the page at a very slanted angle along the direction of the two lines, a third or even fourth line appears as a strong illusion. Such optical effects and illusions appear when two lines or a group of lines intersect at very small angles.

918 You have supervision, just like Superman, since you can close the gap and the bridge simply by looking at it. All you have to do is look squint-eyed at the picture from a distance.

919

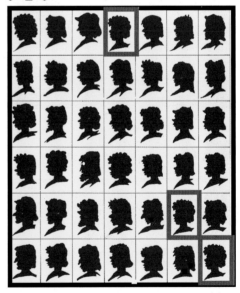

920 A palace guard. If you can't make it out, stand about 1 meter from the picture and squint.
There are more than 120 million photoreceptors that split up the images projected on the retina into point-sized messages—not unlike newspaper pictures printed in halftone dots, computer monitors broken into pixels, and pointillistic paintings.

921 Position number 5 is in direct line with the tank.

922
The missing slice of cake can be found by turning the picture upside-down.

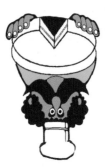

923
When seen with squinting eyes from three or four feet away, the pattern resolves into the famous smile of the Mona Lisa.

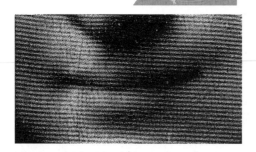

924
The pairs are 1-8, 4-10 and 7-5. The set of three is 2-3-9. The odd one out is 6.

925
The letters in the words at the bottom all have horizontal symmetry. For such an image, a reflection is the same as a 180-degree rotation. The rotation is more easily perceived because the image still spells out recognizable English words.

926
The fly can be in one of three positions:

1. On the outside of the box, on the checkered vertical side facing you.

2. On the outside of the box, on the bottom.

3. On the inside, on the checkered floor.

927
Just turn the picture upside-down.

CHAPTER 14 SOLUTIONS

928
Building 1—Blueprint 11 (top view)
Building 2—Blueprint 9 (top)
Building 3—Blueprint 13 (top)
Building 4—Blueprint 5 (top)
Building 5—Blueprint 7 (top)
Building 6—Blueprint 16 (front view)
Building 7—Blueprint 8 (front)
Building 8—Blueprint 15 (front)

929
The design shown below requires only twelve outlets.

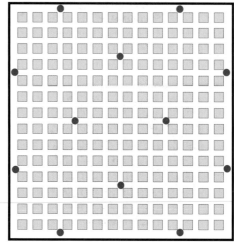

930
Through trial and error, you can determine that the three groups of nine tracks can be arranged 3, 3 and 3 (for 27 intersections), 2, 3 and 4 (for 26 intersections) or the minimal solution, shown, of 2, 2 and 5 (for 24 intersections).

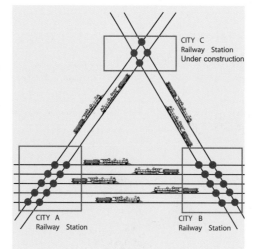

931

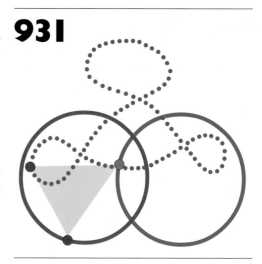

932

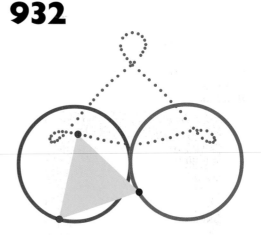

933
It is problematic to solve this sort of problem by looking at the three-dimensional figure; some corners and edges will always be hidden. Instead, one can create a topologically equivalent two-dimensional diagram, such as this one, on which to work out the solution.

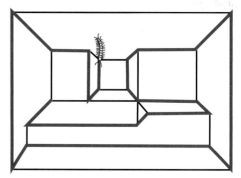

934 A circle can be divided into any number of regions of equal area using a compass and a ruler. Simply divide the diameter into the number of equal divisions required and from those points draw semicircles, as shown.

Ancient Chinese mathematicians knew of this method; the yin-yang is an example.

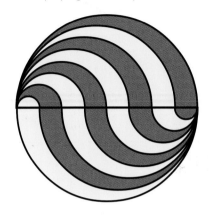

935

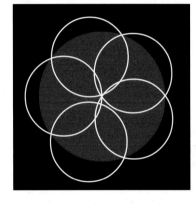

936 This is the best solution found so far.

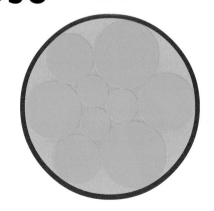

937 One possible answer is shown below. If the puzzle had required you to traverse each line once and only once, it would have been impossible!

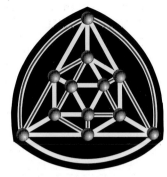

938 One of many solutions.

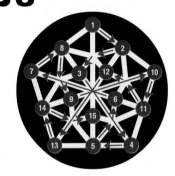

939 The results are independent of the way the smaller shapes intrude on the larger. After all, the overlap is removed from both the red and blue areas. Therefore, one easy method for comparing the red and blue areas is to find the difference between the sum of the areas of the smaller shapes and the area of the largest shape.

Circles ($r^2\pi$): Red and blue areas are equal.

Squares (a^2): Blue area is larger.

Triangles ($\frac{a^2}{4}\sqrt{3}$): Sum of the red areas is larger.

940 To take into account the worst possible scenario (five red, five yellow, five green and one blue), you must grab sixteen wires.

941 These triangles can overlap to form as many as nineteen regions.

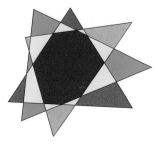

942 For whichever of the seven horses comes in first, there are six different horses that can come in second; for each of the forty-two different combinations of first- and second-place horses, there are five different horses that can come in third. That means there are 7 × 6 × 5, or 210, different combinations of horses.

943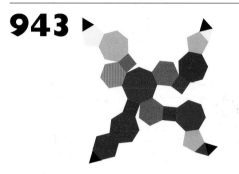

944 The number of nonrepeating three-letter combinations are

26 × 25 × 24, or 15,600

That means his chances are .0064 percent.

945 The red region is two-thirds the area of the original triangle.

946 There must be at least two such boys.

947 The answer can be found by simple multiplication: 26 × 10 × 10 × 10 × 26 × 26 × 26, or 456,976,000.

948 There are fifteen unique pairs of dogs. If the dogs are named, say, A, B, C, D, E and F, the possible pairs are: AB, AC, AD, AE, AF, BC, BD, BE, BF, CD, CE, CF, DE, DF and EF.

949 The eight groups represent the eight possible ways to create different triplets of the numbers 1 through 9 that add up to 15.

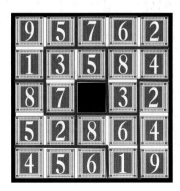

950 These sixteen combinations of four numbers are part of a larger set of eighty-six possible combinations of numbers from 1 through 16 that total 34.

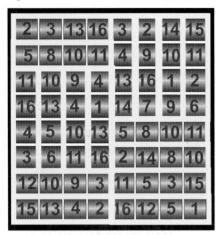

951 Four colors are needed, as shown.

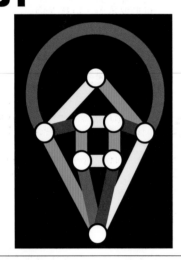

952 Eight.

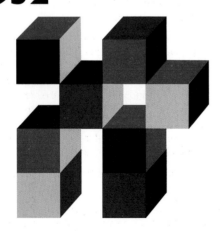

953

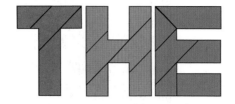

954 The color of each circle is determined by the number of other circles it touches.

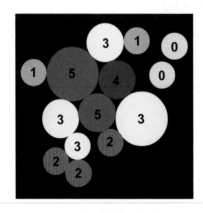

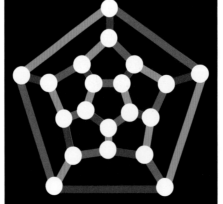

955 Only three colors are necessary, as shown.

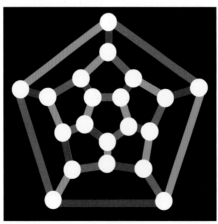

956

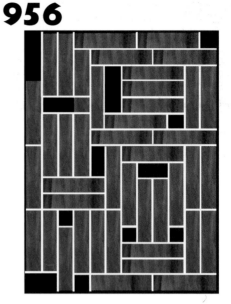

957 Each spot on the robot's electronic display can either show 1, 2, 3 or be blank. That means it can show three different one-digit numbers:

1, 2, 3

nine different two-digit numbers:

11, 12, 13, 21, 22, 23, 31, 32, 33,

and twenty-seven different three-digit numbers:

111, 112, 113, 121, 122, 123, 131, 132, 133, 211, 212, 213, 221, 222, 223, 231, 232, 233, 311, 312, 313, 321, 322, 323, 331, 332, 333

for a total of thirty-nine numbers.
    You can solve this easily with this formula:

$$3 + 3^2 + 3^3 = 39$$

958 The Pythagorean theorem ensures that the areas are exactly equal. Two radii of a pair of touching quarter circles are at right angles to each other, and the radius of the matching quarter circle stretches across the hypotenuse, completing the right triangle.

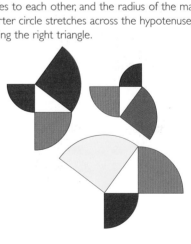

959

As shown, there are fifteen different ways to distribute four pieces of fruit over four plates.

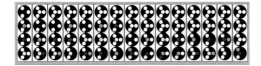

960

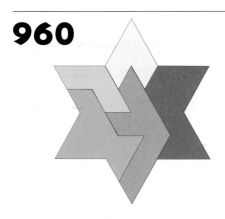

961

This sequence of numbers details the number of new pairs of rabbits produced each month, starting with the first new pair born in January. The total number of pairs is 376.

Jan	Feb	Mar	Apr	May	Jun	Jul	Aug	Sep	Oct	Nov	Dec
1	2	1	3	5	8	13	21	34	55	89	144

962

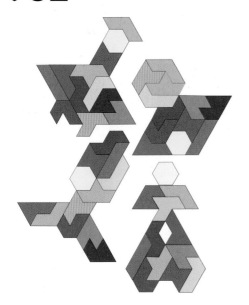

963

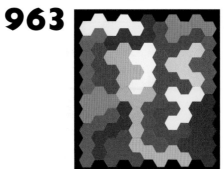

964

COLUMN 1	COLUMN 2
1	3
2	4
5	6

COLUMN 1	COLUMN 2
1	3
2	4
6	5

As you can see in the first diagram, it doesn't matter where player 1 places the 5 because player 2 wins when placing the 6.

COLUMN 1	COLUMN 2
1	3
2	5
4	6
8	7

In the second diagram you can see it is always impossible to place the 9.

965

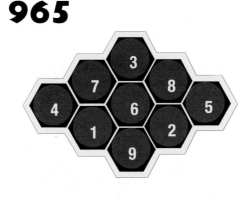

966

The total number of soldiers plus the general must be a square number. The smallest square that is also equal to 1 plus a multiple of eleven is 100, which is $9 \times 11 + 1$.

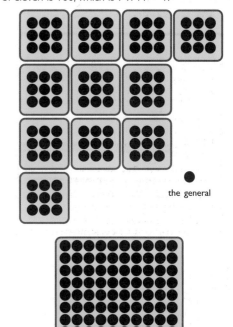

the general

967

The general answer to this problem, called the hailstone problem because of the way the numbers cycle in much the same way as hailstones growing in a thundercloud, is not known. But none of the numbers up to 26 survive for long. Beginning with 7, you get:

7, 22, 11, 34, 17, 52, 26, 13, 40, 20, 10, 5, 16, 8, 4, 2, 1, 4 and so on

The number 27 takes an interesting journey, making it up to 9,232 at step 77 before crashing. It reaches the 1-4-2-1-4-2 loop in step 111. Every number up to a trillion has been tested, and every one eventually collapses into the rut.

968

The area of the one gold square of the first generation is simply ⅑ the area of the original blue. The area of the eight gold squares of the second generation is ⅑ the area of the smaller blue squares, which themselves are ⅑ the area of the original. The third generation finds sixty-four gold squares, each of which is $(\frac{1}{9})^3$ the area of the original blue square. The pattern emerges:

$$1 \times \frac{1}{9} + 8 \times (\frac{1}{9})^2 + 8^2 \times (\frac{1}{9})^3 + 8^3 \times (\frac{1}{9})^4 + \ldots$$

If you carry out the calculation to the twenty-fifth generation, you will find that gold covers an area equal to almost 95 percent of the original blue square. It's clear that the area of the gold will come increasingly close to 100 percent of the original square, but it will never reach total coverage.

969 Counting from the top, the nth plank can have an overhang relative to the plank immediately below it equal to ½n meters. This leads to the sequence ½, ¼, ⅙, ⅛, ⅒, 1/12, 1/14, 1/16; the corresponding overhangs are .500, .250, .167, .125, .100, .83, .71 and .62 meters. The total overhang is then 1.358 meters—just shy of the cheese.

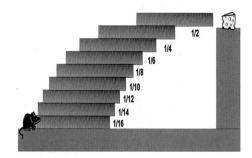

970 I got the inspiration for this puzzle during a lecture by American mathematician and logician Raymond Smullyan. As he explained, the answer is simple: the young man simply asks, "Are you married?"

Regardless of who answers his question, he knows that a "yes" means that Amelia is married and a "no" means Leila is married. Virtuous Amelia will tell him the truth—"yes" if she is, "no" if Leila is—no matter what, and wicked Leila will say "no" if she is married and "yes" if she is single and Amelia is married.

971 You simply move each guest into the room with the number that is twice that of the room he or she is in now. The person in room 1 goes to room 2, the person in room 2 goes to room 4, the person in room 3 goes to room 6 and so on. All the odd-numbered rooms will be vacated, and since there are an infinite number of odd numbers, all your new guests can be accommodated.

972 You should ask him, "Which way to your hometown?"

If he is from Truth City, he'll point to it; if he is from Lies City, he will also point to Truth City.

973

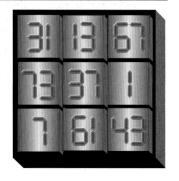

974

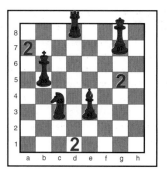

975 You should ask, "Am I in Las Wages?" and "Am I in Las Wages?"

Two yeses will come from a truth teller; two nos from a liar. And a yes and a no will mean that the person alternated between truth and lie.

976 The largest sum you can see on any given die is 15, that is, the sum of 4, 5 and 6. Therefore, the only possible combinations of three different numbers that total 40 are 15 + 14 + 11 and 15 + 13 + 12. But a sum of 13 is impossible to see on the three faces of a real die. (Try it if you doubt this.) That leaves the only answer as 15, 14 and 11, as shown.

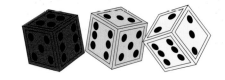

977 This is a classic game, here in a form suggested by Peter Gabor. There are six Fs. The Fs in of are easy to overlook.

978 Although the coin has an equal chance of landing on heads after every throw, the player who tosses first has a decided advantage, no matter how long the game lasts. The probability that the first player will win is the sum of the probabilities that occur at every turn:

$$\tfrac{1}{2} + (\tfrac{1}{2})^3 + (\tfrac{1}{2})^5 + (\tfrac{1}{2})^7 + \ldots$$

This is a series with an infinite number of terms that approaches two-thirds in value. Therefore, the player who tosses first has a chance of winning that is almost twice that of the second player. If you are surprised at this result, play a number of games and keep track of who comes out on top.

979 Simply multiply together the chances that each ball thrown will land in an empty box:

$$\tfrac{4}{4} \times \tfrac{3}{4} \times \tfrac{2}{4} \times \tfrac{1}{4} = \tfrac{6}{64} = 0.09$$

That means there is roughly one chance in ten that each of the four boxes will contain a single ball.

The general formula for this problem is $n!/n^n$.

980 The first spinner is always the best to choose. Against the third spinner, the first spinner will win 51 percent of the time because its 3 will beat the third spinner's 1. The second spinner has a higher average spin (3.33), but the 3 on the first spinner beats the second spinner's 2, which comes up 56 percent of the time.

981

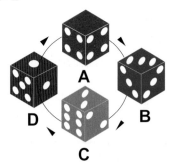

When two six-sided dice are thrown against each other, there are thirty-six possible outcomes. The table below shows the results of die C versus die D: C wins twenty-four times, D wins just twelve. Similar results can be found with D versus A, A versus B, and B versus C. No matter what die your opponent selects, you can pick the die to its immediate left (or D if your opponent chooses A) and win two out of every three times.

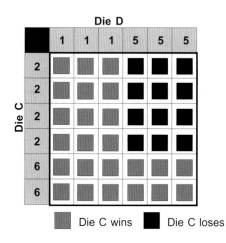

	Die D					
	1	1	1	5	5	5
2						
2						
2						
2						
6						
6						

■ Die C wins   ■ Die C loses

982 The result is two bands—one with a right-hand twist, one with a left-hand twist.

983 You will get an ordinary square "ring"— two sides, two edges and no twists.

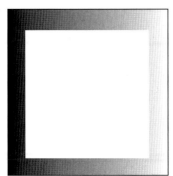

984 The structure is made up of two separate pieces and could be pulled apart.

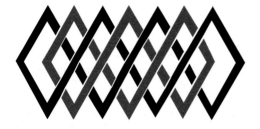

985

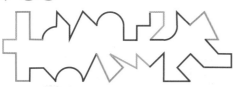

987 The diagram shows all the possible orientations, starting with point 1. As you can see, a right triangle is formed eighteen out of twenty-one times, which means the probability is ⅚.

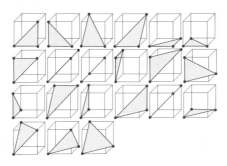

988 The minimal path is a tree—a graph with no closed loops—on which lines are joined together at angles of 120 degrees to one another. For large numbers of points, it is difficult to predict the minimal path. Interestingly, though, a three-dimensional model immersed in a soapy solution will give the solution for even the most complex configurations in an instant.

The five-town solution was provided by Nick Baxter.

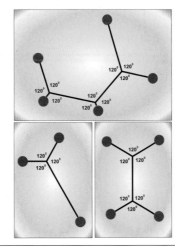

989 As the double cone seemingly rolls "upward," the increasing width of the tracks actually lowers the center of gravity of the cone. In spite of what we think we see, the double cone is actually rolling downhill.

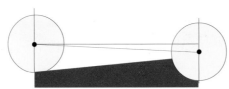

990 If the objects to be weighed are on one pan and the weights on the other, you must have weights of 1, 2, 4, 8, 16 and 32 grams. But if the weights can be on either pan, then a smaller set of masses may be employed: 1, 3, 9 and 27 grams. Claude-Gaspar Bachet first worked out this solution in 1623.

991 The water levels will be as shown here. Where the water flows the fastest, the water pressure will be the lowest and push the water up with the least force. As you can see, the water will flow the fastest in the narrowest part of the pipe.

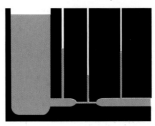

992 In fact, the Pythagorean theorem is valid not only for hexagons and squares but for any set of geometrically similar figures.

Schmerl found a five-piece solution to his problem (shown below, left and right) and American mathematician Greg Frederickson found a "sneaky" four-piece solution. Both are shown.

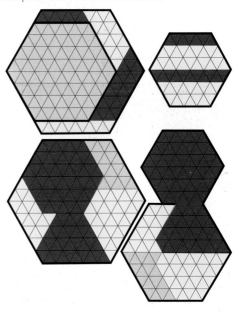

993

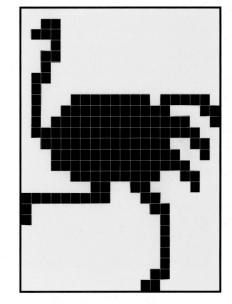

994

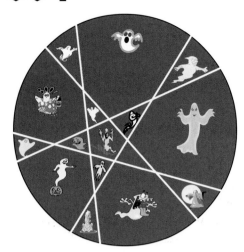

995

There are 21 possible pairs among seven birds. You can use such a list to systematically work out a foraging schedule:

Day 1: 1, 2, 3, involving the pairs 1-2, 1-3 and 2-3

Day 2: 1, 4, 5, involving the pairs 1-4, 1-5 and 4-5

Day 3: 1, 6, 7, involving the pairs 1-6, 1-7 and 6-7

Day 4: 2, 4, 6, involving the pairs 2-4, 2-6 and 4-6

Day 5: 2, 5, 7, involving the pairs 2-5, 2-7 and 5-7

Day 6: 3, 4, 7, involving the pairs 3-4, 3-7 and 4-7

Day 7: 3, 5, 6, involving the pairs 3-5, 3-6 and 5-6

996

In the linked tubes, the water level will be the same. Pressure is independent of the volume or shape of the tube and depends only on the height of the liquid. This is called the hydrostatic paradox.

997

The eleventh square will have sides of 32 units. For every two steps in the progression, the length of the sides doubles.

998

There is less than a 2 percent chance:

$$\tfrac{6}{6} \times \tfrac{5}{6} \times \tfrac{4}{6} \times \tfrac{3}{6} \times \tfrac{2}{6} \times \tfrac{1}{6} = 0.015,$$
or 1.5 percent

999

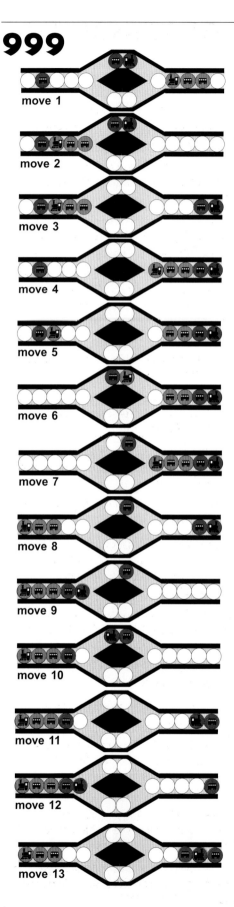

1000

There are exactly eight possibilities for the product of three ages to be 36:

Son 1	Son 2	Son 3	Product	Sum
1	1	36	36	38
1	2	18	36	21
1	3	12	36	16
1	4	9	36	14
1	6	6	36	13
2	2	9	36	13
2	3	6	36	11
3	3	4	36	10

Since Ivan could not solve the problem when he knew the sum of the three numbers—the date of the encounter—that meant the sum must have been 13, for which there are two possibilities. The added information about the youngest son means that one of the possibilities—a nine-year-old and two two-year-olds—can be ruled out, since there is no one youngest son in that case.

That left Ivan with one solution: 1, 6 and 6.

REFERENCES

Ball, W. W.; Rouse, and H.S.M. Coxeter. *Mathematical Recreations & Essays.* New York: Dover Publications, 1987.

Barbeau, Edward J.; Murray S. Klamkin; and William O. Moser. *Five Hundred Mathematical Challenges.* Washington, D.C.: The Mathematical Association of America, 1995.

Barr, Stephen. *Experiments in Topology.* New York: Dover Publications, 1989.

———. *Mathematical Brain Benders: Second Miscellany of Puzzles.* New York: Dover Publications, 1982.

Berlekamp, Elwyn, and Tom Rodgers. *The Mathemagician and Pied Puzzles: A Collection in Tribute to Martin Gardner.* Natick, Mass.: A. K. Peters, 1999.

Berlekamp, Elwyn R.; John H. Conway; and Richard K. Guy. *Winning Ways for Your Mathematical Plays.* Natick, Mass.: A. K. Peters, 2001.

Bodycombe, David J. *The Mammoth Book of Brainstorming Puzzles.* London: Constable Robinson, 1996.

———. *The Mammoth Puzzle Carnival.* New York: Carroll and Graf, 1997.

Brecher, Erwin. *Surprising Science Puzzles.* New York: Sterling Publishing, 1996.

Burger, Edward B., and Michael Starbird. *The Heart of Mathematics: An Invitation to Effective Thinking.* New York: Springer-Verlag, 2000.

Case, Adam. *Who Tells the Truth?: A Collection of Logical Puzzles to Make You Think.* Suffolk, UK: Tarquin Publications, 1991.

Comap. *For All Practical Purposes: Introduction to Contemporary Mathematics.* New York: W. H. Freeman and Company, 1988.

Conway, John H., and Richard K. Guy. *The Book of Numbers.* New York: Copernicus Books, 1997.

Cundy, H. M., and A. P. Rollett. *Mathematical Models.* Suffolk, UK: Tarquin Publications, 1997.

Devlin, Keith. *Mathematics: The Science of Patterns: The Search for Order in Life, Mind, and the Universe.* Scientific American Paperback Library. New York: W. H. Freeman and Company, 1997.

Dewdney, A. K. *The Armchair Universe: An Exploration of Computer Worlds.* New York: W. H. Freeman and Company, 1988.

Dudeney, Henry Ernest. *Amusements in Mathematics.* New York: Dover Publications, 1958.

Epstein, Lewis Carroll. *Thinking Physics: Is Gedanken Physics; Practical Lessons in Critical Thinking.* San Francisco: Insight Press, 1985.

Fomin, Dmitri; Sergey Genkin; and Ilia Itenberg. *Mathematical Circles (Russia Experience).* Providence, R.I.: American Mathematical Society, 1996.

Frederickson, Greg N. *Dissections: Plane & Fancy.* Cambridge, UK: Cambridge University Press, 1997.

Gale, David. *Tracking the Automatic Ant and Other Mathematical Explorations.* New York: Copernicus Books, 1998.

Gamow, George. *One Two Three . . . Infinity: Facts and Speculations of Science.* New York: Dover Publications, 1988.

Gardiner, A. *Mathematical Puzzling.* New York: Dover Publications, 1999.

Gardiner, Tony. *More Mathematical Challenges: Problems from the UK Junior Math Olympiad 1989–95.* Cambridge, UK: Cambridge University Press, 1997.

Gardner, Martin. *Aha! Gotcha: Paradoxes to Puzzle and Delight.* New York: W. H. Freeman and Company, 1982.

———. *Aha! Insight.* New York: W. H. Freeman and Company, 1978.

———. *Entertaining Mathematical Puzzles.* New York: Dover Publications, 1986.

———. *Fractal Music, Hypercards and More: Mathematical Recreations from* Scientific American Magazine. New York: W. H. Freeman and Company, 1991.

———. *Knotted Doughnuts and Other Mathematical Entertainments.* New York: W. H. Freeman and Company, 1986.

———. *The Last Recreations: Hydras, Eggs, and Other Mathematical Mystifications.* New York: Copernicus Books, 1997.

———. *Mathematical Carnival.* New York: Penguin Books, 1965.

———. *Mathematical Circus: More Puzzles, Games, Paradoxes, and Other Mathematical Entertainments.* Washington, D.C.: Mathematical Association of America, 1992.

———. *Mathematical Magic Show.* Washington, D.C.: Mathematical Association of America, 1988.

———. *Mathematical Puzzles of Sam Loyd.* New York: Dover Publications, 1959.

———. *More Mathematical Puzzles and Diversions.* New York: Penguin Books, 1961.

———. *More Mathematical Puzzles of Sam Loyd.* New York: Dover Publications, 1959.

———. *The New Ambidextrous Universe: Symmetry and Asymmetry, from Mirror Reflections to Superstrings.* Rev. ed. New York: W. H. Freeman and Company, 1991.

———. *Penrose Tiles to Trapdoor Ciphers: And the Return of Dr. Matrix.* Washington, D.C.: Mathematical Association of America, 1997.

———. *Perplexing Puzzles and Tantalizing Teasers.* New York: Dover Publications, 1988.

———. *Riddles of the Sphinx: And Other Mathematical Puzzle Tales.* Washington, D.C.: Mathematical Association of America, 1988.

———. *Second Scientific American Book of Mathematical Puzzles and Diversions.* Chicago: University of Chicago Press, 1987.

———. *Time Travel and Other Mathematical Bewilderments.* New York: W. H. Freeman and Company, 1987.

———. *The Unexpected Hanging: And Other Mathematical Diversions.* Chicago: University of Chicago Press, 1991.

———. *Wheels, Life and Other Mathematical Amusements.* New York: W. H. Freeman and Company, 1983.

Gay, David. *Geometry by Discovery.* New York: John Wiley & Sons, 1998.

Golomb, Solomon W. *Polyominoes: Puzzles, Patterns, Problems, and Packings.* Princeton, N.J.: Princeton University Press, 1996.

Gruenbaum, Branko, and G. C. Shephard. *Tilings and Patterns*. New York: W. H. Freeman and Company, 1986.

Gullberg, Jan. *Mathematics: From the Birth of Numbers*. New York: W. W. Norton & Company, 1997.

Higgins, Peter M. *Mathematics for the Curious*. London: Oxford University Press, 1998.

Hoffman, Paul. *Archimedes' Revenge*. New York: Ballantine Books, 1997.

———. *The Man Who Loved Only Numbers: The Story of Paul Erdös and the Search for Mathematical Truth*. New York: Little, Brown and Company, 1999.

Ishida, Non, and James Dalgety. *The Sunday Telegraph Book of Nonograms*. London: Pan Books, 1993.

Konhauser, Joseph D. E.; Dan Velleman; and Stan Wagon. *Which Way Did the Bicycle Go?: And Other Intriguing Mathematical Mysteries*. Washington, D.C.: Mathematical Association of America, 1996.

Kordemsky, Boris A. *The Moscow Puzzles: 359 Mathematical Recreations*. New York: Dover Publications, 1992.

Krause, Eugene F. *Taxicab Geometry*. New York: Dover Publications, 1986.

Lines, Malcolm E. *Think of a Number*. Bristol, UK: Institute of Physics Publishing, 1990.

Madachy, Joseph S. *Madachy's Mathematical Recreations*. New York: Dover Publications, 1979.

Nelsen, Roger B. *Proofs Without Words: Exercises in Visual Thinking*. Classroom Resource Materials, No. 1. Washington, D.C.: The Mathematical Association of America, 1993.

———. *Proofs Without Words II: More Exercises in Visual Thinking*. Washington, D.C.: The Mathematical Association of America, 2000.

Pappas, Theoni. *More Joy of Mathematics: Exploring Mathematics All Around You*. San Carlos, Calif.: Wide World Publishing/Tetra, 1991.

Pentagram. *The Puzzlegram Diary*. London: Ebury Press Stationery, 1994.

Peterson, Ivars. *Islands of Truth: A Mathematical Mystery Cruise*. New York: W. H. Freeman and Company, 1991.

———. *The Mathematical Tourist: New and Updated Snapshots of Modern Mathematics*. New York: W.H. Freeman and Company, 1998.

Pickover, Clifford A. *The Loom of God: Mathematical Tapestries at the Edge of Time*. New York: Perseus Books, 1997.

Salem, Lionel; Frederic Testard; Coralie Salem; and James D. Wuest. *The Most Beautiful Mathematical Formulas*. New York: John Wiley & Sons, 1997.

Schechter, Bruce. *My Brain Is Open: The Mathematical Journeys of Paul Erdös*. Oxford, UK: Oxford University Press, 1998.

Schuh, Fred. *The Master Book of Mathematical Recreations*. New York: Dover Publications, 1969.

Smith, David E. *A History of Mathematics, Volume 1*. New York: Dover Publications, 1978 (reprint).

———. *A History of Mathematics, Volume 2*. New York: Dover Publications, 1972 (reprint).

Smullyan, Raymond. *To Mock a Mockingbird*. Oxford, UK: Oxford University Press, 2000.

Stein, Sherman K. *Strength in Numbers: Discovering the Joy and Power of Mathematics in Everyday Life*. New York: John Wiley & Sons, 1996.

Steinhaus, Hugo. *Mathematical Snapshots*. New York: Dover Publications, 1999.

Stewart, Ian. *Another Fine Math You've Got Me Into . . .* New York: W. H. Freeman and Company, 1992.

———. *From Here to Infinity*. London: Oxford University Press, 1996.

———. *Game, Set and Math*. New York: Penguin Books, 1991.

———. *The Magical Maze: Seeing the World through Mathematical Eyes*. New York: John Wiley & Sons, 1999.

Trigg, Charles W. *Mathematical Quickies: 270 Stimulating Problems with Solutions*. New York: Dover Publications, 1985.

Tuller, Dave, and Michael Rios. *Mensa Math & Logic Puzzles*. New York: Sterling Publications, 2000.

van Delft, Pieter, and Jack Botermans. *Creative Puzzles of the World*. Emeryville, Calif.: Key Curriculum Press, 1995.

Walker, Jearl. *The Flying Circus of Physics*. New York: John Wiley & Sons, 1975.

Wells, David. *Can You Solve These? Series No. 2*. Jersey City, N.J.: Parkwest Publications, 1985.

———. *Can You Solve These? Series No. 3*. Jersey City, N.J.: Parkwest Publications, 1986.

———. *The Guinness Book of Brain Teasers*. London: Guinness Publishing, 1993.

———. *Hidden Connections, Double Meanings*. Cambridge, UK: Cambridge University Press, 1988.

———. *The Penguin Book of Curious and Interesting Geometry*. New York: Penguin Books, 1992.

———. *The Penguin Book of Curious and Interesting Math*. New York: Penguin Books, 1997.

———. *The Penguin Book of Curious and Interesting Puzzles*. New York: Penguin Books, 1993.

———. *You Are a Mathematician*. New York: Penguin Books, 1995.

Wells, David, and Robert Eastaway. *The Guinness Book of Mind Benders*. London: Guinness Publishing, 1995.

DIFFICULTY INDEX

Each puzzle in the book has been assigned a level of difficulty from 1 to 10. Level One puzzles are appropriate for the beginner, Level Ten for the puzzler looking for a challenge.

When you've done a puzzle, mark your accomplishment by putting a check next to the puzzle's name. Boxes have been provided for this purpose, for you and two other *PlayThinks* users.

LEVEL ONE

3	Ahmes's Puzzle	☐ ☐ ☐
666	Anagram	☐ ☐ ☐
927	Before-After	☐ ☐ ☐
918	Broken Bridge	☐ ☐ ☐
469	Egyptian Triangle	☐ ☐ ☐
915	Elusive Spots	☐ ☐ ☐
104	Face It: The Game of Vanishing Faces	☐ ☐ ☐
103	Face It: The Puzzle of Vanishing Faces	☐ ☐ ☐
107	Flatland Playpen	☐ ☐ ☐
625	Gear Chain	☐ ☐ ☐
590	Growth and Size	☐ ☐ ☐
645	Horse Race	☐ ☐ ☐
404	Magic Aliens Square	☐ ☐ ☐
922	Missing Slice	☐ ☐ ☐
708	Möbius Strip 1	☐ ☐ ☐
709	Möbius Strip 2	☐ ☐ ☐
175	Mystery Tracks	☐ ☐ ☐
302	Peg-Board Area	☐ ☐ ☐
10	Pick-up Sticks 1	☐ ☐ ☐
920	Pointillistic Seeing	☐ ☐ ☐
114	Reflection-Reversal	☐ ☐ ☐
661	Roulette	☐ ☐ ☐
9	Sad Clown	☐ ☐ ☐
113	Symmetrical Floor	☐ ☐ ☐
110	Symmetry Squares	☐ ☐ ☐
123	Transclown: Game of a Thousand Faces	☐ ☐ ☐
863	Who Fired the First Shot?	☐ ☐ ☐

LEVEL TWO

595	Amoeba Split	☐ ☐ ☐
96	Another Point of View	☐ ☐ ☐
789	Astronaut on the Moon	☐ ☐ ☐
822	Belt Transmission	☐ ☐ ☐
127	Bilateral Symmetry Game	☐ ☐ ☐
615	Binary Bits	☐ ☐ ☐
835	Bombs Away	☐ ☐ ☐
224	Circle Anatomy	☐ ☐ ☐
243	Circles Coloring	☐ ☐ ☐
820	Clockwork	☐ ☐ ☐
698	Coloring Pattern	☐ ☐ ☐
732	Combination Lock	☐ ☐ ☐
136	Convex or Simple?	☐ ☐ ☐
149	Coordinate Craft	☐ ☐ ☐
573	Counting Animals	☐ ☐ ☐
761	Cube Fold 1	☐ ☐ ☐
778	Cube Fold 2	☐ ☐ ☐
777	Cube Nets	☐ ☐ ☐
765	Distortions	☐ ☐ ☐
759	Distortrix 1	☐ ☐ ☐
764	Distortrix 2	☐ ☐ ☐
766	Distortrix 3	☐ ☐ ☐
570	Flowers Purple and Red	☐ ☐ ☐
571	Flowers Purple, Red and Yellow	☐ ☐ ☐
823	Gear Train 1	☐ ☐ ☐
824	Gear Train 2	☐ ☐ ☐
639	Ghoti	☐ ☐ ☐
322	Hidden Shapes	☐ ☐ ☐
926	Inside-Outside Fly	☐ ☐ ☐
402	Magic Circle 1	☐ ☐ ☐
383	Magic Color Square of Order 3	☐ ☐ ☐
129	Match the Lines Matrix	☐ ☐ ☐
120	Mystery Signs	☐ ☐ ☐
537	Number Cards 1	☐ ☐ ☐
45	Odd Intersection	☐ ☐ ☐
293	Odd Shape	☐ ☐ ☐
635	Parrot	☐ ☐ ☐
98	Pascal's Triangle	☐ ☐ ☐
155	Pixel Craft 1	☐ ☐ ☐
616	Q-Bits	☐ ☐ ☐
31	Scrambled Matchsticks	☐ ☐ ☐
653	Shells Haven	☐ ☐ ☐
569	Soccer Elimination	☐ ☐ ☐
672	Square Count	☐ ☐ ☐
40	Strange Views	☐ ☐ ☐
801	Toppling Box	☐ ☐ ☐
249	Tube Illusion	☐ ☐ ☐
629	Turning Glasses	☐ ☐ ☐
568	Wine Division	☐ ☐ ☐

LEVEL THREE

564	Add a Number	☐ ☐ ☐
611	Add and Multiply	☐ ☐ ☐
866	Air Pressure	☐ ☐ ☐
116	Alphabet 1	☐ ☐ ☐
121	Alphabet 2	☐ ☐ ☐
122	Alphabet 3	☐ ☐ ☐
797	Balls Big and Small	☐ ☐ ☐
95	Blueprint and Solids	☐ ☐ ☐
808	Bottled Volume	☐ ☐ ☐
236	Circle Area	☐ ☐ ☐
391	Clown Fun	☐ ☐ ☐
519	Counting Sheep	☐ ☐ ☐
864	Cracking Route	☐ ☐ ☐
917	Crossing Lines	☐ ☐ ☐
760	Cutting Windows 1	☐ ☐ ☐
769	Cutting Windows 2	☐ ☐ ☐

923	Digits	☐ ☐ ☐
691	Dot Wiggling 1	☐ ☐ ☐
916	Dracula's Coffin	☐ ☐ ☐
638	Facing South	☐ ☐ ☐
357	Factorials	☐ ☐ ☐
791	Falling Stones	☐ ☐ ☐
697	Four-Color Honeycomb	☐ ☐ ☐
913	Green Bird in the Cage	☐ ☐ ☐
806	Halving Mug	☐ ☐ ☐
214	Hamilton Game 1	☐ ☐ ☐
53	Handshakes 1	☐ ☐ ☐
49	Hole in a Postcard	☐ ☐ ☐
525	Horse Count	☐ ☐ ☐
711	Hypercard Ring	☐ ☐ ☐
771	Impossible Rectangles	☐ ☐ ☐
153	Intersect: A Two-Person Game	☐ ☐ ☐
32	Interstellar Greeting	☐ ☐ ☐
566	Jig-Saw	☐ ☐ ☐
523	Lagrange Theorem	☐ ☐ ☐
57	Last Man	☐ ☐ ☐
145	Line Meets Line	☐ ☐ ☐
756	Link Rings	☐ ☐ ☐
776	Linked or Unlinked?	☐ ☐ ☐
641	Marriage	☐ ☐ ☐
272	North Pole Trip	☐ ☐ ☐
538	Number Cards 2	☐ ☐ ☐
295	Odd One Out	☐ ☐ ☐
323	Parallelogram Cut	☐ ☐ ☐
168	Parallelogram Linkage	☐ ☐ ☐
343	Pick-up Polygons	☐ ☐ ☐
693	Pick-up Sticks 2	☐ ☐ ☐
156	Pixel Craft 2	☐ ☐ ☐
700	Polygonal Necklace	☐ ☐ ☐
576	Puppies Galore	☐ ☐ ☐
919	Shadow Profiles	☐ ☐ ☐
407	Square Cascades	☐ ☐ ☐
345	Squares on a Quadrilateral	☐ ☐ ☐
119	Symmetry Alphabet	☐ ☐ ☐
825	Trapdoor	☐ ☐ ☐
87	Traversing Squares	☐ ☐ ☐
644	Truth Tellers	☐ ☐ ☐
228	Why Round?	☐ ☐ ☐
574	Zoo Mix	☐ ☐ ☐

LEVEL FOUR

793	Antigravity	☐ ☐ ☐
527	Apple Pickers	☐ ☐ ☐
393	Balancing Acrobats	☐ ☐ ☐
858	Ball Game Carousel	☐ ☐ ☐
670	Basic Shapes	☐ ☐ ☐
502	Battleships	☐ ☐ ☐
612	Binary Abacus	☐ ☐ ☐
940	Cable Connection	☐ ☐ ☐
6	Chicken or Egg?	☐ ☐ ☐
79	Circle Art Memory Game	☐ ☐ ☐
230	Circle Circumference and Number Pi	☐ ☐ ☐